INTRODUCTION TO HUMAN DISEASE

The Jones and Bartlett Series in Health Sciences

INTRODUCTION TO HUMAN DISEASE

Fourth Edition

Leonard V. Crowley, M.D.

Affiliated Staff Physician
Department of Laboratory Medicine and Pathology
Fairview Riverside Medical Center
Minneapolis, Minnesota

Clinical Assistant Professor
Department of Laboratory Medicine and Pathology
and
Department of Family Practice and Community Health
University of Minnesota, Minneapolis

Professor
Biology Department
Century Community and Technical College
White Bear Lake, Minnesota

Visiting Professor
College of St. Catherine, Minneapolis Campus

JONES AND BARTLETT PUBLISHERS
Sudbury, Massachusetts
Boston   London   Singapore

To my wife,
who was helpful and very understanding

Editorial, Sales, and Customer Service Offices
Jones and Bartlett Publishers
40 Tall Pine Drive
Sudbury, MA 01776
info@jbpub.com
http://www.jbpub.com

Jones and Bartlett Publishers International
Barb House, Barb Mews
London W6 7PA
UK

Library of Congress Cataloging-in-Publication Data
Crowley, Leonard V.
    Introduction to human disease / Leonard V. Crowley.—4th ed.
        p.   cm.
    Includes bibliographical references and index.
    ISBN 0-86720-736-1 (alk. paper)
    1. Pathology.   2. Disease—Causes and theories of causation.
    I. Title.
    [DNLM: 1. Medicine. 2. Disease. WB 100 C953i 1996]
    RB112.C76   1996
    616.07--dc20
    DNLM/DLC
    for Library of Congress   96-24607
                                                                    CIP

Vice President/Editor: Joseph E. Burns
Production Editor: Marilyn E. Rash
Manufacturing Manager: Dana L. Cerrito
Production Service/Typesetting: Publishers' Design and Production Services, Inc.
Cover Design: Marshall Henrichs
Cover Photo: From Figure 13–35, coronary angiograms.
Printing and Binding: Courier Westford
Cover Printing: Henry Sawyer Co.

Printed in the United States of America
00 99 98 97   10 9 8 7 6 5 4 3 2

Contents

8 Communicable Diseases

9 Congenital and Hereditary Diseases

10 Neoplastic Disease

26   The Nervous System

27   The Musculoskeletal System

Preface

The many advances in medicine since publication of the last edition of this book have necessitated the updating and revision of many chapters, as well as the addition of several new illustrations and tables. The growing role of positron emission tomography is covered in Chapter 1. There have been many new applications of recombinant DNA technology to medical practice. New sections dealing with this technology and its applications have been added: gene therapy and prenatal diagnosis of genetic defects by examination of fetal DNA obtained from fetal cells in amnionic fluid. The sections on the immune system and its functions in health and disease have been expanded to include newer concepts dealing with the pathogenesis of autoimmune diseases; and a section on the mechanisms of immunologic injury has been added. The chapter on tumors has been expanded to include recent information on the role of oncogenes and tumor suppressor genes in both hereditary and sporadic tumors. The chapter on coagulation disturbances has been expanded to include information on the interaction of the intrinsic and extrinsic systems that trigger blood coagulation, and a discussion of von Willebrand's disease has been added.

A section on thrombolytic therapy for myocardial infarction has been expanded, and some of the ingeneous newer methods for unblocking coronary arteries are described. Information on several important communicable diseases has been added or expanded, including a more extensive section on AIDS, information on the current resurgence of tuberculosis owing to drug-resistant organisms, a discussion of the pathogenic colon bacillus 0157:H7 and the problems that it causes, and information about the emerging major intestinal parasite that causes cryptosporidiosis.

The sections dealing with the urogenital system consider newer approaches to treating prostatic hyperplasia and the continuing controversy about whether or not to treat prostate cancer. The section on ovarian tumors has been expanded. Other sections consider some of the newer hepatitis viruses. A new section in the chapter on the endocrine system deals with the acute and chronic effects of stress; elsewhere the effects of stress on organ system functions are considered, including a new section on stress-related osteoporosis.

The section on Parkinson's disease has been expanded. New information relating folic acid deficiency to neural tube defects is described, as is the role of the muscle protein dystrophin in muscular dystrophy.

Although the book has undergone considerable updating and revision, I have attempted to retain the same basic format and orientation of earlier editions, emphasizing the major structural and functional changes caused by disease and the basic principles of treatment.

Acknowledgments

Several colleagues reviewed parts of various sections. I would like to thank Dr. Nancy Crowley for reviewing the sections on immunotherapy and Drs. Robert and Jane Naviaux for reviewing several sections dealing with recombinant DNA technology, gene therapy, and related subjects. Dr. Albey M. Reiner kindly reviewed the section on infectious diseases.

I would also like to express my appreciation to Mr. Joseph Burns at Jones and Bartlett Publishers for the many ways he helped during the preparation of this edition.

With each revision there is always a new set of issues, topics, and pedagogical concerns that must be addressed and evaluated. I would like to thank the many people teaching the human disease course who provided the publisher and myself with some very useful suggestions and editorial commentary that helped to improve this edition. Thanks to:

Jerry Adler	Lane Community College
Valerie Baker	Gannon University
Krissa A. Baylor	West Georgia College
Nancy Becker	Lehigh Canon Community College
Julie Boles	Ithaca College
Lennette Burrell	Medical College of Georgia School of Nursing
Joyce Faris	Metropolitan State College of Denver
Kay Fleming	Wytheville Community College
Joanne Gordon	Southwest Missouri State University
Lynda Gordon	Long Beach City College
Paul Hartunian	Montclair State University
Dianne Keelan	Northwestern Michigan College
Mary King	Wharton Community Junior College
Stephen L. Lahr	Ithaca College
Patricia A. Lorenz	Penn Valley Community College
Barbara Odom-Weisley	Texas Woman's University
Patricia Otto	Gateway Technical College
William G. Preston	Cuyahoga Community College
Lisa Seldomridge	Salisbury State University
Patricia Staurakas	East Carolina University
Melinda M. Swenson	Indiana University
Karen Taylor	Chippewa Valley Technical College
Nancy Trimble	Wright State College

Preface to the First Edition

This book is based on courses given for many years to students in nursing and other health professions. It is designed to provide a solid foundation on which students can build for the remainder of their professional careers. A fundamental knowledge of disease requires a clear conception of both the structural and the functional changes caused by disease in tissues and organs, as a basis for understanding the clinical manifestations and principles of treatment. Consequently, to facilitate learning, many illustrations of the salient features of the more important diseases have been included. Photographs of x-ray films, angiograms, and CT scans also are used where appropriate, because such studies are widely used by health professionals to diagnose disease and evaluate response to therapy. A number of brief case studies have been included so that students can more easily relate the clinical manifestations, diagnosis, and treatment of a specific disease to an individual patient.

Purpose and Scope of the Book

The book is organized into two main sections. The first section, comprising the first twelve chapters, deals with general concepts and with diseases affecting the body as a whole. The second section, which includes the remaining fifteen chapters, considers the various organ systems and their diseases.

In the first section, chapter 1 discusses manifestations of disease, classification, diagnosis, and principles of treatment. Chapter 2 considers the organization and basic function of cells and tissues in health and disease. Chapter 3 deals with genes, chromosomes, cell division, and chromosome analysis, as well as the HLA system and its relation to disease. Chapters 4 and 5 consider the body's defenses, the inflammatory reaction and the immune system, and their disorders. Chapters 6 and 7 are concerned with the various pathogenic microorganisms and parasites and the diseases they cause. This material is followed by a discussion of the transmission and control of communicable dis-

Organization

eases in chapter 8 and includes discussion of the clinically important sexually transmitted diseases. Chapter 9 considers congenital and hereditary diseases, and chapter 10 deals with tumors. Chapter 11 describes the coagulation of the blood and conditions in which the blood does not clot normally. Chapter 12 considers conditions in which the blood clots too readily and its attendant complications—thrombosis and embolism.

In the second section, the individual organ systems and their diseases are considered in a systematic manner, with emphasis on the more common and important diseases. Basic pathologic physiology, pathology, and principles of diagnosis and treatment are discussed. Newer diagnostic procedures and methods of treatment are emphasized. Chapter 13 describes diseases of the cardiovascular system and includes an extensive discussion of coronary heart disease, one of the most prevalent diseases in the developed nations of the world. Diseases of the hematopoietic and lymphatic systems are considered together in chapter 14, followed by diseases of the respiratory system in chapter 15. Chapters 16, 17, and 18 should be considered as a unit: diseases of the breast, the female reproductive system, prenatal development, and diseases associated with pregnancy. Chapter 19, diseases of the urinary system, and chapter 20, which is concerned with the male reproductive system, are also best considered as a unit. Chapter 21 describes derangements of the liver and biliary system. This is followed in chapter 22 by diseases of the pancreas, including diabetes mellitus. The upper and lower intestinal tracts and their diseases follow in chapter 23. Chapter 24 departs from the organ system approach and considers disturbances of fluid, electrolyte, and acid-base balance. The material is introduced here rather than in the first section because it is more easily understood and related to specific organ system diseases when considered after chapters 19 through 23. The final three chapters deal, respectively, with diseases of the endocrine glands, nervous system, and musculoskeletal system.

Study Aids and Special Features

Various learning and study aids are included to enhance the usefulness of the book. Learning objectives, review questions, and a detailed outline summary are provided for each chapter. The numbers after the main headings in the outline summary refer to the text pages where the material is covered to facilitate access to the text material for review purposes. Literature for further study is listed at the end of each chapter, and a listing of general references is included at the end of the book. These additional sources should prove useful to students who wish to pursue a subject in greater detail. A glossary with pronunciation guide is appended to the end of the text. This may prove useful to students who have not already had a course in medical terminology and can serve as a convenient reference for other students who wish a quick review of a particular term. Words appearing in the glossary are set in boldface type in the text for easy reference.

Many people helped with the book in various ways, and I would like to acknowledge their assistance. Several colleagues at St. Mary's Hospital in Minneapolis and in the Department of Laboratory Medicine and Pathology at the University of Minnesota made suggestions and comments. Colleagues in the Department of Family Practice and Community Health at the University of Minnesota, at St. Paul–Ramsey Medical Center, and at the West Side Community Health Center in St. Paul also provided helpful comments. Several of the concepts and clinical cases used in the book were based on these clinical contacts and activities.

Acknowledgments

1

General Concepts of Disease
Principles of Diagnosis

Learning Objectives

1. Define the common terms used to describe disease, such as lesions, organic and functional disease, symptomatic and asymptomatic disease, etiology, and pathogenesis.
2. List the major categories of human disease.
3. Explain the approach that a practitioner uses to make a diagnosis and decide on a patient's treatment.
4. Describe the various types of diagnostic tests and procedures that can help the practitioner in making a diagnosis and deciding on proper treatment.

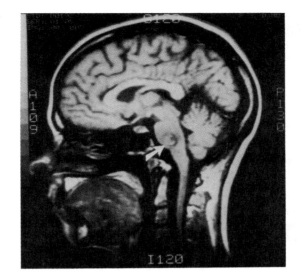

Chapter 1 ▪ Contents

Any disturbance of structure or function of the body may be regarded as **disease.** A disease is often associated with well-defined, characteristic structural changes, called **lesions,** that are present in various organs and tissues. One can recognize lesions by examining the diseased tissue with the naked eye, which is called a *gross examination,* or with the aid of a microscope, which is called a *histologic examination.* A disease associated with structural changes is called an **organic disease.** In contrast, a **functional disease** is one in which no morphologic abnormalities (*morphe* = structure or shape) can be identified, even though bodily functions may be profoundly disturbed. Many nervous and mental diseases are functional. **Pathology** is the study of disease, and a *pathologist* is a physician who specializes in the diagnosis and classification of disease, primarily by examining the morphology of cells or tissues. A *clinician* is any physician or other health practitioner who cares for patients.

A disease may cause various subjective manifestations, such as weakness or pain, in an affected individual: these are called *symptoms.* A disease may also produce objective manifestations, detectable by the clinician, which are called *signs* or *physical findings.* In many diseases, the quantity of blood cells in the circulation may change, and so may the biochemical constituents in the body fluids. These alterations are reflected as abnormal laboratory test results.

A disease that causes the affected individual no discomfort or disability is called an *asymptomatic* disease or illness. A disease is often asymptomatic in its early stages. If the disease is not treated, however, it may progress to the stage where it causes subjective symptoms and abnormal physical findings. Therefore, the distinction between asymptomatic and symptomatic disease is one of degree, depending primarily on the extent of the disease.

The term **etiology** means cause. A disease of unknown etiology is one for which the cause is not yet known. Unfortunately, many diseases fall into this category. If the cause of a disease is known, the agent responsible is called the *etiologic agent.* The term **pathogenesis** refers to the manner by which a disease develops, and a *pathogen* is any microorganism, such as a bacterium or virus, that can cause disease.

Characteristics of Disease

Diseases tend to fall into several large categories, although the diseases in a specific category are not necessarily closely related. Rather, the lesions produced by the various diseases in a category are morphologically similar or have a similar pathogenesis. Diseases are conveniently classified in the following large groups:

1. Congenital and hereditary diseases
2. Inflammatory diseases
3. Degenerative diseases
4. Metabolic diseases
5. Neoplastic diseases

Classifications of Disease

Congenital and Hereditary Diseases

Congenital and hereditary diseases are the result of developmental disturbances. They may be caused by genetic abnormalities, abnormalities in the numbers and distribution of chromosomes, intrauterine injury as a result of various agents, or interaction of genetic and environmental factors. Hemophilia, the well-known hereditary disease in which blood does not clot properly, and congenital heart disease induced by the German measles virus are examples of diseases in this category.

Inflammatory Diseases

Inflammatory diseases are those in which the body reacts to an injurious agent by means of inflammation. Many of the diseases characterized by inflammation, such as a sore throat or pneumonia, are caused by bacteria or other microbiologic agents. Others, such as "hay fever," are a manifestation of an allergic reaction or a hypersensitivity state in the patient. Some diseases in this category appear to be caused by antibodies formed against the patient's own tissues, as occurs in some uncommon diseases classified as autoimmune diseases. The etiology of still other inflammatory diseases has not been determined.

Degenerative Diseases

In degenerative diseases, the primary abnormality is degeneration of various parts of the body. In some cases, this may be a manifestation of the aging process. In many cases, however, the degenerative lesions are more advanced or occur sooner than would be expected if they were age related, and they are distinctly abnormal. Certain types of arthritis and "hardening of the arteries" (arteriosclerosis) are common examples of degenerative diseases.

Metabolic Diseases

The chief abnormality seen in metabolic diseases is a disturbance in some important metabolic process in the body. For example, the cells may not be utilizing glucose normally, or the thyroid gland may not properly regulate the rate of cell metabolism. Diabetes, disturbances of endocrine glands, and disturbances of fluid and electrolyte balance are common examples of metabolic diseases.

Neoplastic Diseases

Neoplastic diseases are characterized by abnormal cell growth that leads to the formation of various types of benign and malignant tumors.

Health and disease may be considered two extremes of a continuum. At one extreme is severe, life-threatening, disabling illness with its corresponding major effect on the physical and emotional well-being of the patient. At the other extreme is ideal good health, which may be defined as a state of complete physical and mental well-being. The healthy person is emotionally and physically capable of leading a full, happy, and productive life that is free of anxiety, turmoil, and physical disabilities that limit activities. Between these two extremes are many gradations of health and disease, ranging from mild or short-term illness that limits activities to some extent through moderate good health that falls short of the ideal state. The midpoint in this continuum may be considered a "neutral" position in which one is neither ill nor in ideal good health. In this continuum, most of us are somewhere between midposition and the ideal state.

The goal of traditional medicine is to cure or ameliorate disease. This is accomplished by various means, ranging from administration of an antibiotic to cure an infection to very complex "high technology" treatments such as kidney transplants and heart surgery. The advances of modern medicine have done much to relieve suffering and advance human welfare, but modern medicine does not guarantee good health. Health is more than an absence of disease; it is a condition in which body and mind function efficiently and harmoniously as an integrated unit. Consequently, we must take an active part in achieving good health by assuming some responsibility for our own physical and emotional well-being. This means practicing such common-sense measures as eating properly, exercising moderately, and avoiding harmful excesses such as overeating, smoking, heavy drinking, or using drugs that can disrupt physical or emotional well-being. Taking responsibility for one's health also requires using one's mind constructively, expressing emotions, and feeling good about oneself. Positive mental attitudes are essential for good health, because negative feelings may be reflected in disturbed bodily functions that are manifested as disease.

Health and Disease: A Continuum

The determination of the nature and cause of a patient's illness by a physician or other health practitioner is called a **diagnosis.** It is based on the practitioner's evaluation of the patient's subjective symptoms, the physical findings, and the results of various laboratory tests, together with other appropriate diagnostic procedures. When the practitioner has reached a diagnosis, he or she can then offer a **prognosis:** an opinion concerning the eventual outcome of the disease. Then, a course of treatment is instituted.

Principles of Diagnosis

The History
The clinical *history* is a very important part of the evaluation. It consists of several parts:

1. The history of the patient's current illness
2. The past medical history
3. The family history
4. The social history
5. The review of systems

The *history of the present illness* elicits details concerning the severity, time of onset, and character of the patient's symptoms. Many diseases have characteristic symptoms. The patient's description of the oppressive substernal pain of a heart attack or the pain and urinary disturbances associated with a bladder infection, for example, may provide very helpful information that suggests the correct diagnosis. The *past medical history* provides details of the patient's general health and previous illnesses. These data may shed light on the patient's current problems as well. The *family history* provides information about the health of the patient's parents and other family members. Some diseases, such as diabetes and some types of heart disease, tend to run in families. The *social history* deals with the patient's occupation, habits, alcohol and tobacco consumption, and similar data. This information may also relate to the patient's general health and current problems. The *review of systems* inquires as to the presence of symptoms other than those disclosed in the history of the present illness; such symptoms might suggest disease affecting other parts of the body. For example, the practitioner inquires about such symptoms as pain or burning on urination, which suggest an abnormality of the urinary tract, and coughing, shortness of breath, or chest pain, which may indicate disease of the respiratory system. In this way, possible dysfunctions of other organ systems are evaluated by systematic inquiry.

The Physical Examination

The *physical examination* is a systematic examination of the patient. The practitioner places particular emphasis on the part of the body affected by the illness, such as the ears, throat, chest, and lungs in the case of a respiratory infection. Any abnormalities detected on the physical examination are correlated with the clinical history. At this point, the practitioner begins to consider the various diseases or conditions that would fit with the clinical findings. Sometimes, more than one possible diagnosis needs to be considered. In a *differential diagnosis,* the practitioner considers a number of diseases that are characterized by the patient's symptoms. For example, if a patient complains of shortness of breath, and abnormalities are detected when the lungs are examined with a stethoscope, the practitioner may consider both chronic lung disease and chronic heart failure in the differential diagnosis.

Often the practitioner can narrow the list of diagnostic possibilities and arrive at a correct diagnosis by using selected laboratory tests or other specialized diagnostic procedures. In difficult cases, the clinician may also wish to obtain the opinion of a medical consultant, who is a physician with special training and experience in the type of medical problem presented by the patient.

Treatment

Once the diagnosis has been established, a course of treatment is initiated. There are two different types of treatment: specific treatment and symptomatic treatment.

A *specific treatment* is one that exerts a highly specific and favorable effect on the basic cause of the disease. For example, an antibiotic may be given to a patient who has an infection that is responsive to the antibiotic, or insulin may be given to a patient with diabetes. *Symptomatic treatment,* as the name implies, makes the patient more comfortable by alleviating symptoms but does not influence the course of the underlying disease. Examples are the treatment of fever, pain, and cough by means of appropriate medications. Unfortunately, there are no specific treatments for some diseases. Consequently, the clinician must be content with treating the manifestations of the disease, without being able to influence its ultimate course.

A wide array of diagnostic tests and procedures are available to help the practitioner make a diagnosis and treat the patient properly. They fall into two classifications: invasive procedures and noninvasive procedures. *Invasive procedures* are so named because the patient's body is actually "invaded" in some way in order to obtain diagnostic information. Such procedures involve introducing needles, catheters, or other instruments into the patient's body. *Noninvasive procedures* are those that entail no risk or minimal risk or discomfort to the patient, such as a chest x-ray or an examination of the urine.

Diagnostic Tests and Procedures

Many diagnostic procedures entail some degree of risk or discomfort to the patient. The risk is greater with invasive procedures, but even some noninvasive procedures are not completely harmless. A chest x-ray, for example, exposes the patient to radiation. Even a relatively simple procedure such as the collection of a blood sample for a laboratory test may be complicated by bleeding around the vein or by formation of a blood clot in the vein at the site of puncture. Therefore, with any diagnostic procedure, the practitioner must balance the possible disadvantages to the patient against the benefits that may be derived from the information obtained by the procedure. Patients also must be fully informed about the possible risks and benefits so that they can make informed decisions as to whether or not to consent to the procedure. It would be unwise to perform a potentially risky diagnostic procedure if the information gained would not contribute significantly to the diagnosis or would not greatly influence the course of treatment. The physician would be much more likely to employ a diagnostic procedure that could provide much useful information at little or no risk to the patient.

Diagnostic tests and procedures can be classified in several major categories:

1. Clinical laboratory tests
2. Tests that measure the electrical activity of the body
3. Tests using radioisotopes (also called radionuclides)
4. Endoscopy
5. Ultrasound procedures
6. X-ray examinations
7. Magnetic resonance imaging
8. Positron emission tomography (PET scans)
9. Cytologic and histologic examination of cells and tissues removed from the patient.

Clinical Laboratory Tests

Clinical laboratory tests have many uses. They can be used to determine the concentration of various constituents in the blood and urine, which are frequently altered by disease. For example, the concentration of a substance in the blood called *urea* is elevated if the kidneys are not functioning properly, because this constituent is normally excreted by the kidneys. The concentrations of hemoglobin and the quantity of red cells are reduced in patients with anemia. One can also determine the concentration (activity) of enzymes in the blood. Sometimes the enzyme level is elevated because (a) enzymes are leaking from diseased or injured organs, (b) enzyme synthesis is increased as a result of disease, or (c) excretion of enzymes is impaired because disease has caused blockage of normal excretory pathways.

Clinical laboratory tests are also used to evaluate the functions of organs. *Clearance tests* measure the rate at which a substance such as urea or creatinine is removed from blood and excreted in the urine. This provides a measure of renal (kidney) function. *Pulmonary function tests* measure the rate at which air moves in and out of the lungs. Determinations of the concentration of oxygen and carbon dioxide in the blood also can indicate pulmonary function. Tests that measure the uptake and excretion of various substances by the liver are used as a measure of *liver function.* One can also detect substances that are likely to be produced by tumors growing within the body and measure their concentration. Serial analyses of these substances can be used to monitor the response of certain tumors to treatment. *Microbiologic tests* detect the presence of disease-producing organisms in urine, blood, and feces. They also determine the responsiveness of the organisms to antibiotics. *Serologic tests* detect and measure the presence of antibodies as an indication of response to infectious agents.

Tests of Electrical Activity

Several different tests measure the electrical impulses associated with various bodily functions and activities. These include the electrocardiogram

(ECG), the electroencephalogram (EEG), and the electromyogram (EMG). The most widely used of these tests is the *electrocardiogram*. Electrodes attached to the arms, legs, and chest are used to measure the serial changes in the electrical activity of the heart during the various phases of the cardiac cycle. The electrocardiogram also identifies disturbances in the heart rate or rhythm and identifies abnormal conduction of impulses through the heart. Heart muscle injury, such as occurs after a heart attack, can also be recognized by means of characteristic abnormalities in the cardiogram. The *electroencephalogram* measures the electrical activity of the brain, often called *brain waves,* by means of small electrodes attached to different areas in the scalp. Brain tumors, strokes, and many other abnormalities of cerebral structure or function may cause altered brain wave patterns that are detected by this examination. The *electromyogram* measures the electrical activity of skeletal muscle during contraction and at rest. Abnormal electrical activity is often encountered in various inflammatory or degenerative diseases involving the skeletal muscles. The test is performed by inserting a needle into the muscle that is being studied. The speed at which a nerve conducts impulses can also be measured by means of electrodes taped to the surface of the skin over the nerve being tested. Abnormal conduction of nerve impulses, encountered in some diseases, can be identified by such studies.

Radioisotope (Radionuclide) Studies

The function of various organs can be evaluated by administering a substance labeled with a radioactive material called a *radioisotope*. Specially designed radiation detectors then measure the uptake and excretion of the labeled substance. For example, in certain types of anemia, one measures the absorption and excretion of radioisotope-labeled vitamin B_{12}, which is a vitamin required for normal blood formation. The ability of the thyroid gland to concentrate and utilize radioactive iodine is used as a measure of thyroid function and can also be used to detect tumors within the thyroid gland. One may administer a radioactive material that is filtered out or concentrated in a tissue or organ and then measure the radioactivity by radiation detectors applied to the exterior of the body and connected to a computer. For example, specially processed albumin labeled with a radioisotope may be administered intravenously as a measure of pulmonary blood flow. The material is filtered out and retained in the lungs as the blood flows through them. If blood flow to a part of the lung is inadequate for any reason, less radioactivity is recorded in that area. This technique is frequently used to detect the presence of blood clots in the lung that impede blood flow to parts of the lung. Phosphorus-containing isotopes are concentrated in the skeletal system. If there are deposits of tumor in bone, the isotopes are concentrated around the tumor deposits and can be easily identified (figure 1–1). Radioactive materials injected intravenously can also be used to evaluate blood flow to heart muscle and to identify areas of damaged heart muscle.

FIGURE 1–1

Radioisotope bone scan of head, chest, and pelvis. Dark areas (*arrows*) indicate concentration of radioisotope around tumor deposits in bone.

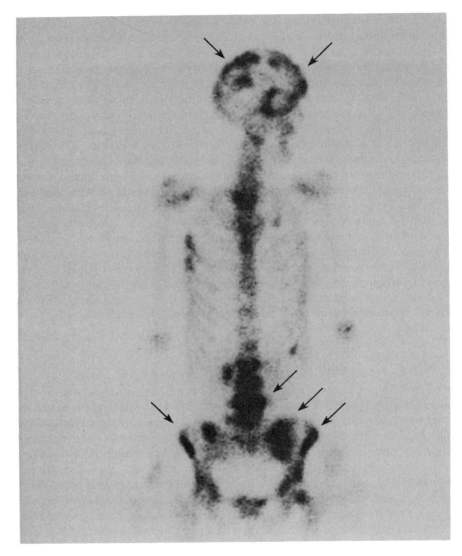

Endoscopy

An **endoscopy,** or endoscopic examination (*endo* = within + *skopeo* = examine), is an examination of the interior of the body by means of various types of rigid or flexible tubular instruments that are named according to the part of the body they are designed to examine. These instruments have a system of lenses for viewing and a light source to illuminate the region being examined. An *esophagoscope,* for example, is used to examine the interior of the esophagus, a *gastroscope* to examine the stomach, and a *bronchoscope* to examine the trachea and major bronchi. An instrument for viewing the interior of the bladder is called a *cystoscope*. A *sigmoidoscope* is a rigid tube used to examine the rectum and the sigmoid colon, and a *colonscope* is a flexible tube that can be used to examine the entire length of the colon. An instrument called a *laparoscope* is used to visualize the pelvic organs. It is inserted into the abdominal cavity through a small incision in the umbilicus.

Ultrasound

Ultrasound is a technique for mapping the echoes produced by high-frequency sound waves transmitted into the body. Echoes are reflected wherever there is a change in the density of the tissue. The reflected waves are recorded on sensitive detectors, and images are produced. This method is widely used to study the uterus during pregnancy, because it does not require the use of potentially harmful radiation and poses no risk to the fetus. The technique can be used to determine the position of the placenta and the fetus within the uterus; it can also identify some fetal abnormalities and detect twin pregnancies (figure 1–2). Ultrasound is also used to study the structure and function of the heart valves. The procedure can detect valve abnormalities and identify blood clots that sometimes form on the heart valves in association with infection of the valve (described in chapter 13). Ultrasound can determine the thickness of the ventricular walls and septum and the size of the ventricular chambers during systole and diastole. Ultrasound can identify gallstones in the gallbladder and abnormalities in the prostate suspicious for prostate cancer. The technique has many other applications in medicine.

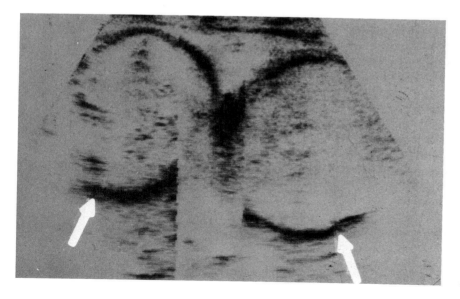

FIGURE 1–2

Ultrasound examination of pelvis late in pregnancy indicating twin pregnancy. Both fetal heads demonstrated (*arrows*).

X-Ray Examination

X-ray examinations are conducted in many ways, but the basic principle is the same for all types of x-ray studies. X-rays are passed through the part of the body to be examined, and the rays leaving the body expose an x-ray film. The extent to which the rays are absorbed by the tissues as they pass through the body depends on the density of the tissues. Tissues of low density, such as the air-filled lungs, transmit most of the rays, and thus the film exposed to x-rays passing through them appears black. Tissues of high density, such as bone, absorb most of the rays; the film remains unexposed and appears white. Tissues of intermediate densities appear as varying shades of gray. The x-ray image produced on the film is called a *radiograph* or *roentgenogram*. The same basic principle is used to obtain x-ray films of the breast. This procedure is called **mammogram.** The applications and limitations of the mammogram procedure are considered in chapter 16 in the section on diseases of the breast.

Although the linings of internal organs such as the intestinal tract, urinary tract, bronchi, fallopian tubes, and biliary tract have little contrast, they can be examined by administering a dense radiopaque substance called *contrast medium*. It coats and adheres to the lining of the structure being examined and enhances its visibility. To examine the interior of the gastrointestinal tract, for example, one gives the patient a suspension of barium sulfate to swallow or administers it as an enema. The opaque barium coats the lining of the intestinal tract, and an abnormality in the lining shows on the film as an irregularity in the column of barium (figure 1–3). The lining of the bronchi can be visualized by instilling a radiopaque oil into the bronchi. The oil forms a thin film on the bronchial mucosa and delineates the contours of the bronchi. This procedure is called a *bronchogram* (figure 1–4).

One uses the same principle to visualize the urinary tract. A radiopaque substance is injected into a vein and is excreted in the urine as the blood flows through the kidney, outlining the contour of the urinary tract. This is called an *intravenous pyelogram* (IVP) (figure 1–5). Another method is to introduce the dye directly into both ureters through tubes that are inserted into both ureters by means of a cystoscope introduced into the bladder. This procedure is called a *retrograde pyelogram*. To visualize the gallbladder, the patient ingests tablets of radiopaque material that is absorbed into the circulation, excreted by the liver in the bile, and concentrated in the gallbladder. Gallstones can be identified because they occupy space in the gallbladder and cause irregularities in the radiopaque material concentrated there (figure 1–6).

One can also use contrast material to study the flow of blood in large arteries and to identify areas of narrowing or obstruction. This procedure is called an **arteriogram** or **angiogram** (*angio* = blood vessel). A small flexible catheter is inserted into a large artery in the arm or leg and advanced into the aorta until it is positioned at the opening of the artery that is to be examined. Radiopaque material is then injected through the catheter. It mixes with the blood, and its flow through the vessel is followed by means of a

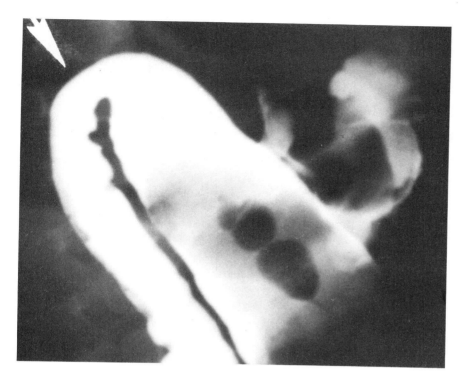

FIGURE 1–3

X-ray film after injection of radiopaque barium sulfate suspension into colon (barium enema), illustrating narrowed a rea (*arrow*) that impedes passage of bowel contents.

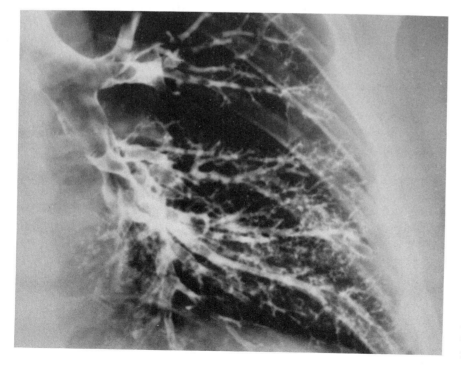

FIGURE 1–4

Bronchogram illustrating normal branching of bronchi and bronchioles that are normal in caliber.

FIGURE 1–5

Intravenous pyelogram (IVP). *Arrows* outline filling defect caused by cyst in kidney that distorts renal pelvis and calyces. Opposite side appears normal.

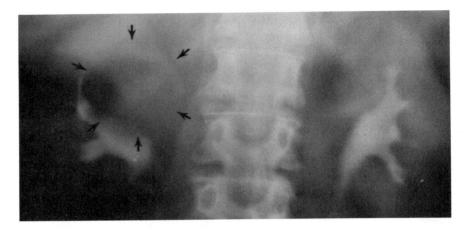

series of x-ray films. If the vessel is narrowed by disease, the film will show areas in which the column of opaque material is narrowed. A complete obstruction of the vessel appears as an interruption of the column. Arteriography is often used to detect narrowing or obstruction of the coronary arteries or of the carotid arteries in the neck, which carry blood to the brain (figure 1–7). Obstruction of the pulmonary arteries by blood clots also can be identified by arteriography. In this case, the catheter used to inject the radiopaque material is inserted into a large vein in the arm, threaded up the vein and through the right side of the heart, and positioned in the pulmonary artery.

This same basic method can be used to study the flow of blood through the heart and can detect abnormal communications between cardiac chambers. This type of study is called **cardiac catheterization.**

Computed Tomographic Scans

A *computed tomographic scan* (**CT scan**) is performed by a highly sophisticated x-ray machine that produces images of the body in cross section by rotating the x-ray tube around the patient at various levels. The x-ray tube is mounted on a movable frame opposite an array of sensitive radiation detectors that encircle the patient. As the x-ray tube moves around the patient, the radiation detectors record the amount of radiation passing through the body (figure 1–8). In computerized scanning, the amount of radiation absorbed is not read directly on an x-ray film. Instead, the data from the radiation detectors are fed into a computer, which reconstructs the data into an image that reproduces the patient's anatomy as a cross-section picture. The image is displayed on a television monitor and can be recorded on film (figure 1–9). As with conventional x-rays, dense substances are white and less-dense substances appear darker in proportion to the amount of radiation they transmit. The individual organs appear sharply separated from one another because the various parts of the body are separated by planes of fat, which have very low density. These separations increase contrast between adjacent organs. Abnormalities of internal organs that cannot be identified by

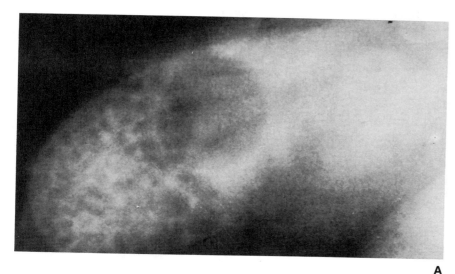

A

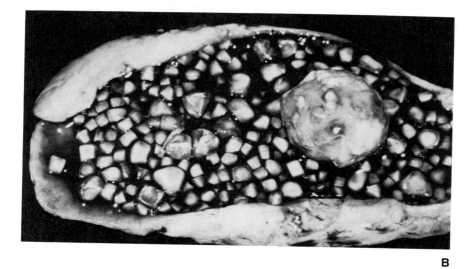

B

FIGURE 1–6

A, Gallstones demonstrated by means of radiopaque material concentrated in bile. Gallstones occupy space in gallbladder and appear as radiolucent (dark) areas within radiopaque (white) bile. Note large radiolucent area, indicating a large gallstone surrounded by smaller radiolucent areas, representing multiple smaller stones. **B,** Opened gallbladder removed surgically from the same patient. Compare appearance and location of stones with x-ray appearance.

means of standard x-ray examinations can often by discovered with CT scans. Figure 1–10 shows a renal cyst located by CT scan.

Magnetic Resonance Imaging

Magnetic resonance imaging (MRI) produces computer-constructed images of various organs and tissues somewhat like CT scans. The device consists of a strong magnet capable of developing a powerful magnetic field, coils that can transmit and receive radiofrequency waves, and a computer, which receives impulses from the scanner and forms them into images that can be interpreted. The MRI scanner with the enclosed magnet and coils

FIGURE 1–7

Narrowing of carotid
artery in neck (*arrow*)
demonstrated by
carotid angiogram.

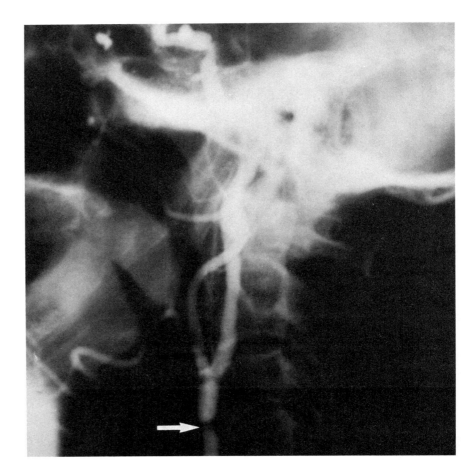

appears similar to a CT scanner. The patient lies on a table that is gradually
moved into the scanner, as is done in CT scans. The principle of MRI, however, is quite different from that of CT scanning, which uses ionizing radiation to construct images based on the density of tissues. MRI scans, in
contrast, depend on the response of hydrogen protons (positively charged
particles in the nucleus around which electrons rotate) contained within
water molecules when they are placed in a strong magnetic field. Hydrogen
protons behave as if they are spinning rapidly about an axis, surrounded by
orbiting negatively charged electrons. When subjected to a strong magnetic
field, the protons become aligned in the direction of the magnetic field.
When a pulse of radiofrequency waves is directed at the protons, they are
temporarily dislodged from their orientation, which causes them to wobble.
As they return to their original positions, they emit a signal (resonance) that
can be measured and used to produce the computer-constructed images.
Body tissues, which have a high water content, are a rich source of protons
capable of excitation. The intensity of the signals produced is related to the

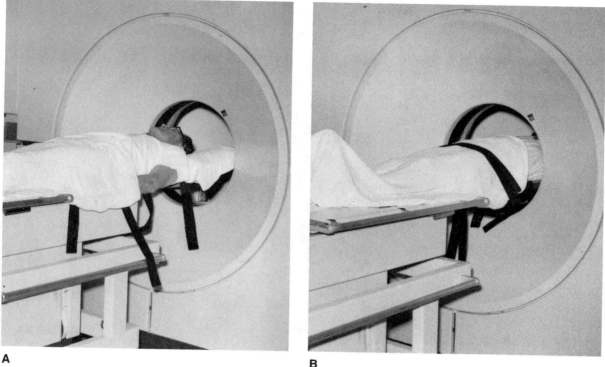

A   **B**

FIGURE 1–8

Computed tomographic (CT) scan. **A,** Patient lies on table. Radiation detectors surround opening in scanner, and x-ray tube rotates around opening. **B,** Patient on table is gradually advanced into scanner, which produces computer-reconstructed cross-section images of patient at multiple levels.

varying water content of body tissues and to the strength and duration of the radiofrequency pulse. Because MRI does not use ionizing radiation, the patient does not receive radiation exposure. MRI does expose the patient to strong magnetic fields and radiowaves, but this appears relatively safe, on the basis of current knowledge.

Applications

MRI detects many of the same types of abnormalities detected by CT, and CT is superior to MRI for many applications. MRI, however, offers distinct advantages over CT in special situations, as, for example, when attempting to detect abnormalities in tissues surrounded by bone, such as lesions in the spinal cord, orbits, or near the base of the skull (figure 1–11). In these locations, bone interferes with scanning because of its density, but it does not produce an image in MRI because the water content of bone is low. MRI also provides a sharp contrast between gray and white matter within the brain and spinal cord, which differ in their water content. For this reason, the technique is useful for demonstrating areas where myelin sheaths of

FIGURE 1–9

CT scan of chest. Mediastinum and heart appear white in the center of scan, with less-dense lungs on either side. *Arrow* indicates tumor, which appears as white nodule, in lung.

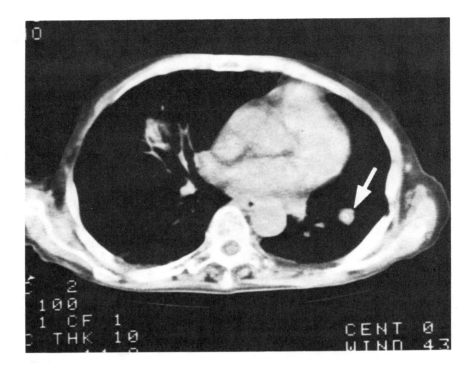

FIGURE 1–10

CT views of abdomen at level of kidneys, illustrating a fluid-filled cyst in kidney (*arrows*). The cyst appears less dense than surrounding renal tissue. Outline of kidney on opposite side appears normal.

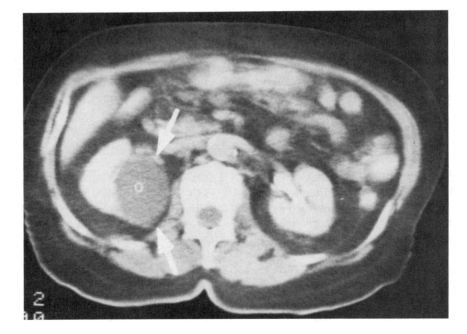

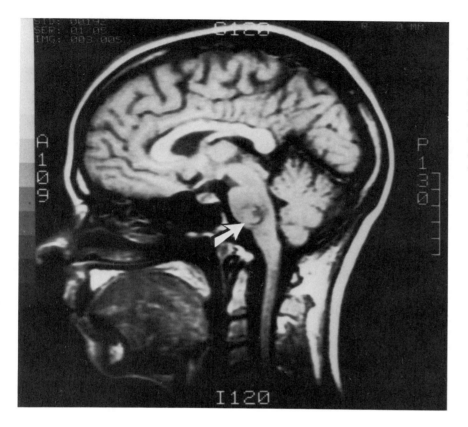

FIGURE 1–11

Magnetic-resonance-imaging view of brain, which is well seen because skull bones are not visualized by MRI. White line surrounding brain represents scalp tissues. Arrow indicates a malformation composed of blood vessels within the brain stem.

nerve fibers have been damaged, as in a neurologic disease called multiple sclerosis (described in chapter 26). Further improvements in equipment will undoubtedly increase the usefulness of this diagnostic procedure.

Positron Emission Tomography

Related to radioisotope studies but much more complex and sophisticated is one of the newest of the diagnostic imaging tests called positron emission tomography (PET), or simply PET scans. Positrons are unique subatomic particles that have the same mass as electrons but carry a positive charge. They are formed when atoms such as carbon, oxygen, or nitrogen are bombarded in a cyclotron with high-energy particles, which breaks down the atomic nuclei and releases the positrons along with other subatomic particles. The positrons escaping from the nuclei collide with negatively charged electrons circling the nuclei, producing radiation that can be detected and measured by means of sensitive radiation detectors.

One uses PET scans to study body functions by injecting into the subject a biochemical compound, such as glucose, that is labeled with a positron-emitting isotope and then assessing the distribution and metabolism of the compound by measuring the radiation produced within the body by the isotope-labeled compound. The radiation output, measured by sensitive radiation detectors, is fed into a computer that constructs computer-generated images similar to those obtained with CT scans. Such studies provide information on the metabolic activities of the organ or tissue being studied, the site within an organ where the compound is being metabolized, and the blood flow to the organ being studied.

Although originally developed for research studies, PET scans are slowly moving from the research laboratory into medical practice. At present, the major clinical applications are to assess biochemical functions within the brain. One can detect and measure changes in brain functions associated with various neurologic diseases such as strokes, brain tumors, Alzheimer's disease, Parkinson's disease, and some hereditary degenerative diseases of the nervous system. The method has also been used to some extent to evaluate changes in blood flow and metabolism in heart muscle after a heart attack. Many other applications of PET scans are being explored and evaluated.

Although PET scans provide useful information, there are some major drawbacks to their widespread application. They are very expensive procedures and are not widely available. Because positron-emitting isotopes must be produced in a cyclotron, the isotopes produced have a very short duration of activity (half-life), and one must have facilities for incorporating the isotope into the biochemical compound required for the PET scan procedure.

Cytologic and Histologic Examinations

Cells covering the surfaces of the body are continually cast off and replaced by new cells. Abnormal cells can often be identified in the fluids or secretions that come in contact with the epithelial surface. This type of examination is called a **Papanicolaou smear,** or simply *Pap smear,* after the physician who developed the procedure. It is widely used as a screening test for recognizing early cancer of the uterus and can be used to detect cancers in other locations as well. The Pap smear is discussed in the section on neoplasms in chapter 10.

Diseased tissues have abnormal structural and cellular patterns that can be recognized by the pathologist. Consequently, it is often possible to determine the cause of a patient's disease by histologic examination of a small sample of tissue removed from the affected tissue or organ. This procedure is called a **biopsy.** Samples of tissue can be obtained from any part of the body. Gastroscopes, bronchoscopes, and other instruments used for endoscopic examination, for example, are constructed so that specimens for biopsy can be obtained while the internal organs are being examined. Biopsy specimens can also be taken directly from internal organs such as the liver or kidney by inserting a thin needle through the skin directly into the organ. Samples of bone marrow are obtained in this way, and bone-marrow biopsy is often performed to diagnose blood disease (figure 1–12).

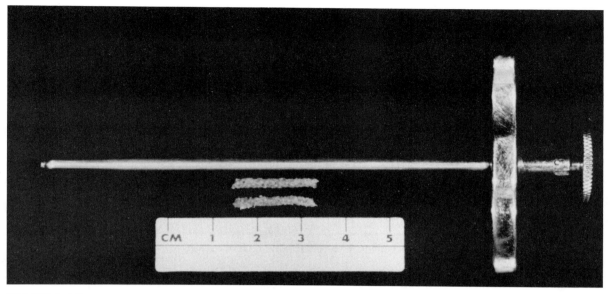

FIGURE 1–12

Two samples of bone marrow (adjacent to scale) obtained from pelvic bones by means of specially designed needle, shown in upper part of photograph.

Questions for Review

1. What are the five major categories of disease?

2. What are the definitions of the following terms: *etiology, symptom of disease, sign of disease, diagnosis,* and *prognosis?*

3. How does an organic disease differ from a functional disease?

4. What principal factors does the physician evaluate in arriving at a diagnosis?

5. What is the difference between specific and symptomatic treatment?

6. What are the major categories of diagnostic tests and procedures that can help the practitioner make a diagnosis? Give some examples.

7. What is the difference between an invasive and a noninvasive procedure?

8. What are the basic concepts on which the following procedures are based? Pap smear, x-ray examinations, ultrasound, electrocardiogram, CT scans.

Supplementary Readings

Chilton, H. M., and Ekstrand, K. E. 1984. Principles and applications of nuclear magnetic resonance imaging. *American Journal of Hospital Pharmacology* 41:763–67. A primer on the physics of MRI imaging and equipment.

Consensus Conference. 1988. Magnetic resonance imaging. *Journal of the American Medical Association* 259:2132–38. Review of practical applications and limitations.

Douglass, B. E. 1981. Examining healthy patients: How and how often? *Mayo Clinic Proceedings* 56:57–60. A review of periodic medical examinations with recommendations of frequency.

Figley, N. M., ed. 1983. Diagnostic imaging and related sciences. *American Journal of Roentgenology* (special section: NMR) 141:1101–1353. A detailed reference on the various applications and limitations of NMR in medical diagnosis.

Jacobson, H. G. 1987. Fundamentals of magnetic resonance imaging. *Journal of the American Medical Association* 258:3417–23. Describes principles and applications of this powerful diagnostic tool.

Kottke, T. E. 1990. Clinical prevention services: How should we define the indications. *Mayo Clinic Proceedings* 65:899–902. Describes applications and limitations of health screening. Intervention must be able to detect, treat, or prevent the condition it has been designed to deal with. We must not harm the patient in our zeal to prevent disease.

Matchar, D. B. 1990. Decision-making in the face of uncertainty: The case of carotid endarterectomy. *Mayo Clinic Proceedings* 65:756–60. Excellent discussion of risks and benefits of therapeutic procedures, as well as biases. The wish to do everything possible for the patient must not lead to misguided actions.

Pritchard, J. W., and Brass, L. M. 1992. New anatomical and functional imaging methods. *Annals of Neurology* 32:395–400. Reviews advantages and disadvantages of various images to evaluate brain anatomy and function. Good review of PET scans.

Chapter 1 ■ Outline Summary

Characteristics of Disease / 3
Disturbance of Structure or Function

Lesions: structural changes identified by gross or microscopic examination.

Symptoms: subjective manifestations.

Signs: objective findings.

Terminology:

Asymptomatic disease: not associated with symptoms or discomfort.

Symptomatic disease: associated with symptoms and abnormal physical findings.

Etiology: cause of disease.

Pathogenesis: manner in which disease develops.

Classifications of Disease / 3

Congenital and hereditary disease: caused by genetic or chromosomal abnormality, intrauterine injury, or interaction of genetic and environmental factors.

Inflammatory disease: associated with inflammation.

Degenerative disease: associated with degeneration of tissues or organs.

Metabolic disease: associated with disturbed metabolic processes.

Neoplastic disease: characterized by various benign and malignant tumors.

Health and Disease: A Continuum / 5
Basic Concepts

Health and disease are two extremes of a continuous spectrum.

Good health is more than absence of disease.

Modern medicine can cure disease but cannot guarantee good health.

Each individual must assume responsibility for achieving good health.

Principles of Diagnosis and Treatment / 5
Diagnosis

Clinical history: information obtained from patient.

Physical examination: objective findings obtained by clinician.

Differential diagnosis: consideration of possible diseases that could be responsible for clinical manifestations.

Treatment

Specific treatment: produces specific curative effect.

Symptomatic treatment: alleviates symptoms but does not alter course of disease.

Diagnostic Tests and Procedures / 7
Categories of Diagnostic Procedures

Invasive procedure: "invades" patient's body to obtain diagnostic information.

Noninvasive procedure: not associated with significant risk or discomfort.

Types of Procedures

Clinical laboratory tests: chemical, serologic, microbiologic tests on blood and body fluids.

Tests that measure electrical activity: ECG, EEG, EMG.

Radioisotope studies: determine uptake and excretion of radioactive materials.

Endoscopy: examines interior of body with specially designed instruments.

X-ray examination:

X-rays absorbed in proportion to density of tissue.

X-rays using contrast media: outline structures that cannot be visualized on standard films.

CT scans: X-rays transmitted to computer produce cross-section views through various levels of the body.

Magnetic resonance imaging: detects same type of abnormalities as CT, but based on movement of protons in magnetic field; has advantages over CT in special situations.

PET scans: measure metabolism of biochemical compounds labeled with positron-emitting isotopes as measure of organ function.

Very expensive procedure not widely available; applications and limitations still being explored.

Major current application is assessment of brain functions in health and disease.

Cytologic and histologic examinations: smears and biopsy samples taken from patient's body have characteristic patterns that permit recognition of disease.

2

Cells and Tissues
Their Structure and Function in Health and Disease

Learning Objectives

1. Make a sketch of the general structure of a typical cell.
2. Explain how cells are organized to form tissues. Diagram the fundamental structure of the four basic types of tissues.
3. Explain how tissues are organized to form organ systems.
4. Write a general description of the three germ layers and their derivatives.
5. Describe how cells utilize the genetic code within DNA chains to convey genetic information to daughter cells during cell division.
6. Explain the process by which the DNA in the nucleus directs the synthesis of enzymes and other proteins in the cytoplasm.
7. Illustrate how materials move in and out of cells. List five processes by which cells adapt to changing conditions.
8. Explain three ways in which an aging cell becomes increasingly vulnerable to injury.

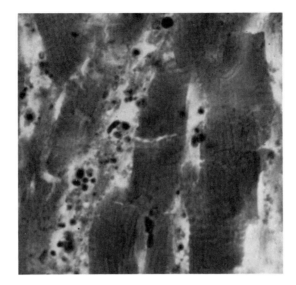

Chapter 2 ▪ Contents

The cell is the basic structural and functional unit of the body. Groups of similar cells arranged to perform a common function form **tissues.** Tissues in turn are grouped together in different proportions to form **organs,** and groups of organs functioning together form **organ systems.** Finally, the various organ systems are integrated to form a functioning organism. Dysfunction at any of these levels of organization can cause disease.

The Cell

Cells having different functions differ somewhat in structure, but all have certain features in common (figure 2–1). Each cell consists of a *nucleus* surrounded by the *cytoplasm.* The nucleus, which contains the genetic information stored in the cell, directs the metabolic functions of the cell, and structures in the cytoplasm carry out these directions. Within the cytoplasm are numerous small structures called **organelles,** which play an important part in the functions of the cell. The cytoplasm also contains filaments of structural protein that form the framework (cytoskeleton) of the cell. Some cells also contain filaments of contractile protein. The cytoplasm, nucleus, and organelles are surrounded by membranes composed of lipid and protein molecules, which separate these structures from one another.

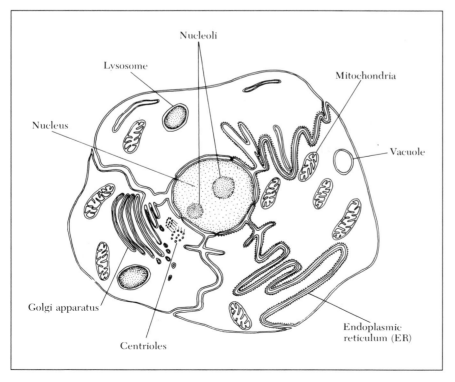

FIGURE 2–1

Structure of a typical cell.

The Nucleus

The nucleus contains two different types of nucleic acid combined with protein. **Deoxyribonucleic acid (DNA)** is contained in the chromosomes, which are long and thin in the nondividing cell and cannot be identified as distinct structures. Instead, they appear as a network of granules called *nuclear chromatin.* **Ribonucleic acid (RNA)** is contained in spherical intranuclear structures called *nucleoli* (singular, *nucleolus*). The nucleus is separated from the cytoplasm by a double-layered nuclear membrane. Small pores in the nuclear membrane permit the nucleus and cytoplasm to communicate.

The Cytoplasm

The cytoplasm of the cell consists of a mass of protoplasm surrounded by a cell membrane, which acts selectively to allow some materials to pass into and out of the cell while it restricts the passage of others. It contains various organelles and may also contain products secreted by the cell, such as glycogen and fat. The most important organelles are the mitochondria, endoplasmic reticulum, Golgi apparatus, lysosomes, and centrioles.

Mitochondria are sausage-shaped structures that contain enzymes capable of converting food materials into energy by oxidizing them. The cell uses this energy to manufacture a high-energy compound called **adenosine triphosphate (ATP)**, the fuel that powers the chemical reactions in the cell.

The **endoplasmic reticulum** is an interconnected network of tubular channels enclosed by membranes. This network communicates with both the nuclear membrane and the cell membrane. *Rough endoplasmic reticulum* (RER) has numerous small nucleoprotein particles called **ribosomes** attached to the external surfaces of its membranes. Its name derives from the knobby appearance that the attached ribosomes give the membranes, and its function is to synthesize protein that will be secreted by the cell. The attached ribosomes synthesize protein molecules that accumulate within the tubules of the RER and are eventually secreted. Digestive enzymes and antibody proteins, for example, are produced in this way. The second type of endoplasmic reticulum lacks ribosomes and is called the *smooth endoplasmic reticulum* (SER). Its membranes contain enzymes that synthesize lipids and some other substances.

The **Golgi apparatus** consists of groups of flattened membranelike sacs located near the nucleus. These sacs are connected with the tubules of the RER. The proteins produced by the ribosomes attached to the RER pass through the RER tubules into the Golgi apparatus, where large carbohydrate molecules are synthesized and combined with the proteins. Then they are formed into secretory granules and eventually discharged from the cell.

Lysosomes digest material (*lysis* = dissolving + *soma* = body) that has been brought into the cell by phagocytosis. A lysosome consists of a cytoplasmic vacuole filled with potent digestive enzymes. When particulate material is ingested by phagocytosis, the particle becomes enclosed within a

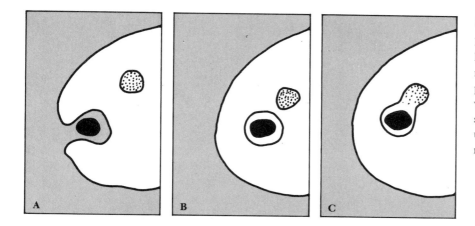

FIGURE 2–2

Digestion of material by lysosomes. **A,** Particulate material is engulfed by cytoplasm of cell. **B,** Phagocytic vacuole is formed. **C,** Lysosome and phagocytic vacuole merge, and engulfed material is then digested.

membrane-lined vacuole called *phagocytic vacuole*. A lysosome then merges with the phagocytic vacuole, and their cell membranes fuse, allowing the digestive enzymes contained in the lysosome to flow into the phagocytic vacuole and digest the engulfed material. Digestion is accomplished entirely within the phagocytic vacuole, which prevents digestive enzymes from leaking into the cytoplasm of the cell and causing injury to the cell (figure 2–2).

Centrioles are short cylindrical structures located adjacent to the nucleus. In cell division, they move to opposite poles of the cell and form the mitotic spindle. The spindle fibers attach to the chromosomes and cause them to separate in the course of cell division.

A tissue is a group of similar cells joined together to perform a specific function. Tissues are classified into four major groups:

The Tissues

1. Epithelium
2. Connective and supporting tissue
3. Muscle
4. Nerve tissue

Epithelium

Epithelium consists of groups of cells closely joined together (figure 2–3). Epithelial cells cover the exterior of the body and line the interior body surfaces that communicate with the outside, such as the gastrointestinal tract, urinary tract, and vagina. Epithelium forms glands such as the thyroid and pancreas and also makes up the functional cells (often called *parenchymal cells* or *parenchyma*) of organs that have excretory or secretory functions, such as the liver and the kidneys. The individual cells may be flat and plate-like (squamous cells), cube shaped (cuboidal cells), or tall and narrow (columnar cells). Many columnar epithelial cells have become specialized to

FIGURE 2–3

Common types of epithelium. **A,** Simple squamous. **B,** Cuboidal. **C,** Columnar. **D,** Pseudostratified columnar (ciliated). **E,** Transitional. **F,** Stratified squamous.

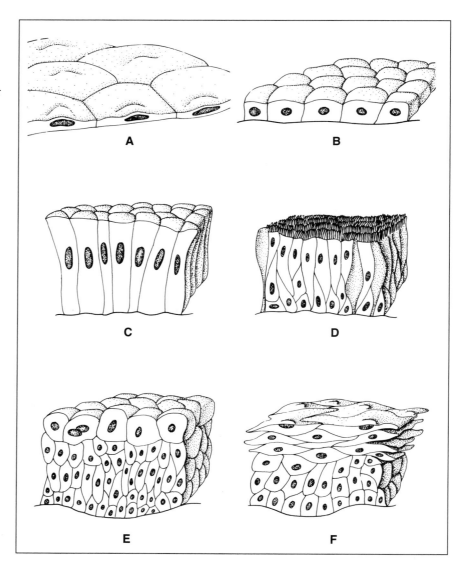

absorb or secrete, and some contain hairlike processes called cilia. Epithelial cells may be arranged in a single layer (simple epithelium) or may be several layers thick (stratified epithelium).

Endothelium and Mesothelium

The interiors of the heart, blood vessels, and lymphatic vessels are lined by a layer of simple squamous epithelium called **endothelium** (*endo* = within). A similar type of epithelium lining the pleural, pericardial, and peritoneal cavities is called **mesothelium** (*meso* = middle). Although these linings are classified as types of epithelium, they arise along with the connective tissues from the embryonic germ layer called the **mesoderm** and are therefore much more closely related to connective tissue than to other types of epithelium. Consequently, they are considered separately and are given distinct names. Moreover, tumors arising from endothelium or mesothelium behave more like tumors originating from connective tissue. They are classified with the connective tissue tumors rather than with tumors arising from surface, glandular, or parenchymal epithelium. This subject is considered in chapter 10.

The Structure of Epithelium

Epithelial cells are supported by a thin basement membrane. The cells are firmly joined to each other, and the deeper layers of epithelium are firmly anchored to the basement membrane; so epithelial cells remain relatively fixed in position. There are no blood vessels in epithelium. The cells are nourished by diffusion of material from capillaries located in the underlying connective tissue.

Simple Epithelium

The distribution of *simple squamous epithelium* is limited. It forms the lining of the pulmonary air sacs. It forms the endothelial lining of the vascular system and the mesothelial lining of the body cavities. *Simple columnar epithelium* lines most of the gastrointestinal tract. *Pseudostratified columnar epithelium* is a type of simple columnar epithelium in which the cells are so tightly packed together that their nuclei appear to lie at different levels. This gives an appearance of stratification. Pseudostratified epithelium is often ciliated. This type of epithelium lines most of the respiratory tract and is present in a few other areas.

Stratified Epithelium

Stratified squamous epithelium forms the external covering of the body and also lines the oral cavity, esophagus, and vagina. Stratified epithelium is named for the appearance of the most superficial cell layer. Consequently, this epithelium is designated "stratified squamous" even though the deeper layers are composed of cuboidal cells. The stratified squamous epithelium that forms the top layer of the skin undergoes a process called *keratinization,* in which the top layers of squamous cells accumulate a fibrous protein called **keratin** (figure 2–4). This fibrous protein forms a dense layer that protects the underlying cells. *Transitional epithelium* consists of a layer of large superficial cells covering a deeper layer of cuboidal cells. It is the characteristic lining of the bladder and other parts of the urinary tract. The superficial cells of transitional epithelium become flattened when the bladder is distended and resume their original shape when the bladder is empty.

Functions of Epithelium

Epithelium performs many different functions. All types of epithelium perform a protective function. Columnar epithelium, such as that lining the intestinal tract, is specialized to absorb and secrete. Other types of epithelium form glands that secrete mucus, sweat, oil, enzymes, hormones, or other products.

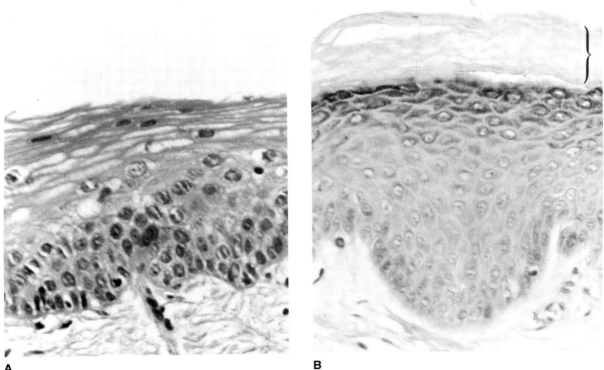

A   **B**

FIGURE 2-4

A, Nonkeratinized squamous epithelium. **B,** Keratinized epithelium. The keratin layer (*bracket*) forms a dense acellular covering that protects the underlying epithelial cells. (Original magnification × 400.)

Glands, such as the pancreas, that discharge their secretions through a duct onto an epithelial surface are called **exocrine glands** (*exo* = out). **Endocrine glands** (*endo* = within), such as the thyroid and adrenals, discharge their secretions directly into the bloodstream.

Connective and Supporting Tissues

Connective and supporting tissues consist of relatively small numbers of cells incorporated in a large amount of extracellular material called **matrix** in which are embedded various types of fibers. The proportions of cells, fibers, and matrix vary greatly in different types of connective tissue. Connective tissue fibers are of three types. *Collagen fibers* are long, flexible fibers composed of a protein called *collagen.* They are strong but do not stretch. *Elastic fibers* are composed of a protein called *elastin.* They are not as strong as collagen but stretch readily and return to their former shape when the stretching force is released. *Reticulin fibers* are very similar to collagen but are quite thin and delicate.

Connective and supporting tissues include various types of loose and dense fibrous tissue, elastic tissue, reticular tissue, adipose tissue, cartilage, and bone. Hematopoietic (blood-forming) tissue and lymphatic (lymphocyte-forming) tissue also are classified as types of connective tissue, primarily because, like other types of connective tissue, they originate from the mesoderm.

Fibrous connective tissue performs a variety of functions that connect and support the various parts of the body. *Loose fibrous tissue,* which is the most widely distributed, forms the tissue just beneath the skin (subcutaneous tissue) and also fills in around organs. *Dense fibrous tissue* forms ligaments and tendons, which reinforce joints and attach muscles to bone.

Elastic tissue forms membranes that are wrapped around the walls of blood vessels and are responsible for the characteristic distensibility of large arteries. Elastic membranes also form part of the walls of the trachea and bronchi.

Reticular tissue is a special type of connective tissue characterized by a fine meshwork of reticulin fibers that form the supporting framework of various organs such as the liver, spleen, and lymph nodes.

Adipose tissue is a variety of loose fibrous tissue containing large numbers of fat cells. Fat is a stored form of energy and also functions as padding and insulation.

Cartilage is a type of supporting tissue in which the cells are dispersed in a dense matrix. There are three types of cartilage. *Hyaline cartilage* is the most common. It is blue and translucent and contains only a few fine collagen fibers suspended in the abundant matrix. Hyaline cartilage covers the ends of bones where they form movable joints, forms the greater part of the laryngeal and tracheal cartilages, and connects the ribs to the sternum. *Elastic cartilage* contains yellow elastic fibers in the matrix and is found in only a few locations, such as the cartilaginous portions of the ears. The elastic fibers impart a flexibility to the cartilage that is lacking in other types of cartilage. *Fibrocartilage* contains many dense collagen bundles embedded in the matrix. It is found in areas where cartilage is subjected to marked weight-bearing stresses. It forms the disks between the vertebral bodies and some of the cartilages in the knee joints; it is also present in a few other locations.

Bone is a highly specialized, rigid supporting tissue in which the matrix containing the bone-forming cells is impregnated with calcium salts.

Muscle Tissue

Muscle cells contain filaments of specialized intracellular contractile proteins called actin and myosin. These are arranged in parallel bundles. During contraction of a muscle fiber, actin filaments slide inward on the myosin filaments somewhat like pistons, causing the fiber to shorten. There are three types of muscle fibers. *Smooth muscle* is located primarily in the walls of hollow internal organs such as the gastrointestinal tract, biliary tract, and reproductive tract and is also present in the walls of the blood vessels. Smooth muscle functions automatically and is not under conscious control. *Striated muscle* moves the skeleton and is under voluntary control. *Cardiac muscle* is found only in the heart. It resembles striated muscle but has some features common to both smooth and voluntary muscle.

Nerve Tissue

Nerve tissue is composed of nerve cells called **neurons,** which transmit nerve impulses, and supporting cells called **neuroglia.** Neuroglial cells are more numerous than neurons. They are of three different types. **Astrocytes** are long, star-shaped cells having numerous highly branched processes that interlace to form a meshwork. Astrocytes form the structural framework of the central nervous system in the way that the connective tissue fibers form the framework of internal organs. **Oligodendroglia** are small cells with scanty cytoplasm that surround individual nerve cells in the central nervous system. **Microglia** are phagocytic cells comparable to the macrophages found in other tissues.

Organs and Organ Systems

An **organ** is a group of different tissues that are integrated to perform a specific function. Generally, one tissue performs the primary function characteristic of the organ, and the other tissues perform a supporting function, such as providing the vascular and connective-tissue framework for the organ. The functional cells of an organ are often called the *parenchymal cells,* and the total mass of functional tissue is called the **parenchyma.** The supporting framework of the organ is called the **stroma.** In the liver, for example, the parenchymal cells are formed by cords of epithelial cells that perform the many metabolic functions characteristic of the liver, such as the synthesis of protein and the excretion of bile. The cord cells are supported by a framework of connective-tissue fibers. Numerous thin-walled blood vessels are interspersed between the cell cords, and the entire liver is surrounded by a capsule composed of dense fibrous tissue.

An *organ system* is a group of organs that are organized to perform complementary functions, such as the reproductive system, the respiratory system, and the digestive system. Finally, the various organ systems are integrated into a functioning individual.

The Germ Layers and Their Derivatives

The highly complex structure of the entire body evolves from a single cell, the fertilized ovum, by a complex process that includes periods of cell multiplication, differentiation, and organization to form organs and organ systems. (Prenatal development is considered in chapter 18 in conjunction with diseases of pregnancy.) As the fertilized ovum grows, its cells differentiate into two groups. The peripheral group of cells is called the **trophoblast.** This forms the placenta and other structures that will support and nourish the embryo. The inner group of cells is called the **inner cell mass.** These are the cells that will give rise to the embryo, and they soon become

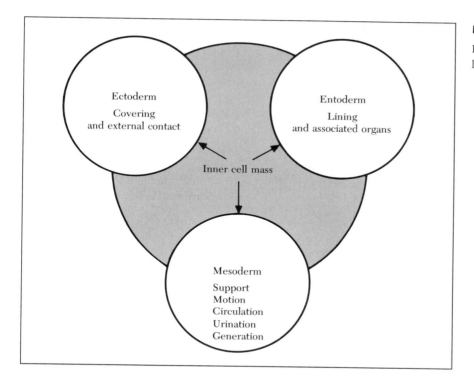

FIGURE 2–5

Derivatives of the germ layers (simplified scheme).

arranged into three distinct layers called the **germ layers.** Each layer will form certain specialized tissues and organs (figure 2–5). The outer layer, called the **ectoderm** (*ecto* = outer + *derm* = skin), forms the external covering of the body and the various organs that bring the individual into contact with the external environment: the nervous system, eyes, and ears. The inner layer, called the **entoderm** (*ento* = within), forms the internal "lining": the epithelium of the pharynx, the respiratory tract, the gastrointestinal tract and the organs closely associated with it (the liver, biliary tract, and pancreas), and some parts of the urogenital tract. The **mesoderm** (*meso* = middle) is the layer of cells sandwiched between the other two layers. From these cells are derived the various supporting tissues (connective tissues, cartilage, and bone), muscle, the circulatory system (heart, blood, and blood vessels), and major portions of the urogenital system. Each normal cell in the body is part of a community of cells and is integrated with its neighbors so that it functions along with other cells to meet the body's needs.

The chromosomes contain a series of messages called the **genetic code.** It is this code that regulates the various functions of the cell. The genetic code is contained within the structure of DNA and is transmitted to each newly formed cell in cell division.

Cell Function and the Genetic Code

The Structure of DNA

The chromosomes are composed of DNA combined with protein. The basic structural unit of DNA, called a *nucleotide,* consists of a phosphate group linked to a five-carbon sugar, *deoxyribose,* which in turn is joined to a nitrogen-containing compound called a **base** (figure 2–6A). There are two different types of DNA bases: a *purine base,* which contains a fused double ring of carbon and nitrogen atoms, and a *pyrimidine base,* which contains only a single ring. There are four different bases in DNA: the purine bases *adenine* and *guanine,* and the pyrimidine bases *thymine* and *cytosine.* Consequently, there are four different nucleotides in DNA, each containing a different base (figure 2–6B). The nucleotides are joined together in long chains, with the nitrogen bases projecting at right angles from the long axes of the chains. A DNA molecule consists of two strands of DNA that are held together by weak chemical attractions between the bases of the adjacent chains. The chemical structure of the bases is such that only adenine can pair with thymine and only guanine can pair with cytosine. Bases that pair in this way are called *complementary bases.* The DNA chains are twisted into a double spiral somewhat like a spiral staircase, with the sugar and phosphate groups forming the two railings and the complementary base pairs forming the steps (figure 2–7A, B, and C).

FIGURE 2–6

General structure of a DNA nucleotide. **A,** Deoxyribose is identical with ribose except for absence of an oxygen atom (location indicated by *arrow*). **B,** Structure of the bases. *Arrows* indicate sites at which bases are joined to deoxyribose.

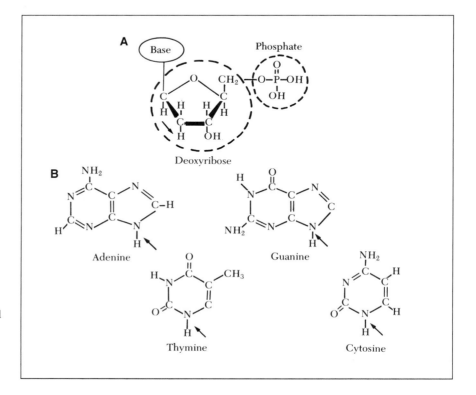

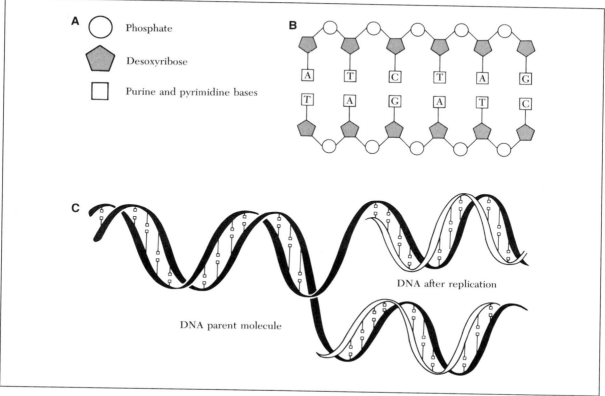

FIGURE 2–7

A, Components entering into the formation of the DNA molecule. **B,** Structure of double-stranded DNA. **C,** Duplication (replication) of the DNA molecule.

Duplication (Replication) of DNA

As a cell prepares to divide, the double strands of DNA duplicate themselves. The two chains separate, and each chain serves as the model for the synthesis of a new chain (figure 2–7C). Because adenine always pairs with thymine and guanine with cytosine, the arrangement of the nucleotides in the original chains determines how the nucleotides will reassemble to form the new chains. The process of duplication forms two double strands, each containing one of the original strands plus a newly formed strand. In this way, each of the two daughter cells produced by cell division receives an exact duplicate of the genetic information possessed by the chromosomes of the parent cell.

The Genetic Code

The DNA in the nucleus "tells the cell what to do" by directing the synthesis of enzymes and other proteins by the ribosomes located in the cytoplasm.

The "instructions" are carried by *messenger RNA* (mRNA), so named because it carries the message encoded in the DNA to the ribosomes in the cytoplasm. Messenger RNA is quite similar to DNA but consists of only a single rather than a double strand. It also differs by containing the five-carbon sugar *ribose* instead of deoxyribose and a base called *uracil* instead of thymine. During synthesis of mRNA, the DNA chains partially separate, and the DNA serves as the model upon which the mRNA is assembled. Therefore, the information transported on the mRNA strand is an exact copy of the genetic information possessed by the nuclear DNA.

The mRNA strand leaves the nucleus through the pores in the nuclear membrane and becomes attached to the ribosomes in the cytoplasm, which are small nucleoprotein particles where enzymes and other proteins are constructed from individual amino acids. The combination of amino acids required to assemble the protein is determined by the information contained in the mRNA strand. The amino acids are transported to the ribosomes by means of another type of RNA called *transfer RNA* (tRNA), so named because it "picks up" the required amino acids from the cytoplasm and transfers them to the ribosomes where they are assembled in proper order, as specified by the mRNA (figure 2–8).

Movement of Materials into and out of Cells

In order for the cell to function properly, oxygen and nutrients must enter the cell and waste products must be eliminated. Materials entering and leaving the cell must cross the cell membrane, which limits the passage of some

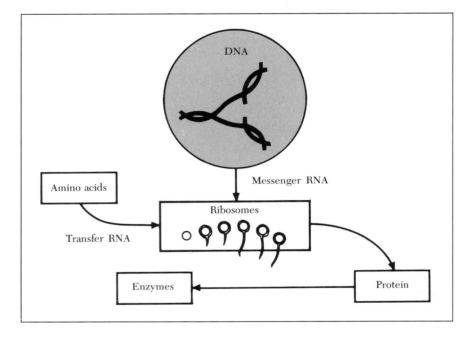

FIGURE 2–8

Role of messenger RNA and transfer RNA in the synthesis of enzymes and other proteins by ribosomes in the cytoplasm.

molecules and is freely permeable to others. Materials cross the cell membrane in three ways:

1. Diffusion and osmosis
2. Active transport
3. Phagocytosis and pinocytosis

Diffusion and Osmosis

Diffusion is the movement of *dissolved particles* (*solute*) from a more concentrated to a more dilute solution. *Osmosis* is the movement of *water molecules* from a dilute solution to a more concentrated solution (figure 2–9). Both are passive processes that do not require the cell to expend energy.

Osmotic Pressure and Osmolarity
The water-attracting property of a solution is called its *osmotic pressure*. The more concentrated the solution, the higher its osmotic pressure. The quantitative expression of the osmotic pressure of a solution is called **osmolarity.** Osmolarity reflects the number of dissolved particles in the solution, not the molecular weight or valence of the particles. For a substance such as glucose, which does not dissociate in solution, 1 g molecular weight dissolved in 1 L of water has an osmolarity of 1 osmole per liter (abbreviated Osm/L). However, 1 g molecular weight of a substance that dissociates in solution into two univalent ions (such as sodium chloride) has an osmolarity

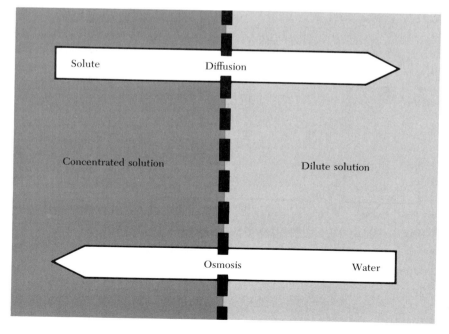

FIGURE 2–9

Processes of diffusion and osmosis across a porous membrane (indicated by *dashed line*).

of 2 Osm/L. One gram molecular weight of a salt containing a divalent ion such as calcium chloride ($CaCl_2$) has an osmolarity of 3 Osm/L because the salt dissociates into three particles: one calcium and two chloride ions. The osmolarity of body fluids is usually expressed in milliosmoles per liter (mOsm/L) because body fluids contain low concentrations of dissolved particles (1 Osm = 1000 mOsm). The term *tonicity* also is sometimes used when referring to the osmotic pressure of a solution. An **isotonic solution** (*iso* = equal + *tonos* = pressure) has an osmolarity that is physiologically equivalent to that of blood plasma and other body fluids. A more concentrated solution is said to be **hypertonic** (*hyper* = above), and a more dilute solution is said to be **hypotonic** (*hypo* = below).

Osmotic Pressure Differences Between Cells and Extracellular Fluids

If the osmolarity of the *extracellular fluid* (ECF) is higher than that within the cells, water flows by osmosis from the cell into the ECF, causing the cell to shrink. Conversely, if the osmolarity of the ECF is lower than that of the cells, water moves by osmosis into the cells, causing the cells to swell. Normally, the osmotic pressures within the cell and in the ECF are equal; so the shape and water content of the cells do not change. In disease, the osmolarity of the ECF may be abnormally low or high, which will lead to secondary changes in the water content of the cells and will impair their function.

Active Transport

Active transport is the transfer of a substance across the cell membrane from a region of *low concentration* to one of *higher concentration*. The process requires the cell to expend energy because the substance must move against a concentration gradient. Many metabolic processes depend on active transport of ions or molecules. For example, in order for the cell to function normally, the intracellular potassium concentration must be higher than the concentration in the ECF, and the intracellular sodium concentration must be much lower. This is accomplished by a mechanism that actively transports potassium into the cell and simultaneously moves sodium out.

Phagocytosis and Pinocytosis

Phagocytosis is the ingestion of particles that are too large to pass across the cell membrane. The cytoplasm flows around the particle and the cytoplasmic processes fuse, engulfing the particle within a vacuole in the cytoplasm of the cell. A similar process called **pinocytosis** consists of the ingestion of fluid rather than solid material.

Cells respond to changing conditions in various ways. Common adaptive mechanisms are:

1. Atrophy
2. Hypertrophy and hyperplasia
3. Metaplasia
4. Dysplasia
5. Increased enzyme synthesis

In many instances, the adaptation enables the cells to function more efficiently. Sometimes, however, the adaptive change may be detrimental to the cell, as occurs in dysplasia.

Atrophy

Atrophy is a reduction in the size of cells in response to diminished function, inadequate hormonal stimulation, or reduced blood supply. The cell decreases in size in order to "get by" under the less-favorable conditions. For example, skeletal muscles are reduced in size when an extremity is immobilized in a cast for long periods, and the breasts and genital organs shrink following menopause as a result of inadequate estrogen stimulation. A kidney becomes smaller if its blood supply becomes insufficient because of narrowing of the renal artery.

Hypertrophy and Hyperplasia

If cells are required to do more work, they may increase either their size or their number in order to accomplish their task. **Hypertrophy** is an increase in the size of individual cells without an actual increase in their numbers. The large muscles of a weight lifter, for example, result from hypertrophy of individual muscle fibers. The number of fibers is not increased. Similarly, the heart of a person with high blood pressure often enlarges as a result of hypertrophy of the individual cardiac muscle fibers. This occurs because the heart must work harder in order to pump blood at a higher-than-normal pressure.

    Hyperplasia is an increase in the size of a tissue or organ caused by an increase in the number of cells. Hyperplasia occurs in response to increased demand. For example, the glandular tissue of the breast becomes hyperplastic during pregnancy in preparation for lactation. Endocrine glands such as the thyroid may enlarge in order to increase their output of hormones.

Metaplasia

Metaplasia is a change from one type of cell to another type that is better able to tolerate some adverse environmental condition. For example, if the lining of the bladder is chronically irritated and inflamed, the normal transitional epithelial lining may assume the characteristic structure of a thick layer of squamous epithelium. The metaplastic epithelium is more resistant to irritation and is better able to protect the bladder wall in the presence of chronic infection.

Dysplasia

Dysplasia (*dys* = bad + *plasia* = formation) is a condition in which the development and maturation of cells is disturbed and abnormal. The individual cells vary in size and shape, and their relationship to one another is also abnormal (figure 2-10). Dysplasia of epithelial cells may result from chronic irritation or inflammation. In some cases, dysplasia may progress to formation of a tumor; this is called **neoplasia.** The epithelium covering the uterine cervix is a common site of dysplasia, and cervical epithelial dysplasia sometimes progresses to cervical cancer. This subject is discussed in chapter 10.

Increased Enzyme Synthesis

Increased synthesis of enzymes is another adaptive change that occurs in cells. Sometimes cells are called upon to inactivate or detoxify drugs or chemicals by means of the enzymes present in the smooth endoplasmic reticulum

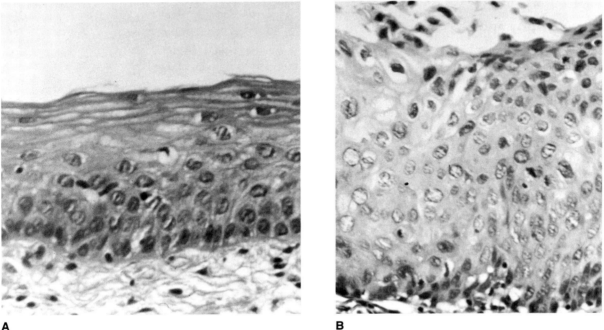

A   **B**

FIGURE 2–10

Comparison of normal squamous epithelium (**A**) with dysplastic epithelium (**B**). Note variations in nuclear polarity and staining reaction. (Original magnification approximately × 400.)

(SER). If increased demands are placed on the cells, they respond by synthesizing more SER enzymes so that drugs or chemicals can be processed more efficiently. Once the cells increase their ability to handle such chemicals or drugs, they can rapidly eliminate other substances that are handled by means of the same enzyme systems. A person accustomed to heavy consumption of alcohol, for example, is able to metabolize the alcohol more efficiently because of this adaptive change. Such an individual may also metabolize and eliminate other drugs at a greatly accelerated rate. Consequently, if a physician administers a medication that is metabolized by the same enzyme systems, the usual therapeutic doses of the medications may be ineffective.

Cell Injury

An injured cell may exhibit various morphologic abnormalities. The two most common changes are cell swelling and fatty change.

Cell Swelling
A normally functioning cell actively transports potassium into the cell and moves sodium out. This process requires the cell to expend energy. If the cell is injured and unable to function normally, the transport mechanism begins to fail. Sodium diffuses into the cell, and water moves into the cell along with the sodium, causing the cell to swell. If the swelling continues, fluid-filled vacuoles may accumulate within the cell, and eventually it may rupture.

Fatty Change
If the enzyme systems that metabolize fat are impaired, leading to accumulation of fat droplets within the cytoplasm, fatty change may occur. This condition is a common manifestation of liver cell injury, because liver cells are actively involved in fat metabolism.

Cell Death and Cell Necrosis

A cell dies if it has been irreparably damaged. Several hours after the cell dies, various structural changes to begin to take place within the nucleus and cytoplasm. Lysosomal enzymes are released and begin to digest the cell. The nucleus shrinks and either dissolves or breaks into fragments. Sometimes calcium is deposited in the dead cells and tissues. These structural changes are termed cell **necrosis**. All necrotic cells are dead, but a dead cell is not necessarily necrotic, because the structural changes that characterize cell death take several hours to develop. Necrotic cells are easily recognized on histologic examination because they appear quite different from normal cells in both their structural and their staining characteristics (figure 2–11).

Cell Injury, Cell Death, and Cell Necrosis

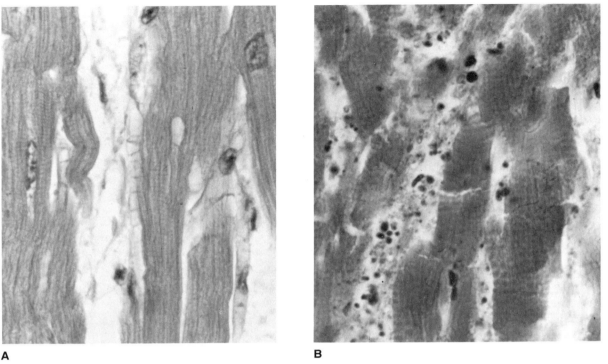

A   B

FIGURE 2–11

Comparison of normal cardiac muscle fibers (**A**) with necrotic fibers (**B**). Note fragmentation of fibers, loss of nuclear staining, and fragmented bits of nuclear debris. (Original magnification × 400.)

Aging and the Cell

All organisms grow old and eventually die, and each species has a predetermined life-span. Although human life expectancy has increased over the years, the increase is chiefly because early deaths from infectious diseases, accidents, and other conditions have been greatly reduced. The causes of aging are not well understood but appear to reside in the cell. Although each type of cell has a definite life-span, under normal circumstances, cell longevity is also influenced by environmental factors. The life-span of an individual in turn reflects the survival of the various populations of cells that together form the individual.

Many investigators believe that aging of cells is genetically programmed and is an inherent property of the cell itself. Examples can be seen in the graying of the hair, which is the result of an eventual failure of the hair cells to produce pigment, and in the menopause, which is a predetermined failure of reproductive function. Aging changes in the brain appear to be caused by the wearing out and eventual death of neurons, which are not capable of cell division. The degenerative changes in the walls of arteries, called arteriosclerosis, are thought to be caused partially by a gradual failure of the endothelial cells lining the blood vessels to prevent fatty substances from seeping into the arterial walls. The common type of arthritis seen in older persons begins as an aging change in the cartilage covering the ends of the bones.

As a cell ages, many of its enzyme systems become less active and the cell becomes less efficient in carrying out its functions. The cell also becomes more susceptible to harmful environmental influences that may shorten its life. For example, the life-span of a red cell is four months, and thus the red cells circulating in the bloodstream vary greatly in age, ranging from newly produced cells to those nearing the end of their life-span. Each red cell contains enzyme systems that generate its energy, enable it to perform its varied metabolic functions, and maintain the hemoglobin in a condition suitable for transporting oxygen. As the red cell ages and its enzyme systems gradually decline, the cell is less able to protect itself from injury than is a young, "vigorous" cell. If the red cells are exposed to harmful drugs or antibodies that damage the cell membranes, it is the older cells that bear the brunt of the damage and die. The younger cells are able to survive and continue to function.

An example of aging change in cells that affects the organism as a whole can be seen in the lymphocytes of which our immune system is composed. These cells help eliminate pathogenic organisms and also eliminate any of our own cells that become abnormal and have the potential of forming tumors. The cells of the immune system become less efficient as they age. Consequently, the aging individual becomes more susceptible to various infectious diseases, which can shorten the life-span. The aging immune system also becomes less able to eliminate abnormal cells that arise sporadically within the body. This may predispose to the formation of malignant tumors, which occur with increasing frequency in older persons.

Aging of cells may also be caused by damage to cellular DNA, RNA, and cytoplasmic organelles that occurs at a pace more rapid than the cell's ability to repair itself. According to this concept, these components become damaged by radiation or other environmental factors or by accumulation of metabolic products within cells. Eventually, the cells begin to malfunction. Some cells can repair the damage and continue to function. Others cannot and die. The more efficient the repair process within the cell, the more likely the cell is to survive.

In summary, cells have a finite life-span. But the less they are exposed to harmful environmental influences, and the more efficient they are in repairing their own malfunctions, the greater their chances for survival to a "ripe old age."

Questions for Review

1. How does the nucleus direct the activities of the cell? What is the genetic code, and what is its role in directing the functions of the cell?

2. What are the functions of the following organelles: rough endoplasmic reticulum, ribosomes, lysosomes, centrosomes?

3. How is epithelium classified, and what are its functions? Why are mesothelium and endothelium considered separately from other types of epithelium?

4. What are the germ layers, and what are their functions?

5. What is the difference between atrophy and hypertrophy, between metaplasia and dysplasia, between cell death and cell necrosis?

6. What morphologic abnormalities are manifested by an injured cell? Why do they develop?

7. What factors cause a cell to age?

Supplementary Readings

Baserga, R. 1981. The cell cycle. *New England Journal of Medicine* 304:453–59. Describes the biology of cell division and its relation to tumor growth and treatment of tumors by cytotoxic drugs.

Fox, S. I. 1993. Cell structure and genetic control. Chap. 2 in *Human physiology*. 4th ed. Dubuque, Iowa: Wm C. Brown Communications. Basic concepts relating to cell structure and function.

Ganong, W. F. 1993. The general and cellular basis of medical physiology. Chap. 1 in *Review of medical physiology*. 16th ed. Norwalk, Conn.: Appleton & Lange. A standard reference dealing with important concepts of cell structure and function.

Hocman, G. 1980. Biochemistry of Ageing—II. *International Journal of Biochemistry* 12:515–22. A summary of the aging process at the cellular level.

Levine, A. J. 1995. The genetic origins of neoplasia (Editorial). *Journal of the American Medical Association*. 273:592. Mutations in three groups of genes contribute to the origins and progression of neoplasms: oncogenes, tumor suppressor genes, and mutator genes. Mutations that convert proto-oncogenes into oncogenes include amplifications, translocations, and point mutations, and they act as dominant mutations. Mutations of tumor suppressor genes are the basis of inherited predisposition to cancer and are inherited in the heterozygous state. A random mutation of the remaining normally functioning allele leads to loss of regulator function that results in malignancy. Mutator genes correct errors in DNA duplication, and loss of mutator gene function increases the mutation rate.

McCord, J. M., and Fridovich, I. 1978. The biology and pathology of oxygen radicals. *Annals of Internal Medicine* 89:122–27. A discussion of an important mechanism of cell injury.

Scarpelli, D. G., and Iannaccone, P. M. 1990. Cell injury and errors of metabolism. In *Anderson's pathology*. 9th ed. Ed. J. M. Kissane. St. Louis: Mosby. A review of essential concepts relating to structural and functional derangements in cells.

Vander, A. J., Sherman, J. H., and Luciano, D. S. 1994. Cell structure; Molecular control mechanisms. Chaps. 3 and 4 in *Human physiology: The mechanisms of body function*. 6th ed. New York: McGraw-Hill. Discusses structural features and control mechanisms of the cell as a basis for understanding structural and functional abnormalities.

Chapter 2 ■ Outline Summary

The Cell / 27
Composition
  Nucleus: contains genetic information and directs activities.

  Cytoplasm: carries out metabolic activities directed by nucleus.

   Mitochondria: oxidize food to form ATP, energy source of cell.

   Endoplasmic reticulum: two types of hollow tubes in cytoplasm. RER has ribosomes and synthesizes protein. SER has enzymes and synthesizes lipids and other materials.

   Golgi apparatus: functions with endoplasmic reticulum to synthesize and package secretory granules, which are eventually discharged.

   Lysosomes: vacuoles containing digestive enzymes.

   Centrioles: short cylinders that form mitotic spindle during cell division.

The Tissues / 29
Epithelium
  Structure:

   Forms coverings and linings.

    Simple: one layer thick.

    Stratified: multiple layers.

   Endothelium and mesothelium: separate category.

   Forms parenchymal cells of excretory or secretory organs.

Function:

   Protection.

   Absorption.

   Secretion.

   Forms glands: exocrine and endocrine.

Connective and Supporting Tissues / 32
Structure and Function

Fibrous connective tissue: connection and support.

Elastic tissue: stretches. Wrapped around blood vessels.

Reticular tissue: framework of liver, spleen, lymph nodes.

Adipose tissue: energy storage, padding, insulation.

Cartilage and bone: support.

Muscle Tissue / 33
Structure and Function

Smooth: in walls of hollow organs and blood vessels. Regulatory.

Striated: moves skeleton under voluntary control.

Cardiac: found only in heart. Properties intermediate between smooth and skeletal muscle.

Nerve Tissue / 34
Structure and Function

Impulse transmission.

Composed of nerve cells and supporting cells: neuroglia.

Organs and Organ Systems / 34
Organs

A group of different tissues integrated to perform a specific function.

Composed of parenchymal (functional) cells and stromal (supporting) cells.

Organ Systems

A group of organs that perform related functions: e.g., reproductive system.

Germ Layers and Their Derivatives / 34
Function

Embryonic cell layers that give rise to specific tissues and organs.

   Ectoderm: external coverings, nervous system, eyes, ears.

   Mesoderm: supporting tissue, muscle, circulatory system, urogenital system.

   Entoderm: lining of body and associated organs.

Cell Function and the Genetic Code / 35
Function

DNA composed of chains of nucleotides containing genetic information.

In cell division, original chain serves as model for building new chain.

Genetic Code

Nucleus directs activities of cytoplasm by means of mRNA, which attaches to ribosomes and directs protein synthesis.

Transfer RNA brings amino acids to ribosomes for assembly as specified by nucleotides in mRNA.

Movement of Materials into and out of Cells / 38
Diffusion and Osmosis: Passive Processes

Diffusion: movement of solute from concentrated to dilute solution.

Osmosis: movement of water from dilute to more concentrated solution.

Osmotic pressure: a measure of concentration.

Depends on number of dissolved particles.

Tonicity often used interchangeably with osmolarity.

Active Transport: Expends Energy

Transfer of materials against a concentration gradient.

Necessary to maintain proper concentration of intracellular and extracellular ions.

Phagocytosis and Pinocytosis: Ingestion by Cell

Phagocytosis: ingestion of particulate material.

Pinocytosis: ingestion of water.

Adaptations of Cells to Changing Conditions / 41
Nature of Adaptations

Atrophy: reduction in size in response to unfavorable conditions.

Hypertrophy: increase in cell size for more efficient function.

Hyperplasia: increase in number of cells to increase functional capabilities.

Metaplasia: change from one type of cell to more-resistant type.

Dysplasia: disturbed development. May proceed to neoplasia.

Increased enzyme synthesis: adaptation in order to inactivate or detoxify materials more efficiently.

Cell Injury, Cell Death, and Cell Necrosis / 43
Cell Injury

Cell swelling: mechanism for transporting sodium out of cell begins to fail when cell is injured. Sodium diffuses into cell along with water, causing cell to swell.

Fatty change: fat metabolism impaired; fat accumulates in cell.

Cell Death and Necrosis

Cell death follows irreparable injury.

Structural changes that follow called cell necrosis.

Aging and the Cell / 44
Basic Concepts

Cells and organisms have predetermined life-span.

Harmful environmental factors damage DNA, RNA, and organelles. This shortens life-span.

Cells are capable of repairing damage. The more efficient the repair process, the greater the likelihood of cell survival.

Chromosomes, Genes, and Cell Division

Learning Objectives

1. Describe how chromosomes are studied. Explain how a karyotype is determined.
2. Compare mitosis and meiosis.
3. Compare spermatogenesis and oogenesis. Explain the implications of abnormal chromosome separations in the course of meiosis in older women.
4. Describe the inheritance pattern of genes and define dominant, recessive, codominant, and sex-linked inheritance.
5. Describe the HLA system and explain its application to organ transplantation and its relation to disease susceptibility.
6. Describe the applications and limitations of gene therapy.

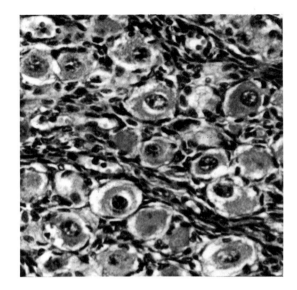

Chapter 3 ▪ Contents

The activities of cells are controlled by the chromosomes present in the nucleus. In the somatic cells (cells other than those giving rise to eggs and sperm), chromosomes exist in pairs. One member of each pair is derived from the male parent and one member from the female parent. Except for the sex chromosomes, both members of the pair are similar in size, shape, and appearance and are called **homologous chromosomes.** In human beings, the normal chromosome component is twenty-two pairs of **auto-somes** (the general term for chromosomes other than the sex chromosomes) and one pair of *sex chromosomes.*

As described in chapter 2, the chromosomes are composed of double coils of deoxyribonucleic acid (DNA) combined with protein. The genes, which are the basic units of inheritance, are segments of the DNA chains that determine some property of the cell. Genes are sometimes described as being arranged along the chromosome like beads on a string.

The sum total of all the genes contained in a cell's chromosomes is called it's **genome** and is the same in all cells, but not all genes are expressed (active) in all cells and not all genes are active all the time. Some genes code for specific enzymes or other proteins that the cell needs in order to function, and others act as regulators to control the activities of neighboring genes. An enzyme or other protein specified by a gene, which is transcribed into messenger RNA and translated through transfer RNA and cytoplasmic ribosomes into protein, is called the **gene product.**

The human genome contains about 3 billion pairs of DNA bases, each pair consisting of an adenine paired with thymine or a guanine paired with cytosine, and there are between 50,000 and 100,000 genes arranged on the various chromosomes. Actually, only about 10 percent of the total DNA in the human genome consists of genes. The functions of the remaining 90 percent of the DNA, which is interspersed between the genes, are not yet known. The parts of the DNA chains that code for specific proteins are called **exons,** and the parts of the DNA chains interspersed between the exons are called **introns.** When parts of the DNA chains are translated into messenger RNA in order to make a gene product in the cytoplasm, both the genes (exons) and the noncoding parts of the DNA chains (introns) are transcribed, but the introns are removed from the messenger RNA before it leaves the nucleus. Only the coding sequences that specify the protein to be constructed are delivered to the ribosomes by the messenger RNA.

The genes that are expressed in a given cell determine both its structure and its functions, which is why a liver cell, for example, has a different structure from that of a blood cell and functions differently as well.

Sex Chromosomes

Genetic sex is determined by the X and Y chromosomes. A person having two X chromosomes is genetically female, whereas a male has one X and one Y chromosome. In the female, the genetic activity of both chromosomes is essential only during the first few weeks of embryonic development. Thereafter, one of the two X chromosomes is inactivated and appears as a

Chromosomes

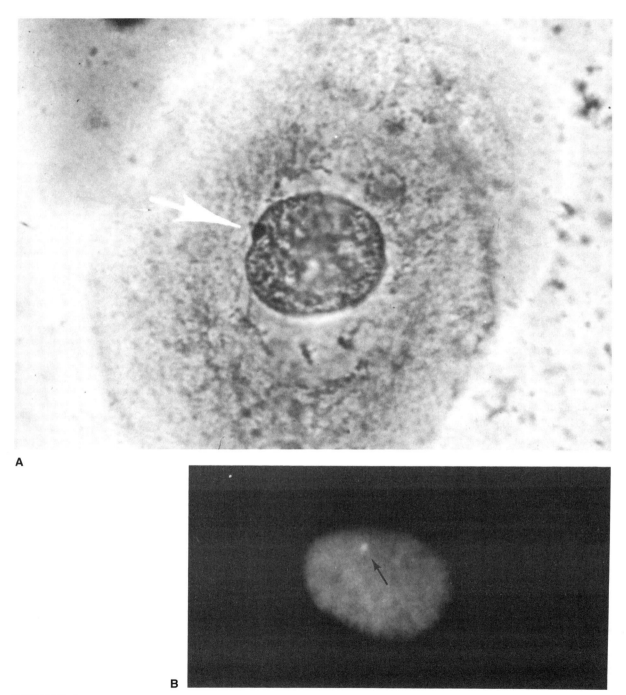

A

B

FIGURE 3–1

A, Characteristic appearance of the sex chromatin body (Barr body) in the nucleus of squamous epithelial cells (*arrow*). **B,** Fluorescent Y chromosome (*arrow*) in intact cell.

small, dense mass of chromatin attached to the nuclear membrane of somatic cells. This structure is called a *sex chromatin body* or **Barr body** (after the man who first described it) and can be identified in stained slides prepared from the cells of a normal female (figure 3–1A).

It is also possible to identify the Y chromosome in the cells of a normal male. The Y chromosome stains intensely with certain fluorescent dyes and appears as a bright fluorescent spot within the nucleus of the intact cell when suitably stained preparations are examined microscopically under ultraviolet light (figure 3–1B).

A combination of staining and ultraviolet light makes it possible to determine the X and Y chromosome composition of intact cells. The cells of the normal male possess the fluorescent spot but lack the sex chromatin body, and the cells of the normal female contain the sex chromatin body but lack the fluorescent spot. Cells for examination are usually obtained by scraping the mucosa of the cheek gently with a tongue depressor and preparing slides from this material. However, cells obtained from any convenient site may be used for examination.

Cell Division

There are two types of cell division: mitosis and meiosis. **Mitosis** is characteristic of somatic cells. **Meiosis** is a specialized type of cell division that occurs during the development of the eggs (ova) and sperm, a process called **gametogenesis.** In mitosis, each of the two new cells (called the **daughter cells**) resulting from the cell division receives the same number of chromosomes that were present in the precursor cell (called the parent cell). In meiosis, the number of chromosomes is reduced, and so that the daughter cells receive only half the chromosomes possessed by the parent cell.

Mitosis

Mitosis is characteristic of somatic cells, but not all mature cells are able to divide. Some mature cells, such as skeletal and cardiac muscle cells and nerve cells, do not divide. Others, such as connective tissue cells and liver cells, divide as needed to replace lost or damaged cells or to heal an injury. And yet others divide continually, such as those lining the testicular tubules that produce sperm cells and those in the bone marrow that continually replace the circulating cells in the blood stream. Regardless of the frequency of cell division, the rate of cell division is controlled closely to match the body's needs, and excess cells are not normally produced.

The stimulus that induces a cell to divide or inhibits its division does not originate within the cell itself but rather comes from neighboring cells. Various soluble growth promoting factors or growth inhibitors that are secreted by neighboring cells bind to receptors on the cell membrane of the target cell and activate the receptors. The activated receptors in turn transmit biochemical signals to the "machinery" inside the cell. Depending on the signal, either the cell is induced to grow and divide or its growth is inhibited.

These intercellular communications allow normal cells to divide often enough to accomplish their functions and replenish cell losses from injury or normal aging but restrain excessive proliferation. Moreover, normal cells cannot continue to divide indefinitely. They are programmed to undergo a limited number of cell divisions, and then they die.

Before a cell begins mitosis, its DNA chains are duplicated to form new chromosome material. Each chromosome and its newly duplicated counterpart lie side by side. The two members of the pair are called **chromatids.** Mitosis is the process by which chromatids separate. (The use of the terms *chromosomes* and *chromatids* may at times be confusing. Each chromosome duplicates itself before beginning cell division. Because there are normally forty-six chromosomes in each somatic cell, just prior to cell division there are actually the equivalent of ninety-two chromosomes in the cell [that is, 46 × 2]. When the chromosomes shorten in the course of cell division, each chromosome can be seen to actually consist of two separate chromosomes that are still partially joined where the spindle fibers attach. The term *chromatids* is applied to the still-joined chromosomes at this stage. As soon as they separate, they are again called chromosomes.)

Mitosis is divided into four stages (figure 3–2): prophase, metaphase, anaphase, and telophase.

Prophase
Each chromosome thickens and shortens. The centrioles migrate to opposite poles of the cell and form the mitotic spindle, which consists of small fibers radiating in all directions from the centrioles. Some of these spindle fibers attach to the chromatids. The nuclear membrane breaks down toward the end of prophase.

Metaphase
The chromosomes line up in the center of the cell. At this stage, the chromatids are partially separated but still remain joined at a constricted area called the **centromere,** which is the site where the spindle fibers are attached.

Anaphase
The chromatids constituting each chromosome separate to form individual chromosomes, which are pulled to opposite poles of the cell by the spindle fibers.

Telophase
The nuclear membranes of the two daughter cells reform, and the cytoplasm divides, forming two daughter cells. Each is an exact duplicate of the parent cell.

Meiosis

Meiotic cell division reduces the number of chromosomes by half and also leads to some intermixing of genetic material between homologous chro-

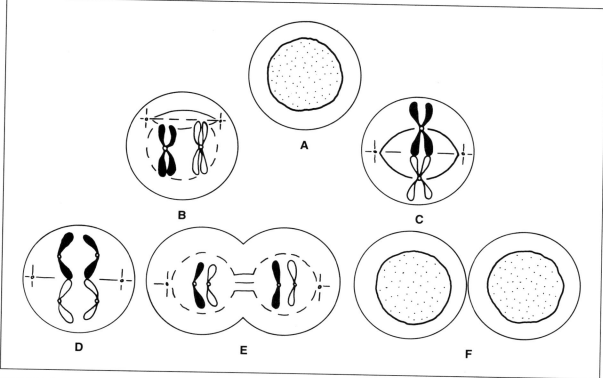

FIGURE 3–2

Stages of mitosis. The behavior of only one pair of chromosomes is shown. **A,** Prior to cell division. **B,** Prophase. **C,** Metaphase. **D,** Anaphase. **E,** Telophase. **F,** Daughter cells resulting from mitosis, each identical with the parent cell.

mosomes. The process entails two separate divisions called the first and second meiotic divisions (figure 3–3).

First Meiotic Division

As in mitosis, each chromosome duplicates itself before beginning cell division, forming two chromatids. During *prophase,* each homologous pair of chromosomes come to lie side by side over their entire length. This association is called a **synapse.** At this stage, there is frequently some interchange of segments between homologous chromosomes, which is called a **crossover.** The pairing of homologous chromosomes and the interchange of genetic material during prophase is the characteristic feature of meiosis. In the female, the two X chromosomes synapse in the same way as autosomes, but, in the male, the X and Y chromosomes synapse end to end and do not exchange segments.

In *metaphase,* the paired chromosomes become arranged in a plane within the middle of the cell. During *anaphase,* the homologous chromosomes separate and move to opposite poles of the cell. Each chromosome

FIGURE 3–3

Stages of meiosis. The behavior of only one pair of chromosomes is indicated. In the first meiotic division, each daughter cell receives only one member of each homologous pair, and the chromosomes are not exact duplicates of those in the parent cell. The second meiotic division is like a mitotic division, but each cell contains only twenty-three chromosomes.

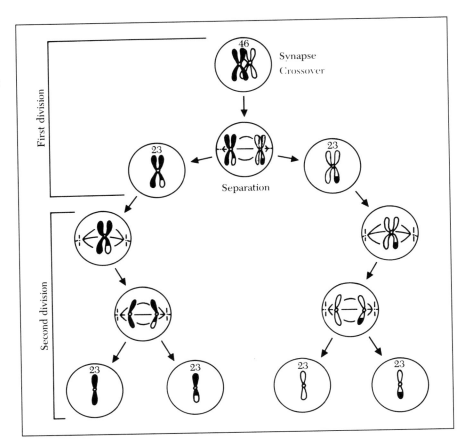

consists of two chromatids, but they do not separate at this stage. In *telophase,* two new daughter cells are formed. Each daughter cell contains only one member of each homologous pair of chromosomes; so the chromosomes in each daughter cell are reduced by half. The chromosomes in the daughter cells are also somewhat different from those in the parent cell because of the interchange of genetic material during synapse.

Second Meiotic Division

The second meiotic division is similar to a mitotic division. The two chromatids composing each chromosome separate, and two new daughter cells are formed, each containing half the normal number of chromosomes.

Gametogenesis

The testes and ovaries, called **gonads,** contain precursor cells called germ cells, which are capable of developing into mature sperm or ova. The mature germ cells are called **gametes,** and the process by which they are formed is **gametogenesis.** The development of sperm (spermatogenesis) and that of ova (oogenesis) are similar in many respects (figure 3–4).

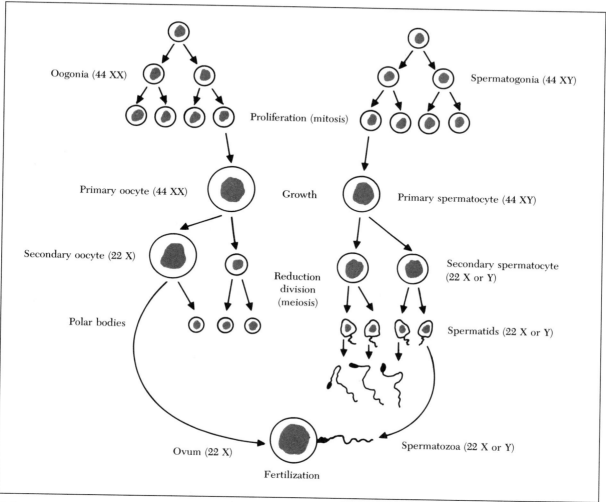

FIGURE 3–4

Sequence of events in gametogenesis. The numbers and letters in parentheses refer to the chromosomes in the cell. *Numbers* indicate autosomes; *letters* designate sex chromosomes.

Spermatogenesis

The precursor cells in the testicular tubules are called *spermatogonia* (singular term, *spermatogonium*). Each contains a full complement of forty-six chromosomes. Spermatogonia divide by mitosis to form *primary spermatocytes,* which, like the precursor cells, contain forty-six chromosomes. The primary spermatocytes then divide by meiosis. In the first meiotic division, each primary spermatocyte forms two *secondary spermatocytes,* each containing twenty-three chromosomes. Each secondary spermatocyte completes the second meiotic division and forms two **spermatids,** also containing twenty-three chromosomes, and the spermatids mature into sperm. The entire process of spermatogenesis takes about two months, and sperm are being produced continually.

Oogenesis

The precursors of the ova are called *oogonia* (singular term, *oogonium*). Each contains forty-six chromosomes. Oogonia divide repeatedly in the fetal ovaries before birth, forming *primary oocytes,* which contain forty-six chromosomes. The oocytes then become surrounded by a single layer of cells called **granulosa cells** or *follicular cells,* forming structures called *primary follicles* (figure 3–5). The primary oocytes in the follicles begin the prophase of the first meiotic division during fetal life but do not carry the division through to completion. A very large number of primary follicles are formed, but many of them degenerate during infancy and childhood. However, about a half million of the primary follicles persist into adolescence. This is a very great excess. Even if 1 egg were released each month over a reproductive span of forty years, only 480 eggs would ever be ovulated and only a few, if any, would ever be fertilized.

The ovaries with their contained primary follicles remain inactive until puberty. Then cyclic ovulation begins under the influence of the pituitary gonadotrophic hormones, follicle-stimulating hormone (FSH), and luteinizing hormone (LH). During each menstrual cycle, a number of primary follicles begin to grow, but normally only one follicle comes to full maturity and is ovulated. When the oocyte is discharged, it completes its first meiotic division and gives rise to two daughter cells, which are unequal in size. One daughter cell, which receives half the chromosomes (one member of each homologous pair) and almost all of the cytoplasm, is called a *secondary oocyte* (twenty-three chromosomes). The other daughter cell, which receives the remaining twenty-three chromosomes but almost none of the cytoplasm, is called the first **polar body** and is discarded. The newly formed secondary oocyte promptly begins its second meiotic division, which will lead to the formation of the *mature ovum* and a *second polar body,* each containing twenty-three chromosomes. The meiotic division is not completed, however, unless the ovum is fertilized.

Comparison of Spermatogenesis and Oogenesis

Spermatogenesis and oogenesis have many similarities, but there are two major differences.

First, four spermatozoa are produced from each precursor cell in spermatogenesis, but only one ovum is formed from each precursor cell in oogenesis. The other three "daughter cells" derived from the meiotic divisions are discarded as polar bodies.

Second, spermatogenesis occurs continually and is carried through to completion in about two months. Consequently, seminal fluid always contains relatively "fresh" sperm. In contrast, the oocytes are not produced continually.

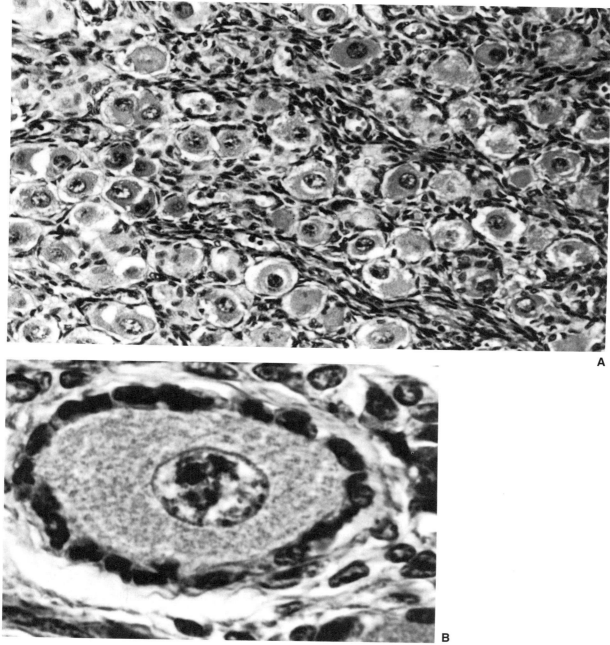

FIGURE 3–5

A, Low-magnification photomicrograph of ovary of newborn infant, illustrating large numbers of primary follicles distributed throughout the ovary. (Original magnification × 100.) **B,** High-magnification photomicrograph illustrating a primary follicle composed of a central oocyte surrounded by a collar of granulosa cells. (Original magnification × 400.)

All the oocytes present in the ovary were formed before birth and have remained in a prolonged prophase of the first meiotic division from fetal life until they are ovulated. This may be why congenital abnormalities that result from abnormal separation of chromosomes in the course of gametogenesis are more frequent in older women. The ova released late in a woman's reproductive life have been held in prophase for as long as forty-five years before they finally resume mitosis at the time of ovulation. These ova have been exposed for many years to potentially harmful radiation, chemicals, or other injurious agents, and this predisposes them to abnormal separation of chromosomes when cell division is resumed. If the chromosomes do not separate normally in meiosis, an ovum may end up with either an excess or a deficiency of chromosomes. If the abnormal ovum is fertilized, a fetus that has an abnormal number of chromosomes may be conceived. This subject is considered in chapter 9.

Chromosome Analysis

The chromosome composition of the human cell can be studied with great accuracy by culturing cells in a suitable medium. The presence of abnormalities in chromosome number or structure also can be detected in this way. Usually, human blood is used as a source of cells for these studies; the blood lymphocytes can be induced to undergo mitotic division. Certain chemicals are added to stop the mitotic division after the chromosomes have become separate and distinct, and so many cells arrested in mitosis accumulate in the culture medium. Additional methods are employed to cause swelling of the cells, which causes the chromosomes to separate. Stained smears are then prepared, and the chromosomes can be examined. Figure 3–6 illustrates the appearance of a swollen cell arrested in mitosis with the chromosomes well separated. A normal dividing cell arrested in mitosis contains forty-six chromosomes, each consisting of two chromatids joined at their centromeres. Chromosomes are classified according to their size, the location of the centromere, the relative lengths of the chromatids that extend outward from the centromere (called the arms of the chromosome), and the pattern of light and dark bands along the chromosome. Each chromosome has its own unique structure. The separated chromosomes from a single cell are photographed, and the individual chromosomes in the photograph are cut out and arranged in a standard pattern called a **karyotype.** Figure 3–7 illustrates the karyotype of a female, as indicated by the two X chromosomes. A male karyotype would contain a single X and single Y rather than two X chromosomes. The karyotype illustrated is not normal: there is an extra chromosome 21. (Chromosomal abnormalities are considered in chapter 9.)

Genes and Inheritance

A gene is a section of the DNA chain that determines some property of the cell. Each gene occupies a specific site on the chromosome; this site is called the **locus** of the gene. Chromosomes exist in pairs except in the ova and sperm. Consequently, genes are also paired, and the members of each pair

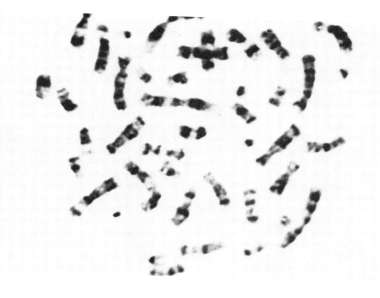

A

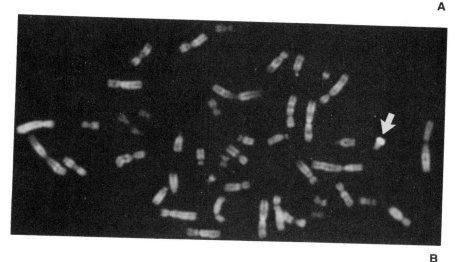

B

FIGURE 3–6

The appearance of chromosomes from a single cell arrested in mitosis, illustrating the banded pattern that facilitates the identification of individual chromosomes. The two chromatids composing each chromosome lie side by side. **A,** Giemsa stain. (Photograph courtesy of Dr. Jorge Yunis.) **B,** Fluorescent stain. *Arrow* indicates intensely fluorescent Y chromosome. (Photograph courtesy of Patricia Crowley.)

are located at corresponding gene loci on homologous chromosomes. Alternate forms of a gene that can occupy the same locus are called **alleles,** and any one chromosome can carry only one allele at a given locus. An individual is **homozygous** for a gene if both alleles are the same and **heterozygous** if the alleles are different.

Genes are responsible for inherited traits, but the effects that they produce (called the expression of the gene) vary with different genes. A **recessive gene** is one that produces an effect only in the homozygous state. A **dominant gene** expresses itself in either the heterozygous or the homozygous state. Sometimes both alleles of a pair are expressed. Such alleles are called *codominant.* For example, each of the alleles that direct hemoglobin syn-

FIGURE 3–7

Karyotype of a female. Karyotype is not normal. There is an extra chromosome 21. (Giemsa stain.)

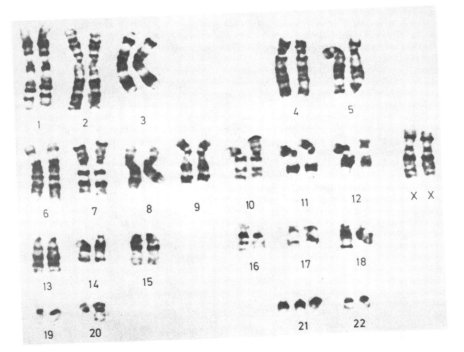

thesis induces the formation of a specific type of hemoglobin in the red blood cells. If two different alleles are present, two different types of hemoglobin are produced.

Genes carried on sex chromosomes are called **sex-linked genes,** and the effects that they produce are called *sex-linked traits.* The small Y chromosome carries few genes other than those that direct male sex differentiation, but the much larger X chromosome carries many genes in addition to those concerned with sexual development. For practical purposes, only X-linked traits are recognized, and most are recessive. The female carrier of a recessive X-linked trait is normal, because the effect of the defective allele on one X chromosome is offset by the normal allele on the other X chromosome. The male, however, possesses only one X chromosome. Consequently, he can be neither heterozygous nor homozygous for X-linked genes and is called **hemizygous** (*hemi* = half) for genes carried on the X chromosome. If the male receives an X chromosome containing a defective gene, the normal offsetting allele possessed by the female carrier is lacking, and the defective X-linked gene functions like a dominant gene when paired with the Y chromosome.

Genes of the Histocompatibility (HLA) Complex

Successful transplantation of organs from one person to another requires that the antigens present on the cells of the organ donor resemble as closely as possible those of the recipient. (Organ transplantation is considered in chapter 5.) The antigens present on cells are determined by a cluster of genes on chromosome 6. This group of genes, which was first identified in laboratory animals in connection with transplantation experiments, is called the **major histocompatibility complex** (MHC complex). In humans, these cell surface proteins (antigens) were first identified on peripheral blood leukocytes. Consequently, they were named **human leukocyte antigens** (HLA antigens), and the human major histocompatibility complex is often called the **HLA system.**

Although the HLA surface proteins are often called HLA antigens, their antigenicity actually depends on whether they are one's own proteins or the HLA proteins of another person. The HLA proteins on a person's own cells (called self-antigens) are unique for the person possessing them and are recognized by the immune system as being part of that person, not as being foreign; but they are foreign proteins (non-self-antigens) in another person in whom they are antigenic and incite an immune response.

Originally MHC proteins were considered of interest only with respect to organ transplantation, because transplantation of cells containing MHC proteins different from those of the transplant recipient was followed by rejection of the transplant unless the immune system was suppressed. However, we know now that they have a much larger role, in that they take part in generating immune responses to foreign antigens of all types. The interaction of the HLA antigens with the various cells of the immune system are considered in chapter 5.

The HLA complex consists of four separate but closely linked gene loci designated *HLA-A, HLA-B, HLA-C,* and *HLA-D,* and there are additional subdivisions within the *HLA-D* locus. Each locus has many alleles. Almost fifty different alleles, for example, have been identified at the *HLA-B* locus alone, and many alleles are identified at other HLA gene loci as well. Each allele is designated by a specific letter to designate the locus and a number to indicate the allele, such as *HLA-B27.* A set of HLA genes on one chromosome is called a **haplotype** and is transmitted as a unit. Because chromosomes are paired, each person has two haplotypes, each consisting of four HLA genes. The two haplotypes together determine a total of eight HLA proteins on the cell. Because of the large number of alleles in the HLA system, the chances of two persons who are not identical twins having the same HLA proteins on their cells is very remote.

The surface proteins within the HLA system fall into two major groups, designated *MHC Class I proteins* and *MHC Class II proteins.* The Class I proteins are determined by the *HLA-A, HLA-B,* and *HLA-C* genes and are present on virtually all nucleated cells and on blood platelets, which are small cytoplasmic fragments of large nucleated bone marrow cells called *megakaryocytes* (described in chapter 14). Class I proteins are not found on the surface of mature red blood cells, however, because these cells lack nuclei. Class II proteins are determined by the *HLA-D* genes and are found on only a few types of cells—those that play very important roles in the immune response: phagocytic cells called macrophages, along with related cells having functions similar to those of macrophages; and some types of lymphocytes (described in chapter 5).

Figure 3–8 illustrates the inheritance of HLA haplotypes. Each child receives one of two possible haplotypes from each parent. Consequently, a child has only one haplotype in common with each parent. Because of the way in which chromosomes are transmitted from parent to child, the child has any one of four different combinations of HLA haplotypes, as shown in the illustration by the haplotypes of the first four children. There is a one in four probability that two children will both possess the same pair of haplotypes. In this example, each of the first four children has a different combination of HLA haplotypes. The fifth child, however, has the same haplotypes as the second child, indicating that organ transplantation between these two children would have a much better chance for success than would transplantation between individuals having different haplotypes.

HLA Types and Susceptibility to Disease

Certain HLA types appear to predispose to specific diseases. The most striking example of such an association is between the HLA-B27 and a particular type of arthritis of the spine and the sacroiliac joints. HLA-B27 is present in about 5 percent of the random white population but is found in about 90 percent of persons affected with this type of arthritis, indicating that a B27-positive individual is much more likely to develop this disease than is a person of a different HLA type. However, the presence of the B27 type indicates only a predisposition to the disease. It does not mean that any given individual will invariably be affected, because no more than about 25 percent of B27-positive persons ever develop this type of arthritis. Predisposition to other diseases also has been associated with this HLA type.

FIGURE 3–8

The possible distribution of HLA haplotypes illustrated in a family of five children. Each haplotype consists of four separate linked HLA genes and is arbitrarily designated by an arabic numeral. The four possible combinations of haplotype are illustrated in the first four children. In this example, the haplotype of the fifth child is the same as those of the second child.

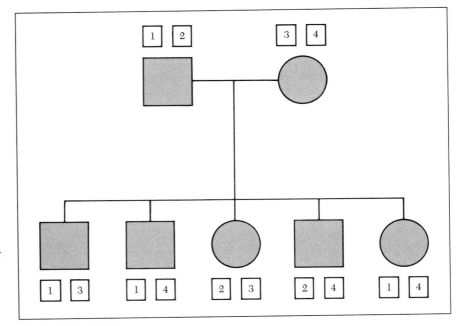

Similar associations exist between certain HLA-D types and specific diseases, which are considered in other chapters. The diseases include a type of diabetes, prone to develop in children and young adults, called *insulin dependent diabetes* (chapter 22) and a type of arthritis called *rheumatoid arthritis* (chapter 27).

The reason for the association of specific diseases with HLA types seems to be related to the relation of the HLA gene complex to genes controlling the immune response. The genes that regulate immunity are closely associated with the HLA genes. Individuals having certain specific HLA types also appear to possess genes that are less capable of regulating their immune responses when subjected to antigenic stimulation. Consequently, they seem prone to develop abnormal immune responses that are directed against their own cells and tissues. This type of abnormal reaction leads to cell and tissue injury or dysfunction, which causes various diseases classified as **autoimmune diseases** (described in chapter 5). In contrast, persons of a different HLA type have immune response genes that regulate responses to antigenic stimulation in a more normal manner.

Genes and Recombinant DNA Technology (Genetic Engineering)

Genes direct the synthesis of gene products—that is, enzymes or other proteins that play a role in the activities of the cells that make the proteins. Cells make many important biologic products, such as insulin, growth hormone, proteins that regulate the immune responses, and proteins that activate the body's clot-dissolving mechanisms. Many of these proteins are used in clinical medicine: insulin to treat diabetes; growth hormone, which allows a child with a growth hormone deficiency to grow normally; and proteins to unplug blocked coronary arteries of patients with heart attacks. Recent advances in DNA technology have led to the development of methods for large-scale production of these and many other important biologic products. The technology that paved the way for these advances has been called by various names: **recombinant DNA technology** (because genes from two different sources are being recombined in a single organism), **genetic engineering** (because genes are being manipulated), or **gene splicing** (because a piece of genetic material is being cut open and another piece of genetic material is being spliced into it).

Whatever name one uses for it, the process requires the insertion of a gene that encodes a desired products, such as insulin, into a bacterium or yeast. If a bacterium is used, the gene is inserted into a small circular DNA segment within the bacterium, called a **plasmid,** which is distinct from the main bacterial chromosome. The circular plasmid is opened by means of an enzyme that "cuts" the plasmid DNA so that the desired gene can be inserted between the cut ends of the plasmid. After the gene has been inserted, the bacterial plasmid contains not only its own genes, but also the new gene, which directs the synthesis of the desired protein. The bacterial-foreign gene combination (recombinant DNA) is now carried along by the bacterium as it divides repeatedly to produce a large population of bacterial cells, each producing large quantities of the desired protein that can be purified and used for various purposes.

Although recombinant DNA technology is relatively simple in concept, the technology is quite complex in practice. One must isolate from human cells the messenger RNA that directs the synthesis of the desired protein. Then, using the enzyme *reverse transcriptase,* one must construct a complementary DNA copy of the messenger RNA. (This is the reverse of the usual flow of genetic information in which DNA is the model on which the complementary messenger RNA is assembled.) The complementary DNA copy of messenger RNA contains the genetic information required to make the desired protein. It is in fact the DNA gene composed entirely of exons without the introns. Finally, the newly made DNA gene is inserted into the bacterial plasmid, and the bacterium with its new gene makes the protein.

Other applications of DNA technology in biology and medicine are based on these same principles. DNA technology has been a source of insight into the molecular basis of genetic diseases by increasing our understanding of normal gene structure and function; it has application in the prenatal diagnosis of genetic diseases by identifying abnormal genes and gene products in fetal cells. When the structure of a normal gene that specifies a gene product is known, it is possible to identify a mutation of the gene in fetal cell DNA obtained from amnionic fluid cells. Prenatal diagnosis of genetic diseases by DNA analysis of fetal cells is considered in chapter 9.

Gene Therapy

One of the most exciting advances in DNA technology—gene therapy—is an extension of the principles of recombinant DNA technology. In recombinant DNA technology, a gene is inserted into a bacterial or yeast cell to make a protein. In gene therapy, a normal gene is inserted into a defective cell lacking an enzyme or structural protein that the cell needs in order to function effectively, and the inserted gene compensates for the missing or dysfunctional gene.

For the successful application of gene therapy, several goals must be achieved:

1. One must identify and select the correct gene to insert into the cell.
2. One must choose the proper cell to receive the gene.
3. One must select an efficient means of getting the gene into the cell.
4. One must ensure that the newly inserted gene can function effectively long enough within the cell to make the therapy worthwhile.

The identification of the gene for insertion involves the same approaches used in recombinant DNA technology. The agent (vector) used to introduce the gene into the selected cell is usually a virus, although sometimes the gene can be coupled to a lipid or other material that is taken into the cell by endocytosis. Gene therapy targets somatic cells, not the germ cells that produce eggs and sperm, and gene therapy directed at germ cells is not considered either feasible or desirable.

The initial gene therapy studies on patients used lymphocytes as target cells. A sample of blood was collected from the patient, and the lymphocytes were grown in culture. Then the lymphocytes were "infected" with a genetically engineered virus containing the desired gene and reinfused into the patient, where they were able to function for as long as two months. A landmark study in 1990 used a similar technique to insert a normal gene coding for an enzyme called adenosine deaminase into the lymphocytes of a patient whose lymphocytes lacked this enzyme. This enzyme deficiency leads to a severe malfunction of the immune system called severe combined immunodeficiency, which renders the patient extremely susceptible to a wide variety of infectious agents. The gene therapy supplied a population of genetically engineered lymphocytes that could produce the required enzyme and the patient improved. The gene therapy treatment had to be repeated periodically as the infused lymphocytes reached the end of their life-span and were removed from the circulation. Eventually, however, it may be possible to target for gene therapy the lymphocyte precursor cells (stem cells) in the bone marrow rather than the circulating lymphocytes. Because the stem cells continue to divide in the bone marrow, they might be able to deliver into the circulation a continuous supply of genetically engineered lymphocytes containing the inserted gene, thereby avoiding the need to reintroduce new populations of gene-treated lymphocytes periodically, as is required at present.

Although many of the current gene therapy studies involve removing the cells for gene therapy from the patient, inserting the gene, and returning the modified cells to the patient, other studies are bypassing the cell-removal–gene-insertion–reinfusion steps, and introducing the gene-carrying agent directly into the patient. Using a selected gene-carrying virus that "attacks" only a specific type of cell, one can target a specific cell for gene therapy because the virus seeks out its target cell and introduces its gene, which corrects the malfunctioning target cell. In some clinical trials, for example, weakened respiratory viruses (adenoviruses) carrying an inserted gene are transported by a nasal spray into the respiratory tract where they carry the desired gene into the respiratory epithelial cells of patients lacking the gene. These patients have a serious genetic disease called cystic fibrosis (described in chapter 22), which causes extremely thick respiratory mucus secretions that plug the small air passages, predisposing the affected persons to repeated bouts of pulmonary infection that gradually destroys pulmonary function.

Various other gene therapy trials are being performed on patients with some types of cancer in an attempt to improve their survival. The aim of these approaches is either to insert a gene into the patient's cells that allows the cells to combat the cancer more effectively or to insert a gene into the tumor cells that will impede their growth or function or make them more susceptible to destruction by the patient's own immune defenses.

Gene therapy has great potential, but it also has limitations. The correct gene must be inserted into the correct cell to substitute for a dysfunctional gene, but the inserted gene must not disrupt the activities of other cellular genes that regulate other cell functions. Gene therapy shows great promise as a powerful tool for fighting against disease, but much work remains to be done before gene therapy can be applied widely in clinical medicine.

Questions for Review

1. What is meant by the following terms: *homologous chromosomes, autosomes, sex chromosome, Barr body, gene, gametogenesis,* and *centrosome?*

2. How does the process of mitosis compare with meiosis?

3. What are the differences between spermatogenesis and oogenesis?

4. What is a chromosome karyotype? How is it obtained? How is it used?

5. What is the major histocompatibility complex? What is its function? What is its relation to disease susceptibility?

6. What is a haplotype? How are haplotypes inherited by children from their parents? What are the chances that two children will have the same haplotype?

Supplementary Readings

Crowley, L. V. 1974. *An introduction to clinical embryology.* Chicago: Year Book Medical Publishers. Basic concepts for students in the health professions. Chapters on cytogenetics and cell division.

Goldman, J. N., and Goldman, M. B. 1981. What the clinician should know about the major histocompatibility complex. *Journal of the American Medical Association* 246:873–76. The major histocompatibility complex is a closely linked group of genes that determine the structure of cell surface antigens and several plasma proteins and also regulate the immune responses.

Levine, F., and Friedman, T. 1993. Gene therapy. *American Journal of Diseases of Children* 147:1167–74. A review article dealing with applications and limitations of the procedure.

Marieb, E. N. 1992. *Human anatomy and physiology.* 2d ed. Redwood City, Calif.: Benjamin/Cummings. A standard text well written with good diagrams.

Morsey, M. A., Kohnosuke, M., Clemens, P., and Caskey, T. 1993. Progress toward human gene therapy. *Journal of the American Medical Association* 270:2338–45. A review article discussing methods of gene delivery and related subjects.

Samara, G. Sawicki, M. P., Hurwitz, M., and Passaro, E. 1993. Molecular biology and therapy of disease. *American Journal of Surgery* 165:720–27. A review article.

Yunis, J. J., and Chandler, M. E. 1977. The chromosomes of man: Clinical and biologic significance. *American Journal of Pathology* 88:466–95. A classic article by a leader in the field.

Chapter 3 ▪ Outline Summary

Chromosomes / 51
Structure

Double coils of DNA combined with protein.

Exist in pairs: autosome and sex chromosomes.

Genes (segments of DNA chain) arranged along chromosome.

Sex Chromosomes

In female: one X inactivated and appears attached to nuclear membrane.

In male: Y chromosome appears as bright fluorescent spot in intact cell.

Cell Division / 53
Mitosis

No reduction in chromosomes; daughter cells identical with parent cell.

Characteristic of somatic cells.

Sequence:

Prophase: chromosomes shorten, nuclear membrane breaks down, and spindle forms.

Metaphase: chromosomes line up in middle of cell.

Anaphase: chromosomes pull apart.

Telophase: two daughter cells reform.

Meiosis

Chromosomes reduced by half and modified by crossover.

Characteristic of germ cells.

Sequence:

First meiotic division: homologous chromosomes synapse and exchange segments.

Homologous chromosomes separate, and daughter cells reform, each containing one member of homologous pair.

Chromosomes reduce by half.

Second meiotic division: like mitosis, but each cell has only twenty-three chromosomes.

Gametogenesis / 56

Spermatogenesis

Spermatogonia (forty-six chromosomes) form primary spermatocytes (forty-six chromosomes).

Each primary spermatocyte forms two secondary spermatocytes (twenty-three chromosomes).

Each secondary spermatocyte forms two spermatids (twenty-three chromosomes).

Spermatids mature into sperm.

Oogenesis

Oogonia (forty-six chromosomes) form primary oocytes (forty-six chromosomes) in fetal ovaries.

Primary oocyte forms primary follicle and begins prophase of meiosis but does not carry it through.

Many follicles degenerate during infancy and childhood. About one-half million persist.

Follicle matures under influence of FSH-LH, and one is ovulated each cycle.

Primary oocyte completes first meiotic division to form secondary oocyte (twenty-three chromosomes) and polar body (twenty-three chromosomes).

Secondary oocyte completes second meiotic division if fertilized to form mature ovum (twenty-three chromosomes) and polar body (twenty-three chromosomes).

Comparison of Spermatogenesis and Oogenesis / 58

Spermatogenesis

Four sperm from each precursor cell.

Continual: always fresh sperm.

Oogenesis

One ovum from each precursor.

All precursors form prior to birth and remain in prophase until ovulated.

Ova ovulated late in reproductive life more prone to abnormal chromosome separation.

Chromosome Analysis / 60

Method of Analysis

Blood cells cultured and lymphocytes induced to divide.

Cells arrested in metaphase and caused to swell.

Stained smears prepared.

Chromosomes cut out and arranged to form karyotype.

Genes and Inheritance / 60

Genes

Exist in pairs (alleles), one on each chromosome.

Homozygous: alleles the same.

Heterozygous: alleles different.

Expression of genes varies.

Dominant: gene expressed in heterozygous state.

Recessive: gene expressed in homozygous state.

Codominant: both alleles expressed.

Sex-linked genes.

Carried on X chromosome.

Female has two X. Either can carry abnormal gene. Not clinically affected if acquires abnormal X because effect offset by chromosome on normal X.

Male has only one X (hemizygous). Acquires hereditary disease if receives X chromosome containing defective gene.

Genes of the Histocompatibility (HLA) Complex / 62

Structure and Function

Important in organ transplantation.

Four linked gene loci on chromosome 6 designated *HLA-A, HLA-B, HLA-C,* and *HLA-D.*

Multiple alleles at each gene locus.

Genes control antigens on cells.

Genes on each chromosome 6 are transmitted as set called a haplotype.

Inheritance

Each child receives one haplotype from each parent.

Four different combinations of haplotype possible in children.

Probability is one in four that two children of same parents will possess same HLA haplotype.

HLA and Susceptibility to Disease

Genes controlling immune response associated with HLA complex.

Certain HLA types less capable of regulating immune response are prone to develop specific types of autoimmune diseases.

Genes and Recombinant DNA Technology / 65

Technique inserts foreign gene into bacterial plasmid or yeast cell.

Microorganism produces desired protein.

Complex technology.

Principles applicable to understanding molecular basis of genetic disease.

Principles applicable to prenatal diagnosis of genetic disease.

Gene Therapy / 66

Gene introduced into cell with genetic defect to compensate for missing or dysfunctional gene.

Gene usually introduced by virus, but other methods can be used to incorporate gene into cell.

Cells can be removed from patient, treated, and reinfused or gene-carrying virus can be introduced into patient to treat cells.

Limited trials on patients with cancer to improve survival.

Inflammation and Repair

Learning Objectives

1. List the characteristics and clinical manifestations of an acute inflammation. Differentiate inflammations on the basis of their component of fluid and inflammatory cells (serous, purulent, fibrinous, and hemorrhagic inflammations).
2. Describe the possible outcomes of an inflammatory reaction.
3. Name the chemical mediators of inflammation. Explain how they interact to intensify the inflammatory process.
4. Describe the harmful effects of inflammation. Explain why it is sometimes necessary to suppress the inflammatory process.
5. Compare inflammation and infection. Name some of the terms used to describe infections.

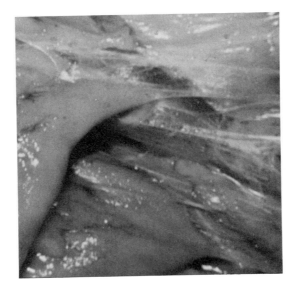

Chapter 4 ▪ Contents

The inflammatory reaction is a nonspecific response to any agent that causes cell injury. The agent may be physical (such as heat or cold), chemical (such as a concentrated acid or alkali or another caustic chemical), or microbiologic (such as a bacterium or virus). The inflammatory reaction is characterized by both local and systemic effects, as indicated diagrammatically in figure 4–1.

The Inflammatory Reaction

Local effects consist of dilatation (expansion) of blood vessels and increased vascular permeability. Leukocytes (white blood cells) are attracted to the site of injury. They adhere to the endothelium of the small blood vessels, force their way through the walls, and migrate to the area of tissue damage (figure 4–2). The characteristic signs of inflammation are heat, redness, tenderness, swelling, and pain. The increased warmth and redness of the inflamed tissues are caused by dilatation of capillaries and slowing of blood flow through the vessels. Swelling occurs because the extravasation (*extra* = out + *vas* = vessel) of plasma from the dilated and more permeable vessels causes the volume of fluid in the inflamed tissue to increase (figure 4–3). The tenderness and pain are secondary to irritation of sensory nerve endings at the site of the inflammatory process.

The polymorphonuclear leukocyte is the cell most important in the acute inflammatory response. It is an actively phagocytic cell that is attracted to the area by the cell injury. Mononuclear cells (monocytes, macrophages) appear later in the inflammatory reaction. One of their major functions is to clean

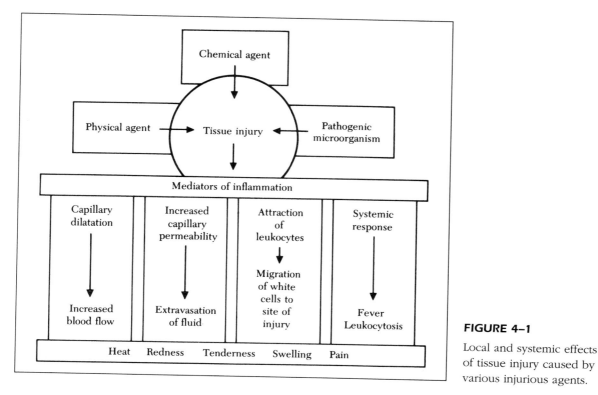

FIGURE 4–1

Local and systemic effects of tissue injury caused by various injurious agents.

FIGURE 4–2

Photomicrograph illustrating leukocytes adherent to capillary endothelium and migrating through wall to site of tissue injury. (Original magnification × 400.)

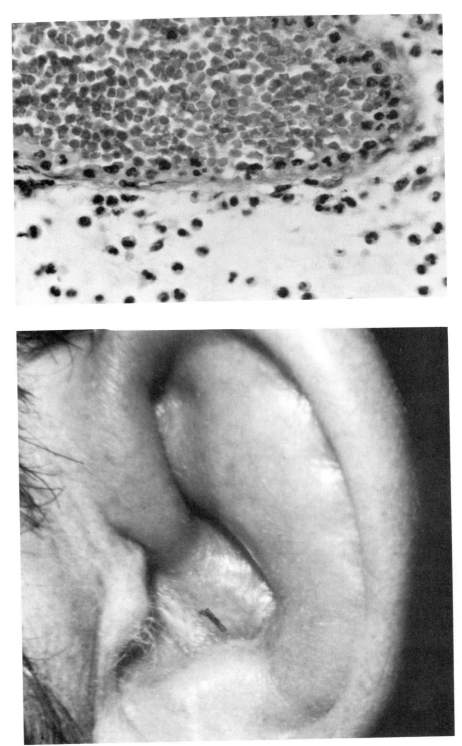

FIGURE 4–3

Marked swelling of ear caused by acute inflammation.

up the debris produced by the inflammatory process. These cells are also active in chronic inflammatory reactions.

The fluid mixture of protein, leukocytes, and debris that forms during the inflammatory process is called **exudate.** Its proportions of protein and inflammatory cells vary. If the exudate consists primarily of fluid containing very little protein, the term *serous exudate* is sometimes used. If a large amount of serous fluid accumulates in injured tissues—as, for example, after a severe burn of the skin—blisters may form (figure 4–4). An exudate consisting largely of inflammatory cells is called a *purulent exudate,* and the creamy yellow exudate is called *pus.* The term *fibrinous exudate* is used if the fluid in the exudate is rich in a blood protein called fibrinogen, which coagulates and forms fibrin, producing a sticky film on the surface of the inflamed tissue (figure 4–5). (The proteins concerned in the coagulation of the blood are considered in chapter 11.)

If a fibrinous exudate involves two surfaces in close proximity, such as adjacent loops of small intestine, the surfaces may stick together. This type of inflammation often heals by ingrowth of fibrous tissue, which binds the adjacent surfaces together by means of fibrous bands called **adhesions** (figure 4–6). A

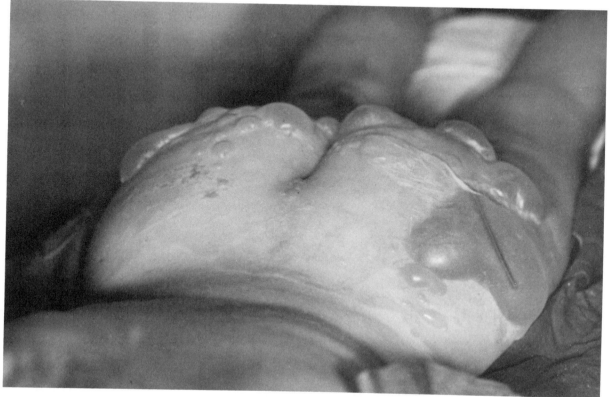

FIGURE 4–4

Extensive burn with marked extravasation of fluid into burned area leading to large blisters.

FIGURE 4–5

Fibrinous inflammation of exterior of heart, which appears rough because fibrin has accumulated on epicardium. *Arrow* indicates a large aggregate of fibrin.

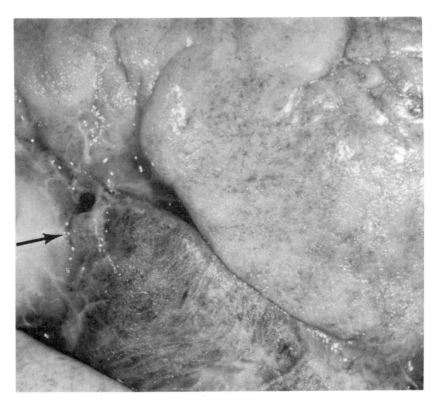

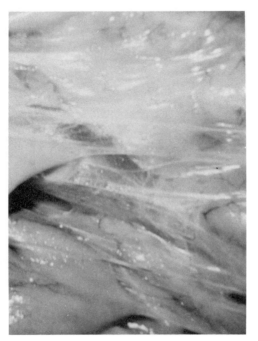

FIGURE 4–6

Adhesions between adjacent loops of small intestine resulting from previous abdominal inflammation.

hemorrhagic exudate occurs when the inflammatory process had ruptured many small capillaries, allowing red blood cells to escape into the tissues so that the exudate appears bloody.

If the inflammatory process is severe, systemic effects become evident. The individual feels ill, and the temperature is elevated. The bone marrow accelerates its production of leukocytes so that the number of leukocytes circulating in the bloodstream increases.

If the inflammation is mild, it soon subsides, and the tissues return to normal. This process is called **resolution.** If the inflammatory process is more severe, tissue is destroyed to some extent and must be repaired (figure 4–7). During healing, damaged cells are replaced and the framework of the injured tissue is repaired as an ingrowth of cells produces connective-tissue fibers and new blood vessels. Scar tissue replaces large areas of tissue destruction (figure 4–8). Sometimes, the scarring subsequent to a severe inflammation is so severe that function is seriously disturbed (figure 4–9).

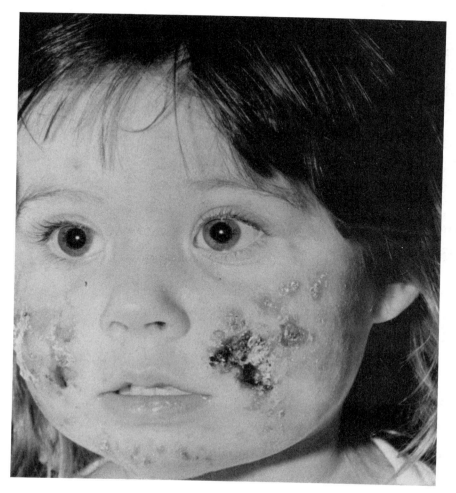

FIGURE 4–7

Acute inflammation of face with superficial necrosis of skin. Crusts of dried exudate (scabs) have formed on skin surface.

FIGURE 4-8

Extensive tissue destruction of lower lip, which is covered with inflammatory exudate. Child chewed an electric light cord, exposing bare wire, and sustained a severe electrical burn of lip.

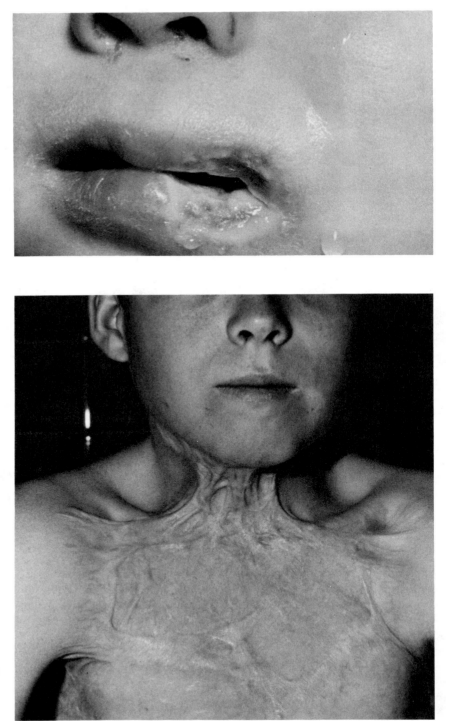

FIGURE 4-9

Marked scarring following healing of severe burn, which has restricted motion of neck and arms. Skin grafting was required to improve function.

Chemical Mediators of Inflammation

The characteristic features of the inflammatory reaction are not caused by the tissue damage itself. They are caused by chemical agents called *mediators of inflammation,* which are formed when tissues are damaged. Some mediators are derived from cells, and others are formed from proteins in the blood plasma that accumulate in the injured area.

Cell-Derived Mediators

Mast cells, a major source of cell-derived mediators, are specialized cells that are widely distributed throughout the connective tissues of the body. Their cytoplasm is filled with granules containing histamine and other chemicals. If tissue is injured, the mast cells discharge their granules, liberating the chemicals to initiate the inflammatory process. Histamine is a potent **vasodilator** (*vaso* = blood vessel + *dilate* = expand) and also greatly increases vascular permeability. *Blood platelets* also contain histamine and another mediator called **serotonin,** which are released when platelets adhere to collagen fragments at the site of tissue injury. Other important cell-derived mediators are a group called **prostaglandins** (so named because compounds of this type were first isolated from the prostate gland) and a group of similar compounds called **leukotrienes.** These biologically active compounds are synthesized by cells from arachidonic acid present in cell membranes in response to stimuli that induce inflammation, and they function as mediators that intensify the inflammatory process.

Mediators from Blood Plasma

Blood plasma contains various protein substances that circulate as inactive compounds and leak from the permeable capillaries into the area of tissue damage where they become transformed (activated) by a complex process into chemical mediators. One important group of mediators formed in this way is called **bradykinins** (or simply kinins). The series of reactions that leads to the formation of bradykinins is triggered by one of the proteins concerned with blood coagulation, which is activated by the tissue injury.

Mediators of inflammation are also formed from another group of blood proteins called **complement.** Complement consists of nine separate protein components, designated C_1 through C_9, that interact in a regular sequence to yield a series of by-products, some of which function as mediators of inflammation. Complement is activated when an antigen combines with an antibody but may also be activated in other ways that do not require antigen-antibody interaction.

Figure 4–10 illustrates how the various mediators interact. The release of mediators from any source not only initiates the inflammatory process, but also induces release of more mediators from other sources, setting off a "chain reaction" that intensifies the inflammatory process.

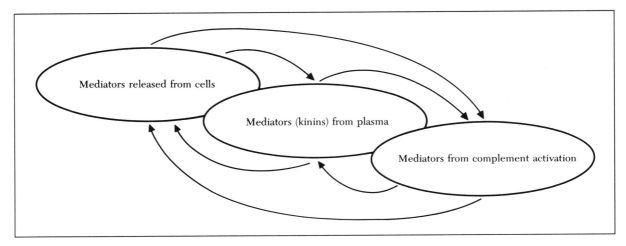

FIGURE 4–10

Interaction of mediators of inflammation. Activation of mediators from any source also leads to formation of mediators from other sources, which intensifies the inflammatory reaction.

The Role of Lysosomal Enzymes in the Inflammatory Process

The cytoplasm of phagocytic neutrophils and monocytes that are attracted to the site of inflammation by chemical mediators contains granules called **lysosomes** (*lysis* = dissolving + *soma* = body). They contain potent enzymes that are capable of digesting the material brought into the cytoplasm of the cells by phagocytosis. During phagocytosis, bacteria or other foreign materials become enclosed within vacuoles in the cell cytoplasm, and the lysosomes dissolve the material by discharging their enzymes into the vacuoles.

In the course of any inflammatory reaction, many neutrophils and monocytes are damaged or destroyed, and their lysosomal enzymes are released. Some lysosomal enzymes also escape from intact leukocytes during phagocytosis. Much of the tissue injury in an area of inflammation is a result of the destructive effect of the lysosomal enzymes released from leukocytes. The tissue injury in turn generates more mediators, and this induces further inflammatory changes.

Inflammation Caused by Antigen-Antibody Interaction

Antibodies are one of the body's defense mechanisms. This is discussed in chapter 5. When antigen and antibody interact, an intense inflammatory reaction with marked tissue necrosis often follows. The interaction of antigen and antibody activates complement, and the mediators generated from complement activation induce the inflammatory reaction. Large numbers of leukocytes are attracted to the site, and the release of potent lysosomal enzymes from the leukocytes is the chief cause of the tissue damage.

Harmful Effects of Inflammation

The tissue injury that results from an inflammation is due in part to the injurious agent and in part to the inflammatory reaction itself. In most cases, the inflammatory process is self-limited and subsides when the harmful agent has been eliminated. At times, however, an inflammatory process may persist and cause extensive, progressive tissue injury. If this occurs, it is sometimes necessary to suppress the inflammatory process by administering adrenal corticosteroid hormones to reduce the tissue damage that would result if the inflammatory process were not restrained. (Suppression of the immune response is considered in chapter 5.)

Terminology of Infection

The term **infection** is used to denote an inflammatory process caused by disease-producing organisms. A number of different terms are used to refer to infections in various sites. Generally, the ending -*itis* is appended to the name of the tissue or organ in order to indicate an infection or inflammatory process. For example, the terms appendicitis (figure 4–11), hepatitis, colitis, and pneumonitis refer to inflammation of the appendix, liver, colon, and lung, respectively. An acute spreading infection at any site is called **cellulitis** (figure 4–12). Usually, this term is used to refer to an acute infection of the skin and deeper tissues. The term **abscess** is used when an infection is associated with

Infection

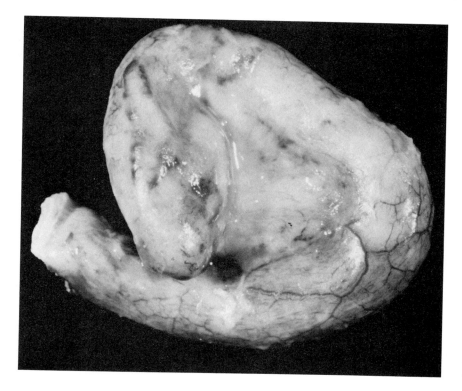

FIGURE 4–11

Acute appendicitis. Marked inflammatory exudate on surface.

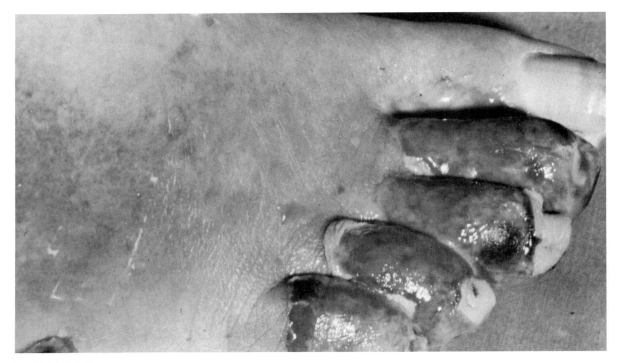

FIGURE 4–12

Cellulitis of foot.

breakdown of the tissues and the formation of a localized mass of pus (figure 4–13). If a localized infection spreads into the lymphatic channels draining the site of inflammation, the term **lymphangitis** is used. **Lymphadenitis** refers to infection in the regional lymph nodes draining the primary site of infection. The term **septicemia** is used to refer to an overwhelming infection in which pathogenic bacteria gain access to the bloodstream.

Factors Influencing the Outcome of an Infection

In any infection, the invading organism is pitted against the defenses of the body. Bacteria and other microbiologic agents vary in their ability to cause disease. Many are not harmful to humans. Others, capable of causing human disease, are called **pathogenic** (*pathos* = disease + *genic* = producing) organisms. The term **virulence** refers to the ease with which a pathogenic organism can overcome the defenses of the body. A highly virulent organism is one likely to produce progressive disease in the majority of susceptible individuals. In contrast, an organism of low virulence is capable only of producing disease in a highly susceptible individual under favorable circumstances.

The outcome of any infection depends upon two factors: the virulence of the organism combined with the numbers ("dosage") of the invading organisms and the resistance of the infected individual (often called the **host**). These

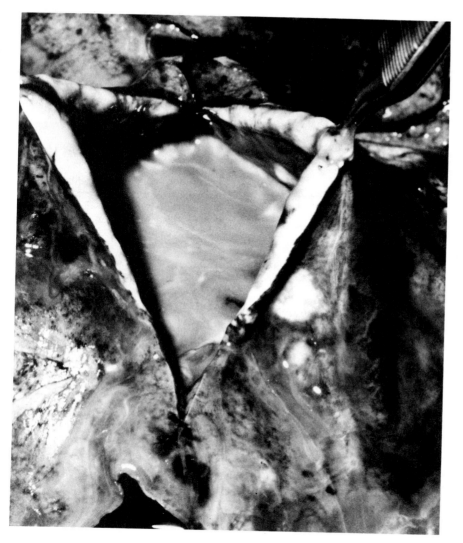

FIGURE 4–13

Lung abscess. Pleural surface has been incised to expose large abscess cavity filled with pus.

may be considered balanced against one another, as indicated diagrammatically in figure 4–14. When large numbers of organisms of high virulence are introduced into the body, especially when host resistance is lowered, the balance is tipped in favor of the invader, and progressive or fatal disease develops. When the virulence or dosage of the organism is low or the body's resistance is high, the balance is tipped in favor of the host. The infection is then overcome, and healing occurs.

Chronic Infection

Sometimes, the organism and host are evenly matched. Neither can gain the advantage; the result is a stalemate. Clinically, this results in a *chronic infection,* characterized by a relatively quiet, smoldering inflammation that

FIGURE 4–14

Factors influencing the outcome of an infection.

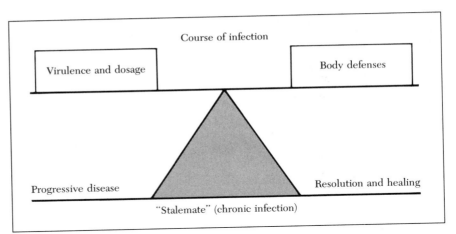

is usually associated with vigorous attempts at healing on the part of the host. The balance between the host and the invader is precarious. The infection may flare up at times when the pathogen obtains a temporary advantage or it may become quiescent at other times when the defenses of the host gain the upper hand. Lymphocytes, plasma cells, and monocytes are the predominant cells in chronic inflammatory processes.

Questions for Review

1. What is the inflammatory reaction? What are its clinical manifestations?

2. What factors influence the outcome of an infection?

3. What are mediators of inflammation? How do they function?

4. What is meant by the following terms: *chronic infection, pathogenic, complement?*

Supplementary Readings

Boxer, G. J., Carnutte, J. T., and Boxer, L. A. 1985. Polymorphonuclear leukocyte function. *Hospital Practice* 20:69–90. Describes phagocytosis and interactions involved in engulfing, killing, and ingesting microorganisms.

Broide, D. 1994. Inflammatory cells, structure and function. In *Basic and clinical immunology*. 8th ed. Ed. D. P. Stites, A. I. Terr, and T. G. Parslow. Norwalk, Conn.: Appleton & Lange. Reviews functions and interactions of cells involved in the inflammatory reaction.

Galin, J. I., ed. 1992. *Inflammation: Basic principles and clinical correlates.* 2d ed. New York: Raven Press. An in-depth treatment of the subject.

Johnston, R. B., Jr. 1988. Monocytes and macrophages. *New England Journal of Medicine* 318:747–53. Describes the structure and function of the mononuclear phagocyte system. Monocytes form in the marrow, have a half-life of about three days in the blood, and then migrate to the tissues where they live for several months. They are activated by lymphokines from T lymphocytes.

Unanue, E. R., and Allen, P. M. 1987. The basis for immunoregulatory role of macrophages and other accessory cells. *Science* 236:551–57. Discusses the immunoregulatory role of macrophages. Basic review article.

See also sections on inflammation in standard textbooks in pathology, listed in the General References.

Chapter 4 ▪ Outline Summary

The Inflammatory Reaction / 73
Characteristics of the Inflammatory Reaction
Dilatation of blood vessels.

Migration of leukocytes through vessel walls to site of inflammation.

Increased capillary permeability.

Extravasation of fluids.

Clinical Manifestations of Inflammation
Heat and redness: dilated blood vessels.

Swelling: accumulation of fluid and exudate.

Tenderness and pain: irritation of nerve endings.

Types of Inflammation Reactions
Serous inflammation: chiefly fluid exudate.

Purulent inflammation: chiefly inflammatory cells.

Fibrinous inflammation: exudate rich in protein, which coagulates.

Hemorrhagic inflammation: many capillaries ruptured, allowing escape of red cells.

Systemic Effects of Inflammation
Patient feels ill.

Elevated temperature.

Leukocytosis.

Outcome of Inflammation
Resolution: inflammation subsides and tissues return to normal.

Repair: replacement of damaged cells and tissues.

Large areas of destruction replaced by scar tissue.

Mediators intensify inflammatory process and generate more mediators.

Role of Lysosomal Enzymes in Inflammation
Lysosomal enzymes released from leukocytes cause tissue injury.

Injury generates more mediators, which promotes further inflammation and tissue injury.

Inflammation Caused by Antigen-Antibody Interaction
Interaction activates complement, leading to formation of mediators. This attracts leukocytes.

Lysosomal enzymes from leukocytes cause tissue injury.

Harmful Effects of Inflammation
Inflammation usually subsides.

Persisting inflammation may cause severe tissue injury.

It may be necessary to suppress inflammatory reaction by corticosteroids to reduce tissue damage.

Chemical Mediators of Inflammation
Mast cells: discharge granules containing mediators.

Kinins form from blood proteins leaking into inflamed area.

Activation of complement generates mediators.

Infection / 81
An Inflammation Caused by a Pathogenic Organism
Terms used to name infections:

Named by adding *-itis* to name of affected organ.

Cellulitis: acute spreading infection.

Abscess: tissue breakdown forming pus pockets.

Lymphadenitis: inflammation of draining lymph nodes.

Septicemia: bloodstream infection.

Factors influencing outcome:

Virulence of organism.

Dosage.

Resistance of host's body.

Chronic Infection
Organisms and host evenly balanced.

Lymphocytes and plasma cells predominate.

5

Immunity, Hypersensitivity, Allergy, and Autoimmune Diseases

Learning Objectives

1. List the basic features of cell-mediated and humoral immunity. Explain the role of lymphocytes in the immune response.
2. Compare immunity and hypersensitivity. Explain why it is sometimes necessary to suppress the immune response and describe how this is accomplished.
3. List the five classes of antibodies and explain how they differ from one another.
4. Describe the pathogenesis of allergic manifestations and the role of IgA in allergy. Compare the methods of treatment.
5. Summarize the theories concerning the pathogenesis of autoimmune disease, the clinical manifestations, and the methods of treatment.

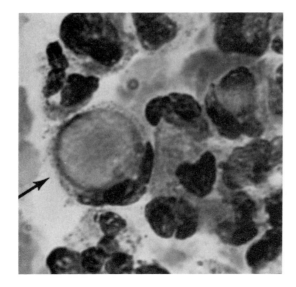

Chapter 5 ■ Contents

The body has two separate defense mechanisms for dealing with pathogenic microorganisms and other potentially harmful substances. One mechanism consists of the *inflammatory reaction,* which is a nonspecific response to any harmful agent and includes phagocytosis of the material by neutrophils and macrophages. The second, which depends on the immune system, consists of the development of an *acquired immunity.* The two mechanisms complement one another and function together to protect an individual from disease.

Acquired immunity, which develops after contact with a pathogenic microorganism, is only one manifestation of a person's capacity to react to a large number of foreign antigens. There are two different types of acquired immunity: humoral immunity and cell-mediated immunity.

Humoral immunity is associated with the production of antibodies that can combine with and eliminate the foreign material. Humoral immunity is the body's major defense against many bacteria and bacterial toxins. **Cell-mediated immunity** is characterized by the formation of a population of lymphocytes that can attack and destroy the foreign material. It is the main defense against viruses, fungi, parasites, and some bacteria. Cell-mediated immunity is the mechanism by which the body rejects transplanted organs and eliminates the abnormal cells that sometimes arise spontaneously in cell division.

Acquired immunity is often associated with a stage of altered reactivity to bacterial products or foreign material, leading to an intense inflammatory reaction at the site of contact with the foreign antigen. This increased responsiveness is called **hypersensitivity.** For example, contact with the tubercle bacillus leads to cell-mediated immunity and is also associated with the development of tissue hypersensitivity to antigens of the tubercle bacillus. An individual who displays hypersensitivity to an organism or its products usually possesses some degree of immunity as well. However, many diseases are associated with the development of an acquired immunity without demonstrable hypersensitivity.

Normally, a person develops an immune response not against cell proteins in his or her own cells and tissues (called self-antigens) but only against foreign antigens (called non-self-antigens), because the body has developed a tolerance to the self-antigens present within it. Any lymphocytes that are inadvertently programmed in the course of prenatal development to react against self-antigens are destroyed or inactivated or their functions are suppressed.

However, there are diseases in which the patient forms antibodies to his or her own cells and tissues, and these antibodies may injure or destroy the patient's cells or tissue components. This type of antibody is called an autoantibody (*auto* = self) and the diseases associated with autoantibodies are called **autoimmune diseases.**

Immunity

The Role of Lymphocytes in Acquired Immunity

The important cells of the immune system are the lymphocytes (figure 5–1), which respond to foreign antigens, and the macrophages and related cells that process the antigen and "present" it to the lymphocytes.

The various cells of the immune system communicate with one another and produce many of their effects by secreting soluble protein (peptide) chemical messengers. Those secreted by lymphocytes are called **lymphokines,** and those secreted by monocytes are called **monokines.** The general term **cytokines** is used to designate any chemical messengers that take part in any function of the immune system, and some cytokines have specific names. Those that act by interfering with the multiplication of viruses within cells are called **interferons.** Those that send regulatory signals between cells of the immune system are called **interleukins.** Cytokines that can destroy foreign or abnormal cells are called **tumor necrosis factors,** so named because they can destroy tumor cells, although their destructive functions are not restricted to tumor cells.

Development of the Lymphatic System

Development of Immune Competence
The precursor cells of the lymphocytes are formed initially from stem cells in the bone marrow, and they eventually develop into either of two groups

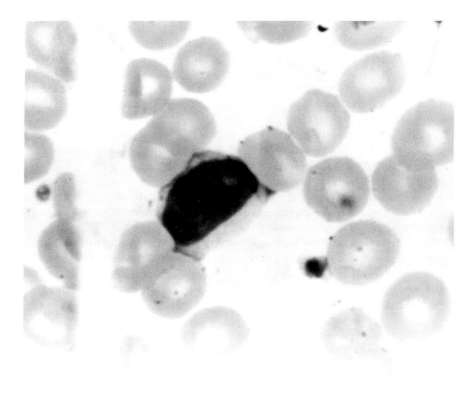

FIGURE 5–1

Structure of a mature lymphocyte in the peripheral blood. (Original magnification × 1000.)

of lymphocytes, depending on where they undergo further development and "learn" their functions—a process called *developing immune competence.* In the fetus, some of these precursor cells migrate from the marrow into the thymus, where they undergo further maturation and develop into cells that are destined to form a specific type of lymphocyte called **T** (*thymus-dependent*) **lymphocytes.** Other lymphoid cells remain within the bone marrow, where they differentiate and develop into cells destined to form a second specific type of lymphocyte called **B** (*bone-marrow*) **lymphocytes.**

The programming process by which lymphocytes acquire immune competence involves a rearrangement of genes within the developing B and T lymphocytes. Each programmed lymphocyte develops antigen receptors on its cell membrane that enable the lymphocyte to "recognize" and respond to a specific antigen. The antigen receptors of B lymphocytes are immunoglobulin (antibody) molecules, each a copy of the antibody that the B lymphocyte will eventually produce when stimulated by the appropriate antigen. T lymphocytes develop somewhat different types of receptors, but they serve the same functions as those on B cells. When the programming process has been completed, many millions of different T and B cells have formed, each programmed to recognize and respond to a different antigen. Although a single lymphocyte can respond to only a single antigen, there is such an enormous population of lymphocytes that some member of the "immunologic response team" can respond to any antigen the individual may ever encounter.

Migration and Circulation of Lymphocytes

Before birth, the precursor cells of both T and B lymphocytes migrate into the spleen, lymph nodes, and other sites. Here they proliferate to form the masses of mature lymphocytes that populate the various lymphoid organs.

T lymphocytes are usually classified into two major groups based on the type of protein molecules, called *CD* (cell differentiation) *antigens,* on their cell membranes. Lymphocytes containing CD4 antigens are usually called T4 lymphocytes, and those with CD8 antigens are called T8 lymphocytes. As will be described later, each group of T lymphocyte has different functions and responds somewhat differently when stimulated by an antigen.

Lymphocytes vary in their life-span. Some have only a short survival time, but others live for many years. Lymphocytes do not remain localized within lymphoid organs. They continually recirculate between the bloodstream and the various lymphoid tissues. T and B lymphocytes are both present in the circulation and can be distinguished by special techniques.

About two-thirds of the circulating lymphocytes are T lymphocytes, and most of the rest are B lymphocytes. From about 10 to 15 percent of the circulating lymphocytes, however, have neither T nor B cell receptors. These cells are called **natural killer cells** or, simply, **NK cells.** Their major targets are virus-infected cells and cancer cells, which they can attack and destroy by secreting destructive lymphokines, even though they have not been previously exposed to the foreign antigens that they are attacking. Furthermore, NK cells can destroy the target cells without the delay as a result of the time that it takes B cells and T cells to become activated and function effectively. Although NK cells are not actually part of either the cell-mediated or the humoral immune-defense systems, their functions are to some extent regulated by the immune system. NK cells are related to cell-mediated immunity because they are activated and function much more effectively when stimulated by lymphokines secreted by T lymphocytes. They are also related to humoral immunity because some types of NK cells possess cell membrane receptors for antibody molecules, which makes it easier for the NK lymphocytes to attach to and destroy target cells coated with antibodies.

Response of Lymphocytes to Foreign Antigens

Figure 5–2 summarizes the role of lymphocytes in acquired immunity. The first step in the immune-defense reaction is the interaction of lymphocytes with the antigen that it has been programmed to recognize. The antigen must first be "processed" and displayed on the cell membrane of the antigen-processing cell before the immune response can be set in motion. When appropriately stimulated, B lymphocytes mature into antibody-forming plasma cells, and T lymphocytes form a diverse population of cells that both regulate the immune response and generate a cell-mediated immune reaction to eliminate the antigenic material.

Initial contact with a foreign antigen is followed by a lag phase of a week or more before an immune response is demonstrated. This lag corresponds to the time required for processing the antigen and for the lymphocytes to respond. Once the body's immune mechanisms have reacted to a foreign antigen, however, some of the lymphoid cells retain a "memory" of the antigen that induced sensitization. They pass this information to succeeding generations of lymphocytes. Consequently, any later contact with the same antigen provokes a renewed proliferation of sensitized lymphocytes or antibody-forming plasma cells.

Role of MHC Proteins in Displaying Processed Antigen   The major histocompatibility (MHC) proteins play an essential role in "presenting" processed antigen to the responding cells of the immune system in order to generate an immune response. The MHC proteins are carbohydrate-protein (glycoprotein) molecules on the surface of cells that distinguish the cells of one person from those of another. As described in chapter 3, there are two major classes of MHC proteins: MHC Class I proteins are present on all nucleated cells; MHC Class II proteins are restricted to B lymphocytes, macrophages and related antigen-processing cells, and some activated T lymphocytes. The main function of the MHC proteins is to serve as a carrier for the processed foreign antigen fragments on the surface of cells, to which the immune system can respond.

B Lymphocyte Response to Antigen   B and T lymphocytes respond differently to foreign antigens. B lymphocytes, which have immunoglobulin molecules on their cell membranes that function as antigen receptors, can

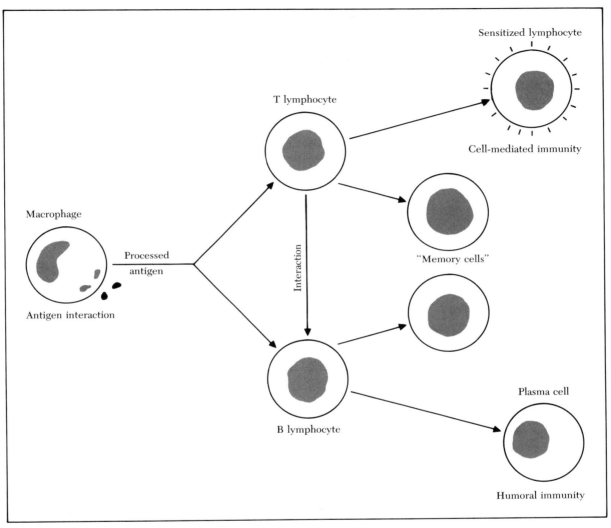

FIGURE 5–2

Interrelations of cell-mediated and humoral immunity.

bind entire antigen molecules to their receptors. The bound antigen is transported across the cell membrane and is processed into fragments within the
cytoplasm of the B lymphocyte; then the processed fragments are displayed
on the cell membrane along with the B lymphocyte's own MHC Class II proteins. T lymphocytes are activated by the displayed antigen–MHC-Class-II
complex on the B lymphocytes, and they secrete lymphokines that induce
the B cells to proliferate, mature into plasma cells, and produce antibodies.
Some of the activated B lymphocytes, however, are set aside as memory cells

and can respond rapidly to generate an intense humoral antibody response if the same antigen is encountered again.

T Lymphocyte Response to Antigen Unlike B lymphocytes, which function as their own antigen-processing cells, T lymphocytes are unable to respond to a foreign antigen until a macrophage or a similar macrophage-like antigen-processing cell has phagocytosed the antigen, digested it, and displayed on its cell membrane the antigen fragments combined with its own MHC Class II proteins. The T lymphocyte having preprogrammed receptors to match the displayed antigen–MHC-Class-II complex responds by proliferating to form a group (clone) of identical T cells, in much the same manner that B cells proliferate when stimulated by antigenic contact. The macrophages are also activated when they process and present antigen to the T cells, and they secrete a cytokine that stimulates the responding T cells.

Major Functions of T Lymphocyte Populations Several different types of T cells are recognized. Their activities are coordinated, and they function together both to regulate the immune response and to act against the foreign antigens. The regulator T cells are *helper T cells,* which are T4 (CD4+) cells, and *suppressor T cells,* which are T8 (CD8+) cells. The effector cells are *cytotoxic T cells,* which are T8 (CD8+) cells, and a group of T4 (CD4+) cells taking part in delayed hypersensitivity reactions and thus often called *delayed hypersensitivity cells* or simply *sensitized T cells.* In addition, a population of long-lived *memory cells* can initiate a rapid cell-mediated immune response upon later contact with the same antigen.

Helper T cells promote the immune response by secreting lymphokines that activate T and B cells, and suppressor T cells dampen the immune response by inhibiting T and B cell functions. Together, these cells control the immune response so that it does not get out of control. They control the rate of antibody formation and regulate the intensity of the cell-mediated immune response. Proper immune system function depends on the correct balance between the helper T lymphocytes that promote immune reactions and the suppressor T lymphocytes that inhibit these reactions (figure 5–3). Deficient or defective suppressor T cell function leads to loss of normal inhibitory control of the immune response and can increase the likelihood of acquiring autoimmune diseases, described in a later section. Conversely, loss or destruction of helper T cells leads to a relative excess of suppressor T cells, which inhibits the immune response and greatly increases the susceptibility to infection. The devastating effect of helper T cell deficiency on the immune system is illustrated by the acquired immune deficiency syndrome (AIDS, described in chapter 8), which is caused by a virus that attacks and destroys helper T lymphocytes.

Cytotoxic T cells attack and destroy body cells infected with viruses or intracellular bacteria. The infected cells are marked for destruction because some of the viral or bacterial antigens are broken down within the infected cells and transported to the cell surface combined with MHC Class I proteins (present on all nucleated cells). The cytotoxic T cells respond to the foreign

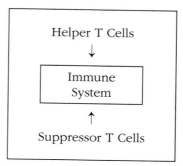

FIGURE 5–3

Interaction of helper and suppressor T lymphocytes, which regulate the immune response.

antigen-MHC complex, and they destroy the infected cells by secreting destructive lymphokines. Cytotoxic T cells can also attack cancer cells, which possess antigens different from those of normal cells, and they are responsible for the rejection of transplanted organs, which also contain foreign antigens.

Delayed hypersensitivity T cells respond to foreign antigens by accumulating at the site of the antigenic material, where they secrete a variety of lymphokines. Some of the lymphokines attract macrophages, activate them, and stimulate them to secrete cytokines, including interferon and tumor necrosis factor. Other lymphokines stimulate cytotoxic T cells and natural killer cells, both of which secrete destructive lymphokines. In this way, the delayed hypersensitivity cells generate an intense inflammatory response directed against the antigen that sensitized them.

Relation of MHC Proteins to Effector T Cell Responses   The two types of effector T cells are restricted in their ability to respond to processed antigens complexed and presented with MHC proteins. Cytotoxic T cells, which are T8 (CD8+) cells, can respond only to antigens complexed with MHC Class I proteins displayed on infected host cells, whereas delayed hypersensitivity (sensitized) T cells, which are T4 (CD4+) cells, can respond only to processed antigen displayed on macrophages or related cells along with MHC Class II proteins. Consequently, the manner in which the processed antigen is displayed determines which type of effector T cell will respond to the complexed antigen. Cytotoxic T cells are "designed" to attack and destroy infected host cells or other antigenically foreign or abnormal cells. Delayed hypersensitivity T cells function by orchestrating an intense inflammatory reaction to any type of foreign antigen, including macroorganisms such as the tubercle bacillus that are phagocytosed by macrophages. Activated macrophages, assisted by lymphoid cells, are the cells that play a major role in eliminating the antigenic material.

Immune-Response Genes   The ability to generate an immune response is under genetic control. Genes called **immune-response genes,** which are closely associated with the HLA complex on chromosome 6 (described in chapter 3), control the immune response by regulating T cell and B cell proliferation. In this way, the genes regulate the intensity of the cell-mediated immune reaction and control the synthesis of antibody molecules. As a result, they influence resistance to infection and resistance to tumors. They also influence the likelihood of acquiring an autoimmune disease.

The Role of Complement in Immune Responses

Complement functions along with the immune system to destroy or inactivate all types of foreign antigens including invading microorganisms. As described in chapter 4, complement can be activated in two ways: *the classical pathway,* which is triggered by antigen-antibody interactions; and the *alternative pathway,* in which complement is activated by bacterial cell wall material or by products generated during the inflammatory reaction. When complement is activated, the complement components interact to accomplish several important functions. Some components function as mediators of inflammation. Other components coat the surface of invading bacteria, which makes them easier for macrophages and neutrophils to phagocytose. Finally, the interaction of the complement components generates a large molecule called an *attack complex,* which destroys the target microorganism or abnormal cell by "punching holes" in its cell membrane.

Antibodies (Immunoglobulins)

Antibodies are globulins produced by plasma cells and are usually called **immunoglobulins** to emphasize their role in immunity. There are five different classes of immunoglobulins:

1. Immunoglobulin M (IgM)
2. Immunoglobulin G (IgG)
3. Immunoglobulin A (IgA)
4. Immunoglobulin D (IgD)
5. Immunoglobulin E (IgE)

Although the immunoglobulins differ somewhat from one another in their chemical composition, molecular weight, and size, they all have the same basic structure: two matched pairs of polypeptide (protein) chains joined by chemical bonds (figure 5–4). One pair is called *heavy chains.* The second pair is only half as long as the heavy chains and is called *light chains.*

The arrangement of the Ig chains somewhat resembles the appearance of a fork. The ends of the Ig chains that combine with the antigen can be compared to its prongs. The "prong" end of the immunoglobulin molecule, which is different in each antibody, is called the *variable part* of the molecule. It is this part that imparts specificity to the molecule. Because of its structure, the antibody can react only with the specific antigen that induced its formation. The *constant part* of the chain, which can be compared to the handle of the fork, is the same for each major class of antibody. The "handle" end does not combine with antigen but determines other properties of

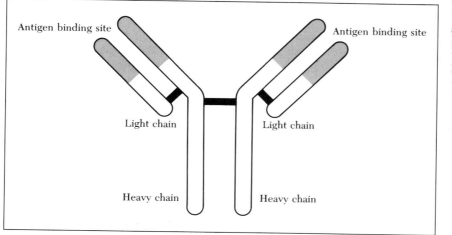

FIGURE 5–4

Structure of an immuno-globulin molecule.

the antibody, such as the ability to activate complement or fix to the surface of cell membranes.

All Ig molecules have the same basic four-chain unit structure, but some immunoglobulins characteristically aggregate to form clusters of two, three, or five individual units. For example, IgM is usually a cluster of five individual units, and IgA is usually a pair of units.

An antibody molecule is not a rigid structure. The junction of its constant and variable parts is quite flexible and is called the *hinge region*. This feature allows the variable end of the Y-shaped molecule to adapt to the configuration of the antigen that it is binding. Treatment with enzymes breaks an immunoglobulin molecule into three fragments. The variable region yields two fragments called the F_{ab} *fragments* (antibody combining fragments), each consisting of a light chain and the associated part of the heavy chain. The other fragment is the constant region of the molecule and is called the F_c *fragment* (constant fragment).

Immunoglobulin M (IgM) is present in the blood as a cluster of five individual molecules (a pentamer) joined together in a star-shaped configuration with the antigen binding ends projecting outward and the opposite ends of the molecules directed toward the center of the cluster. As a pentamer, IgM forms a very large antibody cluster that is very efficient in combining with large particulate antigens such as fungi; it is often called a *macroglobulin* because of its large size and high molecular weight. IgM molecules are also found as single (monomeric) molecules attached, with their antigen binding sites protruding, to the cell membranes of B lymphocytes, where they function as the antigen receptors on the surface of B lymphocytes. *Immunoglobulin G* (IgG) is a much smaller antibody molecule and is the principal type of antibody molecule formed in response to the majority of infectious agents. *Immunoglobulin A* (IgA) is produced by antibody-forming cells located in the respiratory and gastrointestinal mucosa. It is present in secretions of the respiratory and gastrointestinal tracts. IgA apparently functions by combining with potentially harmful ingested or inhaled antigens, forming antigen-antibody complexes that cannot be absorbed. In this way, IgA prevents the antigens from inducing sensitization. *Immunoglobulin D* (IgD) is found on the cell membranes of B lymphocytes, along with the monomeric form of IgM, and is present in only minute quantities in the blood. *Immunoglobulin E* (IgE) is normally present in only small quantities in the blood of most persons, but its concentration is greatly increased in allergic individuals.

Hypersensitivity Reactions: Immune System Related Tissue Injury

The immune system, while protecting us from foreign antigens that could harm us, may also damage the tissues where the immune response occurs. The desirable effect, which eliminates the foreign antigen, is called *immunity*. The undesirable effect, which is the associated tissue damage, is called *hypersensitivity*. Both are manifestations of the same process. The situation could be compared to the successful efforts of fire fighters in putting out a potentially destructive house fire, but at the same time breaking some windows and causing some water damage to the house and furniture.

It is conventional to classify the various types of hypersensitivity reactions based on how the immune system caused the injury (table 5–1). Four different types of hypersensitivity reactions, usually designated by roman numerals, are recognized. The first three types are related to antibodies formed in response to antigenic material and the fourth type is a cell-mediated hypersensitivity reaction. This section deals with the various mechanisms of immunologic injury. Specific examples of immune-mediated organ damage will be considered in connection with the disease of the various organ systems.

Type I. Immediate Hypersensitivity Reactions: Allergy and Anaphylaxis

Type I hypersensitivity reactions follow contact with foreign antigens that induce formation of specific IgE antibodies in the sensitized person. IgE has the unusual property of attaching to the surface of mast cells and similar cells circulating in the blood called basophils. The IgE attaches itself to the cell membrane by means of the F_c end of the molecule (the "handle of the fork"). If the sensitized person is later exposed to the sensitizing antigen, the antigen attaches to the free antibody combining sites (the "prongs of the fork") on the IgE molecules. The union of antigen and antibody causes the cells to release their cytoplasmic granules filled with histamine, prostaglandins, and other potent chemical mediators. Immediate hypersensitivity reactions either may be localized, called *allergic reactions* or may evoke a widespread systemic reaction, called *anaphylaxis*.

Allergy   Individuals who develop localized IgE-mediated reactions are predisposed to form specific IgE antibodies (become allergic) to ragweed, other plant pollens, and various other antigens that do not affect most persons. The

Type	Mechanism	Examples
I: Immediate Hypersensitivity	IgE antibodies fix to mast cells and basophils. Later contact with sensitizing antigen triggers mediator release and clinical manifestations.	Localized response: hay fever, food allergy, etc. Systemic response: bee sting, or penicilin anaphylaxis, etc.
II: Cytotoxic Reactions	Antibody binds to cell or tissue antigen, and complement is activated, which damages cell, causes inflammation, and promotes destruction of antibody-coated cell by phagocytosis	Autoimmune hemolytic anemia Blood transfusion reactions Rh hemolytic disease Some types of glomerulo-nephritis
III: Immune complex disease	Circulating antigen-antibody complexes form, which activate complement and cause inflammatory reaction.	Some types of glomerulo-nephritis Lupus erythematosus Rheumatoid arthritis
IV: Delayed (cell-mediated) hypersensitivity	Sensitized (delayed hypersensitivity) T cells release lymphokines that attract macrophages and other inflammatory cells.	Tuberculosis Fungus and parasitic infections Contact dermatitis

TABLE 5–1

Mechanisms of immunologic injury

allergy-prone individual is called an **atopic person;** the sensitizing antigen is called an **allergen;** and the allergic manifestations are localized to the tissues that are exposed to the allergens—for example, swollen itchy eyes, stuffy nose, and sneezing in a ragweed-sensitive person (figure 5–5).

Because histamine is one of the mediators released from the IgE-coated cells, antihistamine drugs (which block the effects of histamine) often relieve many of the allergic symptoms. A more specific method of treating an allergic individual consists of immunizing the person to the offending allergen by repeated subcutaneous injections of the antigen that induced the allergy, such as an extract of ragweed pollen in a ragweed-sensitive person. This method of treatment, which is called **desensitization,** induces the formation of specific IgA and IgG antibodies against the offending allergen. The IgA and IgG act by combining with the allergen before it can affix to the cell-bound IgE and trigger the release of mediators. In a ragweed-sensitive person, for example, the ragweed-specific IgA present in the secretions of the respiratory tract combines with some of the inhaled ragweed antigen and helps prevent absorption of the allergen. At the same time, the ragweed-specific IgG circulating in the bloodstream combines with much of the absorbed ragweed anti-

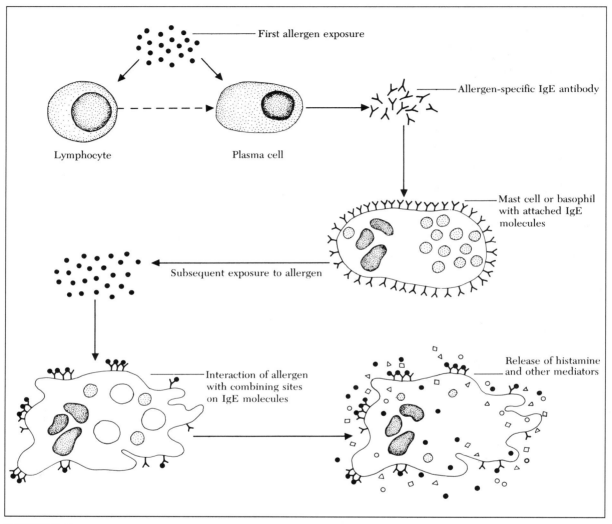

FIGURE 5–5

Pathogenesis of allergy. First exposure to allergen induces production of specific IgE antibody, which binds to mast cells and basophils by nonantigen receptor end of the molecule. Subsequent exposure to allergen leads to antigen-antibody interaction, liberating histamine and other mediators from mast cells and basophils. These mediators induce allergic manifestations.

gen before it can interact with the IgE on the surface of the mast cells and basophils. Because less antigen is available to combine with cell-bound IgE and thereby trigger release of mediators, the allergic manifestations are minimized.

Anaphylaxis   A severe generalized IgE-mediated hypersensitivity reaction may be life threatening and is called **anaphylaxis.** This condition may result, for example, from taking a drug, such as penicillin, to which the person has become sensitized or may result from a bee sting in a highly sensitive person. The sensitizing antigen is carried in the circulation throughout the body and triggers widespread mediator release from IgE-coated mast cells and basophils. This release may lead to a fall in blood pressure with circulatory collapse and is often accompanied by severe respiratory distress caused by mediator-induced spasm of smooth muscle in the walls of the bronchioles, which restricts air flow into and out of the lungs. Prompt treatment of this immunologic catastrophe with epinephrine and other appropriate agents is essential.

Type II. Cytotoxic Hypersensitivity Reactions

In this type of hypersensitivity reaction, antibody formed against a cell or tissue antigen binds to the surface of the target cell or tissue. The antigen-antibody reaction activates complement, and products of complement activation directly or indirectly damage the target. The complement components interact to form a large molecule called an *attack complex* that directly damages the target cell membrane. Inflammatory cells also are attracted and contribute to the tissue injury by releasing destructive enzymes; they may also destroy the antibody-coated target cells by phagocytosis.

Examples of Type II reactions include transfusion reactions caused by administration of incompatible blood, hemolytic disease of newborn infants caused by Rh incompatibility (described in chapter 18), some types of chronic hemolytic anemia associated with autoantibodies directed against red blood cells (chapter 14), and a type of kidney disease caused by autoantibodies directed against basement membranes of glomerular capillaries (chapter 19).

Type III. Tissue Injury Caused by Immune Complexes ("Immune Complex Disease")

In this condition, antigen and antibody form clumps called *immune complexes* within the circulation that are deposited in the tissues. The antigen-antibody complexes activate complement, and the activated complement components, along with the inflammatory cells that they attract, damage the tissues. Sometimes the immunologic reaction within the tissues is quite severe and leads to thrombosis of blood vessels and considerable tissue necrosis.

An example of organ damage caused by immune complexes is a type of kidney disease called immune complex glomerulonephritis (described in chapter 19), in which the complexes are trapped within the glomeruli as the blood flows through the kidneys. Other important diseases in which tissue injury is related to immune complexes include lupus erythematosus, considered in connection with autoimmune disease, and rheumatoid arthritis (described in chapter 27).

Type IV. Delayed (Cell-Mediated) Hypersensitivity Reactions

In delayed hypersensitivity reactions, T lymphocytes rather than antibodies are responsible for the tissue injury. This type of hypersensitivity reaction is commonly encountered in persons who have been infected with the tubercle bacillus and have developed a cell-mediated immune reaction directed against the organism, but some other types of bacteria, as well as fungi and parasites, evoke a similar response. The initial antigenic contact sensitizes the affected individual, and the lymphocytes that generate the cell-mediated immune response are T4 (CD4+) lymphocytes that are often called *delayed hypersensitivity T cells* or, simply, *sensitized T cells*. Once sensitization has occurred, any subsequent contact with the sensitizing antigen induces proliferation of T4 cells that accumulate at the site of antigen contact. The sensitized T cells secrete cytokines that attract and activate macrophages and other lymphocytes and incite an inflammatory reaction.

Delayed hypersensitivity reactions may also follow skin exposure to poison ivy, as well as various drugs, cosmetics, and chemicals. These agents combine with normal skin proteins to form a complex that induces sensitization. Any later skin contact with the offending agent that induced the initial sensitization provokes an intense cell-mediated inflammatory reaction in the skin, a condition called *contact dermatitis*.

Unlike immediate hypersensitivity reactions, which are mediated by antibodies, a cell-mediated inflammatory reaction requires from 24 to 48 hours to develop, the delay being the time necessary for sensitized T cells to accumulate at the site and generate an inflammatory reaction. Because this type of reaction takes place in persons who have been infected with the tubercle bacillus, a delayed hypersensitivity reaction is sometimes called *tuberculin type hypersensitivity*. The commonly used Mantoux skin test to detect infection with the tubercle bacillus is based on the presence or absence of a delayed hypersensitivity reaction to proteins of the tubercle bacillus. If an individual has had a previous contact with the tubercle bacillus, injection of a small test dose of proteins from the tubercle bacillus leads to an inflammatory reaction at the injection site. A positive test, however, only indicates a previous infection with the organism and development of cell-mediated immunity, along with associated hypersensitivity to the tubercle bacillus, but does not necessarily indicate that the person has active tuberculosis.

Suppression of the Immune Response

Reasons for Suppression

Cell-mediated and humoral immune responses protect against potentially harmful microorganisms and other foreign substances. These same immunologic mechanisms may at times have undesirable effects:

1. They may be directed against the individual's own cells or tissue components, leading to autoimmune diseases.
2. They are responsible for the rejection of transplanted organs.
3. They lead to Rh hemolytic disease in newborn infants.

Methods of Suppression

It is sometimes necessary to suppress the immune response to treat certain autoimmune diseases, to perform organ transplants, and to prevent Rh hemolytic disease. The main types of immunosuppressive agents used in clinical medicine are:

1. Radiation
2. Immunosuppressive drugs that impede cell division or cell function
3. Adrenal corticosteroid hormones
4. Gamma globulin preparations containing potent antibodies

Radiation and Immunosuppressive Drugs

Radiation destroys normal cells. It exerts its immunosuppressive effect by destroying lymphoid tissue, which plays a key role in both cell-mediated and humoral immunity. There are several types of drugs that can suppress the immune response. *Cytotoxic drugs* (*cyto* = cell + *toxic* = poisonous) act by suppressing growth and division of lymphocytes. Lymphoid tissue is especially susceptible to the inhibitory effect of these drugs. *Antimetabolites,* as the name implies, inhibit important cellular metabolic functions, thereby inhibiting cell proliferation and suppressing the inflammatory reaction. Another important immunosuppressive drug called *cyclosporine* is often used to suppress the immune response in patients who have received organ transplants. The drug selectively inhibits T lymphocytes by interfering with the formation of a lymphokine called *interleukin-2* which stimulates T lymphocyte proliferation. As a result, cell-mediated immune responses are suppressed with little effect on humoral immune responses or on the inflammatory reaction. (Cytotoxic drugs and antimetabolites are also used to treat some types of leukemia and malignant tumors, as described in chapter 10.)

Corticosteroids

Adrenal corticosteroids act in several ways. They suppress the inflammatory response and impair phagocytosis. They also inhibit protein synthesis, thereby suppressing the growth and division of lymphocytes and inhibiting antibody formation by plasma cells.

Antibodies as Immunosuppressive Agents

Antibodies themselves may act as immunosuppressive agents under certain circumstances. Giving a patient a specific antibody somehow prevents the body's immune mechanisms from reacting to the corresponding antigen. Apparently, the antibody binds to the antigen in such a way that the antigen no longer incites an immune response, but how the antibody exerts this effect is uncertain. Possibly, the antibody covers specific sites on the antigen, and so the antigen can no longer be recognized by the body as foreign. An alternative possibility is that the antibody combines with the antigen after it has been processed by the macrophages, which prevents the antigen from interacting with the lymphocytes and inducing an immune response.

Suppression of the immune response by means of an antibody is widely used in preventing hemolytic disease of newborn infants caused by Rh incompatibility. The administration of Rh immune globulin containing potent

Rh antibody prevents an Rh-negative mother who has given birth to an Rh-positive infant from forming an Rh antibody. Because the mother does not form Rh antibody, Rh hemolytic disease is prevented in subsequent pregnancies. This application is described in connection with diseases of pregnancy (chapter 18).

Tissue Grafts and Immunity

An individual will accept a graft of his or her own tissue or that of an identical twin, but not that of another person, because a graft from another person contains HLA antigens foreign to the recipient. The body "recognizes" the foreign antigens in the transplant, which becomes infiltrated by lymphocytes and macrophages and is eventually destroyed. This process is called **rejection** of the transplanted organ, and it is a manifestation of a cell-mediated immune reaction. Physicians who are treating kidney failure by transplantation can keep a foreign kidney from being rejected by inhibiting the recipient's immunologic defenses, using drugs that suppress the immune response. Transplantation of kidneys and other organs has been successful because it is usually possible to suppress the body's immune responses sufficiently to allow the transplanted organ to survive.

Autoimmune Diseases

The reasons why an individual forms an autoantibody to his or her own cells or tissue components are not well understood. Three major mechanisms have been postulated to explain the pathogenesis of autoimmune diseases:

1. Alteration of the patient's own (self) antigens that causes them to become antigenic and provoke an immune reaction.
2. The formation of cross-reacting antibodies against foreign antigens that also attack the patient's own antigens.
3. Defective regulation of the immune response by regulator T lymphocytes.

The subject's own antigens may be altered by a viral infection or an infection with some other microbiologic agent in such a manner that the immune system no longer recognizes the antigen as a self-antigen. An immune reaction is generated against the altered antigen, which may injure the antigenically similar self-antigen as well. Alternatively, some drug or medication ingested by the patient may change the structure of a self-antigen so that it is perceived as foreign and generates an immune response. Cross-reacting antibodies may induce organ damage when an antibody is formed against a foreign antigen, such as an invading bacterium, that shares antigenic determinants with some of the subject's own cell or tissue antigens. As a result, the antibody that formed against the antigenic determinants in the foreign antigen cross-reacts with similar antigenic determinants in the subjects own tissues, leading to tissue injury (figure 5–6).

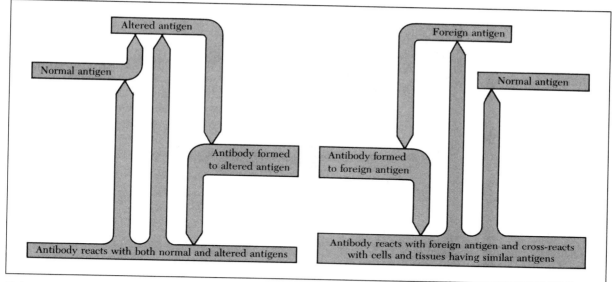

FIGURE 5–6

Mechanisms thought to cause autoantibody formation.

Defective regulation of the immune system by helper-suppressor T lymphocytes may lead to autoimmune disease by permitting lymphocytes directed against self-antigens to become activated and to attack one's own cells and tissues. When lymphocytes are programmed to respond to specific antigens (develop immune competence) in the thymus and bone marrow as the immune system is developing, some lymphocytes are inadvertently programmed to respond to self-antigens. These cell populations are either destroyed, inactivated, or suppressed so that they do not function. As a result, a normally functioning immune system does not attack self-antigens. Not all self-antigen–reacting lymphocytes are destroyed, however. Some are only suppressed and their "attack" functions are held in check by suppressor T lymphocytes. If the regulator function of suppressor T cells is impaired, lymphocytes programmed to recognize self-antigens are freed from suppressor T cell restraint. They become activated and attack one's own cells and tissues. On the other hand, hyperactivity of helper T cells may stimulate the immune system excessively, which may also activate previously suppressed self-reactive lymphocytes and induce autoimmune disease.

Autoimmune Disease Manifestations and Mechanisms of Tissue Injury

The manifestations of autoimmune disease depend on which cells or tissue components are targeted for attack by the immune system. The mechanisms of tissue injury are those described in connection with immune-mediated hypersensitivity reactions and may include humoral mechanisms, cell-mediated mechanisms, or a combination of both. Autoantibody-associated tissue injury results when antibody becomes attached to the cell membrane of the target cells, activating complement and causing complement-mediated destruction of the target, usually assisted by activated macrophages and killer lymphocytes (type II reaction). Alternatively, antigen and antibody may combine to form immune complexes that are deposited in the tissues and induce a similar type of complement-mediated tissue injury (type III reaction). Cell-mediated destruction of target tissues is caused by sensitized T lymphocytes that secrete lymphokines, which generate a destructive inflammatory reaction in the target tissue or organ (type IV reaction).

Not all autoantibodies destroy target tissue. Sometimes they derange the function of the target but do not destroy it. The thyroid gland, for example, may be attacked by two different types of autoantibodies. One type destroys thyroid cells and impairs thyroid function, causing hypothyroidism. Another type stimulates the thyroid cells and makes them hyperfunction, causing hyperthyroidism.

In general, treatment of autoimmune disease is not very satisfactory. Large doses of adrenal corticosteroid hormones may have a beneficial effect. They suppress the inflammatory reaction and impair antibody formation. Various cytotoxic drugs act by depressing the patient's ability to form antibodies.

Table 5–2 summarizes the features of some of the more important diseases in which autoantibody formation appears to play a role. These diseases are considered in greater detail in subsequent chapters.

Connective-Tissue (Collagen) Diseases

The fibrous connective tissue that forms the framework of all tissues in the body is called *collagen.* The term *connective-tissue disease,* or *collagen disease,* is used to describe a group of diseases characterized by necrosis and degeneration of collagen fibers throughout the body. In many instances, autoantibodies directed against antigens present in various cells and tissues can be detected in the serum of affected individuals, and aggregates of antigen combined with antibody (termed *antigen-antibody complexes*) can be identified at the sites of tissue damage. Often, large numbers of lymphocytes and plasma cells accumulate in the affected tissues. These cells are presumed to be responsible for the tissue injury by means of cell-mediated immune reactions and formation of autoantibodies. Therefore, the connective-tissue diseases are usually classified as autoimmune diseases.

The clinical features of a connective-tissue disease depend on the organ system affected and the extent of the injury to the tissues. Involvement of the connective tissue of the joints and periarticular tissues is manifested by swelling, pain, and tenderness in the joints. Figure 5–7 compares the cellular structure of a normal joint lining with a diseased one. Connective-tissue diseases that affect the cardiovascular system cause collagen fibers of the heart valves to swell and degenerate (leading to valve injury). The heart muscle

	Probable pathogenesis	Major clinical manifestations
Rheumatic fever	Antistreptococcal antibodies cross-react with antigens in heart muscle, heart valves, and other tissues	Inflammation of heart and joints
Glomerulonephritis	Some cases caused by antibodies formed against glomerular basement membrane; other cases caused by antigen-antibody complexes trapped in glomeruli	Inflammation of renal glomeruli
Rheumatoid arthritis	Antibodies formed against serum gamma globulin	Systemic disease with inflammation and degeneration of joints
Autoimmune blood diseases	Autoantibodies formed against platelets, white cells, or red cells; in some cases, antibody apparently is formed against altered cell antigens, and antibody reacts with both altered and normal cells	Anemia, leukopenia, or thrombocytopenia, depending on nature of antibody
Lupus erythematosus and related collagen diseases	Various antinuclear antibodies cause widespread injury to several organs	Systemic disease with manifestations in several organs
Thyroiditis	Antithyroid antibody causes injury and inflammatory cell infiltration of thyroid gland	Hypothyroidism
Diffuse toxic goiter	Autoantibody mimicking thyroid-stimulating hormone (TSH) causes increased output of thyroid hormone	Hyperthyroidism

TABLE 5–2

Etiology and clinical manifestations of common autoimmune diseases

becomes inflamed, the connective tissue in the myocardium becomes necrotic, and destructive lesions occur in the small and medium-sized blood vessels. Renal manifestations include inflammation and scarring of the glomeruli, damage to the glomerular basement membrane, and consequent leakage of protein and red blood cells into the urine. Severe glomerular damage impairs renal function and may eventually lead to renal insufficiency. Injury to the connective tissues of the lungs, pleura, and pericardium leads to pleural and pericardial pain, sometimes with accumulation of fluid in the serous cavities. Autoantibodies directed against one of more of the formed elements in the blood may cause anemia, owing to destruction of red blood cells (*hemolytic anemia*), reduction in platelets (*thrombocytopenia*), or a decrease in the number of white blood cells (*leukopenia*).

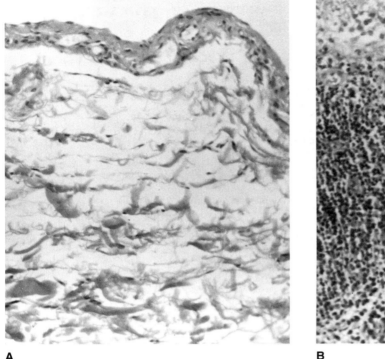
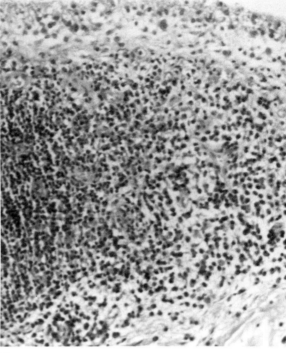

A   B

FIGURE 5–7

Comparison of normal joint lining (**A**) with joint lining in one type of connective-tissue disease (**B**). The lining of the affected joint is heavily infiltrated with lymphocytes and plasma cells, and the joint injury is secondary to the inflammatory reaction. (Original magnification × 100.)

Lupus Erythematosus

One of the more common connective-tissue diseases is called *lupus erythematosus*. This disease is seen most frequently in young women and is characterized by widespread damage to fibrous connective tissue in the skin, articular tissues, heart, serous membranes (pleura and pericardium), and kidneys. Hemolytic anemia, leukopenia, and thrombocytopenia are frequent hematologic manifestations of lupus; these are caused by autoantibodies. Many patients die of renal failure resulting from the severe renal glomerular injury.

A characteristic feature of lupus erythematosus is the presence of antinucleoprotein antibodies in the patient's blood, which can be demonstrated by various methods, as shown in figure 5–8. The original technique consisted of incubating the patient's blood serum with intact white blood cells. The antinucleoprotein antibodies damage many of the leukocytes, causing swelling and loss of structural detail in the cell nuclei. The dam-

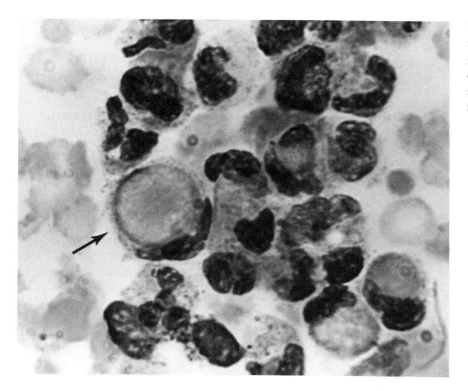

FIGURE 5–8

Positive test for lupus erythematosus. Spherical mass of debris (*arrow*) engulfed by neutrophil. (Original magnification × 1000.)

aged nuclei are converted into large, homogeneous, spherical "blobs" of blue-staining nuclear debris that becomes surrounded and phagocytized by polymorphonuclear leukocytes. The phagocytized spherical mass fills the cytoplasm of the cell and displaces the nucleus to the edge of the cell, resulting in the characteristic appearance called an *LE cell*. This classic method of demonstrating antinucleoprotein antibodies has been superseded by newer and more sensitive techniques, but the method does clearly illustrate the damaging effect of nucleoprotein antibodies on intact cell nuclei.

The pathogenesis of lupus is not well understood. Some investigators have proposed that the disease results from a viral infection or other antigenic stimulation in an individual with a genetically determined abnormal immune response characterized by hyperactive helper T cell function and deficient suppressor T cell function. As a result, the regulatory control of B cell activity is impaired, which leads to excessive stimulation and hyperactivity of B lymphocytes. The intense B cell stimulation may also activate B lymphocytes that have been programmed to respond to self-antigens but are normally suppressed by the immune system. These activated B cells, directed against self-antigens, form injurious autoantibodies that are responsible for the organ damage characteristic of this disease.

Questions for Review

1. What is meant by the following terms: *acquired immunity, cell-mediated immunity, humoral immunity, hypersensitivity?*

2. What is the role of the lymphocyte in acquired immunity? What is the role of the macrophage?

3. How does the physician manipulate the body's immune reaction to allow kidney transplantation?

4. What is meant by the following terms: *B lymphocyte, T lymphocyte, lymphokine?*

5. What are immunoglobulins? What is their basic structure? How do they function?

6. What is meant by the following terms: *light chains, macroglobulin, allergy?*

7. What is an autoantibody? What are some of the postulated mechanisms that result in autoantibody formation? What is the effect of autoantibody directed against the patient's own blood cells?

8. What is a connective-tissue disease? What are its manifestations? What is an LE cell?

9. What are antigen-antibody complexes? How do they cause tissue injury?

10. How can the immune response be suppressed? Why is this sometimes necessary?

Supplementary Readings

Jensen, M. M., and Wright, D. N. 1993. *Introduction to microbiology for the health sciences.* 3d ed. Englewood Cliffs, N.J.: Prentice Hall. Good sections on the immune system.

Nossal, Gustav J. V., et al. 1993. *Life, death, and the immune system. Scientific American* (September Issue). A series of well-written articles on various aspects of the immune system and its functions in health and disease.

Vander, A. J., Sherman, J. H., and Luciano, D. S. 1994.

Human physiology. 6th ed. New York: McGraw-Hill. Good sections on the immune system.

Wallace, D. J., et al. 1981. Systemic lupus erythematosus: Survival patterns. *Journal of the American Medical Association* 245:934–38. A good review of factors influencing prognosis.

Winkelstein, A. 1990. Immune suppression. In *Basic and clinical immunology,* 7th ed. D. P. Stites, A. I. Terr, and T. G. Parslow. Norwalk, Conn.: Appleton & Lange.

Chapter 5 ▪ Outline Summary

Immunity / 90
Characteristics of Immune Response
Depends on lymphocytes and antigen-processing cells.

Specific populations of lymphocytes perform specific functions.

Cells of immune system communicate and produce their effects by secreting cytokines.

Types of Immunity
Autoimmunity
Development of the Lymphatic System
Immature lymphocytes develop immune competence in thymus (T lymphocytes) or bone marrow (B lymphocytes).

Lymphocytes are programmed to develop receptors for the antigens that they will eventually recognize.

T lymphocytes are classified into major groups based on CD antigens on cell membranes.

NK cells lack T or B receptors and can destroy infected or abnormal cells without prior antigenic contact.

Response of Lymphocytes to Foreign Antigens
B lymphocytes can respond to intact antigen and proliferate with T cell help.

T lymphocytes require macrophage-processed antigen in order to respond.

Antigens are presented to responding cells complexed with MHC proteins.

Types of Responding T Cells

Helper T cells: promote immune response.

Suppressor T cells: suppress immune response.

Cytotoxic T cells: attack and destroy infected cells, cancer cells, transplants.

Delayed hypersensitivity cells: attract and activate macrophages, cytotoxic T cells, NK cells.

Memory cells: set aside to respond rapidly if the same antigen is encountered again.

Response of effector T cell is determined by type of MHC protein displayed with processed antigen.

Genetic Control of Ability to Generate Immune Response
The Function of Complement
Antibodies / 96
Structure

Composed of two light and two heavy chains.

Constant part of molecule determines class of antibody.

Variable part of molecule determines specificity.

Five types of immunoglobulins.

IgM: combines with large complex substances.

IgG: principal antibody formed against majority of infectious agents.

IgA: produced by cells in respiratory and gastrointestinal tracts. Combines with antigens to prevent absorption.

IgD: on surface of lymphocytes.

IgE: increased in allergic persons. Attaches to mast cells and basophils.

Hypersensitivity Reactions / 98

Cell-tissue injury resulting from immune response.

Classified on pathogenesis of injury.

Type I. Immediate Hypersensitivity

Localized response: allergy.

Tendency to form IgE antibodies to antigens that do not sensitize most individuals.

IgE attaches to mast cells and basophils.

Subsequent contact with allergen leads to antigen-antibody interaction with release of mediators and allergic manifestations.

Antihistamines block some effects.

Desensitization induces formation of IgA and IgG which combine with allergen before it can interact with IgE.

Systemic response: anaphylaxis.

Generalized mediator release from mast cells and basophils may be life threatening.

Prompt treatment essential.

Type II. Cytotoxic Hypersensitivity

Antibody attaches to cell or tissue antigen.

Complement activated and cell-tissue damage follows.

Type III. Immune Complex Disease

Circulating antigen-antibody complexes deposited in tissues.

Complement activated and cell-tissue injury follows.

Type IV. Delayed Hypersensitivity

Sensitized T lymphocytes secrete cytokines that attract lymphocytes, macrophages, and other inflammatory cells, which produce tissue injury.

Mantoux test based on delayed hypersensitivity response to proteins from tubercle bacillus as indication of previous infection.

Suppression of the Immune Response / 102
Unwanted Effects of Immune Response

Autoimmune disease.

Rejection of transplanted organs.

Rh hemolytic disease in newborn infants (discussed in later chapter).

Methods for Suppressing the Immune Response

Radiation: destroys lymphocytes.

Cytotoxic drugs: suppress growth of lymphocytes.

Adrenal corticosteroids: suppress inflammatory reaction, impair phagocytosis, and inhibit protein synthesis.

Antibodies: prevent body from reacting to corresponding antigen.

Tissue Grafts and Immunity

Graft contains foreign antigens.

Lymphocytes recognize foreign antigen and attempt to eliminate (rejection).

Immune response must be suppressed to prevent rejection of transplant.

Autoimmune Diseases / 104
Pathogenesis

Antibodies formed to altered antigens and react with normal antigens.

Antibodies formed to foreign antigens and cross-react with normal tissue antigens.

Suppressor T lymphocytes abnormal; fail to control immune response.

Treatment

Corticosteroids.

Cytotoxic drugs.

Connective-Tissue (Collagen) Diseases

Clinical Features:

Autoimmune disease characterized by necrosis and degeneration of fibrous connective tissue.

Clinical features depend on organs affected.

Lupus Erythematosus

A connective-tissue disease of young women.

Associated with antinucleoprotein antibodies.

Positive LE test indicates autoantibody damage to leukocyte nuclei that are phagocytosed by neutrophils.

6

Pathogenic Microorganisms

Learning Objectives

1. Explain the characteristics by which bacteria are classified. List and describe the major groups of pathogenic bacteria.

2. Describe the mechanism by which antibiotics inhibit the growth and metabolism of bacteria. Explain the adverse effects of antibiotics.

3. Describe the procedures used in antibiotic sensitivity testing and explain the principles by which the results are interpreted.

4. Explain the mode of action of virus infections and describe how the body's response to viral infection leads to recovery.

5. List the common infections caused by chlamydiae, mycoplasmas, and rickettsiae.

6. Discuss the spectrum of infections caused by fungi. Explain the factors that predispose to systemic infections. Describe the methods used to treat fungus infections.

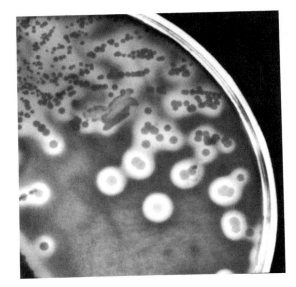

Chapter 6 ■ Contents

The human species coexists with a large number of microorganisms. In most instances, we and our microbiologic associates live in harmony. Of the wide spectrum of organisms found in nature, only a relatively small proportion cause disease in humans. These pathogenic microorganisms are classified into several large groups:

1. Bacteria
2. Viruses
3. Chlamydiae
4. Rickettsiae
5. Mycoplasmas
6. Fungi

In addition, humans serve as host to a number of animal parasites capable of causing illness or disability. The various organisms that are injurious to humans vary in their ability to cause disease. A small number of microbiologic agents are extremely virulent. Others are of very low virulence and are capable of causing disease only when the body's normal defenses have already been weakened by a debilitating illness.

Classification of Bacteria

Bacteria are classified on the basis of four major characteristics:

1. Shape
2. Gram-stain reaction
3. Metabolic and cultural characteristics
4. Antigenic structure

Shape

A bacterium may be spherical (*coccus*) or rod shaped (*bacillus*) or it may have a spiral or corkscrew shape. Cocci may grow in clusters (*staphylococci*), in pairs (*diplococci*), or in chains (*streptococci*).

Gram-Stain Reaction

In the gram-stain method, a dried, fixed suspension of bacteria, prepared on a microscope slide, is stained first with a purple dye and then with an iodine solution. Next, the slide is decolorized with alcohol or another solvent; it is then stained with a red dye. Bacteria that resist decolorization and retain the purple stain are called *gram positive,* whereas those that have been decolorized and accept the red counterstain are termed *gram negative.* By means of the gram-stain method, all organisms may be characterized as either gram positive or gram negative.

Biochemical and Cultural Characteristics

Some bacteria are quite *fastidious* and can be grown only on enriched media under carefully controlled conditions of temperature and acidity (pH). Other

Bacteria

bacteria are hardy and capable of growing on relatively simple culture media under a wide variety of conditions.

Most bacteria grow best in the presence of oxygen (*aerobic* organisms). Some bacteria are able to grow only in the absence of oxygen or under extremely low oxygen tension. These are called *anaerobic* (without oxygen) bacteria. Others grow equally well under either aerobic or anaerobic conditions.

Many bacteria have special structural characteristics. Some bacteria have **flagella:** hairlike processes covering their surface. Flagella give a bacterium its motility; organisms that lack flagella are nonmotile. Some bacteria form **spores:** spherical structures formed within the bacterial cell. Spores can survive under conditions that would kill an actively growing bacterium. They may be considered a dormant, extremely resistant bacterial modification that forms under adverse conditions. Spores can germinate and give rise to actively growing bacteria under favorable conditions.

Most bacteria have distinct biochemical characteristics. Some types of bacteria are capable of fermenting carbohydrates and can bring about many different biochemical reactions under suitable cultural conditions. Each type of bacterium has its own "biochemical profile," which aids in its identification.

Antigenic Structure

Each type of bacterium contains a large number of antigens associated with the cell body, the capsule of the bacterium, and the flagella (in the case of motile organisms). The antigenic structure can be determined by special methods, defining a system of antigens unique for each group of bacteria.

Identification of Bacteria

The methods of classifying bacteria can be applied to the identification of a specific bacterium. Let us assume, for example, that an organism has been isolated from the blood of a patient with a febrile illness. By means of the gram-stain reaction, the organism is identified as a gram-negative bacillus. The cultural characteristics indicate that it is not a fastidious organism and is capable of growing on a wide variety of culture media at various temperatures; moreover, it grows well both in the presence of oxygen and under anaerobic conditions. The organism is motile and does not form spores.

At this point, the number of possible organisms consistent with these characteristics has been reduced to relatively few gram-negative bacteria. The number of possibilities is narrowed still further by various biochemical tests indicating that the bacterium does not ferment lactose but is able to ferment glucose and certain other sugars. These and other biochemical tests support the conclusion that the organism is a type of pathogenic bacterium, called *Salmonella*, found in the gastrointestinal tract and capable of causing a typhoidlike febrile illness. The bacterial antigens within the cell body and flagella of the bacteria can be identified to determine the exact type of Salmonella responsible for the patient's illness.

Once the organism has been identified, the clinician can begin proper treatment and can institute proper isolation and control procedures based on the means by which the disease is transmitted.

Major Classes of Pathogenic Bacteria

This section summarizes important bacteria that infect humans, and the principal diseases that they cause. These major classifications of pathogenic bacteria and their gram-stain reactions are given in table 6–1.

Staphlococci

Staphylococci are normal inhabitants of the skin and the nasal cavity. They are a common cause of boils, other skin infections, and postoperative wound infections. Many cases of toxic shock syndrome in menstruating women associated with tampon use are caused by toxin-producing staphylococci growing in the vagina. The toxin produced by the organism is absorbed from the vagina and causes a skin rash along with a fall in blood pressure and shock.

Occasionally, staphylococci cause serious pulmonary infections and other types of systemic infections. Staphylococcal infections often pose a serious problem in hospitals because the organisms are widely distributed and

Type	Gram-stain reaction	
	Gram positive	Gram negative
Cocci	Staphylococci Streptococci Pneumococci	Gonococci Meningococci

Bacilli	Diphtheria bacillus (aerobic)
	Clostridia (anaerobic)
		Hemophilus
		Gardnerella
		Francisella
		Yersinia
		Brucella
		Legionella
		Salmonella
		Shigella
		Campylobacter
		Cholera bacillus
		Colon bacillus
		  (*Escherichia coli*) and
		  related organisms

Spiral organisms	*Treponema pallidum* *Borrelia burgdorferi*	
Acid-fast organisms	Tubercle bacillus Leprosy bacillus	

TABLE 6–1

Important pathogenic bacteria

many hospitalized patients are unusually susceptible to infection. Many patients have had recent surgical operations; others have various chronic diseases associated with impairment of the body's normal defenses against bacterial infection. Some strains of staphylococci are highly resistant to antibiotics, and infections caused by antibiotic-resistant staphylococci are extremely difficult to treat.

Streptococci

There are many kinds of streptococci, and their pathogenicity varies. These organisms are subdivided into a large number of serologic types on the basis of their antigenic structure. They may also be classified on the basis of the cultural characteristics that they display when grown on a solid medium containing blood. *Alpha hemolytic streptococci* produce green discoloration of the blood immediately around the colony. These organisms are normal inhabitants of the upper respiratory tract and are not normally pathogenic. *Beta hemolytic streptococci* produce a narrow zone of complete hemolysis of blood around the growing colony (figure 6–1). Beta hemolytic strepto-

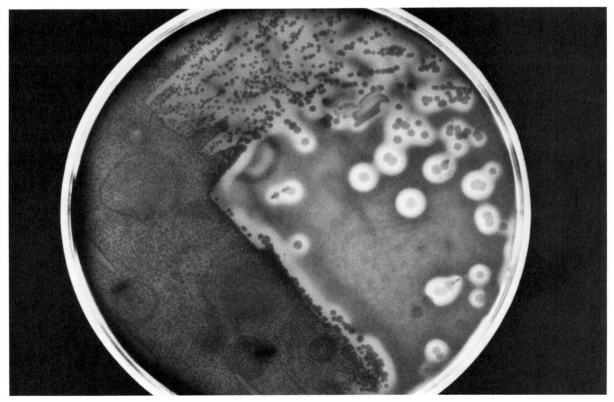

FIGURE 6–1

Bacteriologic culture plate containing colonies of beta hemolytic streptococci. Hemolysis of blood in culture medium causes clear zones around bacterial colonies.

cocci (or, simply, beta streptococci) are further subdivided into eighteen groups designated A through R on the basis of carbohydrate antigens in the streptococcal cell wall. One of the most important members of the beta streptococcal groups is the *group A beta streptococcus.* Many group A beta streptococci are extremely pathogenic, causing streptococcal sore throat, scarlet fever, serious skin infections, and infections of the uterus after childbirth. Some produce a toxin that causes a toxic shock syndrome similar to that caused by toxin-producing staphylococci. One particularly virulent toxin-producing group A beta streptococcal strain causes a rapidly progressive, destructive infection of the subcutaneous tissues and the fibrous tissue (fascia) covering the adjacent muscles. This condition, called *necrotizing fasciitis,* may be complicated by necrosis (gangrene) of the overlying skin and by necrosis of the muscles in the infected area (streptococcal myositis). These organisms cause such rapid and extensive tissue destruction that they have been called "flesh eating bacteria."

In addition to causing infections in various tissues, some strains of group A beta streptococci are capable of inducing a state of hypersensitivity in susceptible individuals, leading to development of rheumatic fever or a type of kidney disease called *glomerulonephritis.* These diseases are considered in greater detail in the sections on the circulatory system (chapter 13) and kidneys (chapter 19). Fortunately, group A beta streptococci still remain quite sensitive to penicillin and other antibiotics.

Other groups of streptococci also are of medical importance. Group B beta streptococci frequently inhabit the genital tracts of pregnant women and may infect newborn infants during delivery. *Gamma streptococci* cause no changes in the blood medium surrounding the bacterial colony; thus, they are often referred to as *nonhemolytic streptococci.* In general, these organisms are nonpathogenic.

Closely related to the streptococci but classified separately are organisms that inhabit the intestinal tract called *enterococci* (*enetron* = bowel). These organisms are often very resistant to multiple antibiotics. Consequently, an enterococcal wound or urinary tract infection may be very difficult to treat.

Pneumococci

Pneumococci are gram-positive cocci that grow in pairs and short chains and have certain biochemical characteristics setting them apart from streptococci. Pneumococci are a common cause of bacterial pneumonia.

Gram-Negative Cocci

Most gram-negative cocci are nonpathogenic members of the genus *Neisseria* and are normal inhabitants of the upper respiratory passages. This group has two pathogenic members. The meningococcus (*Neisseria meningiditis*) causes a type of meningitis (inflammation of the membranes surrounding the brain and spinal cord) that frequently occurs in epidemics. The gonococcus (*Neisseria gonorrhoeae*) causes gonorrhea. This disease is transmitted by sexual contact and is discussed in greater detail in chapter 8.

Gram-Positive Bacilli

Aerobic Non-Spore-Forming Gram-Positive Bacilli Members of this group are called **corynebacteria.** Most are nonpathogenic inhabitants of the upper respiratory passages. However, one member of the group (*Corynebacterium diphtheriae*) causes diphtheria. This organism causes an acute ulcerative inflammation of the throat and produces a potent toxin that can injure heart muscle and nerve tissue.

Anaerobic Spore-Forming Gram-Positive Bacilli Anaerobic spore-forming bacilli are called **clostridia.** These are normal inhabitants of the intestinal tract of humans and animals and are also found in the soil. Members of this group produce potent toxins and cause several important diseases. Some clostridia cause gas gangrene, some cause tetanus (lockjaw), and others cause botulism.

Gas gangrene develops in dirty wounds contaminated with certain species of clostridia. These anaerobic organisms grow in dead or devitalized tissue, especially in wounds where considerable necrosis of muscle has taken place. The clostridia produce large amounts of gas by fermenting the necrotic tissues, and they also release powerful toxins with widespread systemic effects.

One species of clostridia produces a potent toxin that causes spasm of voluntary muscles. The common term "lockjaw" comes from the marked rigidity of the jaw muscles that is a common feature of this disease. Tetanus may be fatal because of respiratory failure resulting from spasm of the muscles concerned with respiration.

The *Clostridium botulinum* produces a potent neuroparalytic toxin. **Botulism** can generally be traced to eating improperly processed or canned foods in which the organism has grown and produced toxin. Botulism is actually a poisoning caused by the ingestion of toxin in food rather than a bacterial infection. Although botulism was more common when home canning was prevalent, outbreaks of botulism have been traced to contamination of canned tuna fish and canned soup prepared in commercial canneries.

Gram-Negative Bacteria

There are many gram-negative organisms of clinical importance. Several different groups of small fastidious organisms cause important diseases in humans. These are named *Hemophilus, Francisella, Yersinia, Brucella,* and *Legionella.* Members of the genus *Hemophilus* are normal inhabitants of the respiratory tract. One member of this group, *Hemophilus influenzae,* sometimes causes meningitis in infants and young children. Occasionally, it produces respiratory infections in patients with chronic lung disease. Another closely related organism was previously classified as *Hemophilus* but has recently been renamed *Gardnerella.* In conjunction with other bacteria, this organism causes a common vaginal infection called *nonspecific vaginitis* (described in chapter 17). One member of the genus *Yersinia* is responsible for bubonic plague. A member of the genus *Francisella* produces a somewhat similar illness called *tularemia.* Members of the genus *Brucella* cause disease in animals that can be transmitted to human beings. Undulant fever, a febrile illness, is contracted by drinking unpasteurized milk obtained from infected animals. *Legionella* is a recently recognized organism that causes a serious respiratory illness called *Legionnaire's disease.*

Other gram-negative organisms of medical importance include a number of closely related organisms that live in the gastrointestinal tract of people and animals. Other members of this group are free-living organisms, widely distributed in nature. Important pathogenic members of the group include *Salmonella, Shigella, Campylobacter,* and the cholera bacillus (*Vibrio cholerae*). These organisms cause various types of febrile illness and gastroenteritis. The organisms are excreted from the gastrointestinal tract in the feces of infected patients and are transmitted by contaminated food or water.

An organism closely related to *Campylobacter* but recently designated *Helicobacter* is of medical importance because it appears to cause chronic inflammation of the stomach lining (chronic gastritis) and stomach ulcers. This organism is considered in connection with the gastrointestinal tract (chapter 23).

Other members of this large group are of only limited pathogenicity but sometimes produce disease when they are outside their normal habitat in the gastrointestinal tract. These organisms may cause wound infections, urinary tract infections, and pulmonary infections in susceptible individuals. The best known enteric bacterium is the colon bacillus (*Escherichia coli*), which is the predominant organism found within the intestinal tract of humans and animals. Some strains of the colon bacillus can produce various toxins that can cause intestinal symptoms ranging from a cholera-like diarrhea to a dysentery-like acute inflammation of the intestinal tract. One well-known pathogenic strain is designated *E.coli 0157:H7,* the numbers referring to the antigens contained in the bacterial cell and its flagellae. This organism's toxin causes an acute inflammation of the colon characterized by bloody diarrhea and abdominal pain. Sometimes there is also an associated destruction of the patient's red blood cells, with marked anemia and impaired renal function with renal failure, called the *hemolytic uremic syndrome.* This pathogenic organism is present in the intestinal tract of infected cattle, and people usually become infected by consuming contaminated, incompletely cooked beef or by drinking raw milk. A recent outbreak of more than five hundred cases, traced to a "fast food" restaurant chain, was caused by consumption of improperly cooked hamburgers prepared from beef contaminated with the organism.

Spiral Organisms

The spiral organisms can cause a wide variety of illnesses. The best-known member of this group is *Treponema pallidum,* which causes syphilis—one of the sexually transmitted diseases. These diseases are considered in chapter 8. Another spiral organism in this group is *Borrelia burgdorferi* which causes *Lyme disease.* Named after a town in Connecticut where the disease was first recognized, it is now widespread in North America, Europe, and Australia. Transmission to humans is by the bite of an infected tick (*Ixodes dammini* and other *Ixodes* species). Most infections occur in the summer when exposure to ticks is frequent. Untreated Lyme disease typically progresses through three stages. In the first stage, a roughly circular, localized skin rash appears at the site of the tick bite and is frequently associated with flulike symptoms of fever, chills, and headaches, along with muscular and joint aches and pain. The rash and other manifestations eventually subside, but, weeks or months later, many patients develop various neurologic, cardiac, and joint manifestations, which characterize the second stage of the disease. The third stage, which eventually develops in some untreated patients, is characterized by chronic arthritis and various neurologic problems. Diagnosis is made by means of various serologic tests, and treatment is by means of appropriate antibiotics.

Acid-Fast Bacteria

Acid-fast bacteria have a waxy capsule, which is stained with difficulty by means of certain red dyes. Once the organism has been stained, the stain-impregnated capsule resists decolorization with various acid solvents. This property, attributable to the capsule, is the reason for the term *acid-fast,* used to refer to this type of organism. Acid-fast bacteria cause a special type of chronic inflammatory reaction, called a *chronic granulomatous inflammation,* rather than the polymorphonuclear inflammatory reaction usually seen with bacterial infections.

The best-known acid-fast bacterium is the tubercle bacillus (*Mycobacterium tuberculosis*) responsible for tuberculosis. Mycobacteria, other than the tubercle bacillus, may at times cause a tuberculosis-like disease affecting lungs, lymph nodes, or skin, and some may cause severe systemic infections in immunocompromised persons. (Disseminated infection caused by *Mycobacterium avium intracellulare* in persons with the acquired immune deficiency syndrome is described in chapter 8.) Another acid-fast bacterium (*Mycobacterium leprae*) causes leprosy.

Antibiotic Treatment of Bacterial Infections

The discovery of antibiotic compounds and their widespread use in the treatment of various types of infections has been one of the great advances in medicine. Antibiotics are substances that destroy bacteria or inhibit their growth. They are useful clinically because of their ability to injure bacterial cells without producing significant injury to the patient.

The bacterial cell is a complex structure containing genetic material, a protein-synthesizing mechanism, numerous enzyme systems concerned with intracellular metabolic functions, a semipermeable cell membrane, and a rigid cell wall. The bacterial genetic material is arranged as a circular DNA molecule that is attached to the cell membrane. Some bacteria also contain smaller circular DNA molecules, called *plasmids,* that contain genes coding for various properties useful to bacteria but often harmful to the persons infected by the bacteria. Such properties include resistance to antibiotics, toxin production, and formation of soluble factors that inhibit growth of normal bacterial flora; so the plasmid-bearing bacterium has a growth advantage

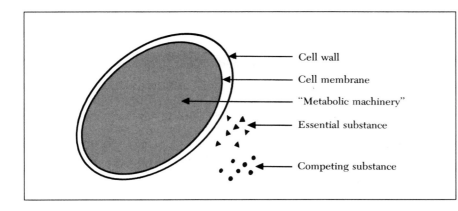

FIGURE 6–2

Various sites of action of antibiotics. Antibiotics may act by disrupting the bacterial cell wall, by disturbing the functions of the cell membrane, or by interfering with the intracellular "metabolic machinery." Some antimicrobial drugs are not directly injurious to the bacterial cell but compete with essential substances required for bacterial growth and multiplication.

over the bacterial flora with which it must compete. Antimicrobial substances act by interfering with the structure or function of the bacterial cell in one or more of the following ways (figure 6–2):

1. Inhibition of cell-wall synthesis
2. Inhibition of cell-membrane function
3. Inhibition of metabolic functions
4. Competitive inhibition

Inhibition of Cell-Wall Synthesis
The bacterial cell has a high internal osmotic pressure, and the rigid outer cell wall maintains the shape of the bacterium. In some respects, the function of the cell wall can be compared to a corset or girdle supporting the enclosed cell. Penicillin and several other antibiotics act by inhibiting the synthesis of the bacterial cell wall so that the cell body is exposed. Because of the high osmotic pressure inside the bacterium, the relatively unsupported cell swells and eventually ruptures.

Inhibition of Cell-Membrane Function
The cell membrane is a semipermeable membrane surrounding the bacterial protoplasm. It controls the internal composition of the cell by regulating the diffusion of materials into and out of the cell. Some antibiotics act by inhibiting various functions of the cell membrane. Loss of the selective permeability of the cell membrane leads to cell injury and death.

Inhibition of Metabolic Functions
Some antibiotics interfere with nucleic acid or protein synthesis by bacteria so that the organisms are unable to carry out essential metabolic functions.

Competitive Inhibition
Some antibiotics resemble important compounds required by bacteria for growth and multiplication. The bacteria are unable to distinguish between

the essential compound and the antibiotic that resembles it, but the antibiotic cannot be substituted for the required compound in the metabolic process. When the bacteria use the "wrong" compound rather than the "correct" substance, bacterial metabolism is disrupted, leading to inhibition of bacterial growth.

Antibiotic Sensitivity Tests

In selecting antibiotics to treat a bacterial infection, the practitioner is aided by laboratory tests called *antibiotic sensitivity tests.* These tests measure, under standardized conditions, the ability of the antibiotic to inhibit the growth of the organism isolated from the patient. One method, called a *tube dilution sensitivity test,* consists of preparing various dilutions of antibiotics in test tubes and inoculating the tubes with the organism to be tested. The tubes are then incubated for a period of time in order to permit growth of the organism. Finally, determination of the highest dilution of antibiotic that inhibits the growth of the organism indicates the sensitivity of the organism to the drug.

Another method of sensitivity testing consists of inoculating the organism on a bacteriologic plate containing a culture medium. One then places several filter-paper disks on the plate, each containing a standardized concentration of a different antibiotic. Next, the plate is incubated to allow the organism to grow. During incubation, the antibiotics in the disks diffuse into the surrounding culture. If the antibiotic is capable of inhibiting the organism, the organism is unable to grow in the area around the disk, and a circular clear zone free of bacterial growth appears (figure 6–3). The organism is said to be *sensitive* to the antibiotic. On the other hand, if the growth of the organism is not influenced by the antibiotic, growth will not be inhibited around the disk, and the organism is said to be *resistant* to the antibiotic. The diameter of the zones of inhibition around the disks is a further indication of the sensitivity of the organism.

A bacteriology laboratory report that the organism is sensitive to a given antibiotic means that the organism probably can be inhibited by giving the patient the usual therapeutic dose of that drug. A report that the organism is resistant to an antibiotic indicates a therapeutic dose of antibiotic is unlikely to inhibit the growth of the organism.

It should be emphasized, however, that the sensitivity of an organism to an antibiotic is only one factor influencing a patient's response to an infection. Other factors include the patient's own resistance and the antibiotic's ability to diffuse in sufficient quantities into the site of the infection.

Adverse Effects of Antibiotics

Toxicity

Antibiotics are useful because they are much more toxic to bacteria than they are to the patient. Antibiotics vary in their effects on people, but all are toxic to some degree. Some injure the kidneys; others injure nerve tissue or the blood-forming tissues. Penicillin and other antibiotics that act by interfering

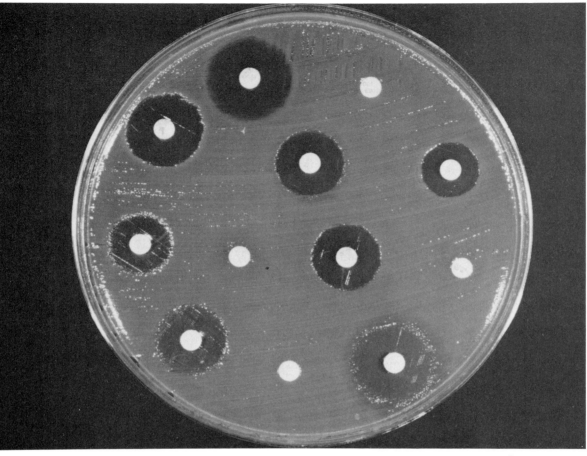

A

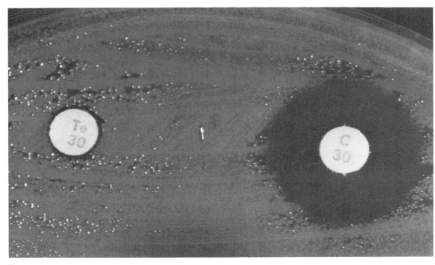

B

FIGURE 6–3

A, Sensitivity test, illustrating antibiotic-impregnated filter-paper disks on surface of culture plate. Clear zones around disks indicate that antibiotic in disk has inhibited growth. **B,** Closer view of two disks on plate. Antibiotic contained in disk on *left* fails to inhibit growth of organism, which is said to be **resistant** to the antibiotic. Clear zone surrounding disk on *right* indicates that the antibiotic in disk inhibits growth of the organism, which is **sensitive** to the antibiotic.

with bacterial cell-wall synthesis are relatively nontoxic, probably because the body cells have no structure comparable to the bacterial cell wall. Some antibiotics that interfere with bacterial metabolic functions can at times produce similar derangements in the patient's own metabolic functions. For example, tetracycline is a relatively nontoxic antibiotic, excreted chiefly by the kidneys. If renal function is impaired, very high blood levels of antibiotic may develop after administration of the usual therapeutic doses of the drug; this may cause severe and often fatal impairment of the patient's own cellular metabolic functions.

Hypersensitivity

Some antibiotics induce a marked hypersensitivity that can lead to a fatal reaction if the drug is later administered to a sensitized patient. Penicillin is capable of inducing extremely severe anaphylactic reactions, although the antibiotic itself has a very low toxicity.

Alteration of Normal Bacterial Flora

The normal bacterial flora in the oral cavity, the colon, and other locations may be altered by antibiotics. If the normal bacteria are destroyed, there may be overgrowth of resistant bacteria and fungi previously controlled by the normal flora. These resistant organisms may cause infections in susceptible patients.

Development of Resistant Strains of Bacteria

Some bacteria that are initially sensitive to antibiotics eventually become resistant. There are two ways in which an organism becomes resistant. It may undergo a spontaneous mutation that conveys resistance or it may acquire a plasmid that contains resistance genes from another bacterium.

Spontaneous mutations do not occur frequently in cell division, but many bacteria divide so rapidly that spontaneous mutations can present a problem if the rapidly dividing bacteria are not quickly eliminated by the antibiotic. Once a mutation that conveys antibiotic resistance occurs, the mutant organism has an advantage over its antibiotic-sensitive counterpart, because it can flourish in the presence of the antibiotic while the antibiotic-sensitive organisms are eliminated.

Plasmid-acquired resistance can be a major problem because the transferred plasmid may convey resistance to multiple antibiotics, and plasmid transfers can take place between bacteria of different types. In this process, a bacterium with antibiotic-resistance genes carried on one of its plasmids (the donor) extends a thin cytoplasmic tube to contact another bacterium (the recipient), "reels in" the bacterium it has contacted, and passes a copy of its plasmid to the recipient bacterium. Now both bacteria possess antibiotic-resistance plasmids, which they in turn can pass to other bacteria.

There are a number of mechanisms by which resistant bacteria can circumvent an antibiotic's effect. Such mechanisms include: (1) developing enzymes to destroy the antibiotic; (2) either changing their cell-wall structure so that the antibiotic is unable to get into the cell or developing mechanisms to expel the antibiotic as soon as it enters the cell and before it can disturb bacterial functions; (3) changing their intracellular "metabolic machinery" so that the antibiotic is no longer able to disturb bacterial functions.

A few examples serve to illustrate the ingeneous adaptations of bacteria that thwart our efforts to eliminate them. A bacterium that is penicillin sensitive may develop an enzyme, penicillinase, that inactivates the antibiotic and allows the bacterium to survive in the presence of the drug. The bacterium may develop an alternative metabolic pathway for carrying out an essential function that has been blocked by an antibiotic. For example, if an antibiotic blocks a single step in a complex metabolic pathway, the bacterium may develop a pathway that detours around the site of the block, allowing the metabolic process to continue by the alternative route (figure 6–4). An antibiotic that acts against an enzyme required for a bacterial function, such as constructing a cell wall, may be rendered ineffective if the bacterium slightly alters the structure of its enzyme so that the antibiotic can no longer bind to the enzyme and inactivate it. An antibiotic that attaches to bacterial ribosomes, preventing protein synthesis, may be rendered ineffective if the bacterium slightly changes the structure of the ribosome so that the antibiotic can no longer act against it.

Widespread use of an antibiotic predisposes to the development of resistant strains. This may complicate the treatment of patients who become infected with antibiotic-resistant organisms. Staphylococci, in particular, have raised this problem, because many strains isolated from hospital patients have been found to be highly resistant to a large number of antibiotics. Treatment of gonorrhea also has been complicated by the development of a high degree of penicillin resistance in many strains of gonococci; so prolonged courses of therapy and much larger doses of antibiotic are required to eradicate the infections. Even the pneumococcus is no longer uniformly sensitive to penicillin, as it was in the past. Some strains are resistant to penicillin and other drugs normally used against them. Resistant strains of tubercle bacilli also have developed, hindering treatment of tuberculosis with antituberculosis drugs. On the other hand, some bacteria still remain quite sensitive to antibiotics. For example, group A beta streptococci remain sensitive to penicillin, despite widespread use of penicillin to treat streptococcal infections. *Treponema pallidum,* the organism responsible for syphilis, also has remained quite sensitive to penicillin, even though the drug has been used to treat syphilis for many years.

FIGURE 6–4

One mechanism by which bacteria become resistant to antibiotics. **A,** A bacterium carries out essential metabolic functions by means of a series of biochemical reactions. In this example, the intermediate step B→C can proceed by two alternative routes, but normally the "direct" route is favored. **B,** If the "direct" route is blocked by the action of an antibiotic, the alternative metabolic pathway is utilized. Eventually the bacterium is able to resume its metabolic processes by "detouring around" the site of the block.

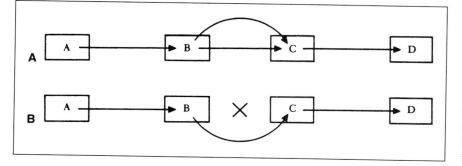

Viruses

Viruses are the smallest infectious agents. A typical virus consists of a molecule of nucleic acid (either DNA or RNA), its *genome,* enclosed within a protein shell called a **capsid.** The capsid is made of subunits called **capsomeres,** which are arranged in a precise geometric fashion around the genome. Many viruses are also covered by an outer lipid envelope acquired from the cytoplasm of the host cell when the virus buds from the cell that it has infected. Projections from the surface of the virus allow the virus to attach to the cell that it will infect. Viruses vary greatly in size. The smallest are only slightly larger than protein molecules, whereas the largest viruses approach the size of a bacterium.

The nucleic acid of the virus genome may be arranged in either a single or a double strand, and the complexity of the viral genome varies. Some viruses have as many as four hundred genes within their nucleic acid structure, whereas others have as few as eight. Viruses have few metabolic enzymes and therefore must rely on the cells of the infected person to carry out their activities. When a virus invades the cell, the viral genome directs the metabolic processes of the cell to synthesize more virus particles. In many respects, the virus may be likened to a criminal who takes over a business, forcing it to function for the criminal's benefit rather than for the benefit of the owner (figure 6–5).

Classification of Viruses

An older classification of viruses was based on the major clinical features of the viral infection, and viruses were classified on the basis of the portion of the body or organ system in which the viral infection produced the most prominent clinical manifestations. A more modern classification categorizes viruses on the basis of their nucleic acid structure, size, structural configuration, and biologic characteristics. In this classification, several large groups of viruses are recognized, and a large number of viruses are identified in each group. Table 6–2 presents a simplified classification of viruses and the diseases they cause.

Mode of Action

A distinction is sometimes made between a viral infection and a viral disease. A condition in which a virus infects a cell without causing any evidence of cell injury is considered a *latent viral infection.* Many viruses are capable of coexisting with normal cells in lymphoid tissue and the gastrointestinal tract, and probably in other sites, without causing cellular injury. Such viruses are able to live for long periods within the cells of the infected host while they continually discharge virus particles. Other viruses are more virulent and regularly produce cell injury, manifested by necrosis and degeneration of the infected cell. This is called a *cytopathogenic* effect. Some cytopathogenic effects are shown in figures 6–6, 6–7, and 6–8. Some viruses induce cell hyperplasia and proliferation rather than cell necrosis. These effects are

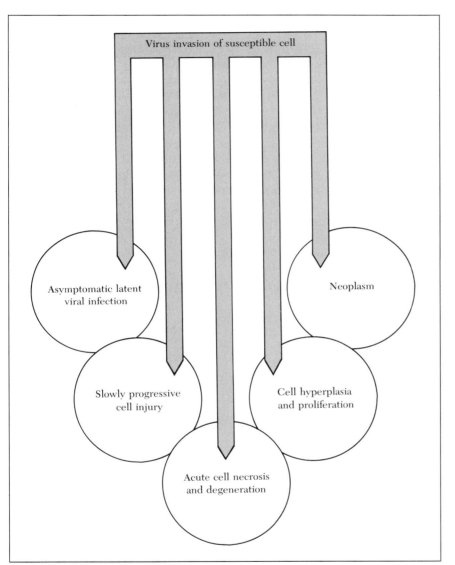

FIGURE 6–5

Summary of possible effects of a virus infection on susceptible cells.

shown in figures 6–9 and 6–10. Many viruses induce various combinations of cell damage and cell hyperplasia.

Under certain circumstances, a latent asymptomatic viral infection may become activated, leading to actual disease. The herpes virus, which infects both the oral cavity and the genital tract, may persist in the tissues of the host for many years. The virus periodically becomes activated and causes crops of painful vesicles that may recur during an intercurrent febrile illness, when the patient's immunologic defenses have been disrupted by a neoplasm or by various other diseases, or sometimes for no apparent reason (figure 6–11).

		Virus	Disease
TABLE 6–2			
Common viruses infecting humans	DNA viruses	Adenoviruses	Respiratory infections
		Hepatitis B virus	Hepatitis B
		Herpes viruses	
		Herpes simplex type I	"Cold sores"
		Herpes simplex type II	Genital herpes
		Epstein-Barr virus	Infectious mononucleosis
		Varicella-zoster virus	Chicken pox, herpes zoster (shingles)
		Cytomegalovirus	Mononucleosis-like illness, hepatitis
		Papilloma virus	Warts, condylomas (benign tumors)
	RNA viruses	Arboviruses	Encephalitis
		Hantavirus (bunyavirus)	Acute respiratory illness
		Hepatitis viruses	
		Hepatitis A virus (picornavirus)	Hepatitis
		Hepatitis C virus (flavivirus)	Hepatitis
		Hepatitis E virus (calicivirus)	Hepatitis
		Myxoviruses	
		Influenza viruses	Influenza
		Parainfluenza viruses	Respiratory infections, croup
		Respiratory syncytial viruses	Respiratory infections
		Measles virus	Measles
		Mumps virus	Mumps
		Picornaviruses	
		Coxsackie viruses	Pharyngitis, myocarditis, pericarditis
		Echoviruses	Respiratory infections, gastroenteritis
		Hepatitis A virus	Hepatitis A
		Polioviruses	Poliomyelitis
		Rhinoviruses	Respiratory infections
		Rabies virus (Rhabdovirus)	Rabies
		Retroviruses	
		HIV virus	AIDS
		HTLV I virus	Adult T cell leukemia
		Rubella virus (Togavirus)	German measles

	Virus	Disease
Incomplete defective and unclassified viruses	Hepatitis D virus (lacks virus coat)	Hepatitis

TABLE 6–2

Continued

Unusual Manifestations of Viral Infection

Some viruses cause tumors in animals, and a few unusual tumors in humans also are caused by viruses. Other viruses produce very slow, progressive diseases that may require many years to develop. These are termed *slow virus infections*. Certain types of neurologic diseases in animals are caused by slow virus infections, and slow virus infections of the nervous system also occur in humans (discussed in chapter 26).

Inclusion Bodies in Viral Disease

Tissues that are infected with virus frequently contain spherical, densely staining structures called **inclusion bodies** (figure 6–12). These are present within the nucleus or the cytoplasm or both locations. Inclusion bodies consist of masses of virus or products of virus multiplication. The presence of inclusion bodies may be of considerable diagnostic aid in recognizing viral infection and determining the type of viral disease present.

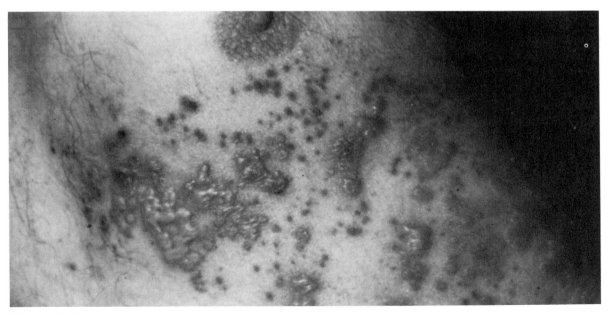

FIGURE 6–6

One type of herpes virus infection (called *herpes zoster* or *shingles*) characterized by clusters of several vesicles that tend to follow the course of a superficial nerve.

FIGURE 6–7

Face of young woman with German measles, illustrating skin rash.

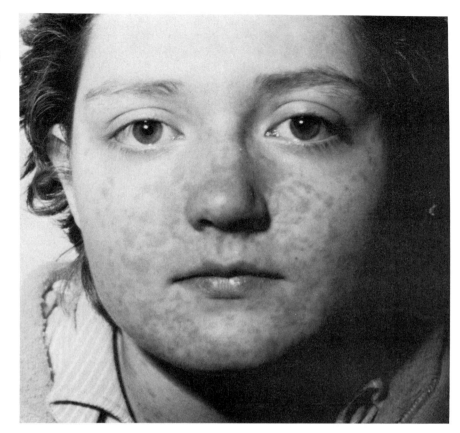

Bodily Defenses Against Viral Infections

The body responds to a viral infection by forming a protein substance called **interferon** and by activating *humoral* and *cell-mediated defense mechanisms.*

Formation of Interferon

Interferon is a general term for a group of carbohydrate-containing proteins produced by cells in response to viral infection and was named from its ability to "interfere" with viral multiplication. Interferon functions as a nonspecific, "broad spectrum" antiviral agent. It inhibits not only the virus that induced its formation, but other viruses as well. This is in contrast with the behavior of a specific antiviral antibody, which reacts only to the virus that induced its formation. Many cells are capable of producing interferon, but monocytes and lymphocytes are the primary sources. Interferon provides a rapid "first line" defense against a viral infection. By slowing viral growth during the early phase of the infection, it allows the infected person time to mobilize humoral and cell-mediated responses directed against the invading virus.

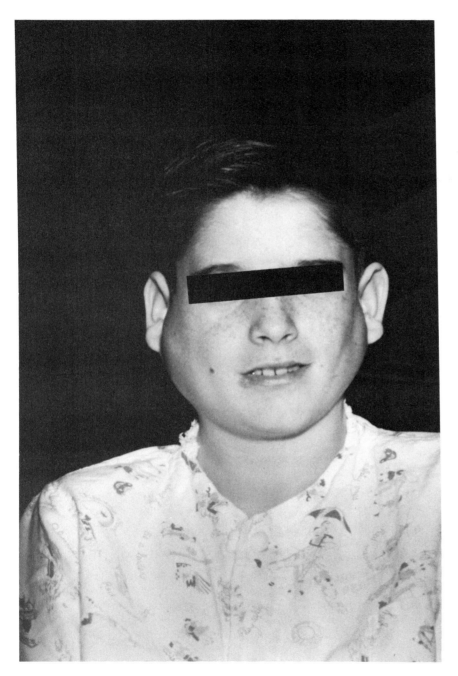

FIGURE 6–8

Noticeable swelling of both parotid glands caused by the mumps virus.

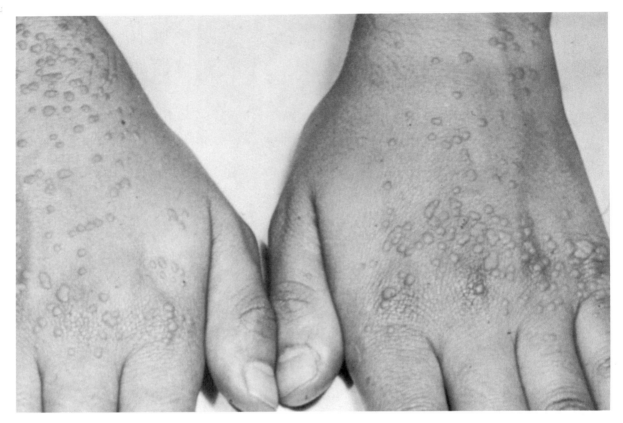

FIGURE 6–9

Multiple warts on skin of hands.

FIGURE 6–10

Multiple papillary lesions called **condylomas** (*arrows*) surrounding anus, caused by a virus. Condylomas also frequently develop around the vulva and on the penis.

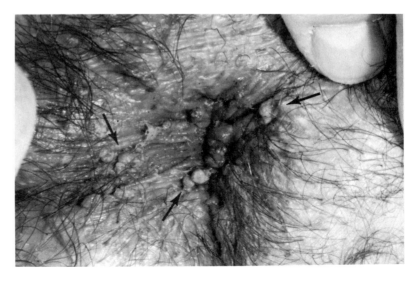

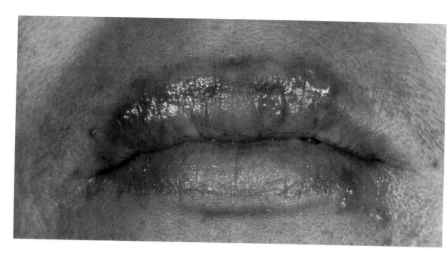

A

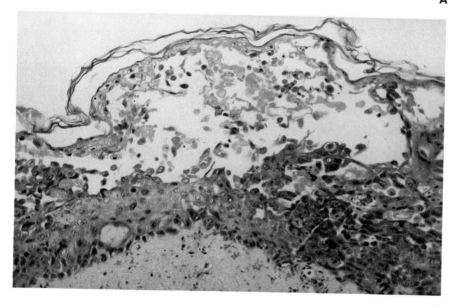

B

FIGURE 6–11

Herpes virus infection. **A,** Recurrent oral herpes caused by herpes virus type I. **B,** Section of small herpes blister (vesicle) caused by virus. The superficial skin layer is almost completely destroyed, and a superficial ulcer will form when the surface epithelium sloughs. (Original magnification × 100.)

In addition to its antiviral activity, interferon has other actions concerned with regulation of the immune system and cell growth. These functions will be considered in chapter 10.

Humoral and Cell-Mediated Immunity in Viral Infections

The body also forms specific antiviral antibodies that are capable of inactivating viruses and may actually destroy virus particles in the presence of complement. Antiviral antibodies cannot combine with the virus, however, unless the virus particles are discharged into the extracellular fluid where

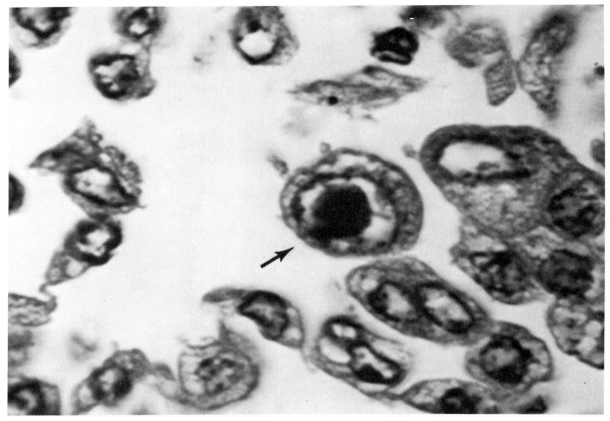

FIGURE 6–12

Intranuclear inclusion body (*arrow*) in lung, characteristic of viral infection. (Original magnification × 1000.)

they are exposed to the action of the antibody. Consequently, antiviral antibodies are relatively inefficient in combating viruses that spread directly from cell to cell, because the virus particles remain within the infected cells and are protected from the antibody. For example, persons who have recurrent fever blisters caused by the herpes virus possess antibodies to the virus, but the antibody is often unable to eradicate the intracellular virus particles.

In addition to producing specific antiviral antibodies, the immune defenses of the host are directed against the virus-infected cells. This occurs because viruses that invade cells often induce the formation of new antigens on the surface of the infected cells. These antigens are recognized as foreign by the host's immune defenses and induce both humoral and cell-mediated immune reactions directed against the virus-infected cells. Antibodies are formed that affix to the infected cells and destroy them in the presence of complement. Sensitized lymphocytes release lymphokines, which damage the cells, and they also produce interferon, which inhibits the multiplication of viruses. Chemical mediators that induce an acute inflammatory reaction also are liberated (see chapter 4). In many viral infections, much of the tissue injury is caused, not by proliferation of the virus within the cells of the host, but to the inflammation and tissue destruction caused by the body's attempts to rid itself of the virus-infected cells.

Treatment with Antiviral Agents

Because viruses are simple structures lacking a cell wall, a cell membrane, and the complex "metabolic machinery" of bacteria, they are not susceptible to the disruptive actions of antibiotics. Some chemotherapeutic agents that are active against viruses have been developed, however. In many cases, their mechanisms of action are similar to those of compounds used to treat cancer (described in chapter 10). Some antiviral agents active against DNA viruses either block synthesis of DNA or induce the formation of an abnormal, nonfunctional DNA, thereby preventing virus multiplication. Another agent active against RNA viruses causes the formation of an abnormal messenger RNA that disrupts viral multiplication. Unfortunately, many compounds that block viral multiplication by such mechanisms also have a similar adverse effect on the host cells and may be as toxic to the host as to the virus. For this reason, antiviral agents have had limited application in clinical medicine.

Newer antiviral agents are being developed, however, that are less toxic and promise to be more useful. One such drug is effective against some infections caused by the herpes group of viruses. The drug is activated within the virus-infected cells by a viral enzyme to yield the active antiviral compound that selectively inhibits synthesis of viral DNA within the cells in which the virus is replicating. It does not interfere with the synthesis of host DNA, and this accounts for its low toxicity. One concern, however, is that extensive use of such antiviral agents may promote the development of resistant strains of virus, in the same way that resistant strains of bacteria have appeared following widespread antibiotic usage.

Interferon is the newest of the antiviral agents being used to treat patients. Large-scale commercial production of interferon has been made possible by advances in recombinant DNA technology, and many clinical studies are underway to evaluate the usefulness of interferon in various virus infections.

Chlamydiae

The chlamydiae are very small, gram-negative, nonmotile bacteria that were once thought to be large viruses. They are deficient in certain enzymes, and so they can live only as parasites inside the cells of the individual that they infect. They are taken into the cells of the host by phagocytosis. Once inside the cell, they divide to form large intracytoplasmic clusters of organisms called **inclusion bodies.** These resemble inclusion bodies formed in some viral diseases. Their growth can be inhibited by various antibiotics that inhibit protein synthesis, such as tetracycline and erythromycin. Some strains of chlamydiae are also inhibited by sulfonamide drugs.

Chlamydiae cause several different types of diseases. The most common chlamydial disease affects the genital tract and is transmitted by sexual contact. In the male, it causes an inflammation of the urethra called *nongonococcal urethritis*. In the female, it causes an inflammation of the uterine cervix that may spread to the fallopian tubes and ovaries as well. If a mother has a chlamydial infection of the cervix, infected secretions may get into her infant's eyes during childbirth and cause an inflammation called *inclusion conjunctivitis*. The name is based on the fact that characteristic inclusions can be demonstrated in the infected cells of the infant's conjunctiva. Other chlamydiae cause pulmonary infections. One species causes a disease of birds called *psitticosis,* which is transmissible to humans and is manifested clinically as a type of pneumonia. Another species of chlamydiae causes an uncommon sexually transmissible disease called *lymphogranuloma venereum*. This disease is characterized by marked enlargement and inflammation of the lymph nodes in the groin and around the rectum.

Rickettsiae

Rickettsiae are very small intracellular parasites. Although they are usually discussed along with the viruses, they are much more closely related to bacteria. They are parasites of insects and are transmitted to humans by insect bites. The organisms multiply in the endothelial cells of small blood vessels, which become swollen and necrotic, leading to thrombosis, rupture, and necrosis. Clinically, a rickettsial infection usually causes a febrile illness, often associated with a skin rash. Typhus and Rocky Mountain spotted fever are the most common rickettsial diseases. These organisms are sensitive to some antibiotics (tetracyclines and chloramphenicol).

Mycoplasmas

The mycoplasmas are very small bacteria that are very fragile because they lack a cell wall. One member of this group causes a type of pneumonia called *primary atypical pneumonia*. Mycoplasmas respond to the antibiotics tetracycline and erythromycin.

Fungi

Fungi are plantlike organisms without chlorophyll and are subdivided into two large groups: yeasts and molds. Yeasts are small ovoid or spherical cells that reproduce by budding. Molds, when grown on suitable media at room temperature, form large colonies composed of multiple branching filamentous structures called **hyphae** (singular, *hypha*) (figure 6–13). The matted mass of hyphae, which is called a **mycelium,** is responsible for the characteristic appearance of the colony (figure 6–14). Some pathogenic fungi exhibit two different growth phases, forming typical mycelial colonies on laboratory cul-

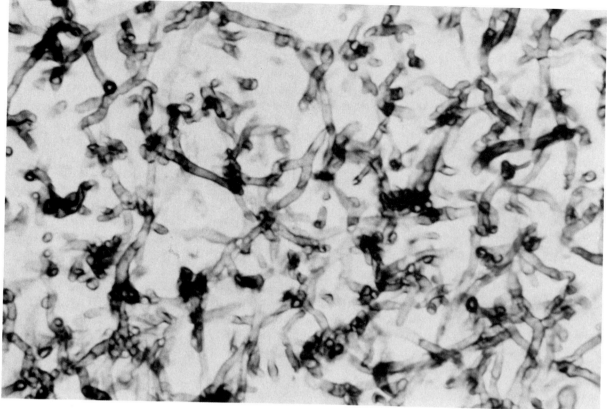

FIGURE 6–13

Low-power photomicrograph illustrating clusters of fungus hyphae. (Original magnification × 160.)

ture media but forming small yeastlike structures in the tissues of the infected individual.

Some fungi live on the skin and only occasionally cause minor discomfort. Others are found in small numbers in the oral cavity, gastrointestinal tract, and vagina, where they live in harmony with the normal bacterial flora. Most fungi have a limited ability to cause disease. Under special circumstances, however, fungi may produce serious localized or systemic infections in susceptible individuals. Two major factors predispose to systemic fungal infections: disturbance in the normal bacterial flora and impaired immunologic defenses.

After intensive therapy with broad-spectrum antibiotics, the normal bacterial flora of the oral cavity, colon, vagina, and other areas may be altered or completely eradicated, disturbing the normal balance between the bacterial flora and fungi. Normally, the predominance of the bacterial flora holds the fungi in check. When the bacteria are eliminated, the fungi may proliferate and cause disease.

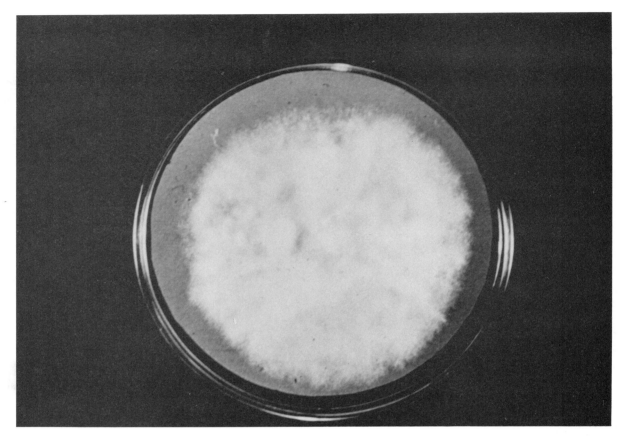

FIGURE 6–14

Appearance of fungus colony growing on laboratory culture medium.

Patients with various types of chronic debilitating diseases may be susceptible to fungal infections. Infections of this type are also encountered in patients whose immunologic defense mechanisms have been depressed by various drugs and chemicals or by radiation therapy. Patients with certain types of cancer, particularly those treated with cytotoxic drugs, may also develop systemic fungal infections.

Superficial Fungal Infections

The common superficial fungal infections of the skin are caused by a group of fungi called **dermatophytes,** which grow on the skin. They cause itchy, scaling skin lesions on the scalp and on other parts of the body. Some have been given such picturesque, popular names as "athlete's foot" and "jock itch." A common superficial fungal infection of the mucous membranes is caused by a yeastlike fungus called *Candida albicans.* This organism is a common cause of vaginal infections, producing symptoms of itching and vaginal discharge (figure 6–15). Pregnant women and women taking oral contraceptive pills seem more susceptible to *Candida* infection, as are persons treated with broad-spectrum antibiotics such as tetracycline. A number of antifungal drugs are available which can be applied locally to treat infections caused by dermatophytes and *Candida*.

Highly Pathogenic Fungi

Although most fungi are at best only potential pathogens of low virulence, two are highly infectious and frequently produce disease in humans. They can be identified by biopsy or by culture of infected tissues. The fungus *Histoplasma capsulatum,* which is found in many parts of the United States, causes the disease *histoplasmosis.* This organism is found in the soil and in the excreta of birds. People become infected by inhaling dust containing dried spores of the fungus. In most cases, the fungus produces an

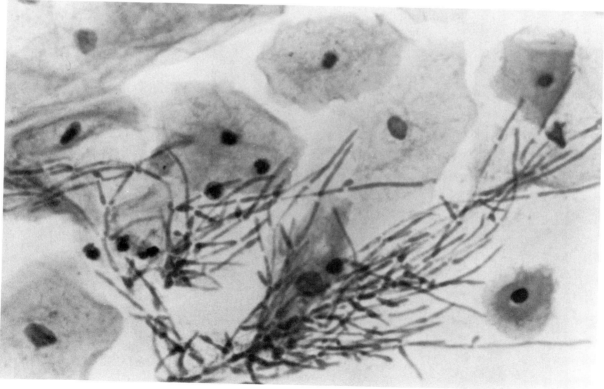

FIGURE 6–15

Cluster of hyphae in vaginal smear from patient with vaginitis caused by *Candida albicans.* (Original magnification × 400.)

acute, self-limited respiratory infection. Less commonly, the organism causes a more chronic pulmonary infection similar to tuberculosis. In some cases, progressive, disseminated, sometimes fatal disease develops. Another fungus, *Coccidioides immitis,* which is found in parts of California and elsewhere in the southwestern part of the United States, causes the disease *coccidioido-mycosis.* As in the case of histoplasmosis, humans become infected by inhaling dust that contains dried spores. The symptoms are similar to those of histo-plasmosis. Coccidioidomycosis is usually manifested as an acute pulmonary infection, but sometimes the fungus causes chronic or severe progressive systemic disease.

Other Fungi of Medical Importance

Two other pathogenic fungi of medical importance are *Blastomyces derma-tiditis,* which causes the disease *blastomycosis,* and *Cryptococcus neofor-mans,* which causes *cryptococcosis.* Infections caused by these organisms are less common than either histoplasmosis or coccidioidomycosis. Both organisms are found in the soil, and infection is caused by inhalation of dust containing the organisms.

Clinically, blastomycosis is similar to histoplasmosis and coccidioidomycosis. Most infections are acute and self-limited. Occasionally, the fungus causes a more chronic pulmonary infection or a widespread systemic disease.

Cryptococcus neoformans is a yeastlike organism that has a large mucoid capsule. The organism initially causes a pulmonary infection but then may be transported in the bloodstream to the meninges of the brain, where it causes a chronic meningitis. The organisms can be identified in smears and cultures of spinal fluid.

Treatment of Systemic Fungal Infections

Acute pulmonary infections caused by fungi frequently subside spontaneously and do not require treatment. Chronic or progressive systemic fungal infections are treated with various antifungal antibiotics, as illustrated by the following cases.

CASE 6–1

A young man who had resided for a short time in the southwestern United States consulted his physician and was found to have a dense infiltrate in the upper lobe of the lung with the formation of a cavity, suggesting tuberculosis. However, cultures of sputum for tubercle bacilli were negative. A specimen from the affected area was obtained by means of a flexible bronchoscope, and material for culture was also obtained. Coccidioides immitis was cultured from the involved area. Biopsy revealed only nonspecific chronic inflammation. No organisms were identified in the biopsy specimen. The patient was treated with an antifungal antibiotic and made an uneventful recovery.

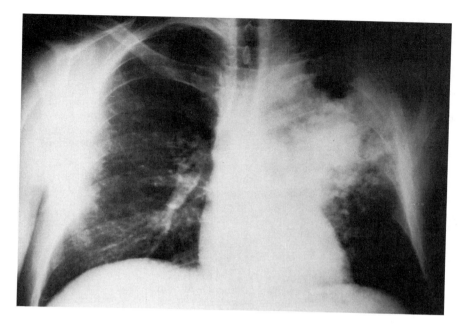

FIGURE 6–16

Chest x-ray illustrating blastomycosis of left lung (right side of photograph), which appears as a dense (white) area occupying the upper part of the lung. Right lung (left side of photograph) appears normal (case 6–2).

A thirty-nine-year-old diabetic man was admitted to the hospital with cough and fever, and chest x-ray revealed a large area of consolidation in the left lung (figure 6–16). Bronchial biopsy revealed nonspecific chronic inflammation, but cultures revealed growth of Blastomyces dermatiditis. The patient responded to treatment with antifungal antibiotics.

CASE 6–2

Questions for Review

1. By what standards are bacteria classified? Name the classifications.

2. What is the gram-stain test procedure? What important diseases are caused by the following bacteria: staphylococci, beta streptococci, pneumococci, gonococci, acid-fast bacteria?

3. What is meant by the following terms: *granulomatous inflammation, gram-positive organism, Legionella?*

4. How do antibiotics inhibit the growth of bacteria? How does penicillin kill bacteria?

5. How do bacteria become resistant to an antibiotic?

6. What are some of the potential harmful effects of antibiotics?

7. What is meant by the following terms: *competitive inhibition, sensitivity test, resistant organism, cell membrane?*

8. How does a viral infection affect a susceptible cell?

9. What is a latent (asymptomatic) viral infection? Give an example.

10. What is meant by the following terms: *inclusion body, chlamydiae, mycoplasma?*

11. What factors render a patient susceptible to an infection by a fungus of low pathogenicity?

12. What are the names of the two highly pathogenic fungi? What type of disease do they produce?

13. A young women receives a course of antibiotics and soon afterwards develops a vaginal infection caused by a fungus. Why?

Supplementary Readings

Bell, B. P., Goldoft, M., Griffin, P. M., et al. 1994. A multistate outbreak of *Escherichia coli* 0157:H7 bloody diarrhea and hemolytic uremic syndrome from hamburgers. *Journal of the American Medical Association* 272:1349–53. More than five hundred people became infected and three died from eating improperly cooked hamburgers prepared by a "fast food" chain.

Brooks, G. F., Butel, J. S., and Ornston, L. N. 1992. *Review of medical microbiology*. 19th ed. Norwalk, Conn.: Appleton & Lange.

Colditz, G. A., Brewer, T. F., Berkey, C. S., et al. 1994. Efficacy of BCG vaccine in the prevention of tuberculosis. *Journal of the American Medical Association* 271:1677–79. BCG vaccination produces cell-mediated immunity against the tubercle bacillus and reduces the risk of infection.

Drutz, D. J. 1979. Urban coccidioidomycosis and histoplasmosis. *New England Journal of Medicine* 301:381–82. A short review of two important and highly infectious fungi.

DuPont, H. L. 1992. How safe is the food we eat? (Editorial). *Journal of the American Medical Association* 268:3240. Discusses the various types of food-borne infections, the relative safety of foods, and the various populations at risk of infection.

Griffin, P. M., et al. 1988. Illnesses associated with *Escherichia coli* 0157:H7 infections: A broad clinical spectrum. *Annals of Internal Medicine* 109:705–12. Describes the hemolytic uremic syndrome and thrombotic thrombocytopenic purpura associated with this toxigenic colon bacillus.

Holmes, K. K. 1981. The chlamydia epidemic. *Journal of the American Medical Association* 245:1718–23. These organisms are assuming greater importance in clinical medicine.

Jogerst, G. J., and Dippe, S. E. 1981. Antibiotic use among medical specialties in a community hospital. *Journal of the American Medical Association* 245:842–46.

Describes utilization of antibiotics and suggestions for improvement.

MacDonald, K. L., et al. 1988. *Escherichia coli* 0157:H7, an emerging gastrointestinal pathogen: Results of a one-year, prospective, population-based study. *Journal of the American Medical Association* 259:3567; 3570. Describes the frequency and clinical manifestations.

Pinner, R. W., Teutsch, S. M., Simonsen, L., et al. 1996. Trends in infectious disease mortality in the United States. *Journal of the American Medical Association* 275:189–93. Between 1980 and 1992 the death rate from infectious diseases increased 58 percent, and infectious disease is now the third leading cause of death after cancer and heart disease. Infectious diseases are still a formidable problem.

Stevers, D. L. 1991. Invasive group A streptococcus infections. *Clinical Infectious Diseases* 14:2–13. A review of the various manifestations of severe toxin-producing group A streptococcal infections including necrotizing fasciitis (the "flesh eating bacteria" of the popular press), myonecrosis, and streptococcal toxic shock syndrome. Describes the toxins produced by these organisms and the methods of treatment.

Stoeckle, M. Y., and Douglas, R. G. 1994. Infectious diseases. *Journal of the American Medical Association* 271:1677–79. A review of recent developments in infectious diseases, including the emergence of antibiotic-resistant pneumococci.

Werner, S. B., et al. 1972. An epidemic of coccidioidomycosis among archeology students in Northern California. *New England Journal of Medicine* 286:507–12. This fungal infection is an occupational hazard in persons exposed to soil and dust in endemic areas; 103 archeology students contracted disease while excavating Indian ruins.

Chapter 6 ▪ Outline Summary

Bacteria / 115
Classification
Shape: coccus, bacillus, spiral.

Gram stain: gram positive and gram negative.

Biochemical and cultural characteristics:

Aerobic and anaerobic.

Spore formation.

Flagella.

"Biochemical profile" aids identification.

Antigenic structure: antigens in cell body, capsule, flagella.

Diseases Caused by Pathogenic Bacteria
Staphylococci: inhabit skin and nasal cavity; cause boils, pulmonary infection.

Streptococci:

Alpha streptococci: normal inhabitants of respiratory tract.

Beta streptococci: cause strep sore throat, scarlet fever, skin infections, uterine infections.

Gamma streptococci: limited pathogenicity.

Pneumococci: pneumonia.

Gram-negative cocci:

Meningococci cause meningitis.

Gonococci cause gonorrhea.

Gram-positive bacilli:

Aerobic: diphtheria bacillus.

Anaerobic: clostridia cause gas gangrene, tetanus, botulism.

Gram-negative bacteria: a large diverse group that causes various systemic and intestinal infections.

Spiral organisms: treponemas cause syphilis.

Acid-fast organisms: tuberculosis.

Antibiotics / 122
Mode of Action
Inhibits cell-wall synthesis: penicillin.

Inhibits cell-membrane function.

Inhibits metabolic functions of bacterium.

Competitive inhibition.

Antibiotic Sensitivity Tests
Tube dilution: measures highest dilution inhibiting growth in test tube.

Disk method: inhibition of growth around disk indicates sensitivity to antibiotic.

Bacterial Resistance to Antibiotics
Bacteria develop enzymes that inactivate antibiotic—e.g., penicillinase.

Bacteria develop alternative metabolic pathways that circumvent effects of antibiotics.

Adverse Effects of Antibiotics
Toxicity: almost all have some toxicity, which varies with the antibiotic.

Hypersensitivity: may cause fatal reaction if given to sensitized patient.

Alteration of normal bacterial flora: disturbs normal bacterial flora and allows overgrowth of pathogens.

Development of resistant strains: may complicate treatment.

Indications for Antibiotic Use
Infection caused by susceptible organisms.

Should not be administered if not indicated because of potential adverse effects.

Viruses / 128
Structure
Either DNA or RNA.

Genome enclosed in capsid.

Size and complexity of genome varies with virus.

Virus lacks metabolic enzymes and relies on metabolic processes of host for survival.

Mode of Action
Invades host cell and produces various effects.

Asymptomatic.

Acute cell necrosis.

Cell hyperplasia and proliferation.

Slowly progressive cell injury.

Neoplasia.

Inclusion bodies formed are caused by masses of viral particles.

Bodily Defenses Against Viral Infection
Formation of interferon: "broad-spectrum" antiviral agent.

Cell-mediated immunity and humoral defenses.

Classification of Viruses
Nucleic acid structure: either DNA or RNA.

Size, structural configuration, and biologic characteristics.

Antiviral Agents
Block viral multiplication or prevent virus from invading cell.

Limited use because of toxicity and limited effectiveness.

Chlamydiae / 137
Characteristics
Gram-negative nonmotile bacteria.

Deficient in enzymes and can only live in host tissue.

Form inclusion bodies in infected cells.

Chlamydial Diseases
Nongonococcal urethritis.

Inclusion conjunctivitis.

Pulmonary infections.

Lymphogranuloma venerum.

Rickettsiae / 138
Characteristics
Intracellular parasite.

Parasite of insects and transmitted to humans by insect bites.

Multiply in endothelial cells of blood vessels.

Cause febrile illness with skin rash.

Respond to some antibiotics.

Mycoplasmas / 138
Characteristics
Fragile bacteria lacking cell wall.

Cause primary atypical pneumonia.

Respond to some antibiotics.

Fungi / 138
Types of Fungal Infection
Superficial fungal infections.

Dermatophytes: athlete's foot, jock itch.

Mucous membranes: *Candida* causes vaginitis.

Highly pathogenic fungi: *Histoplasma* and *Coccidioides* cause acute or chronic pulmonary infection, occasionally progressive systemic infection.

Other systemic fungal diseases of medical importance.

Blastomycosis: similar to histoplasmosis.

Cryptococcus: occasionally causes chronic meningitis.

Treatment of Fungal Infections
Superficial fungal infections respond to various medications.

Acute systemic fungal infections treated with antifungal antibiotics.

7

Animal Parasites

Learning Objectives

List the common parasitic infestations that affect humans. Explain how these infestations are acquired. Describe their clinical manifestations and explain their clinical significance.

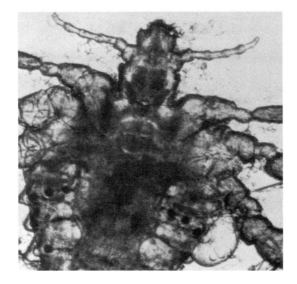

Chapter 7 ▪ Contents

Animal parasites are organisms that have become adapted to living within or on the body of another animal, called the **host.** These organisms are no longer capable of free-living existence. Many animal parasites have a complex life cycle. An immature form of a parasite may spend a part of its cycle within the body of an animal or fish (the intermediate host) before the mature parasite eventually takes up residence within the body of the final host (the definitive host). In general, many animal parasites live within the intestinal tract and discharge eggs in the feces. Transmission is favored by conditions of poor sanitation and by relatively high temperature and humidity, which enhance survival of the parasite in its infective stage. Therefore, many parasitic infestations are common in tropical climates but are much less frequent in cold or temperate climates. Specific drugs are available to effectively treat almost all parasitic infestations.

Animal parasites may be classified into three large groups:

1. *Protozoa,* which are simple, one-celled organisms
2. *Metazoa,* which are more complex, multicellular structures
3. *Arthropods,* which are small insects

Some of the more important protozoal infestations in humans include:

Protozoal Infestations

1. Malaria, caused by various species of *Plasmodium.*
2. Amebic dysentery, caused by a pathogenic ameba, *Entamoeba histolytica.*
3. Genital tract trichomonad infestations, caused by the parasite *Trichomonas vaginalis.*
4. Giardiasis, caused by *Giardia lamblia,* which infests the small intestine.
5. Toxoplasmosis, caused by *Toxoplasma gondii,* which may infect the fetus and cause congenital malformations.
6. Cryptosporidiosis, caused by a newly recognized parasite called *Cryptosporidium parvum,* which parasitizes the intestinal tract and can cause severe diarrhea.
7. Pneumocystis pneumonia, caused by *Pneumocystis carinii,* a parasite that does not cause disease in immunocompetent persons but causes a severe, sometimes fatal pulmonary infection in persons with acquired immune deficiency syndrome (AIDS). This disease is considered in chapter 15.

Malaria

Malaria is caused by several species of the protozoan parasite *Plasmodium,* which has a complicated life cycle. The parasite is transmitted to humans by the bite of the Anopheles mosquito, which breeds in swampy lowland areas. The name *malaria* dates to the time when the disease was thought to be caused by breathing night air near lowland marshes and swampy areas (*malo* = bad + *aria* = air). After the parasite and its mosquito vector were recognized, it became apparent that the marshy areas were mosquito breeding grounds, and the evening hours were the times when the mosquitoes were most active.

The parasites invade the red blood cells of the host. There they multiply, feeding on the hemoglobin, which becomes degraded to a product called malarial pigment. Soon, the rapidly multiplying parasites destroy the red cells that they have invaded, releasing masses of new parasites along with red-cell debris and malarial pigment into the circulation. This event is associated with an elevated temperature and a shaking chill ("chills and fever"). The newly liberated parasites in turn attack other red cells, and the cycles of invasion–multiplication–red-cell destruction continue. The time taken for each species of parasite to complete its cycle is quite constant. Consequently, the episodes of chills and fever tend to occur at regular intervals every forty-eight or seventy-two hours, depending on the species. Besides suffering repeated, periodic chills and fever, infected individuals frequently become anemic because of the excessive red-cell destruction. Often their spleens also enlarge because phagocytic cells in the spleen proliferate and become filled with debris and malarial pigment. In one type of malaria, clumps of parasitized red cells may plug small blood vessels in the brain, heart, or other vital organs. This serious complication impedes blood flow to the affected organs and may be fatal. Diagnosis of malaria is established by demonstrating the parasite in properly prepared and stained slides made from the blood of the infected patient.

Malaria is a major health problem in many parts of the world. It is widespread in many Third World countries, including parts of Africa, Asia, Central America, and South America. More than 100 million people are afflicted at any given time, and about one million people die of the disease each year. Few infectious diseases have had such a profound effect on the social and economic development of countries. Malaria is no longer a problem in the United States, Canada, and Europe. Most cases of malaria in the United States are contracted by persons who have traveled to areas where malaria occurs frequently and become ill after returning home. Malaria is also sometimes transmitted by blood transfusion if the donor carries the parasite. Malarial infections have also been contracted by drug abusers who share contaminated syringes and needles.

CASE 7-1

An American family had been vacationing in a resort outside the United States. After returning to their own country, several members became ill with chills and fever. Examination of the blood smears revealed malarial parasites. The affected family members received a course of antimalarial therapy and made an uneventful recovery.

Amebiasis

Amebiasis is an infection of the intestinal tract by a pathogenic ameba, *Entamoeba histolytica*. The life cycle of the parasite includes an active, motile, vegetative phase (called a *trophozoite*) and a relatively resistant cystic phase. Humans become infected by ingesting cysts of the parasite in contaminated food and water. The motile phase of the parasite develops from the cyst and invades the mucosa of the colon, producing mucosal ulcers and causing symptoms of inflammation of the colon. Occasionally, the amebas are carried to the liver in the portal circulation and may cause amebic hepatitis or amebic liver abscess.

Genital Tract Infections Caused by Trichomonads

The trichomonads are small motile parasites. One species, *Trichomonas vaginalis,* sometimes causes an acute inflammation of the vagina characterized by itching, burning, and a profuse, frothy vaginal discharge. The infection can be transmitted to the male by sexual intercourse and causes an inflammation of the urethra.

> A young woman complained of vaginal itching and profuse vaginal discharge. Examination revealed redness of the vaginal mucosa and abundant yellow vaginal secretions. Microscopic examination revealed large numbers of trichomonads and leukocytes in the secretions. The patient was treated with an antiparasitic drug (metronidazole). Because the disease is transmitted by sexual intercourse, the patient's sexual partner also was treated.

CASE 7–2

Giardiasis

Giardia lamblia is a small pear-shaped parasite that inhabits the duodenum and upper jejunum. The parasite attaches to the mucosa, causing an intestinal inflammation manifested by crampy abdominal pain, distention, and watery diarrhea. Parasites are present in the stools of infected individuals, and the disease is usually transmitted by means of contaminated food and water. The infection is relatively common in certain parts of Russia, and many American tourists traveling there have been infected. Several epidemics of giardia infection caused by contaminated water supplies have occurred in the United States.

Toxoplasmosis

Toxoplasma gondii is a small intracellular parasite that infects a large number of birds and animals, as well as humans. Many cats are infected with the parasite and excrete an infectious form of the organism in their stools. The parasite is frequently present in the flesh of cattle and many other animals. People acquire toxoplasma infections by ingesting raw or partially cooked meat that is infected with the parasite or by contact with cats. Usually the infection does not cause symptoms in healthy adults. About 50 percent of the adult population has had a previous inapparent infection and is immune. The importance of toxoplasmosis is related to its effect on the fetus. If a susceptible (nonimmune) woman acquires a toxoplasma infection during pregnancy, the parasite may be transmitted to the fetus. Infection of the fetus causes severe injury to fetal tissues and often leads to congenital malformations that are described in chapter 9.

Cryptosporidiosis

Cryptosporidium parvum, an organism closely related to *Toxoplasma,* has been recognized recently as a very important cause of severe diarrhea in both immunocompetent and immunocompromised persons. The organism primarily infects cattle and other farm animals. Infected animals excrete in their stool large numbers of the infectious form of the parasite, called an *oocyst,* which can contaminate surface water flowing into rivers and lakes, and oocysts have been identified in from 65 to 85 percent of surface water samples tested throughout the United States. The infectious oocyst has a thick wall and is quite small, only about half the size of a red blood cell. It is highly resistant to chlorination of water supplies and can be removed from municipal water supplies only by filtration. People can become infected by ingesting oocysts in unfiltered municipal water supplies, from oocyst-contaminated water in swimming pools, or by person-to-person fecal-oral transmission in the same way that other intestinal infections are transmitted.

When oocysts are ingested, the cyst wall disintegrates in the intestinal tract, releasing the infectious parasite, which multiplies and infects the intestinal epithelial cells. The parasite is very infectious, and persons with diarrhea excrete large numbers of oocysts in their stool. Persons with normal immune defenses experience an acute self-limited diarrhea when infected with the parasite, but persons with AIDS and other immunocompromised persons develop a severe chronic life-threatening diarrhea. Unfortunately, there is no specific treatment for the infection.

Several large epidemics of cryptosporidiosis have been traced to municipal water supplies where filtration of water to eliminate oocysts either was not performed or was inadequate. Small, swimming-pool–related epidemics also have been reported. In these cases, the oocyst contamination of the pool water was caused by persons with cryptosporidial diarrhea using the pool; oocysts contaminating the perianal skin of these people were released into the pool water and infected other swimmers.

Metazoal Infestations

The three large groups of metazoal parasites are:

1. Roundworms
2. Tapeworms
3. Flukes

Roundworms

The three most important roundworms that parasitize human beings are the *Ascaris,* the pinworm, and the *Trichinella* worm.

Ascaris

The *Ascaris* is a large roundworm, about the size of an earthworm, that lives within the intestinal tract and discharges eggs in the feces. Humans become infested by ingesting material contaminated with *Ascaris* eggs. The worms hatch within the intestinal tract, and the small larval worms burrow through the intestine, enter the circulatory system, and are carried in the circulation throughout the body. They are then filtered out in various organs and tissues. The larvae that lodge in the lung burrow through the alveolar walls and migrate into the bronchi, are coughed up, and eventually are swallowed, finding their way again into the small intestine where they grow to maturity. The stage characterized by the passage of *Ascaris* larvae through the lungs and other tissues is called *the phase of larval migration* and may be associated with fever, cough, and inflammation of the lungs. Adult worms living in the small intestine may at times wander from their usual location. They may migrate upward and be coughed up or vomited or they may pass out through the nose. At times they may enter and block the bile ducts or plug the appendix. Rarely, a large mass of worms may completely block the lumen of the small intestine.

Dogs and cats may be infested with a similar type of roundworm; the animal worm occasionally causes disease in humans. Infestation by the animal worm is most common in children who are in close contact with an infected animal. The children transfer the eggs to their mouths by means of contaminated hands, toys, or other objects. The eggs hatch within the intestinal tract, and the larvae invade the tissues of the host, undergoing a phase of larval migration, which may be associated with systemic symptoms. However, the larvae that have been ingested by a foreign host are eventually destroyed within the tissues of the host and never reach maturity within the intestinal tract.

> A young woman complained of a "funny feeling" in the back of her throat and coughed up a large Ascaris worm. The organism, which normally inhabits the small intestine, had migrated through the stomach and esophagus into the pharynx and was subsequently expelled (figure 7–1).

CASE 7–3

Pinworms

Infestation by the small roundworm called the *pinworm* is frequent in children, and the infestation often spreads throughout a family. The worm measures less than 1 cm in length and lives in the colon. The parasite frequently migrates out of the colon through the anus while the infected individual is asleep and deposits its eggs on the perianal skin. Sometimes the worm migrates into the vagina, through the fallopian tubes, and into the peritoneal cavity, but this is uncommon. The main symptoms of pinworm infestation are intense anal and perianal itching caused by irritation resulting from the migration of the worm. A person becomes infected with the worm by ingesting eggs, which are transferred to the hands from contaminated bedclothes or other objects. The disease is more a nuisance than a threat to life.

Trichinella

Another small roundworm, *Trichinella spiralis,* causes a severe parasitic infestation called *trichinosis.* The organism parasitizes not only humans, but

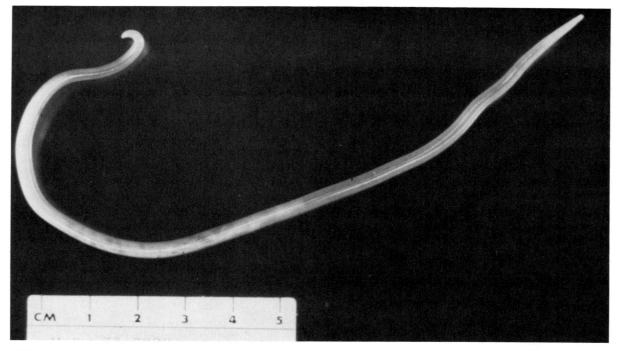

FIGURE 7–1

Large *Ascaris* that migrated into back of a patient's throat and was coughed up (case 7–3).

also a wide variety of animals. Larval forms of the *Trichinella* are encapsulated as small cystic structures within the muscles of the infected human or animal host. People usually become infected by eating improperly cooked pork. After the infected meat has been ingested, the larvae are released from their cysts and develop into mature parasitic worms in the small intestine. The worms then burrow into the intestinal mucosa and produce larvae, which gain access to the circulation and are carried throughout the body. They are filtered out in various tissues, where they incite an intense inflammatory reaction. The parasites that lodge in the muscles of the infected individual become encapsulated, forming small cysts within the muscle. These cysts are the infectious form of the parasite. The phase of larval migration is associated with severe systemic symptoms, and there may also be symptoms referable to disturbed function of organs that have been heavily infiltrated by the parasites. Extremely heavy parasitic infestations may be fatal.

Tapeworms

Tapeworms are long, ribbonlike worms that sometimes grow to a length of several feet. They inhabit the intestinal tract. In general, tapeworms cause no great inconvenience to the individual carrying them except for depriving the host of the food that nourishes the worm. Three species of tapeworms are recognized: the pork tapeworm, the beef tapeworm, and the fish tapeworm. Humans become infected by eating the flesh of an infected animal that contains the larval form of the parasite.

Flukes

Flukes are thick, fleshy, short worms that are provided with suckers for the attachment to the host. They have a complex life cycle involving one or more intermediate hosts. Flukes are classified according to the area of the body in which the development of the adult flukes is completed and the eggs are deposited. Some species of flukes live within the intestinal tract; others live within the liver; one species lives within the lung. Some flukes called *Schistosomes,* or blood flukes, live within the portal venous system and its tributaries or within the veins draining the bladder, where they cause serious damage to the surrounding tissues. Fluke infestations are an important cause of illness and disability in some Asiatic countries, but human fluke infestations are not seen in the United States or Canada.

Although human fluke infestations do not occur in North America, some animal schistosomes can infect humans but are more a nuisance than a cause of serious illness. Birds and mammals, infected with their own specific species of schistosomes, excrete them in their droppings into lakes and other bodies of water, where they develop into the infectious form of the parasite. People who swim in bird or animal schistosome-infested lakes may be "attacked" by the parasites, which can penetrate the skin of the swimmers. The parasites cause discrete areas of acute pruritic inflammation at the site where they entered the skin. They cannot cause a systemic infection, however, because humans are not the normal host for the parasite, and the parasites are destroyed in the skin by the body's immune defenses. The condition is called *schistosome dermatitis* but is more commonly referred to as "swimmers itch." Many lakes in North America and some saltwater beaches are infested with bird or animal schistosomes.

Arthropods

There are two common parasitic skin infestations: scabies and lice. Both are transmitted by close physical contact and are often spread by sexual contact. Both infestations respond promptly to treatment with antiparasitic medications applied to the skin.

Scabies is caused by a small parasite called *Sarcoptes scabiei,* which burrows in the superficial layers of the skin, where it lays eggs that hatch in a few days. The infestation causes intense itching. The tracks made by the parasites as they burrow in the skin appear as fine, wavy, dark lines in the skin measuring from 1 mm to 1 cm in length. Common sites of involvement are the base of the fingers, the wrists, the armpits, the skin around the nipples, and the skin around the beltline.

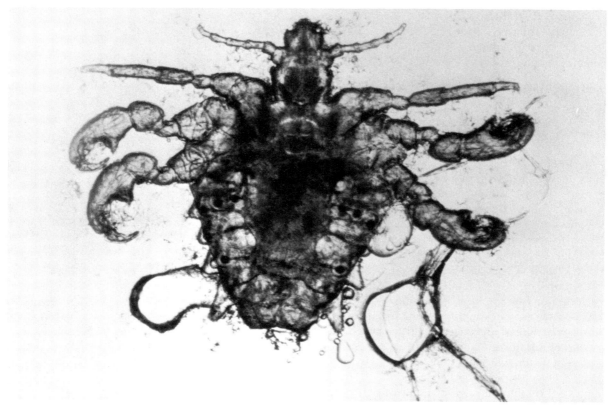

FIGURE 7–2

Appearance of crab louse, illustrating turtle-shaped body with three pairs of claws. Size about 1 mm.

Of the various types of lice that may infest the body, the most common and best known is the *crab louse* (*Pediculosis pubis*), which lives in the anal and genital hairs (figure 7–2). The organism also causes intense itching. The louse lays eggs that become attached to the hair shafts. Diagnosis is established by identifying either the parasite or the eggs.

CASE 7–4

A young man complained of intense itching in the pubic area. Examination revealed small crab lice in the pubic hair and numerous eggs attached to the hair shafts. Both the patient and his sexual partner were treated with an antiparasitic drug (Kwell).

Questions for Review

1. What are some of the more important protozoal infections?

2. How is malaria transmitted?

3. What is trichinosis? How is it transmitted?

4. What are the more important worm infestations? What are their manifestations?

5. What are "crabs"? What symptoms do they cause? How are they acquired?

Supplementary Readings

Barrett-Connor, E. 1978. Latent and chronic infections imported from Southeast Asia. *Journal of the American Medical Association* 239:1901–6. A number of parasitic infestations occur in refugees and in U.S. citizens exposed in Southeast Asia.

Blumenthal, D. S. 1977. Intestinal nematodes in the United States. *New England Journal of Medicine* 297:1437–39. Worm infections are common in rural communities in the southeastern United States and among immigrants from tropical countries. Manifestations, diagnosis, and treatment are described.

Centers for Disease Control and Prevention. 1994. *Cryptosporidium* infections associated with swimming pools—Dane County, Wisconsin, 1993. *Morbidity and Mortality Weekly Report* 43:561–63. Members of swim team became infected from a swimming pool. Measures to prevent such infections are discussed.

Hayes, E. B., Matte, T. D., O'Brien, T. R., et al. 1989. Large community outbreak of cryptosporidiosis as a result of contamination of filtered water supply. *New England Journal of Medicine* 320:1372–76. Parasites in municipal supply caused large community outbreak.

Joklik, W. K., Willett, H. P., Amos, D. B., and Wilfert, C. M. 1992. *Zinsser microbiology*. 20th ed. Norwalk, Conn.: Appleton & Lange. Excellent section on medical parasitology, section VII.

Krick, J. A., and Remington, J. S. 1978. Toxoplasmosis in the adult: An overview. *New England Journal of Medicine* 298:550–52. Asymptomatic toxoplasmosis occurs in a large percentage of the population. It may cause an illness resembling infectious mononucleosis, and it can cause a fatal infection in an individual whose immune defenses have been suppressed. An important cause of congenital abnormalities caused by intrauterine infection.

MacKenzie, W. R., et al. 1994. A massive outbreak in Milwaukee of *Cryptosporidium* infection transmitted through the public water supply. *New England Journal of Medicine* 331:161–67. Documents a huge outbreak with some deaths related to this parasite in unfiltered water.

Olliaro, P., Cattani, J., and Wirth, D. 1996. Malaria: The submerged disease. *Journal of the American Medical Association* 275:230–33. Malaria is an increasing worldwide problem and is becoming harder to control because the organisms are becoming resistant to antimalarial drugs. About one thousand new cases are reported annually in the United States, usually acquired outside the country by travelers, military personnel, and immigrants from malaria-endemic countries, but a small number of cases are acquired in the United States.

Rubenstein, E., and Sederman, D., eds. 1995. *Scientific American medicine*. New York: Scientific American, Inc. Good section on helminthic infections, section XXXV.

Volk, W. A., Benjamin, D. C., Kadner, R. J., and Parsons, J. T. 1991. *Essentials of medical microbiology*. 4th ed. Philadelphia: Lippincott. Very good section on medical parasitology, unit six.

Wolfe, M. S. 1975. Giardiasis. *Journal of the American Medical Association* 233:1362–65. A very common infection of both humans and animals. Organisms cause considerable irritation of small bowel, causing an acute diarrhea and distention. Methods of diagnosis and treatment discussed.

Chapter 7 ▪ Outline Summary

Animal Parasites / 147
Classification
  Protozoa: simple one-celled organisms.

  Metazoa: complex, multicelled.

  Arthropods: small insects that infest skin.

Protozoal Infestations / 149
Malaria
  Transmission by mosquito, occasionally by blood transfusion or hypodermic syringes of illicit drug users.

  Parasites red blood cells and causes febrile illness with red-cell destruction.

Amebiasis
  Transmission by contaminated food or water.

  Invades colon with mucosal ulcers.

  Occasionally causes liver abscesses.

Trichomonads
  Cause vaginal infection.

  Transmission by sexual intercourse.

Giardia
  Transmission by contaminated food and water.

  Causes inflammation of small intestine with crampy pain and diarrhea.

Toxoplasma

Parasite in flesh of animals.

Infection acquired by eating incompletely cooked meat or from contact with cats who excrete infectious form of parasite.

Toxoplasma infection of pregnant women may be transmitted to fetus and cause intrauterine injury.

Cryptosporidia

Animal parasite excreted in stool and contaminates surface water.

Infectious oocysts resistant to chlorination. Can be eliminated only by water filtration.

People infected from ingestion of unfiltered water from municipal water supplies, swimming pool water, or direct person-to-person spread. Organisms infect small intestine and cause diarrhea, which can be chronic and severe in AIDS patients.

No specific treatment available.

Metazoal Infestations / 152
Roundworms

Ascaris

Ingested eggs hatch in intestine.

Larvae migrate into circulation and migrate through tissues.

Worms lodging in lung are coughed up, swallowed, and mature in intestine.

Pinworms

Worms live in colon.

Migrate out of anus and lay eggs.

Cause itching as a result of worm migration.

Transmitted by ingestion of eggs on hands and in bedclothes.

Trichinella

Parasite in flesh of pigs and other animals.

Human beings usually infected by eating improperly cooked pork.

Worms hatch in intestine; larvae enter circulation and are filtered out in tissues.

Worm migration causes systemic symptoms, eosinophilia, and evidence of disturbed organ function.

Tapeworms

Live in intestinal tract and consume nutrients ingested by host.

Flukes

Short fleshy worms that live in liver, intestine, or lung.

Human fluke infestations not seen in United States and Canada.

Bird or animal flukes (schistosomes) may cause skin inflammation (dermatitis) in people who swim in schistosome-infested water.

Arthropods / 155
Scabies

Small parasite burrows in skin, lays eggs, and causes severe itching.

Spread by close physical or sexual contact.

Responds to antiparasitic medications.

Crab Louse

Lives in pubic hair and lays eggs that are attached to hair shafts.

Causes intense itching.

Spread by close physical and sexual contact.

Responds to antiparasitic medications.

8

Communicable Diseases

Learning Objectives

1. Explain how communicable diseases are transmitted and controlled.
2. List the common sexually transmitted diseases. Describe their major clinical manifestations, complications, and methods of treatment.
3. Describe the symptoms of herpes infection in men and women. Explain the effects on sexual partners. Describe how herpes may affect a fetus or newborn infant of an infected mother.
4. Understand the pathogenesis of human immunodeficiency virus infections, the groups affected, and the effects of the virus on the immune system. List the major clinical manifestations of the infection, the significance of a positive test for antibody to the virus, and methods of preventing spread of the infection.

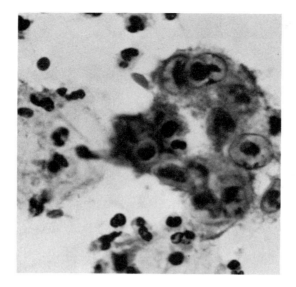

Chapter 8 ▪ Contents

An infectious disease that is readily transmitted from person to person is considered a *communicable disease*. Such a disease is said to be **endemic** (*en* = within + *demos* = population) if small numbers of cases are continually present in the population. It reaches **epidemic** proportions (*epi* = upon + *demos* = population) when relatively large numbers of people are affected. Sometimes an endemic disease may flare up and assume epidemic proportions.

A communicable disease may be transmitted from person to person by either direct or indirect methods. Direct transmission is either by direct physical contact or by means of droplet spread, such as by coughing or sneezing. Indirect transmission of an infectious agent is accomplished by some intermediary mechanism, such as transmission in contaminated water or by means of insects. A few communicable diseases are primarily diseases of animals and are transmitted to humans only incidentally.

Methods of Transmission

For a communicable disease to perpetuate itself, there must be a continuous transmission of the infectious agent from person to person by either direct or indirect methods. Therefore, in order to eradicate or control the disease, the chain of transmission must be broken at some point (figure 8–1).

This section deals with some of the methods that can be applied to the control of a communicable disease. In practice, multiple methods of control are applied whenever possible.

Methods of Control

Immunization

If a large proportion of the population can be immunized against a communicable disease, the disease will eventually die out, because there will be very few susceptible persons in the population. Smallpox is an example of a disease that has been eliminated worldwide because of widespread immunization. Poliomyelitis is another disease that has been eradicated in the United States as a result of widespread immunization of persons at risk.

Immunization can also be used to protect susceptible persons entering a foreign country where a communicable disease is endemic. The immunized person will no longer be susceptible to the disease, even though the disease is widespread in the native population.

Identification, Isolation, and Treatment of Infected Persons

The sick person is identified and treated promptly in order to shorten the time during which he can infect others. Isolation of the infected person prevents contact with susceptible persons and stops the spread of the disease. Identification, isolation, and treatment are the primary methods used to con-

FIGURE 8–1

Methods of eradicating or controlling a communicable disease. **A,** Unimpeded direct or indirect transmission of a communicable disease from person to person. **B,** Immunization protects susceptible person by conferring resistance to infection. **C,** Isolation and prompt treatment of infected individual prevent spread of disease to susceptible persons. **D,** Control of means of indirect transmission blocks spread of the infectious agent.

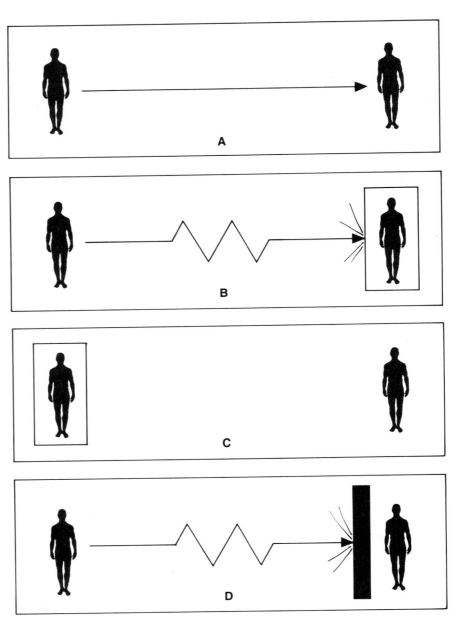

trol diseases when effective methods of immunization are not available. In some cases, these measures are difficult to accomplish, because some diseases produce relatively few symptoms in the infected individual. For example, the person infected with tuberculosis or a sexually transmitted disease may spread the disease to others, but his own disease may not be recognized and treated because he does not feel ill and does not seek medical treatment.

Control of Means of Indirect Transmission

Various control measures can be instituted, depending upon the manner by which the infectious agent is transmitted. Where the transmission is by means of contaminated food or water, methods of control include chlorination of water supplies and establishment of effective sewage treatment facilities, control of food handlers, and standards for monitoring the manufacture and distribution of commercially prepared foods. When a disease is transmitted by insects, either between people or between infected animals and people, it is necessary to eradicate or control the insects that transmit the disease. When a disease is spread from animals to people, control of the animal source of infection also is required.

Requirements for Effective Control

Application of effective control measures requires a knowledge of the cause of the disease and its method of transmission. If this information is not available, control measures are often ineffective. For example, bubonic plague, the "black death" of the Middle Ages, decimated entire populations because the people understood neither the cause of the disease nor how it was transmitted and therefore were unable to protect themselves from its ravages. We now know that plague is primarily a disease of rats and other rodents, that it is caused by a bacterium, and that it is transmitted to people by insects. In some cases, the plague bacillus causes a pulmonary infection in people. When this occurs, direct transmission from person to person can be through droplet spread, causing an extremely contagious and highly fatal pulmonary infection called *pneumonic plague*. In some parts of the United States, plague infection still persists in some rodent populations, but plague is no longer a serious problem, because the disease can be largely prevented in people by control of the infected animal population and by instituting measures that prevent close contact between potentially infected rodents and people. Transmission from person to person is prevented by prompt isolation and treatment of infected persons.

Sexually transmitted diseases, formerly called venereal diseases, are communicable diseases that spread primarily by sexual contact and have reached epidemic proportions. They can be transmitted by sexual relations between heterosexual partners and by sexual acts between individuals of the same sex. The four major sexually transmitted diseases are syphilis, gonorrhea, genital herpes infection, and genital chlamydial infections (see table 8–1). In a class by itself because of its devastating consequences and high mortality is the *acquired immune deficiency syndrome* (AIDS), which is transmitted by both homosexual and heterosexual contacts and by blood and secretions from infected persons.

Other common but less serious sexually transmitted diseases are anal and genital warts (condylomas) caused by the papilloma virus (see figure 6–10),

Sexually Transmitted Diseases

TABLE 8–1

Comparison of four major sexually transmitted diseases

	Syphilis *Treponema pallidum*	**Gonorrhea** Gonococcus (*Neisseria gonorrhoeae*)	**Herpes** Herpes virus	**Chlamydia** *Chlamydia trachomatis*
Organism				
Major clinical manifestations	Primary: chancre Secondary: systemic infection with skin rash and enlarged lymph nodes Tertiary: late destructive lesions in internal organs	Urethritis Cervicitis Pharyngitis Infection of rectal mucosa (proctitis)	Superficial vesicles and ulcers on external genitalia and in genital tract Regional lymph nodes often enlarged and tender	Cervicitis Urethritis
Tests used to establish diagnosis	Demonstration of treponemas in chancre Serologic tests	Culture of organisms from sites of infection	Demonstration of intranuclear inclusions in infected cells Virus cultures Serologic tests in some cases	Detection of chlamydial antigens in cervical/urethral secretions Fluorescence microscopy Cultures
Major complications	Damage to cardiovascular system and nervous system in tertiary syphilis may be fatal	Disseminated bloodstream infection Tubal infection with impaired fertility Spread of infection to prostate and epididymides	Spread from infected mother to infant	Tubal infection with impaired fertility Epididymitis
Treatment	Antibiotics	Antibiotics	Antiviral drug shortens infection but not curative	Antibiotics

nonspecific vaginitis caused by *Gardnerella* in conjunction with anaerobic vaginal bacteria (chapter 6), and trichomonal vaginitis, caused by the protozoan parasite *Trichomonas vaginalis* (chapter 7). Other diseases including scabies and crabs (chapter 7), hepatitis (chapter 21), and some intestinal infections (chapter 23) are also sometimes transmitted sexually.

Syphilis

Syphilis, caused by the spirochete *Treponema pallidum,* is a very serious sexually transmitted disease because it may cause severe damage in almost any organ of the body. If the disease is not treated, it progresses through three stages called primary, secondary, and tertiary syphilis. Each stage has its own characteristic clinical manifestations.

Primary Syphilis

Contact with an infected partner enables the treponemas to penetrate the mucous membranes of the genital tract, oral cavity, or rectal mucosa, or to be introduced through a break in the skin. The organisms multiply rapidly and spread throughout the body. After an incubation period of several weeks, a small ulcer called a *chancre* develops at the site of inoculation. It is easily seen if it is on the penis or vulva, but it may be undetected if it is within the vagina, oral cavity, or rectum.

The chancre, which is swarming with treponemas and is highly infectious, persists for about four to six weeks and eventually heals even if the disease is untreated. Even though the chancre has healed, however, the treponemas are widely disseminated through the body and continue to multiply.

Secondary Syphilis

The secondary stage of syphilis begins several months after the chancre has healed. The infected individual develops manifestations of a systemic infection characterized by elevated temperature, enlargement of lymph nodes, a skin rash, and shallow ulcers on the mucous membranes of the oral cavity and genital tract. This stage of the disease also is extremely infectious because the skin and mucous-membrane lesions contain large numbers of treponemas. The secondary stage persists for several weeks and, like the chancre, eventually subsides even if no treatment is administered. Some subjects experience one or more recurrences of secondary syphilis, but each recurrence subsides spontaneously.

Tertiary Syphilis

After the second stage subsides, the infected individual appears well for a variable period of time, but the organisms are still active and may cause irreparable damage to the cardiovascular and nervous systems and to other organs as well. Chronic inflammation and scarring of the aortic valve lead to valve malfunction and heart failure. Often the aortic wall just above the aortic valve also is damaged by the treponemas. This weakens the aortic wall, causing it to balloon out and eventually rupture. Degeneration of fiber tracts in the spinal cord caused by syphilis impairs sensation and disturbs walking. Damage to the brain by the treponemas causes mental deterioration and eventual paralysis. The late manifestations of the disease, which can appear as long as twenty years after the initial infection, are called *tertiary syphilis*. This stage is not generally communicable because the organisms are relatively few and are confined to the internal organs.

Diagnosis and Treatment
Two different types of laboratory tests are used to diagnose syphilis:

1. Demonstration of treponemas, by means of microscopic examination, in fluid squeezed from the ulcerated surface of the chancre. Specialized techniques and equipment are required.
2. Blood tests, called serologic tests for syphilis, that detect the various antibodies produced in response to a treponemal infection. The serologic tests become positive soon after the chancre appears and remain positive for many years.

Both types of tests are widely used; each has specific applications and limitations. Microscopic examination of material from a suspected chancre establishes the diagnosis of syphilis several weeks before a blood test will show positive results. On the other hand, if the chancre is in an inaccessible location and escapes detection, a positive blood test may be the only indication of syphilis in an individual who does not exhibit symptoms of active infection.

Syphilis can be treated successfully by penicillin and some other antibiotics. Treatment stops the progression of the disease and prevents serious late complications.

Congenital Syphilis
A syphilitic mother may transmit the disease to her unborn infant. The intrauterine infection may cause death of the fetus or the infant may be born with congenital syphilis. The treponemas are not able to pass through the placenta to infect the fetus until after the fourth month of pregnancy because the placental villi are impermeable to the organisms during the early part of pregnancy. Consequently, treatment of the infected mother early in pregnancy prevents infection in the fetus.

Gonorrhea

Gonorrhea, caused by the gonococcus *Neisseria gonorrhoea*, is one of the most common communicable diseases (figure 8–2). The organism primarily infects mucosal surfaces: the linings of the urethra, genital tract, pharynx, and rectum. Symptoms of infection appear about a week after exposure, and the clinical manifestations differ in the two sexes.

Gonorrhea in the Female
In the female, the gonococci infect chiefly the mucosa of the uterine cervix and the urethral mucosa. The gonococcal infection may also spread into Bartholin's

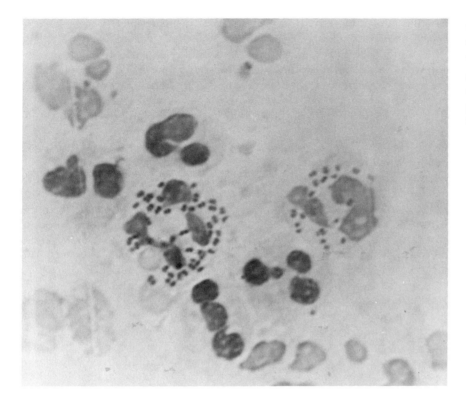

FIGURE 8–2

Gram stain of pus from urethra, illustrating many gram-negative intracellular diplococci characteristic of gonorrhea. (Original magnification × 1000.)

glands, which are located adjacent to the vaginal orifice. The cervical infection usually causes profuse vaginal discharge; the urethral involvement is manifested by pain and burning on urination. Some women, however, have few or no symptoms of infection but are nevertheless capable of transmitting the disease to their sexual partners.

The gonococcal infection may also spread upward from the cervix through the uterus into the fallopian tubes, where it causes an acute salpingitis (*salpinx* = tube). Sometimes the tubal infection is followed by the formation of an abscess within the fallopian tube or an abscess involving both the tube and the adjacent ovary.

Gonococcal salpingitis is manifested by abdominal pain and tenderness together with elevated temperature and leukocytosis. Scarring following the tubal infection may obstruct the lumen of the tube. Blockage of both tubes by scar tissue prevents transport of ova through the tubes and leads to sterility.

Gonorrhea in the Male
In the male, gonococci cause an acute inflammation of the mucosa of the anterior part of the urethra. The infection is usually manifested by a purulent urethral discharge and considerable pain on urination, but occasionally the infected male may have relatively few symptoms although he is still

capable of infecting others. However, gonorrhea is less likely to be asymptomatic in men than in women.

From the anterior urethra, the infection often spreads by direct extension into the posterior urethra, prostate, seminal vesicles, vasa deferentia, and epididymides. An infection in both epididymides and vasa deferentia may lead to sterility because the scarring following the infection may obstruct the duct system and thus block transport of sperm into the seminal fluid.

Extragenital Gonorrhea
Recently, the incidence of gonococcal infection in extragenital sites has increased. Gonoccocal infection of the rectal mucosa causes anorectal pain and tenderness associated with purulent bloody mucoid discharge from the rectum. Rectal infection results from contamination of the rectal mucosa either by infected vaginal secretions or from anal intercourse. Gonococcal infection of the pharynx and tonsils results from oral-genital sex acts. The infection may be asymptomatic but often causes a sore throat.

Disseminated Gonococcal Infection
In a small proportion of infected patients, the organism gains access to the bloodstream and spreads throughout the body. This serious complication is characterized by elevated temperature, joint pain, multiple small abscesses in the skin, and sometimes infections of the joints, tendons, heart valves, and covering of the brain (*meninges*).

Diagnosis and Treatment
Diagnosis of gonorrhea is established by culturing gonococci from suspected sites of infection: urethra, cervix, rectum, and pharynx. Gonococci may also be cultured from the bloodstream in disseminated gonococcal infection.

Most infections respond to penicillin, and various other antibiotics also are effective. Some strains, however, are quite resistant to treatment. Recently, penicillinase-producing strains have appeared that inactivate the antibiotic and are completely penicillin resistant.

Herpes

The herpes simplex virus is one of several herpes viruses that infect people. There are two forms of the herpes simplex virus, designated type I and II. Type I herpes usually infects the oral mucous membrane, where it causes the familiar fever blisters. Most individuals are infected in childhood, and most adults have antibodies to the virus, indicating a previous infection. Type II herpes virus usually infects the genital tract, and infections usually occur after puberty. However, the two types are not restricted in their distribution. Type I virus may cause genital infections, and type II virus may infect the oropharyngeal mucous membrane.

Genital herpes virus infection has increased significantly in recent years. Most genital infections (80 percent) are caused by type II virus. Genital tract infections caused by type I virus also have become more common (20 percent), probably because more people are engaging in oral-genital sexual practices.

The lesions caused by the viral infection usually appear within a week after sexual exposure. They consist of clusters of very small, painful blisters (*vesicles*) that soon rupture, forming painful shallow ulcers that often coalesce. The lesions contain large quantities of virus and are infectious to sexual contacts. Usually the lymph nodes draining the infected areas are swollen and tender. In men, the vesicles usually appear on the glans or shaft of the penis (figure 8–3). In women, the lesions may be quite extensive (figure 8–4). They may be on the vulva, in the vagina, or on the cervix. Vulvar lesions are quite painful, but those deep in the vagina or on the cervix may cause little discomfort because these regions are relatively insensitive. The ulcers heal slowly in a few weeks. However, the virus persists in the tissues of the infected person and may flare up periodically, causing recurrent infections. Some patients have repeated flare-ups for several years after the initial infection.

Active herpetic ulcers shed large amounts of virus, and sexual partners of patients with active lesions are readily infected. Unfortunately, patients without active lesions also may excrete small amounts of virus periodically and infect their sexual partners even though they have no lesions or symptoms of infection.

Diagnosis and Treatment

Herpes can usually be suspected from the clinical appearance of the lesions and can be confirmed by smears obtained from the lesions, which reveal the characteristic intranuclear inclusions in infected cells (figure 8–5). The most reliable diagnostic test is culture of the virus from the ulcers and vesicles, and

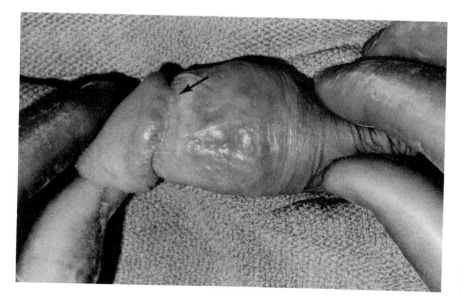

FIGURE 8–3

Several small superficial herpetic ulcers on shaft of penis behind glans (*arrow*).

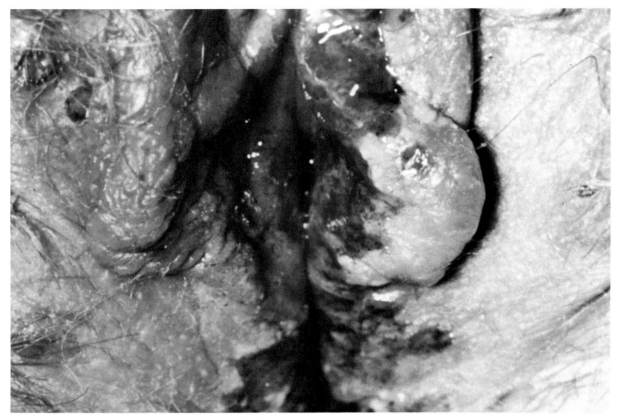

FIGURE 8–4

Multiple confluent ulcers of vulva as a result of herpes.

facilities for virus culture are now widely available. If the patient has not had a previous herpes infection, serologic tests will also reveal formation of antibodies to the herpes virus.

Until recently, little could be done to treat the infection. Cold compresses applied to the affected areas and pain-relieving medications reduced discomfort. Now, an antiviral drug is available (Acyclovir) that shortens the course and reduces the severity of an acute infection but does not eradicate the virus. Depending on the severity of the infection, the drug can be administered intravenously, orally, or applied as an ointment to the lesions. Patients with frequent and disabling recurrent infections sometimes benefit from long-term oral treatment, which seems to reduce the frequency and severity of recurrences.

Herpes Infection and Pregnancy

A pregnant women with a genital herpes infection may infect her infant. If the mother has active herpetic lesions in her genital tract, the infant may

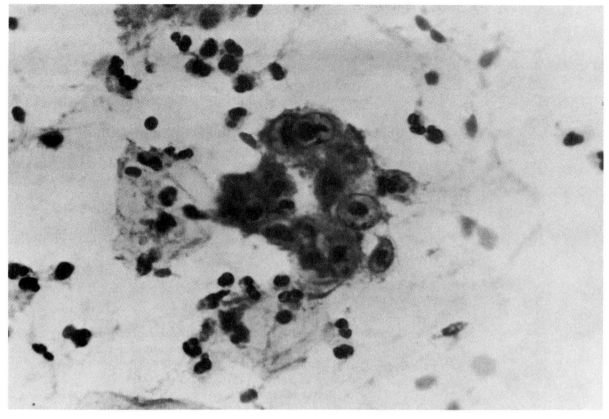

FIGURE 8–5

Vaginal smear illustrating cluster of herpes-infected epithelial cells containing intranuclear inclusions. (Original magnification × 400.)

acquire the virus when passing through the genital tract during delivery. Consequently, a mother with an active infection is usually delivered by cesarean section in order to prevent infection of the newborn infant, which is likely if the infant is delivered vaginally.

Occasionally, the fetus is infected by the herpes virus while still within the uterus. Prenatal infection may cause intrauterine fetal death or may disturb fetal development and lead to congenital malformations.

Genital Chlamydial Infections

Genital tract infections caused by *Chlamydia trachomatis* (described in chapter 6) are now the most common sexually transmitted disease, and it has been estimated that there are between three million and four million new cases each year. Part of this increase reflects the availability of new diagnostic tests that enable the physician to recognize chlamydial infections in patients who have few symptoms, and whose cases probably would previously have gone undetected.

Chlamydia causes much the same type of inflammation and clinical symptoms as gonorrhea. In women, the initial infection is usually in the uterine cervix and is associated with moderate vaginal discharge. Men often develop acute inflammation of the urethra associated with frequency and burning on urination, which is called *nongonococcal urethritis*. Like gonorrhea, the chlamydial infection may spread to the fallopian tubes in women, followed by scarring and impaired fertility, and may cause acute epididymitis in men. As in gonorrhea, many infected persons may have no symptoms of infection but are still able to infect their sexual partners, and may develop complications related to the spread of the infection to other parts of the genital tract.

Diagnosis and Treatment

Diagnosis of chlamydial infection was hampered previously by lack of rapid and reliable diagnostic laboratory tests. Cultures for chlamydia were expensive, time consuming, and not widely available. Recently, highly sensitive specific tests have become available that can detect chlamydial antigens in cervical secretions and secretions from the male urethra. Positive tests have been found in from 10 to 20 percent of young sexually active women attending family planning clinics and from 17 percent to as high as 46 percent of clients attending sexually transmitted disease clinics. Chlamydia can also be detected in smears that are prepared from secretions, stained by special techniques, and examined microscopically. The infection responds to treatment by appropriate antibiotics.

Human Immunodeficiency Virus Infections and AIDS

The acquired immunodeficiency syndrome (AIDS) is a devastating disease that cripples the body's immune system by attacking and destroying helper T lymphocytes, making the affected persons susceptible to a number of unusual infections and malignant tumors. AIDS is the end stage and most serious manifestation of an infection caused by a virus called the *human immunodeficiency virus* or simply the *HIV virus*. Although HIV infection may be regarded as a sexually transmitted disease, many HIV infections are transmitted in other ways. Consequently this disease is considered separately here not only because of the various ways that it can be transmitted, but also because of the devastating effects of the virus on the people who are infected.

The first cases of the disease that we now call AIDS were identified in 1981 in a small group of homosexual men with an unusual opportunistic lung infection. The HIV virus was identified in 1983, and a blood test to detect HIV virus infection became available in 1985. Today we know a lot about the virus and how it damages the immune system, and we know how to avoid becoming infected. Unfortunately, the disease continues to spread because we do not know how to eradicate the virus or stop the progression of the disease that it causes. Worldwide, more than fifteen million persons are infected, and the numbers continue to increase.

The HIV Virus and Its Target

The HIV virus is an RNA virus that belongs to a class of viruses called *retroviruses*. The viral RNA and an important enzyme called *reverse transcriptase* are enclosed within a protein coat (capsid), forming the core of the virus. The core is surrounded by an envelope, composed of a double layer of lipid molecules, that was acquired from the cell membrane of the infected cell when the virus budded from the cell. Projecting from the viral envelope are glycoprotein molecules (designated gp 41 and gp 120). The target of the HIV virus is the CD4 protein present on the cell membranes of helper T lymphocytes, as well as on monocytes, macrophages, and similar macrophage-like cells in the skin, lymph nodes, and within the central nervous system. The CD4 protein functions as a receptor for the virus, to which the virus attaches by means of its gp 120 surface protein. When the virus binds to the cell, the virus envelope fuses with the cell membrane, and the virus enters the cell. Once inside the cell, the virus makes a DNA copy of its own RNA genetic material by means of its reverse transcriptase enzyme, and the DNA copy is inserted into the genetic material of the infected cell, where the virus genes direct the synthesis and assembly of more virus. The newly formed virus particles bud from the infected cells and attack other susceptible cells within the lymphoid tissue throughout the body, where the virus replicates (proliferates) and releases more virus particles to infect still more susceptible cells. Helper T lymphocytes, which are the primary targets for the virus, are damaged and many are killed. Monocytes, however, which are also attacked, are quite resistant and survive, but the virus continues to replicate within the monocytes, releasing virus particles that infect other cells. In addition, the monocytes function as vehicles to transport the virus throughout the body and into the nervous system to infect the brain.

Early Manifestations of HIV Infection

During the early stages of the infection, large amounts of virus can be detected in the blood and body fluids of the infected person, and large numbers of virus-infected lymphocytes are present in lymph nodes and other lymphoid tissue throughout the body. During this phase, many infected persons develop a mild febrile illness. The body responds to the infection by forming anti-HIV antibodies and by generating cytotoxic T lymphocytes. The amount of virus in the blood and body fluids declines as the acute phase of the infection subsides, but unfortunately, the body's defenses are not able to eliminate the virus, and the infection enters a chronic phase. Although the virus continues to replicate and infect other cells, the functions of the immune system are preserved for a time and the subject appears well. Generally, anti-HIV antibodies appear from one to as long as six months after the initial infection. Unfortunately, the antibodies cannot eradicate the virus or reduce its infectivity. Nevertheless, a confirmed positive test for virus antibodies is a useful test to indicate that a person has been infected with the HIV virus, is infectious to others, and is at risk of damage to the immune system from the infection.

There are many different strains of HIV virus. Some appear to be quite aggressive, given that the disease in some infected persons appears to progress relatively rapidly. In contrast, a few strains appear to be relatively benign, because some fortunate individuals who have been infected with the HIV virus for many years do not show any evidence that their immune systems have been damaged.

Late Manifestations of HIV Infection

In most cases, after an interval ranging from a few years to as long as ten years, most infected persons develop manifestations of immune deficiency. The early manifestations, which in the past were designated *AIDS related complex (ARC)*, are characterized by generalized enlargement of lymph nodes, fever, chronic fatigue, weight loss, and sometimes a decrease in blood platelets (thrombocytopenia). These early manifestations gradually progress to more serious late manifestations characterized by various opportunistic infections, neoplasms, and central nervous system damage. The neurologic manifestations of AIDS result not only from direct damage to the nervous system by the virus, but also from various opportunistic infections that target the nervous system. During the late stages of the infection, large amounts of virus can be detected in blood and body fluids, released as a result of widespread destruction of the infected lymphocytes within lymph nodes. Table 8–2 summarizes the sequence of events in HIV infection and their significance.

TABLE 8–2 Sequence of events in HIV infections and their significance	Event	Significance
	HIV invades CD4+ cells and becomes part of cell DNA	Individual is infected for life
	Virus proliferates in infected cells and sheds virus particles	Virus present in blood and body fluids
	Body forms anti-HIV antibody	Antibody is a marker of infection but is not protective
	Progressive destruction of helper T cells, with relative excess of suppressor T cells	Compromised cell-mediated immunity
	Immune defenses collapse	Opportunistic infections Neoplasms

T Lymphocyte Counts as an Index of Disease Progression

Although most of the HIV virus is replicating in lymph nodes and not in the blood, a determination of the number of helper T lymphocytes in the blood allows one to estimate the extent of damage to the immune system. Normally, there are from about 800 to 1200 helper T (CD4+) lymphocytes per microliter of blood, but this number declines progressively as the disease advances. When this number falls to about 500 cells per microliter of blood, the patient becomes at risk of opportunistic infections and, by the time the helper T lymphocyte count falls below 200 per microliter, the infected person is at very high risk of major complications from the disease. It is also possible to monitor the progression of the infection by measuring the amount of virus in the circulation.

In the past, it was customary to assess the extent of damage to the helper T lymphocyte population by expressing the ratio of helper T cells (which are CD4+) to suppressor T cells (which are CD8+). Because the proper function of the immune system depends on the correct balance between helper and suppressor T cells (described in chapter 3), the loss of helper T cells leads to a relative excess of suppressor T cells, which inhibit cell-mediated immunity. Humoral immunity, which depends on B lymphocyte function, is not significantly impaired.

Complications of AIDS

The impaired cell-mediated immunity leads to two very serious problems: a greatly increased susceptibility to infection and a predisposition to various malignant tumors. One or both of these complications eventually proves fatal to most patients.

Infections

Many of the viruses, fungi, parasites, and other pathogens that attack AIDS patients do not usually cause disease in healthy persons. (Infections of this type are often called *opportunistic infections* because the pathogens normally do not have an *opportunity* to cause serious disease in persons whose immune systems are intact.) One of the most common AIDS-related opportunistic infections is pneumonia caused by the protozoan parasite *Pneumocystis carinii* (described in chapter 15). Another relatively common and often fatal systemic infection is caused by a normally nonpathogenic acid-fast bacterium called *Mycobacterium avium-intracellulare.*

AIDS patients are also at risk for acquiring widespread, rapidly progressive tuberculosis or histoplasmosis, infections that normally are held in check by persons with normal immune systems. Many of the symptoms exhibited by patients with AIDS such as fever, cough, shortness of breath, weight loss, and enlarged lymph nodes are the result of the severe infections that afflict these unfortunate individuals. Table 8–3 lists some of the more common, severe, and often life-threatening infections in AIDS patients.

TABLE 8–3 Common infections in AIDS patients	Viruses	Herpes, cytomegalovirus, Epstein-Barr virus (infectious mononucleosis)
	Fungi	Histoplasmosis, coccidioidomycosis, aspergillosis, candida infections
	Protozoa	*Pneumocystis carinii* pneumonia, amebiasis, cryptosporidiosis
	Mycobacteria	Tuberculosis, *Mycobacterium avium-intracellulare* infections

Malignant Tumors

The malignant tumors common in AIDS patients also are related to failure of the immune system, which helps to protect persons from tumors as well as infections (described in chapter 10). The most common malignant tumor in AIDS patients, which is rare in other persons, is *Kaposi's sarcoma*. This tumor, which is composed of immature connective-tissue cells (fibroblasts) and blood capillaries intermixed with inflammatory and phagocytic cells, forms hemorrhagic nodules in the skin, mouth, lymph nodes, and internal organs (figure 8–6). Malignant tumors of B lymphocytes also are common, as are cancers of the mouth, rectum, and uterine cervix.

Prevalence of HIV Infection and AIDS in High-Risk Groups

The distribution of AIDS cases among the various high-risk groups is indicated in table 8–4. Most AIDS cases are found in homosexual or bisexual males and intravenous drug abusers, and these two groups make up about 87 percent of all AIDS cases. Heterosexual contacts of HIV-infected persons make up another 6 percent of the total. Persons with hemophilia who received antihemophiliac globulin, persons who received a blood transfusion, and persons with other sources of infection make up the balance. The percentages of asymptomatic HIV-positive infected persons in these groups are similar to the percentages of AIDS patients in these groups, as would be expected. There are, however, regional variations in the prevalence of HIV infections among these various risk groups. For example, in San Francisco, which has a large homosexual population, about 68 percent of HIV-positive persons are male homosexuals, whereas only 9 percent are heterosexual intravenous drug abusers. In contrast, the largest group of HIV-infected persons in New York City consists of intravenous drug abusers, with a correspondingly much lower number of infected male homosexuals.

There are also some striking ethnic differences in the prevalence of HIV infections and AIDS. There is a disproportionately large number of AIDS cases in minority groups. African Americans and Hispanics comprise about 23 percent of the U.S. population, but they account for about 50 percent of all AIDS cases.

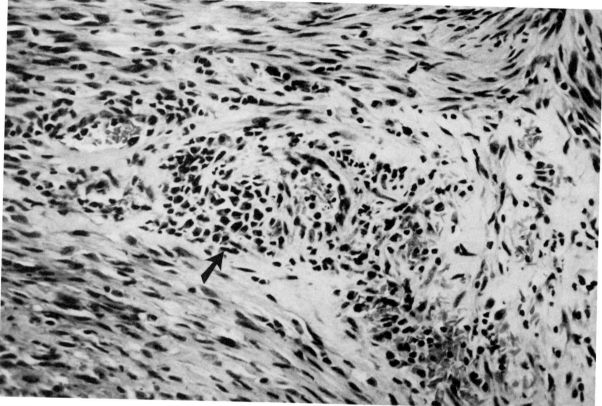

FIGURE 8–6

Kaposi's sarcoma, illustrating proliferating, spindle-shaped, immature connective-tissue cells (fibroblasts). A cluster of lymphocytes and plasma cells (*arrow*) occupies the center of the field. (Original magnification × 100.)

Transmission of the virus is by means of virus-infected blood and body fluids, and the virus is primarily contained within infected lymphocytes and monocytes in the fluids, rather than floating freely as extracellular virus particles. The amount of virus in body fluids varies with the stage of the disease and the source of the body fluids. Blood, seminal fluid, cervical and vaginal secretions, and breast milk generally contain large amounts of virus and are considered quite infectious, whereas urine, stool, saliva, tears, and perspiration contain little virus and are not highly infectious. Transmission of the virus is usually either by sexual contact or by means of infected blood or blood products, but the virus may also be passed from an infected mother to her newborn infant.

Sexual Transmission   Among male homosexuals and bisexuals, transmission of the virus is chiefly by anal intercourse, which injures anal tissues and permits intermixing of infected blood and seminal fluid. Heterosexual

TABLE 8–4

Distribution of AIDS cases by risk group

Risk group	Percentage of total AIDS cases
Homosexual and bisexual men	58
Homosexual and bisexual men who are also IV drug abusers	6
Heterosexual drug abusers	23
Heterosexual contacts of HIV infected persons	6
Hemophiliacs	1
Blood transfusion recipients	2
Other sources of infection	4

Source: H. Fan, R. F. Conner, and L. P. Villarreal. 1994. *The Biology of AIDS,* 3rd ed. Boston: Jones and Bartlett Publishers.

partners of infected persons become infected by sexual intercourse, because semen of infected males and vaginal secretions of infected women contain the virus. Many prostitutes of both sexes are infected, either from drug abuse or sexual contacts, and sexual contacts with prostitutes are very risky. Many Haitians of both sexes, as well as persons from central Africa, are infected. In these countries, the infection is transmitted chiefly by heterosexual intercourse, and both sexes are equally affected.

Transmission by Blood and Blood Products   Intravenous drug abusers become infected by sharing needles and syringes contaminated with blood from an infected person. Hemophiliacs acquired the infection from blood products administered to treat their coagulation defect. Transfusion recipients were infected from contaminated blood received before laboratory tests were available to screen donors for evidence of infection.

Mother-to-Infant Transmission   Infected maternal blood or cervical-vaginal secretions are the source of infection of newborn infants born to infected mothers. The infection may occur during the pregnancy, during labor and delivery, or soon after birth, and about 30 percent of infants born to HIV-infected mothers also are infected. The infected mother is also put at additional risk by the pregnancy. Pregnancy normally is associated with suppression of cell-mediated immunity, and pregnancy seems to increase the likelihood of an asymptomatic maternal HIV infection progressing to AIDS within a few years after delivery. Preliminary data suggest that treatment of an HIV-infected mother during pregnancy with Zidovudine (AZT), which inhibits viral replication, reduces the risk that the infant will become infected. However, we do not yet know whether the Zidovudine taken during pregnancy will have any adverse effects on the growth and development of the infants born to these mothers.

1. Homosexual or bisexual men
2. Present or past intravenous drug abusers
3. Persons with clinical or laboratory evidence of AIDS virus infection
4. Persons born in countries where heterosexual transmission plays the major role in spreading the infection
5. Male or female prostitutes and their sexual partners
6. Sexual partners of infected persons
7. Persons with hemophilia who have received blood products
8. Newborn infants of infected or high-risk mothers

TABLE 8–5

Groups at high risk of immunodeficiency virus infection

Prevention and Control of HIV Infection

Individuals infected with the virus are at risk of late complications, which eventually occur in a significant number of persons. Infections and tumors in AIDS patients can be treated, but treatment of the underlying viral infection has been hampered by lack of a drug that can eliminate the virus. Several drugs are available that can impede viral replication and slow the progression of the disease. Much effort is being directed toward finding ways to control or eradicate the virus, and toward developing a vaccine to immunize against the virus, but at present there are no major breakthroughs on the horizon. The only really effective way to control the disease is to prevent further spread of the infection. This means that each individual must assume responsibility for his or her own behavior if the relentless spread of the disease is to be contained.

1. Uninfected persons should avoid sexual contacts with persons in high-risk groups or known to be infected with the virus (table 8–5).
2. Members of high-risk groups should limit their number of sexual partners, practice "safe sex," which requires the use of condoms to reduce the risk of transmitting the infection, and avoid sexual practices such as unprotected anal intercourse and oral-genital contact, which can spread the virus.
3. Persons at high risk of infection should not donate blood, in order to prevent transmission of the virus by blood transfusion. Blood banks now screen donor blood for antibodies to the AIDS virus (as well as the hepatitis virus) and reject the blood for transfusion if antibodies are detected. The screening tests, however, will not reliably exclude all infected donors, because some persons who have been recently infected may not have yet formed antibodies.
4. Infected women should avoid pregnancy, which increases their risk of AIDS and often leads to the birth of an infected infant.

Case Studies

The following cases illustrate some of the clinical features and medical problems encountered in AIDS patients.

CASE 8–1

A thirty-eight-year-old homosexual man consulted his physician because of recent onset of fatigue, weakness, and shortness of breath that had progressed to such an extent that he was barely able to get out of bed without feeling exhausted. He had had multiple sexual partners in the preceding seven years but was not aware of any health problems in his partners. He had been married but was divorced about twelve years ago and has one daughter who lives with his former wife.

Chest x-ray revealed patches of pneumonia throughout both lungs and a blood test revealed antibodies to the AIDS virus. A number of diagnostic possibilities were considered, including mycoplasmal, chlamydial, or Legionella pneumonia. Because of the patient's homosexuality and positive antibody test, an opportunistic lung infection was considered likely. A small biopsy of lung tissue obtained by means of a bronchoscope was interpreted as *Pneumocystis carinii* pneumonia. The patient was treated with appropriate antibiotics but did not improve significantly, and he acquired additional infections and other complications while in the hospital. After a four-month hospitalization, the patient was cared for at home, where he eventually died.

In this case, pulmonary infection in a homosexual male with a positive antibody test for the AIDS virus suggested pneumocystis pneumonia as a likely possibility, which was confirmed by lung biopsy. This is the most common opportunistic infection in AIDS patients and has a high mortality.

CASE 8–2

A sixty-two-year-old woman, whose husband has hemophilia and had been treated with antihemophiliac globulin, was hospitalized because of low-grade fever, cough, sweating, and a thirty-five-pound weight loss over the previous six weeks. Chest x-ray revealed a bilateral pneumonia. A blood test for antibodies to the AIDS virus was positive, and lung biopsy obtained by bronchoscopy revealed Pneumocystis carinii pneumonia. The patient was treated with appropriate antibiotics but did not respond and died in the hospital three weeks after admission.

This patient had been infected with the AIDS virus through sexual intercourse with her husband, who had become infected previously from blood products used to treat his hemophilia. Although the husband had no symptoms of infection, his wife developed AIDS and died of pneumocystis pneumonia, the most common opportunistic infection in AIDS patients.

CASE 8–3

A thirty-year-old, married homosexual male with a positive antibody test for the AIDS virus and an abnormally low helper/suppressor T lymphocyte ratio had been intermittently ill for the past several years. On previous occasions, he consulted his physician because of fever and weakness, diarrhea, and oral Candida infections. Recently, he was treated for an opportunistic pulmonary infection caused by a gram-negative bacteria (Pseudomonas), which responded to antibiotics. Because of these numerous problems, he had been diagnosed as having AIDS-related complex.

Recently, the patient experienced recurrent fever, fatigue, and weight loss. Physical examination revealed many large lymph nodes in the neck, armpits, and groin. A chest x-ray revealed no evidence of pneumonia.

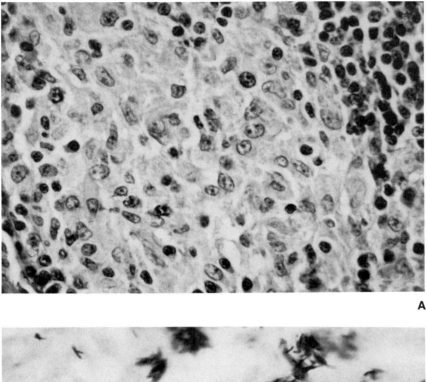

A

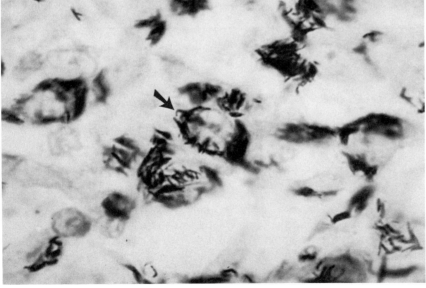

B

FIGURE 8–7

Disseminated *Mycobacterium avium-intracellulare* infection (case 8–3). **A,** Lymph node illustrating clusters of large mononuclear phagocytes (pale staining cells in center of field) surrounded by normal lymphocytes (small dark cells). (Original magnification × 400.) **B,** Acid-fast organisms demonstrated in lymph node by special stains. Nucleus of mononuclear phagocyte (*arrow*) surrounded by masses of organisms in the cytoplasm appears in center of field. Large clumps of organisms fill the cytoplasm of other phagocytes in the field, obscuring the nuclei of the cells (case 8–3).

The lymph node enlargement suggested the possibility of an infection or malignant tumor (B cell lymphoma) involving the lymph nodes. A lymph node biopsy revealed large numbers of mononuclear phagocytic cells filling the lymph node. Special stains revealed that the phagocytes were packed with acid-fast organisms (figure 8–7). Biopsy of the bone marrow revealed similar focal clusters of mononuclear cells within the marrow, and marrow culture yielded Mycobacterium avium-intracellulare. Treatment with appropriate antibiotics was instituted but had little effect on the course of his infection. His prognosis for eventual recovery was poor.

This patient's infection slowly progressed from AIDS-related complex to AIDS, and he developed a disseminated opportunistic infection caused by a normally nonpathogenic acid-fast bacterium.

CASE 8–4

A thirty-nine-year-old homosexual male with multiple sexual partners and a positive test for antibodies to the AIDS virus had been treated on several occasions for Candida infections of the mouth and intermittent chronic diarrhea. Recently, he developed a red vascular nodule in his oral cavity that was biopsied and interpreted as Kaposi's sarcoma. The implications of this diagnosis were explained to the patient, and he was advised of the precautions necessary to prevent spread of the AIDS virus infection to others. He was referred to another physician for further treatment.

Questions for Review

1. How are communicable diseases transmitted? How are they controlled?

2. What is meant by the following terms: *epidemic disease, endemic disease, immunization, sexually transmitted disease?*

3. How is syphilis transmitted? What are its clinical manifestations?

4. How is gonorrhea transmitted? What are its clinical manifestations? What is nongonococcal urethritis?

5. What are the manifestations of herpes infection of the genital tract?

6. What are the manifestations of chlamydial infection of the genital tract? How are chlamydial infections diagnosed and treated?

7. What is AIDS? What is its cause? What are its clinical manifestations? What groups are at high risk of infection and how do they become infected? How can spread of the infection be prevented or minimized?

8. What is the significance of a positive test for antibody to the human immunodeficiency (AIDS) virus?

Supplementary Readings

Centers for Disease Control and Prevention. 1993. 1993 Sexually transmitted diseases treatment guidelines. *Morbidity and Mortality Weekly Report* 42:1–102. A detailed reference to the diagnosis and management of sexually transmitted diseases.

Centers for Disease Control and Prevention. 1994. Birth outcomes following Zidovudine therapy in pregnant women. *Morbidity and Mortality Weekly Report* 43:409–16. Preliminary studies do not indicate an increase or unusual pattern of birth defects in infants of treated HIV-infected mothers.

Centers for Disease Control and Prevention. 1994. Zidovudine for the prevention of HIV transmission from mother to infant. *Morbidity and Mortality Weekly Report* 43:285–87. Zidovudine given to HIV-infected mothers reduced the frequency of infections in the infants. Long-term side effects of treatment are unknown.

Centers for Disease Control and Prevention. 1994. Human immunodeficiency virus transmission in household settings: United States. *Morbidity and Mortality Weekly Report* 43:347–56. The report documents two persons who developed HIV infections from caring for HIV-infected family members.

Centers for Disease Control and Prevention. 1995. First 500,000 AIDS cases: United States 1995. *Morbidity and Mortality Weekly Report* 44:849–53. As of October 31, 1995, 501,310 persons with AIDS have been reported to the Centers for Disease Control and 62 percent have died. Proportion among women has increased to 18 percent in past two years. Proportion among blacks has increased from 25 percent to 38 percent; among Hispanics, from 14 percent to 18 percent. During 1994, the number of AIDS-infected persons per 100,000 population was 101 for blacks, 51 for Hispanics, 17 for whites, 12 for American Indians and Alaskan natives, and 6 for Asians.

Centers for Disease Control and Prevention. 1995. U.S. Public Health Service recommendations for human immunodeficiency virus counseling and voluntary testing of pregnant women. *Morbidity and Mortality Weekly Report* 44 (No. RR-7):1–15. All pregnant women should be counseled and encouraged to be tested for HIV infection both for their own sakes and to reduce the risk of prenatal HIV transmission.

Centers for Disease Control and Prevention. 1995. USPHS/IDSA guidelines for prevention of opportunistic infections in persons infected with human immunodeficiency virus: A summary. *Morbidity and Mortality Weekly Report* 44 (No. RR-8):1–34. Describes current recommendations for preventing exposure, prevention of diseases, and prevention of recurrences of opportunistic infections in HIV-infected persons.

Cooper, D. A., Maclean P., and Finlayson, R. 1985. Acute AIDS retrovirus infection: Definition of a clinical illness associated with seroconversion. *Lancet* 1:537–40. Describes clinical features of acute infectious mononucleosis-like illness caused by the AIDS virus.

Corey, L. 1985. Genital herpes virus infection: Viral shedding during remission. *Journal of the American Medical Association* 254:2147–48. About 1 percent of women have asymptomatic herpes infection of cervix or vulva or both, which may become activated periodically and cause recurrent lesions.

Corey, L. 1985. The natural history of genital herpes. In *The Herpes Virus*. Ed. B. Roizman. Vol. 4, pp. 1–36. New York: Plenum Press. A review article.

Fan, H., Conner, R. F., and Villarreal, L. P. 1994. *The biology of AIDS*. 3d ed. Boston: Jones and Bartlett Publishers. A well-written survey of current knowledge on this subject.

Greene, J. B., et al. 1982. *Mycobacterium avium-intracellulare:* A cause of disseminated life threatening infection in homosexuals and drug abusers. *Annals of Internal Medicine* 97:539–46. Systemic infections as a result of normally nonpathogenic *Mycobacterium* may occur in persons with AIDS and are resistant to most commonly used antimycobacterial drugs.

Greene, W. C. 1993. AIDS and the immune system. In *Scientific American* (September Issue): 99–105. A detailed presentation.

Handsfield, H. H., et al. 1986. Criteria for selective screening for *Chlamydia trachomatis* infection in women attending family planning clinics. *Journal of the American Medical Association* 255:1730–34. Chlamydia was isolated from the cervix of 9.3 percent of women attending family planning clinics. Screening of sexually active women for chlamydia infection strongly recommended.

Kaplan, J. E., Masur, H., Jaffe, H. W., and Holmes, K. K. 1995. Reducing the impact of opportunistic infections in patients with HIV infection: New guidelines. *Journal of the American Medical Association* 274:347–48. One million in this country are infected and 250,000 have severe immunosuppression as measured by CD4+ lymphocyte counts. The various measures to prevent and control opportunistic infections are discussed.

McArthur, J. C. 1987. Neurologic manifestations of AIDS. *Medicine* 66:407–37. Reviews the neurologic complications in 186 patients with HIV infection and biologic properties of the human immunodeficiency virus.

Rooney, J. F., Felser, J. M., Ostrove, J. M., et al. 1986. Acquisition of genital herpes from an asymptomatic sexual partner. *New England Journal of Medicine* 314:1561–64.

Stone, K. M., Grimes, D. A., and Magder, L. S. 1986. Primary prevention of sexually transmitted diseases. *Journal of the American Medical Association* 255:1763–66. Persons at risk for sexually transmitted diseases should modify their sexual behavior and should use barrier methods and spermicides in order to protect themselves.

Chapter 8 ▪ Outline Summary

Methods of Transmission / 161
Direct: Physical contact or droplet spread.

Indirect: Contaminated food or water; insects.

Methods of Control / 161
Immunization
Renders population nonsusceptible.

Disease incidence declines or disease dies out because no susceptible host.

Identification, Isolation, and Treatment of Infected Persons
Identification shortens time of infectivity.

Isolation often not effective because infected persons not recognized.

Control of Means of Indirect Transmission
Control of food and water supplies.

Control of food handlers.

Control of insect population.

Control of animal sources.

Requirements for Effective Control
Know cause.

Know method of transmission.

Sexually Transmitted Diseases / 163
Syphilis
Primary stage: chancre at site of infection will eventually heal without treatment.

Secondary stage:

Follows primary after several months.

Characterized by fever, rash, and large lymph nodes.

Subsides without treatment.

Tertiary stage: late destructive lesions in nervous system and heart.

Congenital:

Acquired by newborn infant of infected mother.

May cause fetal death or live-born infected infant.

Treatment of mother early in pregnancy prevents fetal infection.

Gonorrhea
A surface infection of mucous membranes: genital tract, rectum, pharynx.

May spread to upper genital tract in both sexes.

Extragenital gonorrhea occurs frequently.

Occasional systemic infection affects joints, skin, heart valves, brain.

Herpes
Clinical features:

May be caused by either type I or type II herpes virus.

Causes vesicles that form ulcers in genital tract.

Recurrences occur frequently.

No specific treatment.

Diagnosis of herpes:

By clinical features.

Smears reveal inclusions.

Virus cultured from lesions.

Serologic tests reveal antibodies.

Herpes in pregnancy: may infect infant during delivery. Rarely causes intrauterine infection leading to congenital abnormalities.

Herpes and cervical cancer: increased incidence in women with evidence of previous herpes infection.

Chlamydial Infections
Clinical features:

Most common sexually transmitted disease.

Many patients asymptomatic.

Infects uterine cervix. May spread to fallopian tubes followed by scarring and impaired fertility.

Causes nongonococcal urethritis in men; may spread to cause epididymitis.

Diagnosis and treatment:

Rapid tests detect chlamydial antigens in infected secretions.

Chlamydia can be demonstrated in specially stained smears of secretions by microscopy.

Cultures available but expensive, time consuming, and not widely available.

Infection responds to antibiotics.

Human Immunodeficiency Virus Infections and AIDS
Nature of the disease:

Virus cripples immune system.

AIDS is most devastating manifestation of infection.

Asymptomatic or milder infections in many persons.

Effect of the virus on T cells:

RNA virus invades helper T lymphocytes and monocytes.

Virus makes DNA copy of its own RNA genetic material.

Viral DNA copy inserted into DNA of infected cell and directs production of virus particles in cell.

Virus buds from cell and infects other helper T lymphocytes.

Virus particles appear in blood and body fluids, which are infectious to others.

Antibody response to virus:

Antibodies formed within one to six months.

Antibodies are evidence of infection but do not eradicate virus.

Early manifestations of infection:

Most have no symptoms initially.

Some have brief illness resembling infectious mononucleosis.

Late manifestations of infection: AIDS-related complex and AIDS

AIDS-related complex:

Generalized lymph node enlargement.

Nonspecific symptoms: fever, weakness, fatigue, weight loss.

AIDS:

Pathogenesis:

Destruction of helper T cells with relative excess suppressor T cells.

Reversed helper/suppressor ratio.

Impaired cell-mediated immune defenses.

Humoral immunity relatively unaffected.

Complications of AIDS:

Infections:

Opportunistic infections—Pneumocystis carinii, Mycobacterium avium-intracellulare, and others.

Widespread infections caused by organisms usually controlled by normal persons.

Malignant tumors:

Kaposi's sarcoma.

Malignant tumors of B lymphocytes.

Cancers of oral cavity and rectum.

AIDS in high-risk groups:

Homosexual/bisexual males.

Intravenous drug abusers.

Hemophiliacs.

Heterosexual partners of infected persons.

Children born to infected mothers.

Small percentage of infected persons do not fit into high-risk groups.

Manner of virus transmission in high-risk groups:

Sexual contact:

Primarily anal intercourse and oral-genital contact in homosexuals or bisexuals.

Heterosexual partners of infected persons infected by sexual intercourse.

Prostitutes frequently infected.

Spread primarily by heterosexual contacts in Haiti and central Africa. Both sexes equally infected.

Blood and blood products:

Intravenous drug abusers infected by contaminated needles and syringes.

Hemophiliacs infected from blood products.

Transfusion recipients infected from blood prior to routine screening of blood for AIDS virus.

Mother-to-infant transmission:

Infected maternal blood and/or cervicovaginal secretions infect newborn.

Mother at increased risk of AIDS-related complex of AIDS from pregnancy.

Prevention and control of immunodeficiency virus infection:

Avoid sexual contact with high-risk persons.

High-risk groups should practice "safe sex" and limit number of sexual partners.

High-risk groups should not donate blood, because screening tests to exclude infected blood cannot detect infected persons who have not yet formed antibody to virus.

Infected women should avoid pregnancy.

9

Congenital and Hereditary Diseases

Learning Objectives

1. List the common causes of congenital malformations and their approximate incidence.
2. List four abnormalities of sex chromosomes and describe their clinical manifestations.
3. Describe some of the common genetic abnormalities and explain four methods of transmission.
4. Compare the methods of transmission and clinical manifestations of phenylketonuria and hemophilia.
5. Describe some of the more important malformations resulting from intrauterine injury.
6. Explain the process of amniocentesis.
7. Explain multifactorial inheritance. Give an example of a multifactorial defect and describe the relevant factors.
8. List the causes of Down syndrome and describe its clinical manifestations. Give reasons why it is important to identify a carrier of a 14/21 chromosome translocation.
9. Understand the various methods available to make a diagnosis of a congenital abnormality in the fetus.

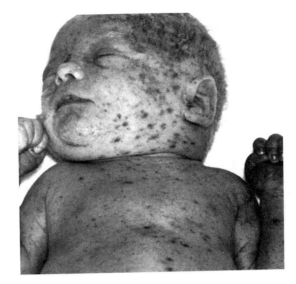

Chapter 9 ▪ Contents

There are many congenital and hereditary diseases. Their clinical manifestations range from minor inconsequential defects to severe malformations that are incompatible with extrauterine life. A *hereditary* or *genetic* disease may be defined as one resulting from a chromosome abnormality or a defective gene. The term **congenital** disease or malformation refers to any abnormality that is present at birth (*congenitus* = with birth), even though it may not be detected until some time after birth; this broad category encompasses all abnormalities caused by disturbed prenatal development, regardless of their nature. Congenital defects are recognized in about 2 to 3 percent of all newborn infants. In an additional 2 to 3 percent, developmental defects are not recognized at birth but become apparent as the infants grow older. Major malformations are also found in from 25 to 50 percent of spontaneously aborted embryos and fetuses and in stillborn infants.

Four major factors are known to induce congenital malformations:

1. Chromosomal abnormalities
2. Abnormalities of individual genes
3. Intrauterine injury to the embryo or fetus by drugs, radiation, maternal infection, or other harmful environmental factors
4. Environmental factors acting on a genetically predisposed embryo

Chromosomal Abnormalities

Occasionally, homologous chromosomes in germ cells fail to separate from one another in either the first or the second meiotic division. This is called *nondisjunction.* It causes abnormalities in the distribution of chromosomes between germ cells (figure 9–1). One of the two germ cells derived from the abnormal chromosome division has an extra chromosome, and the other cell lacks a chromosome. Nondisjunction may involve either the sex chromosomes or the autosomes. If it occurs during gametogenesis, one daughter cell will have twenty-four chromosomes and the other will have twenty-two. If a gamete having an abnormal number of chromosomes fuses with a normal gamete during fertilization, the resulting zygote will either have an extra chromosome or be lacking one of the homologous pair of chromosomes. The presence of an extra chromosome in a cell is called a **trisomy** (*tri* = three + *soma* = body) of the chromosome present in triplicate. Absence of a chromosome is called a **monosomy** (*mono* = one) of the missing chromosome.

Sometimes a chromosome breaks in the course of meiosis, and the broken piece is lost from the cell. This is called a *chromosome deletion.* In some cases, the broken piece is not lost but becomes attached to another nonhomologous chromosome with which it is carried along during meiosis. A misplaced chromosome or part of a chromosome attached to another chromosome is called a **translocation** (*trans* = across + *locus* = place). In *reciprocal translocation,* pieces of chromosomes (containing different sets of genes) are reciprocally exchanged between two nonhomologous chromosomes. Such an accident does not disturb the function of the cell, because there is no loss or gain of genetic material. However, if the translocation occurs in a germ cell, an egg or sperm containing either a deficiency or an excess of

FIGURE 9–1

Effects of nondisjunction in meiosis, leading to formation of gametes with an extra or missing chromosome. Only the chromosome pair involved in nondisjunction is illustrated.
Left, Nondisjunction at second meiotic division.
Right, Nondisjunction at first meiotic division.

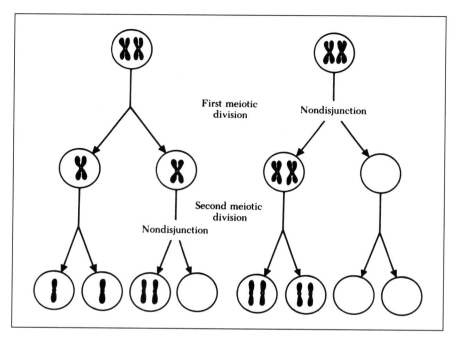

chromosomal material may form during meiosis. If such a chromosomally abnormal gamete unites with a normal gamete during fertilization, the fertilized ovum (*zygote*) contains an abnormal amount of chromosomal material. Many abnormal zygotes are spontaneously aborted, but some survive and give rise to defective fetuses, as illustrated by the following case from the medical literature.

CASE 9–1

A mother gave birth to an infant with multiple congenital abnormalities and had two subsequent pregnancies. Both terminated in spontaneous abortions about eight weeks after conception. Chromosome studies were performed on both parents, the liveborn infant, and the two aborted fetuses. The mother's karyotype was normal. The father's karyotype revealed that a piece of one chromosome 7 had been translocated to chromosome 21. In the offspring with the congenital abnormalities, one chromosome 21 was normal. The other chromosome 21 was abnormal, containing a translocated piece of chromosome 7 that had been transmitted from the father. The karyotypes of both aborted fetuses also were abnormal and were similar. One chromosome 7 was normal, but the other was lacking a piece of chromosome material. This abnormal chromosome also had been transmitted from the father.

In this case, the father was the carrier of a chromosomal abnormality that did not disturb the function of his own cells because all the genetic material was normal. However, it did result in the formation of chromosomally abnormal gametes, which led to spontaneous abortions and congenital abnormalities in the offspring. When the father's chromosomes separated and were distributed to the sperm in meiosis, the sperm could contain any of the following possible combinations of chromosomes 7 and 21 (figure 9–2):

1. Figure 9–2A: Normal chromosomes 7 and 21 (normal chromosomes and normal genetic material)
2. Figure 9–2B: Normal chromosome 7 with chromosome 21 containing the translocated piece (excess genetic material)
3. Figure 9–2C: Deficient chromosome 7, with normal chromosome 21 (deficient genetic material)
4. Figure 9–2D: Deficient chromosome 7 with chromosome 21 containing the translocated piece (abnormal chromosomes but normal genetic material)

In this case, the liveborn infant was derived from fertilization of a normal ovum by sperm B containing excess genetic material, and the two aborted fetuses resulted from fertilization of a normal ovum by sperm C lacking a normal complement of genetic material. The offspring probably would have been normal if the fertilization had been accomplished by chromosomally and genetically normal sperm A or by sperm D, which was chromosomally abnormal but contained a normal amount of genetic material. In the latter case, however, the offspring would be a carrier of the translocated chromosome like the father and would be capable of transmitting an abnormal component of genes to his or her own children. Such an individual is called a *translocation carrier.*

The literature contains many descriptions of clinical abnormalities that are associated with extra chromosomes, chromosome translocation, or loss of entire chromosomes or portions of chromosomes. Identification of chromosomal abnormalities is possible when the chromosomes are abnormal in size or configuration or when an abnormality is identified in the band pattern on the arms of the chromosomes.

Sex Chromosome Abnormalities

Variations from the normal number of sex chromosomes are often associated with some reduction of intelligence. The Y chromosome directs masculine sexual differentiation, and its presence is almost invariably associated with a male body configuration regardless of the number of X chromosomes present. An extra Y chromosome does not cause any significant changes in the appearance of the affected individual, because the Y chromosome carries little genetic material other than genes concerned with male sexual differentiation. If the Y chromosome is absent, the body configuration is female.

The effect of extra X chromosomes depends on the sex of the individual. The presence of one or more extra X chromosomes adversely affects masculine development but has very little effect on the female, because the additional X chromosomes are inactivated and appear as extra sex chromatin bodies attached to the nuclear membrane of the cell.

Several syndromes result from abnormalities in the number or structure of the sex chromosomes. The two most common that occur in the female are (1) *Turner's syndrome,* which usually results from an absence of one X chro-

FIGURE 9–2

Possible offspring produced when one parent is a carrier of a chromosome translocation, as described in case 9–1.

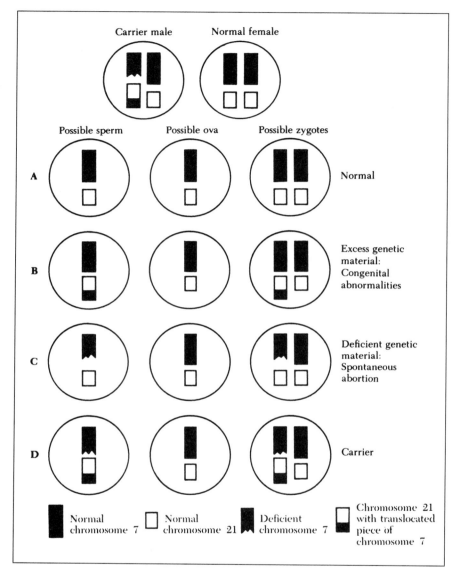

Carrier male   Normal female

Possible sperm   Possible ova   Possible zygotes

A — Normal

B — Excess genetic material: Congenital abnormalities

C — Deficient genetic material: Spontaneous abortion

D — Carrier

■ Normal chromosome 7 □ Normal chromosome 21 ■ Deficient chromosome 7 □ Chromosome 21 with translocated piece of chromosome 7

mosome (genotype XO), and (2) *triple X syndrome,* which results from an extra X chromosome (genotype XXX).

The two most common syndromes in the male are (1) *Klinefelter's syndrome,* which results from extra X chromosomes (usual genotype XXY), and (2) *XYY syndrome,* which results from an extra Y chromosome.

The principal characteristics of these syndromes are summarized in table 9–1.

TABLE 9–1

Syndromes resulting from an abnormal complement of sex chromosomes

	Usual genotype	Approximate incidence	Unusual number of Barr bodies	Usual number of Y fluorescent bodies	Fertility
Turner's syndrome	XO	1:2500 females	0	0	Sterile
Triple X syndrome	XXX	1:850 females	2	0	Usually not impaired
Klinefelter's syndrome	XXY	1:750 males	1	1	Usually sterile
XYY syndrome	XYY	1:850 males	0	2	Usually not impaired

Turner's Syndrome

Because most embryos of XO genotype are aborted spontaneously, Turner's syndrome occurs less often than some other sex chromosome abnormalities. The reported incidence of about 1 in 2500 female births represents only the very small proportion of XO embryos surviving to be born alive. Individuals of XO genotype are called sex-chromatin negative, because their cells lack sex chromatin (Barr) bodies. Figure 9–3 illustrates the appearance of a girl with Turner's syndrome. The body configuration is female but abnormal, and secondary sex characteristics have not developed. Characteristic features include short stature, broad neck with prominent lateral skin folds, broad chest lacking breast development, and widely spaced nipples. The uterus is small, and the ovaries consist only of bands of fibrous tissue. Sometimes congenital abnormalities of the cardiovascular system are also present.

Triple X Syndrome

The presence of an extra X chromosome in the cells of the female is a relatively common abnormality. It has an incidence of about 1 in 850 female births. Usually there are no specific abnormalities of body form because the extra X chromosome is inactivated and appears on the nuclear membrane of the cell as an extra sex chromatin (Barr) body. Sexual development is generally normal. Fertility and intelligence may be either normal or somewhat decreased.

Klinefelter's Syndrome

Having an incidence of about 1 in 750 male births, Klinefelter's syndrome results from the presence of extra X chromosomes in the male (usual genotype XXY). Figure 9–4 illustrates the characteristic appearance of a subject with this chromosomal abnormality. The external genital organs are male but the testicles are atrophic. Usually, no spermatozoa are produced and the individual is sterile. The body configuration is somewhat feminine, and

FIGURE 9–3

Child with Turner's syndrome, illustrating the broad neck resulting from prominent lateral skin folds, broad chest with widely spaced nipples, and short stature. Secondary sex characteristics do not develop. (Photograph courtesy of Dr. Jorge Yunis.)

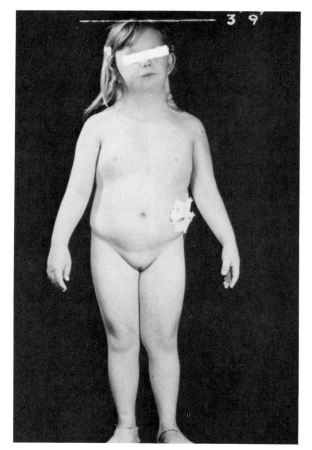

there may be moderate breast hypertrophy. Intelligence tends to be subnormal, but many men with Klinefelter's syndrome function reasonably well in society, and some are able to hold responsible positions. Because of the extra X chromosome, the cells contain a sex chromatin body (Barr body) as well as a Y fluorescent body.

XYY Syndrome

The sex chromosomal abnormality known as XYY syndrome has an incidence of about 1 in 850 male births. It may be associated with some reduction of fertility and intelligence. The individuals are usually taller than normal, but there are no specific abnormalities of body configuration. Some persons of this genotype exhibit aggressive and antisocial behavior.

The Fragile X Syndrome (X-Linked Mental Deficiency)

This condition, while not related to an excess or deficiency of a sex chromosome, is associated with a characteristic abnormality of the X chromosome. The condition is called the *fragile X syndrome* or *X-linked mental*

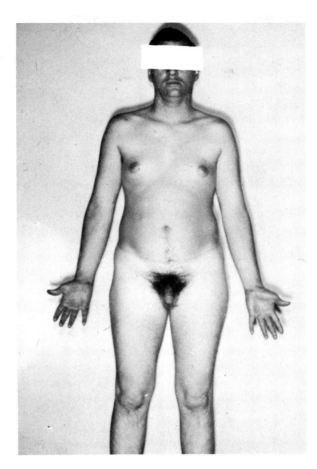

FIGURE 9–4

Characteristic appearance of a subject with Klinefelter's syndrome. This patient's body configuration is male, although there is slight hypertrophy of the breasts. (Photograph courtesy of Dr. Robert Gorlin.)

deficiency and is second only to Down syndrome as a major cause of mental deficiency. The X chromosome abnormality is a constricted area on the long arm of the chromosome near its tip, and so the tip of the long arm looks like a small round knob connected to the rest of the chromosome by a narrow stalklike constriction. The constricted area is quite fragile compared with the rest of the chromosome and is often broken in the course of preparing a chromosome karyotype, which is how the designation "fragile X chromosome" originated.

Molecular genetic studies of this part of the X chromosome have revealed that, in normal persons, the DNA chains in this region normally contain groups (sequences) of the three nucleotides cytosine-guanine-guanine arranged in that order from six to as many as about fifty times (CGG repeating sequences). In contrast, persons with fragile X syndrome have more than the normal number of repeating sequences. In some persons, the number of repeats is only slightly increased, whereas in other, more severely affected persons, the number of repeating CGG sequences may vary from 250 to 4000 or more. The large number of CGG repeats is apparently responsible for the constriction on the X chromosome and the fragility of this site in persons with the fragile X syndrome.

In general, the number of CGG repeats correlates roughly with the degree of mental retardation. Moreover, the number of CGG repeats in the fragile X tends to increase progressively, and the mental deficiency becomes progressively more pronounced, as the fragile X chromosome is passed from parent to offspring in successive generations.

Because the fragile X syndrome follows an X-linked pattern of inheritance, women carrying the fragile X can pass it to both daughters and sons, but men carrying it can pass it only to their daughters. The effect of the fragile X on the offspring depends on which parent transmitted it. When a woman transmits the fragile X, the number of CGG repeats in the transmitted X chromosome becomes greatly increased (amplified), and the degree of mental deficiency in the offspring who received the chromosome may be more marked than that of the mother who transmitted the fragile X. In contrast, when a man carrying the fragile X passes it to his daughter, the number of CGG repeating sequences in the fragile X that the daughter receives does not increase significantly, and the severity of the mental deficiency in the daughter may be no greater than that of the father. The reason why there is an amplification of the CGG repeats in the fragile X chromosome transmitted from the mother but not from the father is related to the behavior of the fragile X chromosome during gametogenesis. The amplification of the CGG sequences in the fragile X chromosome occurs during oogenesis, and the X chromosome with its amplified CGG sequences is in turn transmitted to the daughter. In the male, there is no comparable amplification of CGG repeats during spermatogenesis, and so the number of CGG repeats in the fragile X passed to the daughter does not increase as it does when the mother transmits the fragile X. We still do not understand how the number of repeating CGG sequences is related to the mental deficiency. Future molecular genetic studies should shed more light on this problem.

Autosomal Abnormalities

Absence of an autosome results in the loss of so many genes that development is generally not possible and the embryo is aborted. Deletion of a small part of an autosome may be compatible with development, but it usually results in multiple severe congenital abnormalities in the infant. The most common autosomal trisomy seen in newborn infants is that of the small chromosome 21, which causes *Down syndrome* (*mongolism*). Trisomy of a larger chromosome, such as chromosome 13 or chromosome 18, is less frequent and is associated with multiple severe congenital malformations. Trisomy of other large autosomes is almost invariably lethal.

Down Syndrome (Mongolism)

Down syndrome is the most common chromosomal abnormality, having an incidence of about one in six hundred births. It is characterized by mental deficiency and a characteristic facial expression caused by the upward-slanting eyes and the prominent skin folds extending from the base of the nose to the inner aspects of the eyebrows (figure 9–5). Other abnormalities of body form also are seen. Congenital cardiac malformations occur frequently, as do major congenital defects in other organ systems. The reported incidence of one in six hundred births represents only the proportion of abnormal fetuses surviving to term. About 70 percent of trisomy 21 fetuses are aborted early in pregnancy.

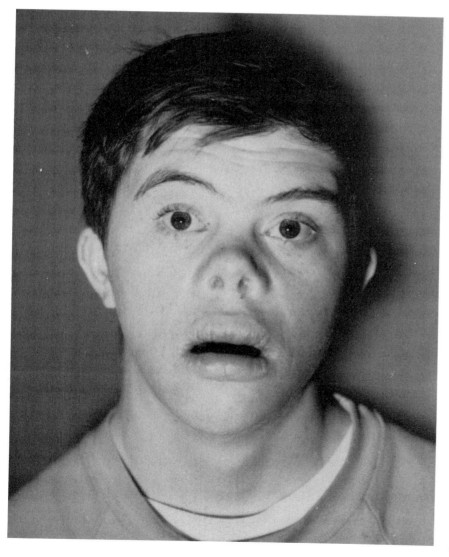

FIGURE 9–5

Young man with Down syndrome, illustrating characteristic facial appearance. (Photograph courtesy of Dr. J. Cervenka.)

Down syndrome may arise as a result of three possible conditions:

1. Nondisjunction during gametogenesis, leading to the formation of an abnormal gamete containing an extra chromosome 21
2. An extra chromosome 21 acquired as part of a translocation chromosome (*translocation Down syndrome*).
3. Nondisjunction occurring in the zygote

Nondisjunction during Gametogenesis   In about 95 percent of cases, Down syndrome results from nondisjunction of chromosome 21 during oogenesis, which causes the formation of an ovum containing an extra chromosome 21. Fertilization by a normal sperm produces a zygote containing forty-seven chromosomes, with chromosome 21 being present in triplicate. Down syndrome resulting from nondisjunction during oogenesis increases in frequency with advancing maternal age. The incidence is as high as one in fifty in the offspring of women over forty.

Translocation Down Syndrome   In a small number of persons with Down syndrome, the extra chromosome 21 is attached to another chromosome, usually chromosome 14. Although the total number of chromosomes is not decreased in these individuals, one of the chromosomes is actually a composite chromosome resulting from the fusion of chromosome 21 with another chromosome; so the affected person has genetic material that is equivalent to forty-seven chromosomes. Chromosome studies performed on the parents of children with translocation Down syndrome often reveal normal chromosomes in the cells of both parents. In these instances, the translocation apparently occurred as an accident in the germ cells of one parent during gametogenesis and is not present in other germ cells or in somatic cells. In other instances, the translocation chromosome can be identified in the karyotype of one of the parents, who is a carrier of the abnormal chromosome. The carrier parent has only forty-five chromosomes, because one chromosome is represented by a fusion of chromosome 21 with another chromosome.

The recognition of a translocation carrier is important, because the carrier is capable of transmitting the abnormal chromosome to his or her children, resulting in translocation Down syndrome. Figure 9–6 illustrates the possible outcome of a pregnancy involving a female carrier of a 14/21 translocation chromosome. As indicated, the ova of the carrier parent can possess any one of four chromosome types, depending upon how chromosomes 14 and 21 are distributed in the reduction divisions of the oocyte. Because there is only one chromosome 14 that can be distributed to the ovum independent of chromosome 21, an ovum can receive either the normal chromosome 14 (ova A and C) or the translocation chromosome (ova B and D). Because only one chromosome 21 can be distributed to the ovum (the other being carried with chromosome 14 as the translocation chromosome), some ova will receive the single chromosome 21 (ova A and D), but

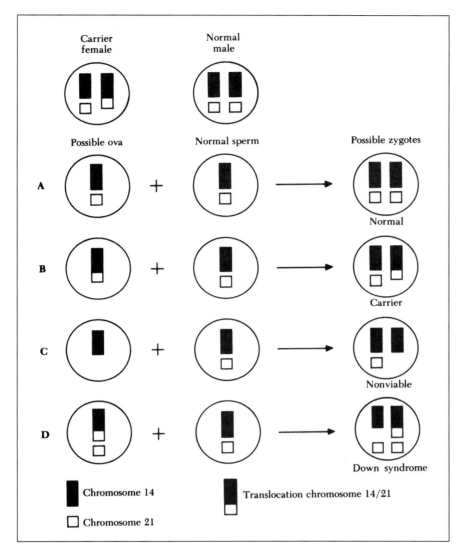

FIGURE 9–6

Possible ova produced by a female carrier of a 14/21 translocation chromosome and possible zygotes that could result from fertilization by normal sperm.

others will fail to receive this chromosome (ova B and C). The consequences of fertilization of these various possible ova by normal spermatozoa are indicated. In the first example (A), union of a normal ovum with a normal sperm produces a normal zygote containing forty-six chromosomes. In the second example (B), a zygote containing forty-five chromosomes results from fertilization, one chromosome being represented by the translocation chromosome. The individual derived from this zygote will be normal but will be a carrier of the translocation chromosome. In example C, the zygote lacks one chromosome 21 and is unable to survive. Fertilization of the ovum containing the translocation chromosome (example D) produces a zygote containing an excess of chromosome 21 material, resulting in a translocation Down syndrome.

Nondisjunction in the Zygote   In a few individuals with Down syndrome, only some of the cells exhibit the characteristic trisomy 21. Other cells have a normal component of chromosomes. This type of Down syndrome results from nondisjunction of chromosome 21 in a cell during the early divisions of the zygote. The cell in which nondisjunction occurs gives rise to one daughter cell lacking the chromosome. The cell monosomic for chromosome 21 fails to survive, but the trisomic cell continues to divide, forming more trisomic cells that multiply along with the normal cells of the zygote. As a result, the zygote eventually becomes composed of a population of normal cells and a population of trisomic cells (figure 9–7). A person composed of two or more types of cells containing different numbers of chromosomes is called a *chromosomal mosaic* or, simply, a *mosaic*. (A mosaic is a picture constructed of tiles or stones of different colors and shapes. By analogy, the term is also applied to persons who are "constructed" of different kinds of cells.) Individuals with mosaic Down syndrome suffer less disability than those in whom all the cells contain an extra chromosome 21.

Trisomy of Other Autosomes
Trisomy of chromosome 13 is associated with multiple severe developmental abnormalities, the most conspicuous being cleft lip and palate, abnormal development of the skull and brain, abnormal eye development, congenital

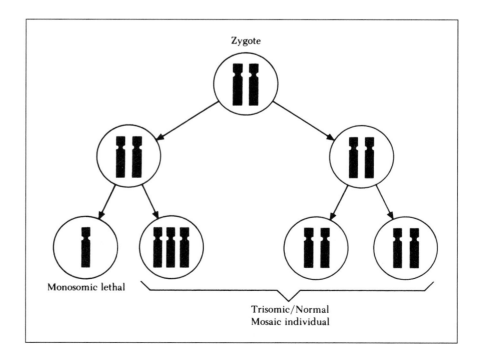

FIGURE 9–7

Pathogenesis of mosaic Down syndrome.

heart defects, and polydactyly (extra fingers and toes). Trisomy of chromosome 18 also is associated with multiple severe congenital malformations. Both chromosomal trisomies are usually fatal in the neonatal period or in early infancy.

Genetically determined diseases are the result of abnormalities of individual genes on the chromosome. The chromosomes themselves appear normal, and the chromosome karyotype is normal. Transmission of the abnormal gene is from parent to offspring, following the well-established patterns of inheritance described in chapter 3.

Genetically Determined Diseases

Genes direct many functions within the cell. Some genes direct the synthesis of proteins. These may be proteins that form the structure of the cell (*structural proteins*) or enzymes that are necessary for cell function. Other genes function by regulating the activity of the genes that direct protein synthesis. Normally, genes are stable and are passed without change from parent to offspring. Occasionally, a gene undergoes a change called a **gene mutation,** which may occur spontaneously or as a result of exposure to chemicals or radiation. Once a mutation has occurred in a germ cell, it can be transmitted from parent to offspring.

Sometimes a gene mutation that induces only a minor change in the structure of a protein may cause a serious change in its properties. For example, sickle hemoglobin (hemoglobin S) differs from normal hemoglobin (hemoglobin A) only in a single amino acid but undergoes crystallization within the red blood cell when the oxygen content of the blood is reduced.

If a mutation involves genes that control the synthesis of an enzyme, the enzyme may be defective and may lack functional activity. Metabolic processes regulated by the enzyme are disturbed, and the cell is unable to function normally.

The traditional diagnostic approach to genetic disease, based on the principles of *classic genetics,* is directed toward first identifying the abnormality in the patient, then identifying the gene product that is responsible for the disease, such as an abnormal hemoglobin or an enzyme deficiency, and finally attempting to identify the gene responsible for the abnormal gene product that caused the cell dysfunction. More recently, as a result of the many advances in recombinant DNA technology that were described in chapter 3, there has been a shift toward molecular genetics, in which one first identifies the mutant gene and determines how it differs from the normal gene, then determines the product of the gene, and finally evaluates how the abnormal gene and its gene product disrupt the functions of the cell. Because this method is the reverse of the classic genetic approach, it is often called *reverse genetics* and has lead to great advances in the prenatal diagnosis of many genetic diseases, as will be described later in the chapter.

Most hereditary diseases are transmitted on autosomes. A few are carried on sex chromosomes (table 9–2).

TABLE 9–2

Mode of inheritance, pathogenesis, and major manifestations of some common genetic diseases

Abnormality	Mode of inheritance	Defect	Manifestations
Phenylketonuria	Recessive	Phenylalanine hydroxylase deficiency	Mental retardation
Tay-Sachs disease	Recessive	Hexosaminidase A deficiency	Mental retardation, motor weakness, blindness
Cystic fibrosis of pancreas	Recessive	Dysfunction of mucous and sweat glands, thick mucus obstructs bronchioles, pancreatic ducts, and bile ducts	Chronic broncho-pulmonary infections as a result of bronchial obstruction by mucus; pancreatic and liver dysfunction as a result of thick mucous obstruction of excretory ducts
Achondroplasia	Dominant	Disordered bone growth at ends of long bones (epiphyses)	Dwarfism with disproportionately short limbs
Congenital polycystic kidney disease (one type)	Dominant	Maldevelopment of nephrons and collecting tubules causes formation of multiple cysts in kidneys	Renal failure
Multiple neuro-fibromatosis	Dominant	Multiple tumors arise from peripheral nerves	Disfigurement and deformities caused by tumors; predisposition to malignant change in tumors
Sickle cell trait	Codominant	Red cells contain mixture of normal (A) and sickle (S) hemoglobin	None
Sickle cell anemia	Codominant	Red cells contain no normal hemoglobin	Severe anemia and obstruction of blood flow to organs by masses of sickled red cells
Hemophilia	X-linked recessive	Deficiency of protein required for normal coagulation of blood	Uncontrolled bleeding into joints and internal organs following minor injuries

Autosomal Dominant Inheritance

A dominant gene expresses itself in the heterozygous state. If either parent carried an abnormal dominant gene, either the abnormal gene or the corresponding normal allele may be passed to the offspring. Consequently, there is one chance in two that the offspring will receive the abnormal gene and will be affected with the hereditary disease. A common example of a genetic disease transmitted in this manner is *achondroplasia,* a type of dwarfism in which the limbs are disproportionately short (described in chapter 27). A second example is one type of *congenital polycystic kidney disease,* which is characterized by the formation of multiple cysts throughout both kidneys that progressively enlarge and eventually destroy renal function (described in chapter 19). A third genetic disease of this type is *multiple neurofibromatosis,* a condition characterized by the formation of multiple tumors that arise from peripheral nerves (see chapter 26).

Autosomal Recessive Inheritance

A trait transmitted as an autosomal recessive is expressed only in the homozygous individual. Many diseases characterized by an enzyme deficiency within the cell are transmitted in this manner. The hereditary disease results only if both alleles are abnormal and no enzyme is produced. Therefore, in order for the offspring to be affected, both parents must carry the abnormal gene, and both must transmit the gene to the offspring. Consequently, when both parents carry an abnormal recessive gene, there is one chance in four that the mother will give birth to an abnormal infant who is homozygous for the defective gene. If only one parent transmits the recessive gene, the infant will be a carrier of the abnormal gene but will be normal because the normal allele will direct the synthesis of enough enzymes to keep the cell functioning normally. The many recognized types of genetically determined enzyme defects are sometimes called *inborn errors of metabolism.* Two of the more important ones are *phenylketonuria* and *Tay-Sachs disease.*

Phenylketonuria

A deficiency of the enzyme *phenylalanine hydroxylase,* which is required for normal metabolism of the amino acid phenylalanine, causes a disease called phenylketonuria. The enzyme deficiency causes no difficulty while the infant is still within the uterus being nourished by the mother. Soon after birth, however, the infant begins to drink milk. Because milk protein contains abundant phenylalanine, which the infant is unable to metabolize, this amino acid accumulates in the infant's blood and is excreted in the urine. The affected infant is able to convert some phenylalanine into phenylpyruvic acid (and other metabolites) by means of other metabolic pathways that do not require phenylalanine hydroxylase (figure 9–8). Phenylpyruvic acid accumulates in the blood and is excreted in the urine along with phenylalanine. Permanent mental deficiency results from the disturbed phenylalanine metabolism, but it can be prevented by restricting the dietary intake of phenylalanine.

FIGURE 9–8

Metabolic defects in phenylketonuria. Infants with this disorder lack the enzyme phenylalanine hydroxylase, and their bodies are unable to hydroxylate phenylalanine to form tyrosine. Some phenylalanine is converted into phenylpyruvic acid (substitution of a keto group for the amino group in the molecule) by other metabolic pathways. Permanent mental deficiency results from disturbed phenylalanine metabolism and can be prevented by restricting dietary intake of phenylalanine.

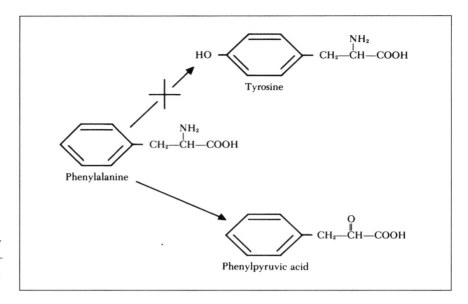

Phenylketonuria can be detected in the newborn infant by means of a screening laboratory test capable of detecting the elevated level of phenylalanine in the blood. It can be confirmed by more detailed testing to detect the presence of phenylpyruvic acid and other metabolites that also are derived from the disturbed metabolism of phenylalanine. This disease is a cause of preventable mental deficiency; thus a routine screening test to detect phenylketonuria is an important requirement for all newborn infants.

Tay-Sachs Disease

Tay-Sachs disease occurs primarily in the offspring of Jewish parents who carry the defective gene. The clinical manifestations result from absence of an enzyme called *hexosaminidase A*. The enzyme deficiency causes a type of lipid called a *ganglioside* to accumulate within the nerve cells of the brain, spinal cord, autonomic nervous system, and retina of the eye, causing cell dysfunction and, eventually, degeneration of the affected nerve cells. Clinically, the disease is characterized by progressive mental deterioration, neurologic dysfunction, and blindness. Onset of symptoms begins by about six months of age, and the disease is invariably fatal by the time the child is three or four years old.

Carriers of the abnormal gene can be detected by means of the low levels of hexosaminidase A in their serum and in their leukocytes. Tests for this enzyme can be used for screening. Surveys have indicated that the carrier rate is relatively high in some Jewish populations (those of Eastern European origin). In these groups, about one in thirty individuals carries the abnormal gene.

Tay-Sachs disease can be diagnosed prenatally by examination of fetal cells obtained by amniocentesis. The applications and limitations of this diagnostic procedure are described later in this chapter.

Other Genetic Diseases

Another relatively common and important genetic disease that is transmitted by autosomal recessive inheritance is called *cystic fibrosis of the pancreas.* The disease, manifested by dysfunction of mucous and sweat glands, is considered in chapter 22 in conjunction with diseases of the pancreas.

Codominant Inheritance

If both alleles of a pair are fully expressed in the heterozygous state, the genes are said to be *codominant.* This type of transmission is illustrated by the genes responsible for the synthesis of **sickle (S) hemoglobin** and other abnormal hemoglobins. These genes are alleles of the gene that directs the synthesis of normal (A) hemoglobin. An individual heterozygous for the sickle hemoglobin gene will have approximately equal quantities of sickle hemoglobin and normal hemoglobin in the red cells. This condition is called *sickle cell trait* and causes no difficulties. Significant clinical manifestations are apparent, however, if the individual is homozygous for the sickle cell gene, and no normal hemoglobin is formed. This leads to a serious hereditary anemia called *sickle cell anemia.* This subject is considered in chapter 14.

X-Linked Inheritance

A few hereditary diseases are transmitted on the X chromosome. *Hemophilia,* caused by a deficiency of a protein required for normal blood coagulation, is the best-known example (described in chapter 11). The female parent carries the defective gene on one of her X chromosomes and can transmit either the normal X chromosome or the one containing the defective gene to her offspring. The child will be born normal if the normal X chromosome is received. If the mother transmits the abnormal X chromosome, its effect depends on the sex of the offspring. A female child will appear normal because the defective gene on the X chromosome is paired with a normal allele on the other X chromosome. However, she will be a carrier of the abnormal gene and can transmit it to her own children. In contrast, a male child will have hemophilia. Because a male has only one X chromosome, he lacks the normal allele possessed by a female carrier. Consequently the abnormal X-linked gene functions like a dominant gene when paired with the Y chromosome.

The embryo or fetus may be injured by drugs, radiation, or an infection that disrupts prenatal development and leads to congenital malformations. The effects of the injury inflicted on the developing embryo vary, depending on the nature of the harmful agent and the stage of gestation. The embryonic period from the third to the eighth week after conception, when the organ systems are forming, is the time when the embryo is most vulnerable to the injurious effects of environmental agents.

Intrauterine Injury

Harmful Drugs and Chemicals

Many drugs are known to harm the developing embryo. The classic example is the tranquilizer thalidomide, which was widely used in Europe in the 1960s but was never marketed in the United States. The drug produced a highly characteristic malformation in which the bones of the extremities were much reduced or absent, the hands or feet arising from the trunk (figure 9–9). Either upper or lower limbs or all four extremities were affected, depending on the time when the drug was taken during pregnancy. In addition to causing limb defects, the drug also caused malformations of the heart, gastrointestinal tract, eyes, and ears. The correlation between thalidomide and congenital malformations was eventually determined because of the unusual type of limb malformations produced by the drug, but unfortunately not until thousands of infants had been damaged by this drug. The thalidomide tragedy clearly demonstrated to the medical profession the disastrous effects of a supposedly innocuous drug taken by a mother during a critical phase of embryonic development. Many other drugs, although less hazardous than thalidomide, may also cause congenital malformations. Currently, all drugs used in the United States are rated in five categories by the U.S. Food and Drug Admin-

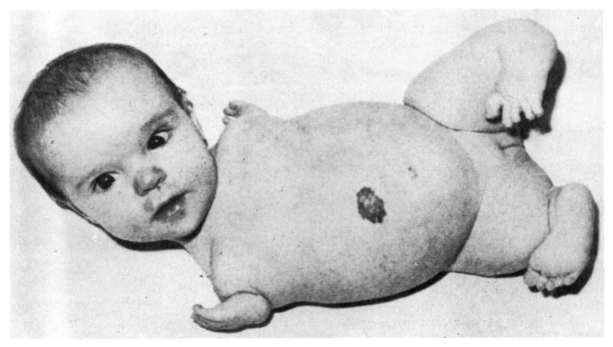

FIGURE 9–9

Characteristic limb deformities caused by thalidomide. (*From:* Tausig, H. B. 1962. Study of German outbreak of phocomelia: Thalidomide syndrome. *Journal of the American Medical Association* 180:1106–1114. Copyright 1962, American Medical Association. Used by permission.)

istration according to the degree of possible risk to the fetus balanced against the drug's potential benefit to the patient (table 9–3). Ratings range from "A" for drugs that are generally considered safe for use in pregnancy through "D" for drugs that may injure the fetus but are of enough benefit to the patient that the benefit of the drug to the patient outweighs the risk to the fetus. "X"-rated drugs are contraindicated in pregnancy because the severe risk to the fetus outweighs any possible benefit to the patient.

Even cigarettes, alcoholic beverages, and caffeine are not without risk. Cigarette smoking leads to retarded intrauterine growth with birth of smaller than normal infants and premature births. Heavy alcohol consumption during pregnancy can result in a characteristic pattern of developmental abnormalities called the *fetal alcohol syndrome*. Affected infants are both physically and mentally retarded, exhibit abnormal cranial and facial development, and often have other congenital malformations affecting the genital tract and cardiovascular system. Consequently, women with severe drinking problems should be cautioned not to become pregnant until their alcoholism is controlled. Even small amounts of alcohol may put the fetus at risk, and it is generally considered that it is unsafe for a pregnant woman to consume any alcohol during pregnancy. Caffeine is known to produce congenital malformations in experimental animals, and there is some concern that caffeine may also be harmful to the human fetus.

Drugs such as heroin, methadone, and cocaine used by a pregnant woman impair fetal growth and development and may lead to congenital malformation, as well as to addiction in both the fetus and the mother. The infant born to an addicted mother may experience narcotic withdrawal symptoms within a few days after delivery. Maternal cocaine use may also disturb blood flow through the placenta, leading to intrauterine fetal death, as described in chapter 18.

Category	Interpretation
A	No risk to fetus demonstrated in well-controlled studies in humans.
B	No evidence of risk to fetus. Either animal studies show risk but human studies do not or there are no adequate human studies but animal studies do not indicate risk.
C	Risk to fetus cannot be ruled out. No human studies available to assess risk. Animal studies either are not available or indicate possible risk.
D	Positive evidence of risk to fetus, but drug is needed to treat patient and no safer alternative drug is available. Potential benefit to patient outweighs risk to fetus.
X	Absolutely contraindicated in pregnancy. Severe risk to fetus greatly outweighs any possible benefit to patient.

TABLE 9–3

Five categories of all drugs used in the U.S. rated by the FDA according to degree of possible risk to the fetus

Some drugs that are well tolerated by the mother may cause manifestations of drug toxicity in the fetus because the fetus lacks an efficient means of detoxifying and excreting these drugs. Some drugs may slow the growth rate of the fetus (*intrauterine growth retardation*), resulting in the birth of a smaller than normal infant. Other drugs retard fetal growth and cause congenital malformations as well.

Some drugs may leave their mark on the developing fetus even though the harmful effects are not immediately apparent. The antibiotic *tetracycline,* when taken by a pregnant woman, is deposited in the developing teeth of the fetus, causing yellow-brown discoloration of the enamel and sometimes, also disturbing the development of the enamel. The abnormality is not apparent until the teeth erupt (described in chapter 23). An even more disturbing late effect of a drug taken during pregnancy has recently been identified. An unusual type of cancer of the cervix and vagina sometimes develops in the daughters of women treated during pregnancy with a synthetic nonsteroid estrogen, diethylstilbestrol (DES), and some other synthetic estrogens that are chemically very similar to DES. From about 1946 to 1970, these drugs were widely used to treat patients prone to spontaneous abortion and some other obstetric problems. These synthetic estrogens, when given to the mother during pregnancy, caused a developmental abnormality in the epithelium of the lower genital tract of the female fetus, which predisposed it to the development of cancer from fifteen to twenty years later. Fortunately, this late complication occurs in only a relatively small proportion of the daughters of women who were treated with these drugs.

Because of the established relation between drugs and congenital defects, most physicians recommend that pregnant women refrain from indiscriminate use of drugs or other medications, especially during the early part of pregnancy when the embryo is especially vulnerable. Many new drugs and antibiotics are not recommended for use in pregnancy because the possible effects of the drugs on the developing embryo are not known.

Radiation

Exposure of a pregnant woman to radiation may harm the fetus. Consequently, x-ray examinations or diagnostic tests using radioactive materials are avoided during pregnancy.

Maternal Infections

Some infections acquired by a pregnant woman may injure the developing fetus. Three infectious agents are known to be important causes of congenital malformations and may also cause a chronic systemic infection of the fetus:

1. The virus of German measles (*rubella*)
2. The virus of cytomegalic inclusion disease (*cytomegalovirus*)
3. The protozoan parasite *Toxoplasma gondii*

Rubella

Rubella is a mild illness that is usually acquired in childhood; 90 percent of women of childbearing age have already had the disease and are immune. If a susceptible woman acquires rubella during pregnancy, the virus may infect the embryo, leading to either spontaneous abortion of severely affected embryos or congenital malformations in many of the embryos that survive. Common malformations resulting from prenatal rubella infection include congenital cataracts, cardiac malformations, deafness, and neurologic disturbances. The earlier in the pregnancy, the greater the hazard to the developing embryo. In cases in which the mothers contract rubella in the first month of pregnancy, as many as 50 percent of their infants develop congenital malformations. The incidence declines to about 25 percent when infection occurs in the second month, and to about 10 percent when the infection occurs later in pregnancy. The virus may also cause a chronic progressive infection in the fetus. When this occurs, the affected infant is born with evidence of an active systemic disease characterized by enlargement of the liver and spleen, anemia, and reduced numbers of platelets in the blood (*thrombocytopenia*). The low platelet levels usually lead to multiple small hemorrhages in the skin (called *thrombocytopenic purpura*). Rubella virus can be isolated from the tissues and secretions of the infected infants. It may persist in the infant's tissues for six months or longer after delivery.

Cytomegalic Inclusion Disease

The name of the cytomegalovirus (*cyto* = cell + *megalos* = large) derives from its characteristic property of producing marked enlargement of the cells it infects. The infected cells also contain characteristic large, basophilic, intranuclear inclusions, causing the virus-infected cell to have a distinctly characteristic histologic appearance (figure 9–10). Cytomegalovirus infection is very common and is usually asymptomatic. More than 50 percent of women of childbearing age have had a previous cytomegalovirus infection and have formed antibodies against the virus, but latent cytomegalovirus persists within the tissues of the infected woman and may become reactivated during pregnancy, leading to intermittent excretion of virus in cervical and vaginal secretions throughout the pregnancy. The fetus may become infected either from a new maternal infection acquired during pregnancy or from reactivation of a prior maternal infection. A newly acquired maternal infection poses the greatest risk to the fetus. The virus may cause severe fetal damage characterized by injury to the brain and eyes, leading to failure of the brain to develop normally (*microcephaly*), mental retardation, and blindness. The cytomegalovirus may also cause a chronic systemic infection of the fetus similar to that caused by the rubella virus, and the virus can be identified in the tissues of the infected infant.

A reactivation of a previous maternal infection is less hazardous to the fetus and may produce only relatively mild symptoms. The fetus may be infected within the uterus prior to delivery, at the time of delivery from virus in cervical and vaginal secretions, or during nursing from virus excreted in breast milk.

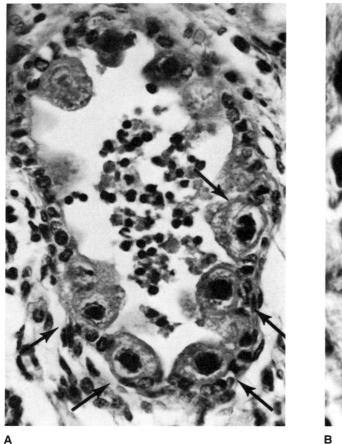

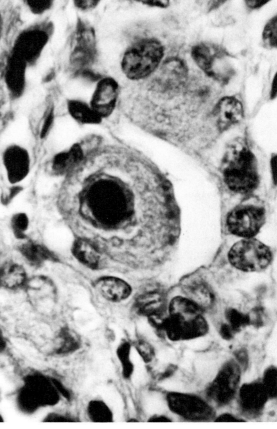

A   B

FIGURE 9–10

Characteristic appearance of cells infected by cytomegalovirus. **A,** Kidney tubule containing several swollen, virus-infected cells. (Original magnification × 400.) Several intranuclear inclusion bodies are seen in cells at lower part of photograph (*arrows*). **B,** Higher magnification of inclusion body, which almost completely fills nucleus of infected cell. (Original magnification × 1000.)

Other Virus Diseases in Pregnancy

The herpes simplex virus, the same virus that causes fever blisters, may at times cause congenital infections similar to those produced by cytomegalovirus, leading to malformations of the nervous system. Some other viruses may occasionally be transmitted to the fetus and cause disease in the fetus, but they are not usually associated with congenital malformations.

Toxoplasmosis

Toxoplasma gondii is a small, ovoid, intracellular parasite described in chapter 7. Adults acquired the infection by eating raw or partially cooked meat that is infected with the parasite or by contact with infected cats, which excrete an infectious form of the organism (oocysts) in their feces. As with cytomegalovirus infection, more than 50 percent of women of childbearing age have had a previous inapparent infection and have formed antibodies to the parasite. These women are immune, and the prior infection does not put the fetus at risk.

A hazard to the fetus exists if a susceptible mother acquires the infection during pregnancy. In the fetus, the parasite causes severe injury to the brain and eyes, leading to abnormal development of the brain (*microcephaly*); obstruction of the ventricles of the brain, causing *hydrocephalus* (described in chapter 26); and visual disturbances or blindness. The infected fetus may be born with evidence of a systemic *Toxoplasma* infection that is clinically quite similar to that caused by rubella and the cytomegalovirus.

It is possible to determine by laboratory tests if a pregnant woman is susceptible to *Toxoplasma*. A susceptible pregnant woman should avoid eating incompletely cooked meat and should exercise caution in contact with cats. Pregnant women with cats are generally advised to adopt the following precautions.

1. Wash hands after handling cats, especially before eating.
2. Have the cat-litter box emptied daily by someone else (to avoid contact with oocysts).
3. Do not permit indoor cats to go outside (because cats allowed to roam outdoors have a higher risk of acquiring a *Toxoplasma* infection).
4. Do not allow outdoor cats or stray cats to enter the house (because they are very likely to be infected with toxoplasma).
5. Do not feed cats raw meat products (because they may become infected in this way).

The following case illustrates the clinical features of a systemic infection of the fetus that resulted from an inapparent infection of the mother during pregnancy (figure 9–11).

> The patient was an infant girl at thirty-six weeks' gestation. The skin was covered with numerous small hemorrhages, and the abdomen was markedly distended because of extreme enlargement of both the liver and the spleen. The infant was moderately anemic, and the platelet count was significantly reduced, which accounted for the widespread hemorrhages in the skin. The infant was considered to be seriously ill as a result of a prenatal infection acquired from the mother. Diagnostic possibilities considered were congenital rubella, cytomegalic inclusion disease, systemic herpes virus infection, or toxoplasmosis. The infant died of the widespread infection about five hours after examination, before further diagnostic studies could be undertaken. The autopsy revealed the infection was caused by the cytomegalovirus.

CASE 9–2

Rubella virus, cytomegalovirus, *Toxoplasma,* and occasionally the herpes virus all produce a similar type of infection in the fetus, and it may not be possible to determine clinically which agent caused the disease unless the infectious agent can be identified by histologic examination, culture, or serologic methods.

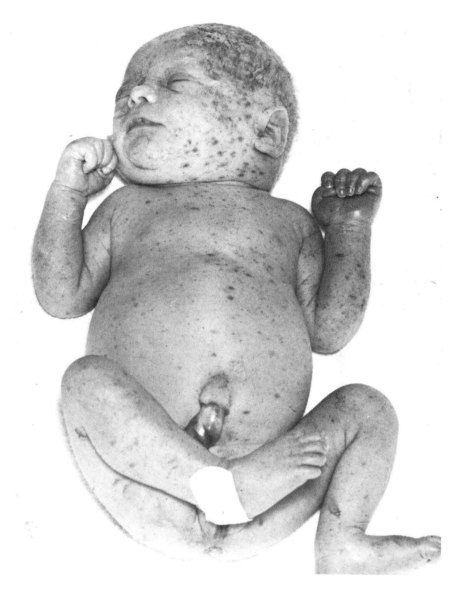

Multifactorial Inheritance

Many congenital defects do not result from single gene abnormalities and are
not entirely caused by environmental factors. Rather, they result from the
combined effects of multiple genes interacting with environmental agents.
This type of inheritance is called **multifactorial inheritance.**

Many of the phases of embryologic development, such as the formation
of the heart or palate, are regulated by multiple genes. Because embryos differ in their genetic makeup, they also vary somewhat in the rates at which
the various organs and other embryonic structures are formed. These genetic

variations will influence the susceptibility of an embryo to drugs or other environmental factors that disturb the normal process of development. Susceptible embryos are likely to develop congenital malformations if they are exposed to harmful environmental agents, whereas genetically resistant embryos remain unaffected under similar circumstances.

In order to understand how multiple genes and environmental factors interact, consider a developmental process such as the formation of the palate, which separates the nasal from the oral cavity. Most of the embryos in a given group will complete this phase of their development within about the same period of time. Some will take a bit longer than the average, and others will complete the process in a shorter-than-average time. The normal variations in the rate of development within the group, which are genetically determined, can be plotted as a graph. When the times taken by each embryo to complete the process are designated on the horizontal axis and the number of embryos who complete the process during each time interval are indicated on the vertical axis, a bell-shaped curve is obtained (figure 9–12). The embryos in the group, defined in terms of the time it takes to complete a specific phase of their development, form a continuous series. They range from embryos with very fast development times at the left end of the bell curve to those with very slow times at the right end, with most embryos falling close to the center of the curve. The mean (average) development time for the entire group is represented by a vertical line drawn through the midpoint of the curve. The mean divides the curve into left and right halves. The embryos to the left of the mean complete this phase of development faster than the average of the entire group, and those to the right of the mean are slower than the average.

Many congenital malformations caused by multifactorial inheritance result because a developmental sequence fails to reach a certain point at an appropriate time. One such abnormality, failure of the palate to close normally, is called *cleft palate*. For a malformation of this type, the concept of a *threshold* is often used. The threshold for a given malformation is the "cut-off line" that separates normally developing embryos from those with congenital malformations. It corresponds to the maximum delay in a developmental process that can be tolerated without producing congenital malformations. As figure 9–12 illustrates, the developmental times of the embryos at the extreme right end of the curve are so prolonged that the threshold is exceeded and malformations occur. The developmental times of all the other embryos fall below the threshold, and all develop normally.

If a drug or other harmful environmental factor slows the developmental process in this hypothetical group of embryos, all the embryos will be affected to roughly the same extent. The average time required for the entire group to complete the developmental process also is prolonged correspondingly. In effect, the entire bell curve is shifted to the right (figure 9–13). As a result, more embryos with slower than average developmental times (right side of bell curve) will now exceed the threshold and will develop congenital malformations. Other embryos whose developmental times are closer to the mean are shifted closer to the threshold of malformation. They can still complete the

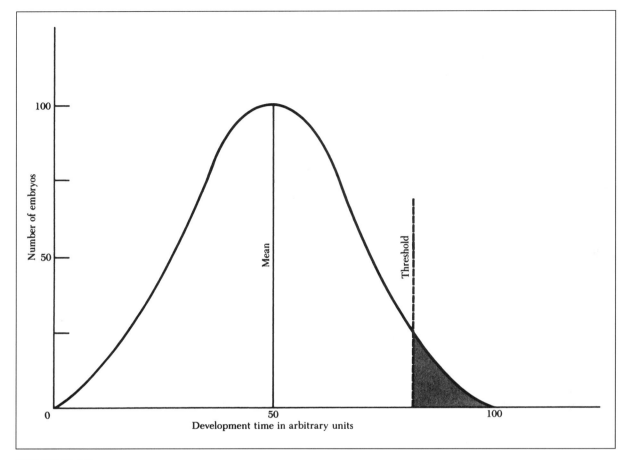

FIGURE 9–12

Graph illustrating genetically determined variation in rate at which a group of embryos complete a phase of development. Threshold (*dashed line*) separates normal from abnormal embryos.

developmental process within the required time, however, despite the slowing, in which case they are not harmed. Embryos whose developmental times are much faster than normal (far left side of curve) are extremely resistant to malformations induced by environmental factors that slow development; their developmental times are so far from the threshold for the malformation that even a relatively marked slowing of the developmental process is not sufficient to exceed the threshold.

How genetic and environmental factors interact to produce congenital abnormalities can be readily demonstrated in animal subjects by experimentally produced cleft palate (figure 9–14). When the palate is formed in the embryo, processes growing inward from the developing face shift from a vertical to a horizontal position as they move toward the midline to fuse. The

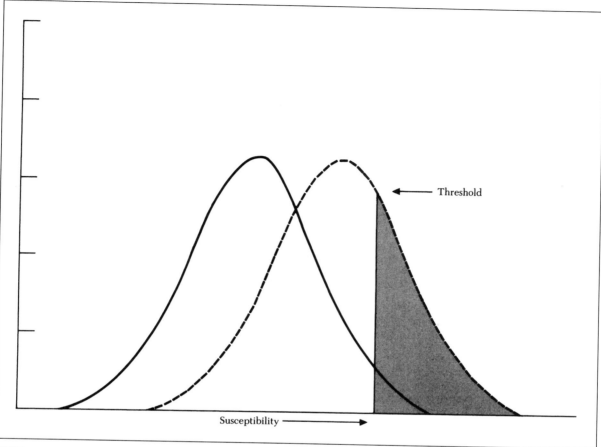

FIGURE 9–13

Effect of harmful environmental agents on susceptibility to congenital malformations. *Vertical line* indicates threshold for malformation. Normal genetic variation in developmental sequence is illustrated by left curve. A small number of embryos exceed threshold (*shaded*) and develop malformations. Curve is shifted to right (*broken line*) by environmental agent, causing more embryos to exceed threshold and develop malformations.

growth and movement of the palatal processes are controlled by multiple genes, each making a small contribution to the total effect. While the palatal processes are growing inward, the head is also growing and carrying the palatal processes farther apart. In some strains of experimental animals ("early-fusion strains"), the processes meet and fuse early in the course of development. In other strains ("late-fusion strains"), the closure occurs somewhat later. If both strains of experimental animals are exposed to a drug that causes a slight delay in the movement of the palatal processes, the delay will have little effect on the embryos whose palates normally fuse early. But in the late-fusion embryos, the continued growth of the head will have carried the palatal processes so far apart during the delay that, by the time they are

FIGURE 9–14

Interaction of genetic predisposition and environmental
factors in experimentally
produced cleft palate.
A, Delay in movement of
palatal processes has no
effect on embryo whose
palate fuses early in development. **B,** Delay causes
cleft palate in late-fusion
strain because growth of
head has carried palatal
processes too far apart to
permit fusion.

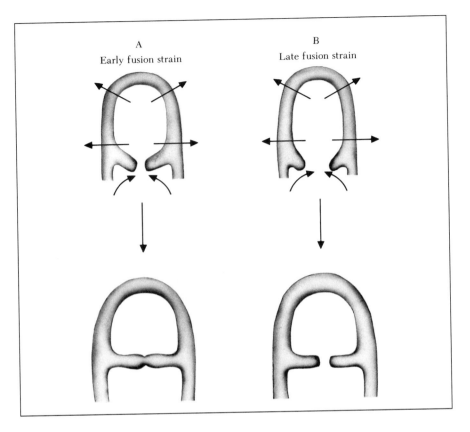

sufficiently horizontal to fuse, they cannot meet in the midline. Cleft palate results. The late-fusion embryos have inherited a genetic predisposition to cleft palate because of their relatively slow rate of palatal fusion, and the predisposition becomes manifest if any environmental factor further slows the process of fusion. In contrast, the early-fusion embryos are quite resistant because of their genetic background.

Some of the common defects in which inheritance is multifactorial include cleft lip and palate, some congenital cardiac malformations, clubfoot, congenital dislocation of the hip, and certain congenital abnormalities of the nervous system called *anencephaly* and *spina bifida*. These multifactorial malformations have an incidence among newborn infants of from one in five hundred to one in two thousand, depending on the malformation. The incidence is much higher, approximately one in twenty-five, if one parent has the same type of congenital malformation or if other children born to the same parents have the malformation. This is because the genes that the parents are transmitting render their offspring more susceptible to disturbances in embryologic development, leading to specific types of congenital abnormalities.

A wide variety of approaches are available to identify congenital abnormalities in the fetus. They fall into three groups:

1. Examination of fetal cells for chromosomal abnormalities and for genetic abnormalities that can be identified by determination of biochemical abnormalities in fetal cells or by analysis of DNA obtained from fetal cells.
2. Examination of amnionic fluid for products secreted into the fluid by the fetus that may indicate a congenital fetal abnormality.
3. Ultrasound examination of the fetus when some specific types of congenital malformations are suspected. Ultrasound examination, described in chapter 1, can detect major structural abnormalities of the nervous system called neural tube defects (anencephaly and spina bifida) and congenital hydrocephalus. These conditions are described in chapter 26. Other structural abnormalities also can be identified, including such defects as congenital obstruction of the urinary tract, failure of the kidneys to develop, or failure of the limbs to form normally.

Fetal cells can be obtained easily from amnionic fluid because the cells in the fluid are of fetal origin. The cells can be grown in the laboratory by tissue culture techniques, and the karyotype of the cells can be determined. In this way, abnormalities in the number or structure of the fetal chromosomes can be determined. Special biochemical studies can detect deficiencies of specific enzymes in amnionic fluid cells, and this approach has been used to diagnose some diseases characterized by intracellular enzyme deficiencies, although many of these biochemical approaches have been superseded by direct examination of DNA in fetal cells, as described later in this chapter. One can also determine the concentration in amnionic fluid of a protein called *alpha fetoprotein,* which is high when the fetus has a neural tube defect. This subject is considered in chapter 26.

Amnionic fluid for study is obtained by a technique called *transabdominal amniocentesis,* which is usually performed between the fourteenth and eighteenth week of pregnancy, although amniocentesis as early as the twelfth to thirteenth week of pregnancy is available in some medical centers. A needle is inserted through the mother's abdominal wall directly into the amnionic sac and a small amount of amnionic fluid is withdrawn. Table 9–4 summarizes the main indications for the procedure. At present, the main use of amniocentesis is for the prenatal detection of a fetus with a chromosome abnormality in a pregnant woman over age 35 because the incidence of Down syndrome and other chromosome abnormalities is relatively high in the offspring of older women. Amniocentesis should also be performed if the woman has previously given birth to an infant with Down syndrome or other chromosomal abnormality. It should also be performed if the woman is a carrier of a translocated chromosome 21 because of the very high incidence of Down syndrome in the offspring of a translocation carrier. The procedure is also indicated if one of the parents has some other type of chromosomal abnormality, such as in case 9–1. Amniocentesis should be performed if

TABLE 9–4

Main indications for amniocentesis

1. Maternal age
2. Previous infant born with Down syndrome or other chromosomal abnormality
3. Known translocation chromosome carrier
4. Other chromosomal abnormality in either parent
5. Risk of genetic disease in the fetus that can be detected prenatally
6. Previous infant born with neural tube defect

there is a history of an inherited disease that can be identified by examination of fetal cells. For example, examination of fetal DNA is indicated when both parents are carriers of an abnormal gene, such as the gene responsible for Tay-Sachs disease, the thalassemia gene associated with defective hemoglobin synthesis, or the hemoglobin gene responsible for sickle cell anemia. (Diseases characterized by defective or abnormal hemoglobins are considered in chapter 14). In these cases, examination of fetal DNA from cells obtained by amniocentesis can determine whether both parents have transmitted their abnormal genes to the fetus, who will be affected with the disease, or whether only one parent has transmitted the abnormal gene, in which case the fetus will carry only one abnormal gene, like the parents, but will not have the hereditary disease. Amniocentesis is also recommended if the mother has previously given birth to an infant with a neural tube defect because the defect follows a multifactorial inheritance pattern, and there is an approximately 5 percent risk that another fetus will also be affected. In this case, the amniocentesis identifies a higher-than-normal concentration of alpha fetoprotein in amnionic fluid when a neural tube defect is present. Ultrasound examination of the fetus also can be used to demonstrate the nervous system malformation.

If an abnormal fetus is identified by means of a prenatal amnionic fluid study, the parents are advised of the nature of the abnormality and its possible effects on the offspring. They must then reach a decision as to whether to terminate the pregnancy or allow it to continue to term.

Chorionic villus sampling also can be used to obtain fetal cells for evaluation and in general provides the same type of information as does amniocentesis, although no amnionic fluid is obtained for chemical examination. (Chorionic villi are frondlike structures that form part of the placenta and attach to the lining of the uterus, described in chapter 18.) The procedure involves passing a small catheter through the cervix to the site where the villi are attached to the uterus and drawing out a small quantity of villi. The procedure has some advantages over amniocentesis because it can be performed at eight to ten weeks gestation, which is earlier than amniocentesis can be performed, and results can be obtained earlier. If a congenital abnormality is detected and the patient wants to terminate the pregnancy, the abortion can be performed earlier in pregnancy, which carries less risk than one performed midway through the pregnancy. There are disadvantages, however. Chorionic villus sampling is technically more difficult than amniocentesis, and complications from the procedure leading to spontaneous abortion are more frequent than with amniocentesis. Moreover, in some instances, chorionic villus sampling may injure the embryo. There appears to be a slight increase of limb deformities in fetuses that have undergone chorionic villus sampling early in pregnancy.

Methods of Fetal DNA Analysis

Sophisticated DNA analysis techniques stemming from advances in recombinant DNA technology have greatly expanded our ability to diagnose genetic abnormalities in the fetus. Many ingenious analytic methods have been developed. One method uses enzymes that cut the fetal DNA into short segments at specific sites in the DNA chains, the sizes of the cut segments depending on the arrangement of the nucleotides in the DNA chains. In some diseases, the DNA fragments produced by enzyme treatment of the abnormal DNA are different from those obtained from normal DNA, and the differences may be sufficiently characteristic to indicate a specific genetic abnormality. This is the case in sickle cell anemia, in which the DNA fragments produced by enzymatic treatment of DNA from an affected fetus are different from normal DNA.

Another approach to fetal DNA analysis is to prepare short single-strand DNA segments called *DNA probes* that have the same complementary arrangement of nucleotides as those in the mutant DNA gene that one is attempting to identify. Such a probe can be used to identify a specific mutant gene because the DNA probe will bind to the mutant gene but will not bind to a normal DNA segment, because the nucleotides are different in the normal DNA segment.

Approaches such as those described have expanded the scope of prenatal diagnosis to the extent that it is now possible to identify a large number of genetic diseases by analyzing DNA obtained from fetal cells by amniocentesis or chorionic villus sampling. Most of the common genetic diseases listed in table 9–2 can be diagnosed in this way, and many other, less-common genetic diseases also can be diagnosed by fetal DNA studies. The list of genetic diseases that can be identified prenatally continues to grow along with the rapid advances in the field of molecular genetics.

Questions for Review

1. What are the consequences of chromosome nondisjunction? What is Down syndrome?

2. What is the karyotype of an individual with Down syndrome? Klinefelter's syndrome? Turner's syndrome?

3. What is the approximate incidence of congenital abnormalities? What are the major causes of congenital abnormalities? What types of maternal infections may cause congenital abnormalities in the infant?

4. What is amniocentesis? How is it used in prenatal diagnosis of congenital malformations? What type of congenital malformations may be detected by this method? In which group of patients is amniocentesis most widely used?

Supplementary Readings

Bass, H. N., et al. 1973. Two different chromosome abnormalities resulting from a translocation carrier father. *Journal of Pediatrics* 83:1034–40. Describes the transmission of abnormal sets of genes to offspring from father who is a carrier of a balanced translocation.

Caskey, C. T. 1994. Fragile X syndrome: Improving understanding and diagnosis (Editorial). *Journal of the American Medical Association* 271:552. Describes the fragile X mental retardation gene and the CGG triplet repeat enlargement.

Centers for Disease Control and Prevention. 1995. Chorionic villus sampling and amniocentesis: Recommendations for prenatal counseling. *Morbidity and Mortality Weekly Report* 44 (No. RR-9):1–11. Chorionic villus sampling carries a small risk of limb deformities probably caused by disruption of the blood supply to the limbs related to the procedure. Risk is from 0.03 to 0.10 percent, with greater risk if the procedure is performed prior to ten weeks gestation. The procedure also carries a greater risk of spontaneous abortion than does amniocentesis.

Clarren, S. K. 1981. Recognition of fetal alcohol syndrome. *Journal of the American Medical Association* 245:2436–39. Heavy maternal alcohol consumption causes characteristic congenital malformations in the offspring, which are described in the article.

Erbe, R. W. 1994. Medical genetics. In *Scientific American Medicine*. Ed. E. Rubenstein. New York: Scientific American, Inc. Updated monthly. A well-written in-depth review of the subject.

Herbst, A. L., et al. 1972. Clear-cell adenocarcinoma of the genital tract in young females. *New England Journal of Medicine* 287:1259–64. The classic article that called attention to the relation between ingestion of DES by mothers and an unusual type of cervicovaginal cancer in their daughters.

Kaback, M., Lim Steele, J., Dabholkar, D., et al. 1993. Tay-Sachs disease: Carrier screening, prenatal diagnosis, and the molecular area. *Journal of the American Medical Association* 270:2307–14. An update on the international experience with carrier screening and prenatal diagnosis.

Little, B. B., et al. 1989. Cocaine abuse during pregnancy: Maternal and fetal implications. *Obstetrics and Gynecology* 73:157–60. A review article outlining major problems and complications from cocaine abuse.

Milunsky, A. 1986. *Genetic disorders and the fetus: Diagnosis, prevention, and treatment.* 2d ed. New York: Plenum Press. A textbook on prenatal diagnosis.

Ouellette, E. M., et al. 1977. Adverse effects on offspring of maternal alcohol abuse during pregnancy. *New England Journal of Medicine* 297:528–30. Describes fetal alcohol syndrome.

Rosengren, J. 1990. Alcohol: A bigger drug problem. *Minnesota Medicine* 73:33–34. Describes the harmful effects of alcohol on the fetus.

Stagno, S., et al. 1986. Primary cytomegalovirus infection in pregnancy. *Journal of the American Medical Association.* 256:1904–8. Primary CMV infection during pregnancy poses a significant risk of intrauterine transmission, and an adverse outcome is more likely when the infection occurs within the first half of gestation.

Weatherall, D. G. 1985. *The new genetics and clinical practice.* Oxford: Oxford University Press. Deals with molecular diagnosis of genetic disorders.

Chapter 9 ▪ Outline Summary

Pathogenesis of Congenital Malformation / 189

Chromosomal Abnormalities

Nondisjunction leading to trisomy, deletions, and translocations.

Sex chromosome abnormalities:

Turner's syndrome: genotype XO lacking sex chromatin body. Abnormal body configuration.

Triple X syndrome: genotype XXX with extra sex chromatin body. No specific somatic abnormalities.

Klinefelter's syndrome: genotype XXY with sex chromatin body. Infertility, testicular atrophy, breast hypertrophy.

XYY syndrome: reduced intelligence and aggressive behavior.

Fragile X syndrome: important cause of mental deficiency.

Abnormalities of autosomes:

Down syndrome:

Mental deficiency, characteristic facial expression, often congenital cardiac malformation.

Owing to nondisjunction during gametogenesis, chromosome translocation, or nondisjunction in zygote.

Genetically Determined Diseases

Gene mutation involving structural protein or enzyme: phenylketonuria and sickle hemoglobin disorders.

Transmission:

Autosomal: dominant, recessive, or codominant.

Sex-linked: male affected if carrying X chromosome containing defective gene. Female may be carrier but is unaffected.

Intrauterine Injury

Harmful drugs, (e.g., thalidomide).

Radiation.

Maternal infections: German measles (rubella), cytmegalovirus, other viral diseases, toxoplasmosis.

Interaction of Genetic and Environmental Factors

Susceptible embryo develops malformation if exposed to environmental agents. Resistant embryo unaffected. Parents are transmitting sets of genes that increase susceptibility to embryologic disturbances.

Prenatal Diagnosis / 217

Application

Detect chromosomal abnormalities and some genetic abnormalities.

Analysis of fetal DNA an important diagnostic test when indicated.

Detect nervous system defects (alpha fetoprotein analysis).

Technique

Perform amniocentesis as early as twelve weeks.

Culture amnionic cells (of fetal origin) and determine karyotype.

Biochemical analysis where indicated.

Alpha fetoprotein analysis where indicated.

Analysis of fetal DNA when indicated.

Chorionic villus sampling: provides same information as amniocentesis. Has some advantages and some disadvantages compared with amniocentesis.

10

Neoplastic Disease

Learning Objectives

1. Compare the general characteristics of benign and malignant tumors. Explain how tumors are named. List the common exceptions to standard terminology.
2. Summarize the features of the principal types of lymphoma.
3. Differentiate between infiltrating and in situ carcinoma. Explain the role of the Pap smear in early diagnosis of neoplasm.
4. Explain how leukemias are classified. Describe the clinical manifestations of each type and its response to treatment.
5. Differentiate myeloma from leukemia, describe its clinical manifestations, and explain how it is diagnosed.
6. Explain the mechanisms of the body's immunologic defenses against tumor.
7. Summarize the principal modalities of tumor treatment, including advantages, disadvantages, and common side effects of each technique.
8. Describe the applications and limitations of tumor-associated antigens in the diagnosis and treatment of patients with tumor.
9. Compare the incidence and survival rates for various types of malignant tumors. Explain the mechanisms of late recurrence. Define the role of adjuvant therapy in preventing late recurrence.
10. Understand the role of activated oncogenes and disturbance in suppressor gene function in the pathogenesis of tumors.

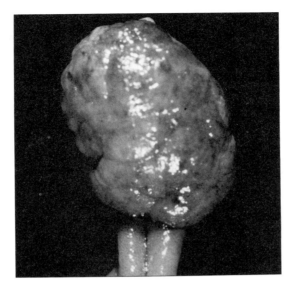

Chapter 10 ■ Contents

Normal life processes are characterized by continuous growth and maturation of cells, and all cells are subject to control mechanisms that regulate their growth rate. This ongoing growth process serves the purpose of replacing cells that have been injured or have undergone degenerative changes. In contrast, a neoplasm (*neo* = new + *plasm* = growth) is an overgrowth of cells that serves no useful purpose. Neoplasms appear not to be subject to the control mechanisms that normally regulate cell growth and differentiation.

Classification and Nomenclature

The terms *neoplasm* and *tumor* have essentially the same meaning and may be used interchangeably. There are two large classes of neoplasms:

1. Benign tumors
2. Malignant tumors

Table 10–1 compares the major characteristics of the two classes.

Comparison of Benign and Malignant Tumors

Generally, a benign tumor grows slowly and remains localized. Although it pushes surrounding normal tissue aside, it does not infiltrate surrounding tissues or spread by blood and lymphatic channels to distant sites. Usually, a benign tumor can be completely removed surgically without difficulty (figures 10–1, 10–2, and 10–3). Histologically, the cells in a benign tumor appear mature and closely resemble the normal cells from which the tumor was derived.

In contrast to the benign tumor, a malignant neoplasm is composed of less well differentiated cells, grows more rapidly, and infiltrates the surrounding tissues rather than growing by expansion (figures 10–4, 10–5, and 10–6). Frequently, the infiltrating strands of tumor find their way into the vascular and lymphatic channels. Bits of tumor may be carried in the lymphatics to reach the lymph nodes, where they establish secondary sites of tumor growth not connected with the original tumor (figure 10–7). Eventually, the tumor may spread widely throughout the lymphatic channels. Tumor cells may also gain access to the bloodstream and be carried to distant sites, lead-

Tumors

	Benign tumor	Malignant tumor
Growth rate	Slow	Rapid
Character of growth	Expansion	Infiltration
Tumor spread	Remains localized	Metastasis by bloodstream and lymphatics
Cell differentiation	Well differentiated	Poorly differentiated

TABLE 10–1

Comparison of benign and malignant tumors

FIGURE 10–1

Well-circumscribed benign tumor. Capsule of tumor is held by clamp. Surrounding normal tissues have retracted, indicating absence of infiltration.

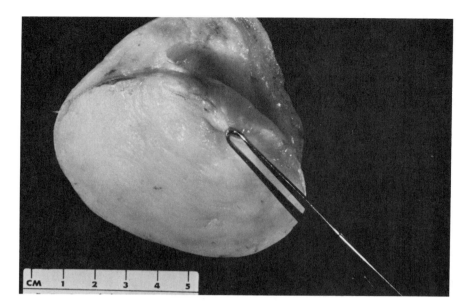

ing to secondary tumor deposits throughout the body. The process by which a tumor spreads some distance from the primary site is called **metastasis** (*meta* = beyond + *stasis* = standing), and the secondary deposits are called *metastatic tumors* (figure 10–8). If a malignant tumor is not eradicated promptly, it may eventually become widely disseminated throughout the body and may kill the patient. Benign tumors do not metastasize.

Tumors are named and classified according to the cells and tissues from which they originate. Therefore, understanding the primary tissue classifications explained in chapter 2 is helpful in understanding the names of tumors. Tumor nomenclature is not completely uniform, but certain generalizations are possible.

TABLE 10–2

Common prefixes used to name tumors

Prefix	Meaning
Adeno-	Gland
Angio-	Vessels (type not specified)
Chondro-	Cartilage
Fibro-	Fibrous tissue
Hemangio-	Blood vessels
Lymphangio-	Lymph vessels
Lipo-	Fat
Myo-	Muscle
Neuro-	Nerve
Osteo-	Bone

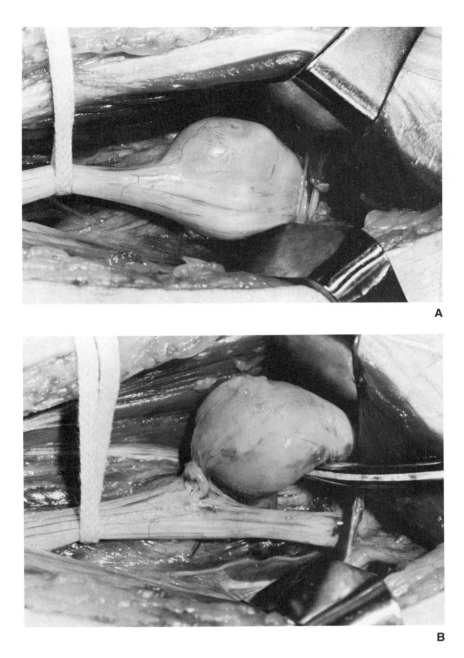

A

B

FIGURE 10–2

A, Benign tumor (neuroma) arising from sciatic nerve. **B,** Tumor dissected from surrounding nerve. Cleavage plane is easily established, indicating that the tumor is sharply circumscribed and does not infiltrate the adjacent nerve.

Benign Tumors

A benign tumor that projects from an epithelial surface is usually called a **polyp** or **papilloma** (figure 10–9). Most other benign tumors are named by adding the suffix *-oma* to the prefix that designates the cell of origin, as shown in table 10–2. For example, a benign tumor arising from glandular epithelium

FIGURE 10–3

Low-magnification photomicrograph of benign breast tumor (fibroadenoma). Note sharp demarcation between tumor and surrounding breast tissue (*arrow*).

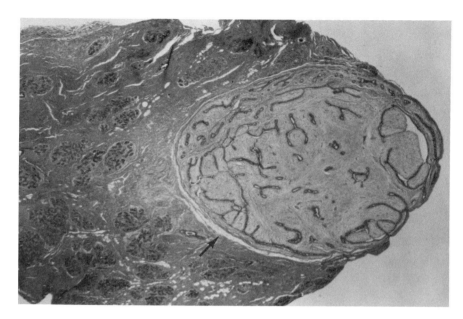

FIGURE 10–4

Biopsy of bronchus from patient with lung carcinoma, illustrating normal respiratory epithelium (*arrow*) and clusters of neoplastic cells from a lung carcinoma. Cancer cells grow in haphazard pattern and exhibit great variation in size and structure. (Original magnification × 400.)

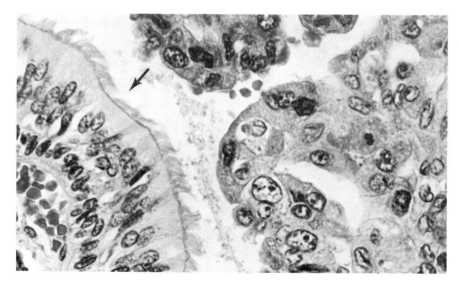

is called an *adenoma*. A benign tumor of blood vessels is an *angioma* (figure 10–10), and one arising from cartilage is designated a *chondroma*.

Malignant Tumors

There are many types of malignant tumors, but all can be classified into three groups: (1) carcinomas, (2) sarcomas, or (3) leukemias. The term *cancer* is a word used to indicate any type of malignant tumor.

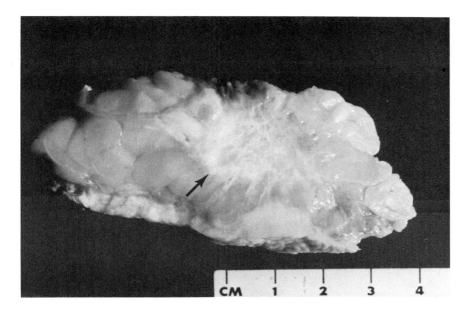

FIGURE 10–5

Breast biopsy illustrating carcinoma (*arrow*) infiltrating adjacent fatty tissue of breast. There is no distinct demarcation between tumor and normal tissue.

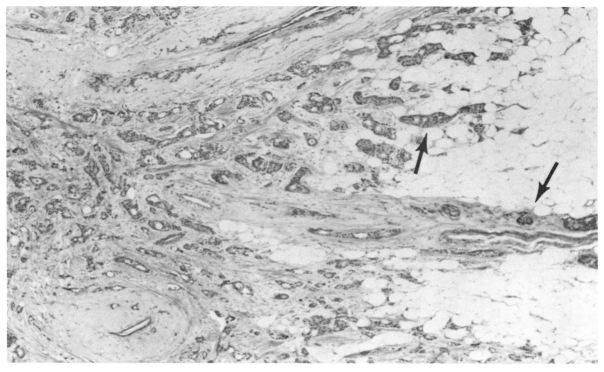

FIGURE 10–6

Low-magnification photomicrograph illustrating margin of breast carcinoma. Small clusters of tumor cells (*arrows*) infiltrate adipose tissue of breast. (Original magnification approximately × 20.)

FIGURE 10–7

Cluster of tumor cells in lymphatic vessel. (Original magnification × 400.)

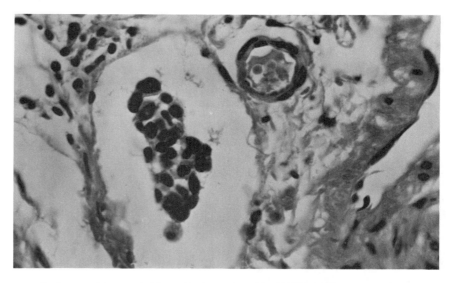

FIGURE 10–8

Multiple nodules of metastatic carcinoma in spleen.

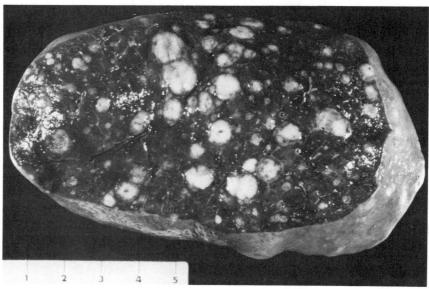

It is generally agreed that a malignant tumor starts from a single cell that has sustained some type of damage to its genome that causes it to proliferate abnormally, forming first a clone of identical cells and, if unchecked, eventually developing into a distinct tumor. Cells of malignant tumors exhibit behavior that is quite different from that of normal cells. They do not respond to normal growth regulatory signals from other cells, and they continue to proliferate when there is no need to do so. Indeed, some cancer cells actually secrete growth factors to stimulate their own growth. As they grow, they acquire properties that allow them to flourish at the expense of the sur-

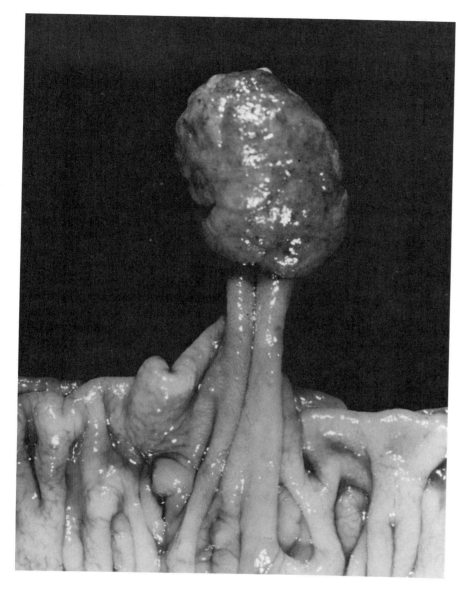

FIGURE 10–9

Benign polyp of colon.

rounding normal cells. They secrete enzymes that break down normal cell and tissue barriers, which allows them to infiltrate into adjacent tissues, invade lymphatic channels and blood vessels, and eventually spread throughout the body. Moreover, the proliferating tumor cells do not "wear out" and die after a specific number of cell divisions, as normal cells do. They become "immortal" and can proliferate indefinitely.

A **carcinoma** is any malignant tumor arising from surface, glandular, or parenchymal epithelium. (The term is not applied, however, to malignant tumors of endothelium or mesothelium, which behave more like malignant connective-tissue tumors.) A carcinoma is classified further by designating the type of epithelium from which it arose. For example, a malignant tumor arising from the transitional epithelium of the urinary bladder is called a *transitional cell carcinoma of the bladder*. A carcinoma arising from the glandular epithelium of the pancreas is termed an *adenocarcinoma of the pancreas* (*aden* = gland), and a tumor arising from the squamous epithelium of the esophagus is called a *squamous cell carcinoma of the esophagus.*

Sarcoma is a general term referring to a malignant tumor arising from primary tissues other than surface, glandular, or parenchymal epithelium. The exact type of sarcoma is specified by prefixing the term designating the cell of origin. For example, a malignant tumor of cartilage is designated as a *chondrosarcoma. Fibrosarcoma, liposarcoma, myosarcoma, osteosarcoma,* and *angiosarcoma* indicate respectively malignant tumors of fibroblasts, fat cells, muscle cells, bone-forming cells, and blood vessels.

The term **leukemia** is applied to any neoplasm of blood-forming tissues. Neoplasms arising from the precursors of white blood cells usually do not form solid tumors. Instead, the abnormal cells proliferate diffusely within the bone

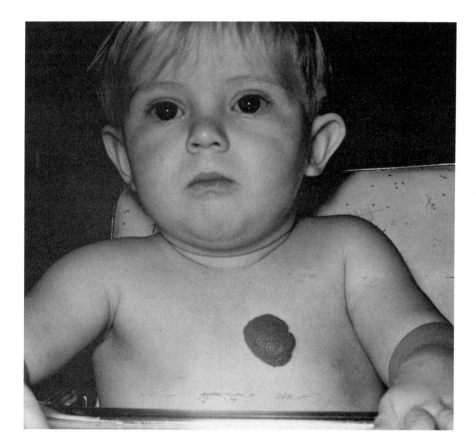

FIGURE 10–10

Benign blood-vessel tumor (angioma) of skin.

marrow, where they overgrow and crowd out the normal blood-forming cells. The neoplastic cells also "spill over" into the bloodstream, and large numbers of abnormal cells circulate in the peripheral blood.

Table 10–3 summarizes the general principles used to name both benign and malignant tumors.

Variations in Terminology

There are some inconsistencies and exceptions to the general principles of nomenclature. Exceptions are encountered in the naming of lymphoid tumors, skin tumors arising from pigment-producing cells within the epidermis, certain tumors of mixed cellular components, and certain types of embryonic tumors seen in children. There are other cases in which names of tumors seem to follow no rules or general principles. The student should not be unduly concerned about the exceptions or unusual situations but should attempt to grasp the general principles of naming tumors.

Lymphoid Tumors

All neoplasms of lymphoid tissue are called **lymphomas.** With extremely rare exceptions, these tumors are malignant (figure 10–11). Therefore, the term *lymphoma* without qualification refers to a malignant, not a benign, tumor. Often, to avoid confusion, the term *malignant lymphoma* rather than simply lymphoma is used.

Lymphomas are generally subdivided into two major groups: Hodgkin's disease and non-Hodgkin's lymphomas. *Hodgkin's disease* is a type of lymphoma that has a variable histologic appearance consisting of large cells called *Reed-Sternberg cells* intermixed with lymphocytes, plasma cells, eosinophils, and fibrous tissues. The Reed-Sternberg cell is a large cell with abundant cytoplasm that characteristically contains two nuclei appearing as mirror images of each other. Each nucleus contains a large nucleolus surrounded by a clear halo (figure 10–12). Four different histologic types of Hodgkin's disease are

General term	Meaning
Polyp, papilloma	Any benign tumor projecting from surface epithelium.
___ + oma (suffix)	A benign tumor. Prefix designates primary tissue of origin.
Carcinoma	Malignant tumor arising from surface, glandular, or parenchymal epithelium (but not endothelium or mesothelium).
Sarcoma	Malignant tumor of any primary tissue other than surface, glandular, and parenchymal epithelium.
Leukemia	Neoplasm of blood cells.

TABLE 10–3

General principles of naming tumors

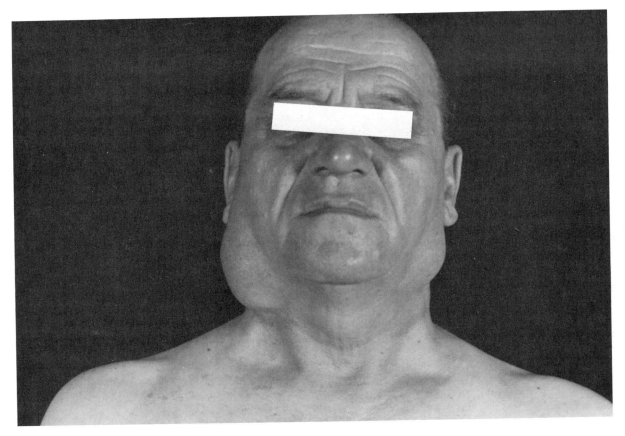

FIGURE 10–11

Severe enlargement of cervical lymph nodes as a result of malignant lymphoma.

recognized, and they differ somewhat in their clinical behavior and prognosis. All other lymphomas are generally grouped together under the general term of *non-Hodgkin's lymphomas* and are classified on the size, shape, and growth pattern of the lymphoma cells. A lymphoma in which the cells resemble small mature lymphocytes is called a *small cell lymphoma,* and one composed of large lymphoid cells is called a *large cell lymphoma;* one in which both types of cells are represented is called a *mixed small and large cell lymphoma.* If the lymphoma cells have irregular nuclear shapes with deep grooves in their nuclear membranes, they are called *cleaved cells,* and those with uniform round or oval nuclei are called *noncleaved cells.* Further classification is based on whether the lymphoma cells infiltrate the lymph node diffusely, which is called a *diffuse growth pattern,* or form cohesive follicle-like clusters that impart a nodular appearance to the affected node, which is called a *follicular growth pattern.* In classifying a lymphoma, all three characteristics are specified. For example, one may speak of a *malig-*

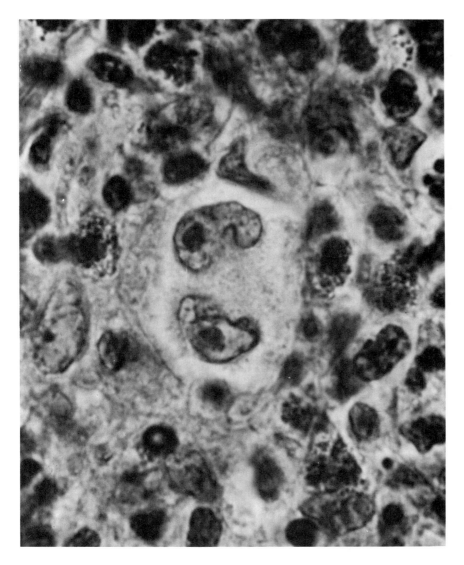

FIGURE 10–12

Characteristic appearance of Reed-Sternberg cell. Note "mirror-image" nuclei with prominent nucleoli. (Original magnification × 400.)

nant lymphoma, small cleaved cell type, follicular pattern, or *malignant lymphoma, mixed small and large noncleaved cell type, diffuse pattern.* This classification provides information on prognosis and helps determine the type of treatment used to control or cure the lymphoma. In general, lymphomas having a follicular growth pattern have a better prognosis than do diffuse lymphomas, and those composed of small noncleaved cells have a more favorable prognosis than do lymphomas composed of large cleaved or noncleaved cells.

Lymphomas can also be classified into prognostic groups. Three categories are recognized: low-, intermediate-, or high-grade lymphoma. Based on the cytologic and histologic growth patterns previously described, the lymphoma is assigned to one of these three groups. Patients with low-grade lymphomas generally have a favorable prognosis and long survival. Those with intermediate-grade lymphomas do not do nearly as well, and those with high-grade lymphomas do poorly.

The characteristics of the cell membrane of the lymphoma cell also can be determined by specialized techniques, thereby determining the type of lymphocyte that gave rise to the lymphoma. About 75 percent of lymphomas arise from B lymphocytes, and most of the remainder originate from T lymphocytes. A small percentage lack distinctive membrane characteristics, and their cells of origin cannot be determined.

Skin Tumors

Most skin tumors arise either from the keratin-forming cells or from the pigment-producing cells of the epidermis. The keratin-forming cells are called **keratinocytes.** The deepest layer of keratinocytes adjacent to the dermis consists of cuboidal cells called *basal cells* that proliferate and give rise to the upper layers of cells, which are called *squamous cells*. Interspersed among the keratinocytes are the skin cells that normally produce pigment and are responsible for normal skin color. These are called **melanocytes,** and the black pigment that they produce is called *melanin.* The common benign pigmented skin lesion that is derived from melanin-producing cells is called a *nevus,* a Latin word which means "birthmark" (figure 10–13). The malignant counterpart is called a **melanoma** (or *malignant melanoma*), the name being derived from the pigment elaborated by the cells.

Keratinocytes can give rise to benign proliferations, called *keratoses,* and two types of skin carcinomas. One type, called a *basal cell carcinoma,* is composed of clusters of infiltrating cells that resemble the normal basal cells of the epidermis. It is a rather indolent, slowly growing tumor that can be locally destructive but rarely metastasizes. The other type, composed of abnormal infiltrating squamous cells, is called a *squamous cell carcinoma* and is a more aggressive tumor that sometimes metastasizes. Both types generally can be cured by complete surgical excision and carry a very good prognosis. Excessive sunlight exposure predisposes to the development of all types of skin cancer, including the potentially lethal melanoma, and also predisposes to the development of some types of keratoses, as well as causing skin damage and premature aging of the skin (figure 10–14).

Tumors of Mixed Components (Teratomas)

A **teratoma** is a tumor derived from cells that have the potential of differentiating into many different types of tissue (bone, muscle, glands, epithelium, brain tissue, hair). Frequently, such tumors consist of poorly organized mixtures of many tissues. Teratomas often arise in the reproductive tract but may also develop in some other locations. Because a teratoma may be either benign or malignant, one must specify the type, calling the tumor either a

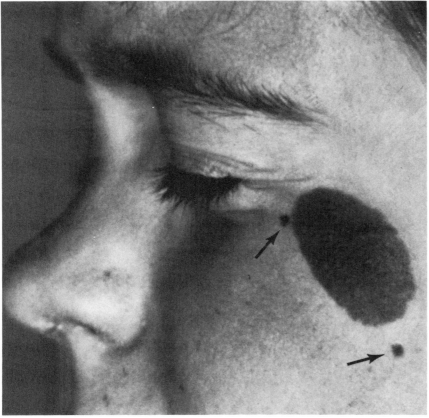

FIGURE 10–13

Benign nevi of skin. Large nevus near eye and two smaller adjacent nevi (*arrows*).

benign teratoma or a *malignant teratoma* (figure 10–15). A common type of cystic benign teratoma arising in the ovary is usually called a **dermoid cyst** (figure 10–16).

Embryonic (Embryonal) Tumors

Certain unusual tumors encountered in children are apparently derived from persisting groups of embryonic cells that have undergone neoplastic change. These tumors may arise in the brain, retina of the eye, adrenal gland, kidney, liver, or genital tract. Embryonic tumors of this type are named from the site of origin, with the suffix *-blastoma* added (*blast* = a primitive cell + *oma* = tumor). Thus, an embryonic tumor arising from the medulla of the brain would be called a *medulloblastoma*. One arising from the retina of the eye is a *retinoblastoma* (figure 10–17). An embryonic tumor of hepatic origin is called a *hepatoblastoma*. An embryonic tumor of the kidney, however, is usually called a *Wilms's tumor* rather than a nephroblastoma.

FIGURE 10–14

Common skin cancers caused by excessive sun exposure. **A,** Cancer arising from keratinocytes (basal cell carcinoma). **B,** Cancer arising from melanocytes (malignant melanoma).

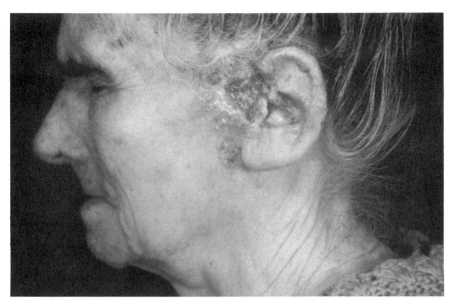

A

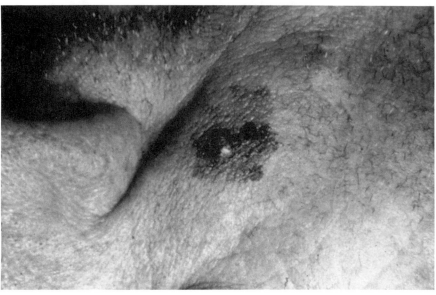

B

Necrosis in Tumors

Tumors derive their blood supply from the tissues they invade. Malignant tumors frequently induce new blood vessels to proliferate in the adjacent normal tissues to supply the demands of the growing tumor. However, a malignant tumor may outgrow its blood supply. When this occurs, the parts of the

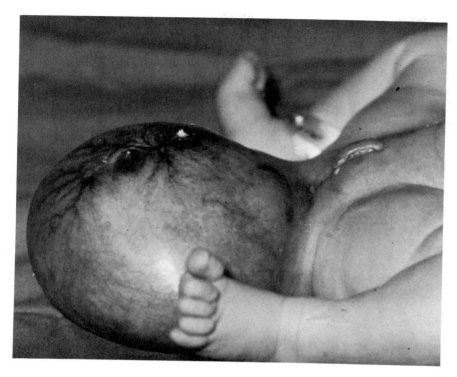

FIGURE 10–15
Large, bulky teratoma of
sacral region in female infant.

tumor with the poorest blood supply undergo necrosis. If the tumor is growing within an organ such as the lung or kidney and is surrounded by normal
tissue, the blood supply is best at the junction of tumor and adjacent normal
tissue, and poorest in the center of the tumor, which often degenerates. In
contrast, if the malignant tumor is growing outward from an epithelial surface,
such as the colon, the best blood supply is at the base of the tumor. The poorest blood supply is at the surface, which frequently becomes necrotic and
sloughs, leaving a shallow crater covered with degenerated tissue and inflammatory exudate (figure 10–18). Often, small blood vessels are exposed in the
ulcerated base of the tumor. Blood may ooze continuously from these vessels, eventually leading to anemia from chronic blood loss. Sometimes, the
ulcerated tumor may be the source of a severe hemorrhage.

Noninfiltrating (in Situ) Carcinoma

Infiltration and metastasis are two characteristic features of malignant tumors.
However, we now know that many carcinomas arising from surface epithelium remain localized within the epithelium for many years before evidence
of infiltration into the deeper tissues or spread to distant sites becomes apparent. This has been well documented for squamous cell carcinoma of the
cervix (figure 10–19). Noninfiltrating tumors have also been recognized in

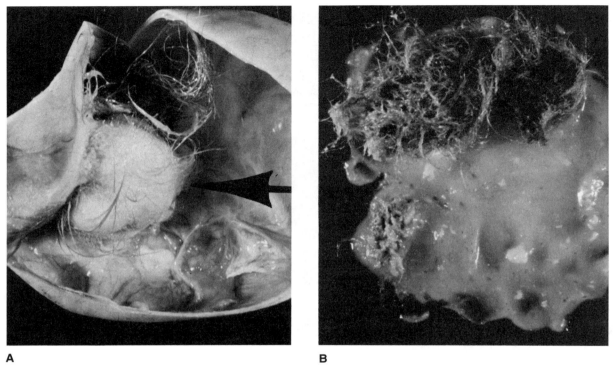

A   B

FIGURE 10–16

A, Cystic teratoma (dermoid cyst) of ovary. Cyst is lined by skin containing sweat and oil glands, and skin surface is covered with hair. *Arrow* indicates a nodule in cyst wall containing fat, muscle, and bone. **B,** Contents of cyst, consisting of matted hair and oil derived from the skin lining the cyst.

many other locations, including the breast (described in chapter 16), urinary tract, colon, and skin. The term *carcinoma in situ* (in-site carcinoma) is used for this type of neoplasm. In situ carcinoma can be completely cured by surgical excision or other treatment that eradicates the abnormal epithelium, and this is the stage most favorable to successful treatment.

Precancerous Conditions

Sometimes the term *precancerous* is used when referring to conditions that have a high likelihood of eventually developing into cancer. Prolonged exposure to sunlight, for example, not only causes premature aging of the skin, but also causes small, crusted, scaly patches to develop on sun-exposed skin, called **actinic keratoses** ("actinic" refers to sun rays). Untreated, many keratoses eventually develop into skin cancers. Another precancerous condition resulting from prolonged sun exposure is a frecklelike proliferation of

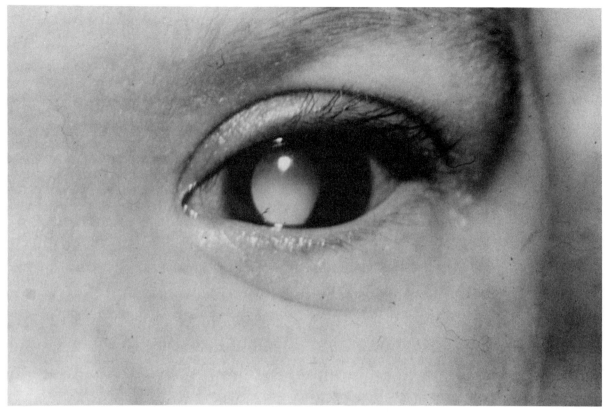

FIGURE 10–17

Retinoblastoma of eye that appears as a pale mass of tissue seen through the dilated pupil.

melanin-producing cells in the skin called **lentigo maligna** (a Latin term meaning "malignant freckle"). They are so named because many eventually become transformed into melanomas. Precancerous, thick white patches descriptively called **leukoplakia** (*leuko* = white + *plakia* = patch) may develop in the mucous membranes of the mouth as a result of exposure to tobacco tars from pipe or cigar smoking or from use of smokeless tobacco (snuff and chewing tobacco) and may give rise to squamous cell cancers of the oral cavity. Somewhat similar precancerous changes may take place in the epithelium of the vulva (described in chapter 17) and may eventuate into vulvar cancer. Some types of colon polyps that are prone to malignant change also are considered precancerous. There are many precancerous conditions, of which these are only a few examples. Precancerous conditions should always be treated appropriately in order to prevent malignant change, which occurs in many, but not all, cases.

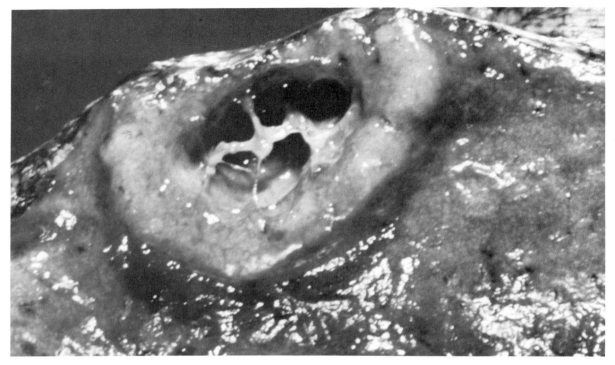

A

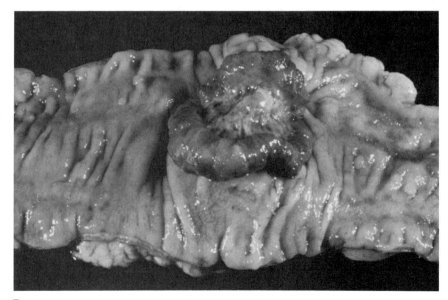

B

FIGURE 10–18

A, Carcinoma of lung with central necrosis. **B,** Carcinoma of colon exhibiting superficial ulceration.

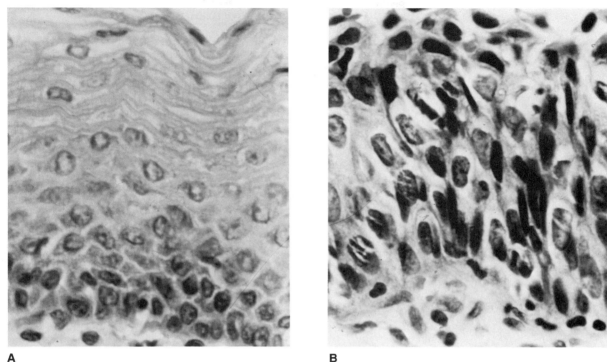

A   B

FIGURE 10–19

Normal cervical squamous epithelium (**A**) compared with in situ carcinoma of cervix (**B**). Note nuclear abnormalities characteristic of carcinoma. The tumor has not yet infiltrated the underlying tissues. (Original magnification × 400.)

Viruses

Many types of tumors in animals are caused by viruses and can be readily transmitted by appropriate methods to animals of the same or a different species. In some instances, a single type of virus is capable of producing many different types of tumors in various species of animals. At least some of the cancers in humans also appear to be caused by viruses. Some unusual types of leukemia and lymphoma are caused by a virus called the *human T cell leukemia-lymphoma virus* (HTLV-I), which is related to the virus that causes the acquired immune deficiency syndrome (AIDS). Some strains of the papilloma virus that cause genital condylomas (described in chapter 17) appear to predispose to cervical carcinoma. Chronic viral hepatitis (described in chapter 21) predisposes to primary carcinoma of the liver. Some types of nasophyngeal carcinoma and some types of lymphoma appear to be related to Epstein-Barr virus infections, the virus that causes infectious mononucleosis.

Etiologic Factors in Neoplastic Disease

Gene and Chromosomal Abnormalities

The basic process common to all neoplasms is an alteration of the genes on the chromosomes of a cell so that the cell no longer responds to normal control mechanisms and proceeds to proliferate without regard for the needs of the body. In the body, many billions of cells are dividing all the time. They are also continually subjected to radiation, various chemical carcinogens (cancer-producing substances), or other agents that can alter the structure of genes. A change in the gene's structure is called a **mutation** (*muto* = change), and the mutated gene may function differently from a normal gene.

Two large groups of genes play important roles in regulating cell functions, and derangements of these genes are associated with formation of tumors. One group comprises **proto-oncogenes,** and the other group **tumor suppressor genes.**

A third group of genes called *mutator genes* also is concerned with cell function. They monitor and correct any errors that may occur during DNA duplication in the course of cell division. Mutator gene dysfunction is associated with an increased mutation rate in the affected cells.

Proto-Oncogenes   Human chromosomes contain a number of normal "growth genes" that promote some aspect of cell growth, differentiation, or mitotic activity. They are called **proto-oncogenes;** they are closely related to genes carried by viruses that cause tumors in experimental animals, and they are named from the tumor viruses that they resemble. A proto-oncogene is a normal gene that regulates some normal growth function in a cell, but a proto-oncogene can undergo a mutation or become translocated to another chromosome where its functions are deranged. Either event can convert a normally functioning proto-oncogene into an **oncogene** (*onkos* = tumor), an abnormally functioning gene that stimulates cell growth excessively and leads to unrestrained cell proliferation. An oncogene is a "gene that causes cancer."

Conversion of a proto-oncogene into an oncogene (activation of an oncogene) may consist of a change in only a single nucleotide in the DNA of the gene, which is called a *point mutation,* or the mutation may generate multiple copies of the same gene, called *gene amplification,* which greatly increases the activity of the gene. Translocation to another chromosome activates an oncogene because of the way in which genes are related on individual chromosomes. A specific gene, such as one that regulates some aspect of cell growth or mitotic activity, is influenced by other nearby genes that either suppress or stimulate its activities. Cell growth and differentiation are normal when the proto-oncogene ("growth gene") and its neighbors function together in an orderly manner, but may be deranged if this relation is disturbed. For example, the translocation may bring the proto-oncogene to a new location on another chromosome where it is freed from the inhibitory genes that formerly controlled its activities. Alternatively, the translocation may bring the proto-oncogene to a new location on another chromosome adjacent to another gene that stimulates its functions.

Tumor Suppressor Genes   These are groups of different genes that function to suppress cell proliferation. Loss of suppressor gene function by mutation or other event disrupts cell functions and can lead to unrestrained cell growth. Suppressor genes exist in pairs at corresponding gene loci on homologous chromosomes, and both suppressor genes must cease to function before the cell malfunctions.

Tumor suppressor genes may also play a role in determining how many times a cell can divide before it involutes and dies. In some cases, loss of a tumor suppressor gene function may allow the cell to proliferate indefinitely rather than dying after a predetermined number of cell divisions, as normal cells do.

Loss of function of specific tumor suppressor genes has been correlated with specific tumors, and the suppressor genes are often named from the tumors with which they have been associated.

Mutator Genes   Mutator genes are part of the cell's DNA "quality control" and repair system. These genes regulate the processes that monitor and repair any errors in DNA duplication that may occur when the cell's chromosomes are duplicated in the course of cell division; they are also concerned with the repair of DNA that has been damaged by radiation, chemicals, or other environmental agents. Any change in the normal arrangement of DNA nucleotides on the DNA chain constitutes a DNA mutation. Consequently, failure of mutator gene function increases the likelihood of DNA mutations within the affected cell. A high mutation rate within cells predisposes to tumors because some mutations may affect cell functions that promote unrestrained cell growth.

Multistep Progression of Genetic Changes Leading to Cancer   In most cases, cancers do not result from mutation of a single gene, but rather are the result of multiple genetic "insults" to the genome characterized by activation of oncogenes along with loss of function of one or more tumor suppressor genes. The transition, for example, from a benign polyp of the colon to an invasive colon cancer requires activation of an oncogene (called *ras*) and inactivation of three distinct tumor suppressor genes (designated *APC, DCC,* and *p53*).

Once a cell has been deregulated and has formed a tumor, additional random genetic changes may take place in the tumor cells, which is indicative of the instability of the tumor cell genome. Often, individual genes may undergo additional mutations or they may reduplicate themselves by gene amplification, forming multiple copies of a single gene. Chromosomes may fragment; pieces of chromosomes may be lost from the cells or be translocated to other chromosomes. Some of these mutations in the unstable tumor cell genome may produce new mutant cells that exhibit more aggressive growth than the original tumor cells, and the new mutant may eventually outgrow the other cells in the tumor. Clinically, this event may be manifested by more rapid growth and aggressive behavior of the tumor, and often the tumor may become less responsive to the anticancer drugs that formerly could control it.

Chromosomal Abnormalities   Not all gene alterations that activate oncogenes or inactivate tumor suppressor genes can be identified from examination of the tumor cell chromosomes. Point mutations do not change chromosome structure, but translocations relocate large pieces of chromosomes and change their structure, as do deletions of chromosome material and amplification of individual genes. Some chromosomal abnormalities occur quite frequently in specific tumors and may be of diagnostic value. Others may give some indication of how aggressively a tumor may behave. The best-known neoplasm-associated chromosomal abnormality, which is called *Philadelphia* or *Ph¹ chromosome* (named after the city where it was discovered), can be demonstrated in the white cells of patients with chronic granulocytic leukemia (described in the section on leukemia). The abnormality is a reciprocal translocation of broken end pieces between chromosomes 9 and 22. In this translocation, a proto-oncogene (designed *abl*) on chromosome 9 is moved to a position on chromosome 22. There it becomes fused with another gene (called *bcr*) to form a composite gene (*abl/bcr*) coding for an abnormal protein that stimulates the unrestrained proliferation of white blood cells characteristic of chronic granulocytic leukemia.

Failure of Immunologic Defenses

The basic processes common to all neoplasms are gene mutations within a cell that deregulate the cell, causing it to proliferate abnormally. Many environmental factors can induce mutations. A mutant cell often produces different cell proteins not present in a normal cell. These mutant-gene encoded proteins are recognized as abnormal by the immune system, which attempts to destroy the abnormal cell by means of various cell-mediated and humoral mechanisms. Apparently, mutations leading to neoplastic transformation of cells are relatively common, but the body recognizes the altered cells as abnormal and destroys them as soon as they are formed. Only a tiny percentage of abnormal cells ever develop into clinically apparent tumors. Therefore, one may consider a tumor to manifest in part a failure of the body's immune defenses. This concept is supported by evidence that individuals with congenital deficiencies of immunologic defense mechanisms have a higher than expected incidence of tumors. Tumors also occur frequently in persons whose immune responses have been deliberately suppressed by drugs or other substances.

Figure 10–20 illustrates the interrelation of the factors concerned with the defense against tumors. On the one hand, abnormal cells arise and tend to proliferate, leading to tumors. On the other hand, the immune-defense mechanisms destroy these abnormal cells before they can prove hazardous to the body. Tumors result when the defense mechanisms fail. Fortunately, in most instances the immune surveillance system eliminates the "bad" cells as soon as they appear. Although the immune-defense mechanisms are quite efficient

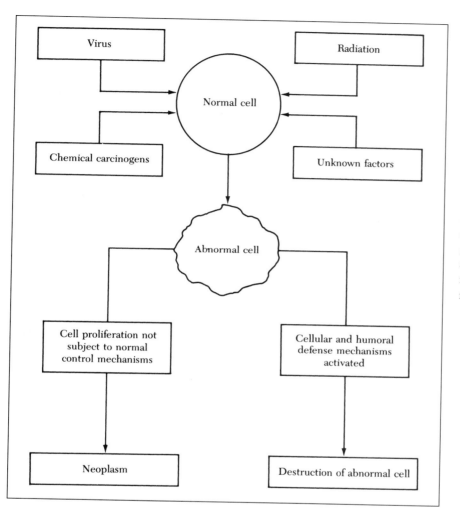

FIGURE 10–20

Factors leading to neoplastic transformation of cells counterbalanced by immunologic defense against neoplasm. Conversion from a normal cell into an abnormal one by various agents requires activation of oncogenes and inactivation of tumor suppressor genes, which renders the cell unresponsive to normal control mechanisms that regulate cell growth. Generally, multiple step-by-step mutations are required to transform a normal cell into a cancer cell.

in eliminating abnormal cells before they develop into a tumor, they are much less effective in eliminating an established tumor.

Heredity and Tumors

Although there is no strong hereditary predisposition to most common malignant tumors, hereditary factors do play a small role in some common tumors. A person whose parent or sibling has been afflicted with a breast, colon, or lung carcinoma has about a three times greater risk of developing a similar tumor than do other people. The predisposition is apparently the result of a multifactorial inheritance pattern in which the individual at risk has inherited sets of genes that influence some hormonal- or enzyme-regulated biochemical process within the body that slightly increases the susceptibility to a specific cancer. The increased risk may be caused by genetic differences in various biochemical or physiologic activities that influence cell functions, such as:

1. Differences in circulating hormone levels that could influence cell growth rates
2. Variations in the rate at which the cell can metabolize and inactivate cancer-causing chemicals to which the cells are exposed
3. Variations in the ability to repair DNA that has been damaged by injurious agents
4. Variations in the efficiency of the immune system in eliminating abnormal cells as they arise

Possibly, women with a slightly higher-than-normal risk of breast carcinoma have different genetically determined patterns of ovarian and pituitary hormone secretions, which may account for the slightly increased susceptibility.

Hereditary factors do play a major role in a small percentage of breast carcinomas. Some of these cases can be traced to an inherited breast carcinoma susceptibility gene designated the *BRCA1* (breast carcinoma 1) gene, which has been localized to chromosome 17 and is a mutant tumor suppressor gene. Women who inherit the mutant gene are at a greatly increased risk of developing ovarian cancer as well. Other, similar cases not related to *BRCA1* appear to be related to another mutant suppressor gene, designated the *BRCA2* (breast carcinoma 2) gene, which has been localized to chromosome 13.

A few relatively rare tumors also are inherited. Some cases of retinoblastoma (see figure 10–17) are hereditary, and this tumor also is a classic example illustrating how tumor suppressor genes control cell function and how loss of control can cause a tumor. Retinoblastoma is a malignant tumor of primitive retinal cells occurring in infants and children that is caused by loss of function of tumor suppressor genes called *RB* genes. Normal *RB* genes exist in pairs, one on each of the homologous pair of chromosome 13, and both *RB* genes must be nonfunctional in a retinal cell before a tumor arises. About half the retinoblastomas are hereditary; the rest occur sporadically, without any hereditary predisposition. The hereditary form of retinoblastoma is prone to occur if a child inherits a defective nonfunctional *RB* gene from a parent. The affected child has only a single functioning *RB* gene in all body cells, including those in the retina, but the single functioning *RB* gene is sufficient to maintain control of cell functions. However, if a chance mutation occurs in the remaining single functional *RB* gene within a retinal cell, all *RB* gene function in the affected cell is lost. The affected cell then proliferates to form a clone of unregulated cells and eventually a malignant retinal tumor. Hereditary retinoblastomas may occur in both eyes, because retinal cells in both eyes are equally vulnerable to similar random *RB* gene mutations in other single functioning *RB* genes. In the sporadic form of retinoblastoma, both *RB* genes in the same retinal cell must undergo mutation in order to deregulate cell function and give rise to a retinoblastoma. Figure 10–21 summarizes the pathogenesis of this tumor. The hereditary form of neuroblastoma is considered to be transmitted as a Mendelian dominant trait,

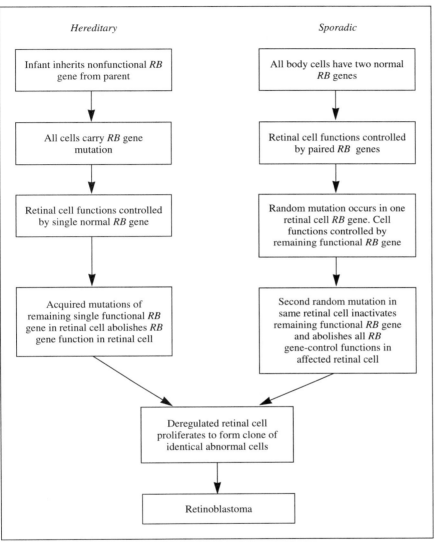

FIGURE 10–21

Pathogenesis of retino-
blastoma.

because the transmission of a single defective *RB* gene from parent to child places the child at very high risk of developing this tumor, even though the second *RB* gene must become nonfunctional in a retinal cell before the neoplasm actually arises.

A condition called *multiple polyposis of the colon,* also a dominant trait, is characterized by the formation of multiple polyps throughout the colon, and usually one or more of them eventually becomes malignant. Another condition transmitted as an autosomal dominant trait is called *multiple neurofibromatosis* (described in chapter 26). Many of the nerves throughout the body give rise to benign tumors called neurofibromas, and often one of these tumors eventually undergoes malignant change. Still another hereditary tumor syndrome, also an autosomal dominant transmission, is called *multiple endocrine adenomatosis* and is characterized by formation of adenomas arising in several different endocrine glands, as the name indicates.

These are some examples of tumors having a well-established pattern of hereditary transmission. Other hereditary tumors have been identified and their inheritance patterns have been determined. It is important to remember, however, that they make up only a minute fraction of all the benign and malignant tumors afflicting humans.

Diagnosis of Tumors

Early Recognition of Neoplasms

The American Cancer Society publicizes a number of signs and symptoms that should arouse suspicion of cancer (table 10–4). In general, any abnormality of form or function may be an early symptoms of a neoplasm and should be investigated by a physician. For example, a lump in the breast, an ulcer on the lip, or a change in the character of a wart or mole may be considered an abnormality of form. Menstrual bleeding in a postmenopausal woman or a change in bowel habits manifested by constipation or diarrhea is an abnormality of function.

A complete medical history and physical examination by the physician are the next steps in evaluating suspected abnormalities. The physical examination may include special studies such as an examination of the rectum and colon by means of a special instrument, vaginal examination and Pap smear in women, examination of the esophagus and stomach with special devices, and various types of x-ray studies.

If a tumor is discovered, exact diagnosis requires biopsy or complete excision of the suspected tumor. Histologic examination of the tissue by the pathologist will provide an exact diagnosis and serve as a guide to further treatment. If the tumor is benign, simple excision is curative. If the tumor is malignant, a more extensive operation or another kind of treatment may be required.

TABLE 10–4

American Cancer Society warning signals

1. Change in bowel or bladder habits
2. A sore that does not heal
3. Unusual bleeding or discharge
4. Thickening or lump in breast or elsewhere
5. Indigestion or difficulty in swallowing
6. Obvious change in wart or mole
7. Nagging cough or hoarseness

Cytologic Diagnosis of Neoplasms

Tumors shed abnormal cells from their surfaces, and these cells can be recognized in the body fluids and secretions that come into contact with the tumor (figure 10–22). Often the abnormal cells can be recognized when the neoplasm is only microscopic in size and is still confined to the surface epithelium. These observations have been applied to the cytologic diagno-

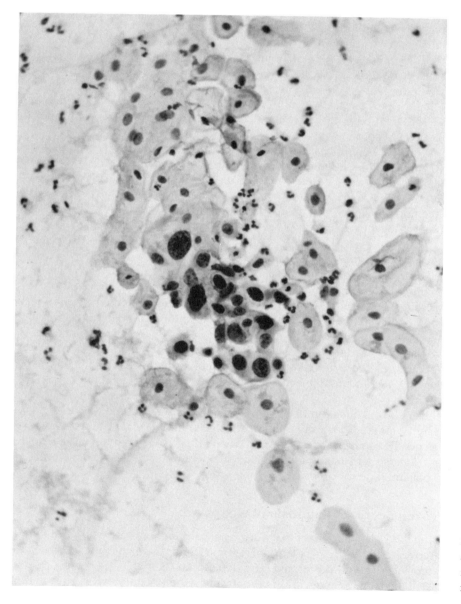

FIGURE 10–22

Photomicrograph of Pap smear illustrating cluster of abnormal cells from in situ carcinoma of cervix. Cells appear much different from the adjacent normal squamous epithelial cells in the photograph. (Original magnification × 150.)

sis of tumors. The method is named after the physician who played a large part in developing and applying cytologic methods, Dr. George Papanicolaou. The microscopic slides of the material prepared for cytologic examination are called **Papanicolaou smears** or, simply, *Pap smears.*

In carcinoma of the uterine cervix, abnormal cells can often be found in the vaginal secretions. They are more readily identified, however, in smears prepared from material that has been gently scraped from the epithelium of the cervix surrounding the cervical opening (*external os*) by means of a small, disposable wooden spatula. Usually, secretions for study are also obtained from the cervical canal at the same time. Widespread application of cytologic methods has led to much earlier detection of cervical carcinoma than had previously been possible and has played a significant role in reducing mortality from carcinoma of the uterine cervix. Cytologic methods can also be applied to the diagnosis of neoplasms in other locations by examining sputum, urine, breast secretions, and fluids obtained from the pleural or peritoneal cavities. However, cytology has been most valuable in the early diagnosis of cervical cancer. This subject is considered further in chapter 17.

It should be emphasized that an abnormal Pap smear indicates only that the epithelium is shedding abnormal cells. It does not necessarily indicate a diagnosis of cancer, because some benign diseases are occasionally associated with the desquamation of atypical cells. A Pap smear should be considered a screening procedure, and an abnormal smear should be followed by a biopsy and histologic examination of the tissue to establish an exact diagnosis.

Cytologic Diagnosis by Fine Needle Aspiration

Cells for cytologic study can also be obtained by aspirating material from organs or tissues by means of a fine needle attached to a syringe and preparing slides from the aspirated material. This technique is often used to evaluate nodules in the thyroid or breast, and often one can determine whether the nodule is benign or malignant from the appearance of the aspirated cells, avoiding the need for a biopsy. Suspected tumors in the lung, liver, pancreas, kidney, and other internal organs also can be examined by fine needle aspiration. When attempting aspiration from internal organs, one must precisely determined the location of the suspected tumor by means of a CT scan or other x-ray examination or by ultrasound and insert the needle into the suspected tumor under x-ray guidance. In general, the diagnostic accuracy of fine needle aspiration is not as good as an actual biopsy but often is adequate for diagnosis and avoids a major surgical operation, which would be required to obtain tissue for biopsy.

Frozen-Section Diagnosis of Neoplasms

Many times, it is important that a surgeon learn immediately whether a tumor discovered in the course of an operation is benign or malignant, because the extent of resection performed may depend on the nature of the neoplasm. Often, the surgeon must also find out during the operation whether a tumor has been excised completely or whether it has spread to lymph nodes or distant sites. A pathologist can provide the surgeon with a rapid histologic diagnosis and other information by means of a special technique called a **frozen section.** In this method, a portion of the tumor or other tissue to be examined histologically is frozen solid at subzero temperature. A thin section of the frozen tissue is cut by means of a special instrument called a *microtome,* and slides are prepared and stained. The slides can then be examined by the pathologist, and a rapid histologic diagnosis can be made. The entire procedure takes only a few minutes.

Tumor-Associated Antigen Tests

Some cancers secrete substances called **tumor-associated antigens.** These are either absent from normal mature tissues or present only in trace amounts. Most tumor-associated antigens are carbohydrate-protein complexes (*glyco-proteins*) that are secreted as a coating on the surface of the cancer cells. Some of the glycoprotein gains access to the circulation, where it can be detected by means of specialized laboratory tests performed on the blood of patients with cancer.

A well-known tumor-associated antigen is a substance called **carcinoem-bryonic antigen** (CEA), so named because it resembles a glycoprotein antigen secreted by the cells lining the fetal intestinal tract. It has been postulated that cancer cells elaborate CEA because they are immature and have acquired some properties of fetal cells that adult cells do not have (figure 10–23).

Not all malignant tumors secrete CEA. Moreover, elevation of CEA levels is not specific for any one type of cancer. CEA is produced by most malignant tumors of the gastrointestinal tract and pancreas, but it is also secreted

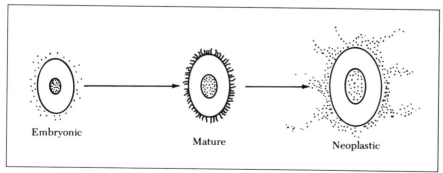

Embryonic

Mature

Neoplastic

FIGURE 10–23

Relation of carcinoembryonic antigen (CEA) to embryonic cells. Embryonic cell (*left*) produces a specific type of carbohydrate-protein coating on its surface. Coating is replaced by a different type in the mature cell (*center*). Neoplastic cell (*right*) reverts to more primitive state and resumes production of embryonic coating material, which enters circulation and can often be detected in the blood of patient with invasive cancer.

by many cancers of the breast and lung and by other cancers as well. The amount of CEA secreted is related to the size of the tumor. CEA is usually not elevated in the blood of persons with small, early cancers, but the levels are often quite high in persons with large tumors or tumors that have metastasized. When CEA is elevated in a patient with cancer, the level falls after the tumor has been removed and often rises again if the tumor recurs or metastasizes (figure 10–24). Many physicians perform serial determinations of CEA to monitor the course of patients with CEA-secreting tumors. If CEA falls after surgical resection of the tumor and later becomes elevated, this usually means that the tumor has recurred and is an indication for additional treatment. Slight elevations of CEA are sometimes detected in patients with diseases other than cancer. This does not detract from the usefulness of the CEA test, however, because the CEA levels are usually much lower than in patients with malignant tumors.

Other products secreted by tumor cells that can be used to monitor tumor growth are discussed in chapter 20. They include *alpha fetoprotein,* a protein produced by fetal tissues but not normally produced by adult cells, and *human chorionic gonadotropin,* the hormone normally produced by the placenta in pregnancy, which are often elevated in patients with testicular carcinoma. Alpha fetoprotein is also frequently elevated in patients with primary carcinoma of the liver. *Acid phosphatase,* an enzyme secreted by prostatic epithelial cells, is often high in patients with prostatic carcinoma, as is *prostatic-specific antigen,* which also is secreted by prostate epithelial cells. Many other tumor markers have been identified and are used to monitor patients with various types of lung, breast, and ovarian carcinoma.

FIGURE 10–24

Use of CEA to monitor response to therapy. Elevated CEA level falls after resection of colon cancer and rises when tumor recurs, indicating need for additional treatment.

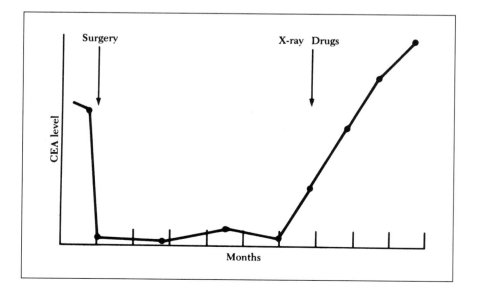

Benign tumors are completely cured by surgical excision. Malignant tumors are much more difficult to treat. Four major forms of treatment are directed against malignant tumors:

1. Surgery
2. Radiotherapy
3. Hormones
4. Anticancer drugs (chemotherapy)

The method of treatment depends upon the type of tumor and its extent, and sometimes several methods are combined. In many cases, treatment eradicates the cancer, and the patient is cured. In less-favorable cases, cure is no longer possible, but the growth of the cancer is arrested and life is prolonged.

Surgery

Many malignant tumors are treated by wide surgical excision of the tumor and the surrounding tissues, usually with removal of the regional lymph nodes that drain the tumor site. This treatment is successful if the tumor has not already spread to distant sites. Unfortunately, many cancers have already metastasized when first detected and may no longer be curable by surgery alone. Other methods of treatment must be used, frequently in combination with surgery.

Radiotherapy

Malignant lymphomas and some epithelial tumors are quite radiosensitive and can be destroyed by radiotherapy rather than by surgical excision. In some cases, radiation and surgery are combined. For example, radiation may be administered preoperatively to reduce the size of a tumor, thereby facilitating its surgical resection; in other instances, radiotherapy is given after a malignant tumor has been resected (cut out) in order to destroy any cancer cells that may have been left behind. Radiotherapy is also used to control the growth of widespread tumors and to treat deposits of metastatic tumor that cause pain and disability. The treatment relieves symptoms and makes the patient more comfortable, even though the cancer is not curable.

Hormone Therapy

Some malignant tumors require hormones for their growth and are called *hormone responsive*. They regress temporarily if deprived of the required hormone. For example, many prostate tumors require testosterone and are inhibited by removal of the testes (eliminating the source of testosterone) or by administration of estrogens (which suppresses testosterone secretion). Many breast carcinomas in postmenopausal women are estrogen responsive and can be controlled by drugs that block estrogen so that the tumor cells are no longer stimulated by estrogen.

Adrenal cortical hormones (*corticosteroids*) also inhibit the growth of many malignant tumors. Corticosteroids inhibit protein synthesis, thereby suppressing the growth and division of the tumor cells. Tumors of the lymphatic tissues are especially susceptible to the effects of corticosteroids.

Anticancer Drugs

Cancer cells, like normal cells, synthesize deoxyribonucleic acid (DNA) from various precursors. The DNA directs the production of the various forms of ribonucleic acid (messenger RNA, transfer RNA, and ribosomal RNA), and the RNA in turn takes part in the synthesis of enzymes and other proteins that are necessary for cell function. Anticancer drugs impede the growth and division of cells by disrupting some phase of this complex process.

The various drugs differ in their mechanisms of action. Some inhibit the synthesis of either DNA or RNA. Others alter the structure of DNA or disturb its function. Still others inhibit protein synthesis or prevent the mitotic spindle from forming, so the cell cannot divide. Frequently, several different anticancer drugs are administered simultaneously, each drug blocking a different phase in the cell's metabolic processes.

Most anticancer drugs work best against fast-growing tumors that contain large numbers of actively growing and dividing cells. They are usually less effective against slowly growing tumors because only relatively small numbers of the tumor cells are in the stages of cell growth or division that are susceptible to the injurious effects of the drugs.

One important group of anticancer drugs is called **alkylating agents.** These drugs interact with both strands of the paired DNA chains in the nucleus and bind them together so that they cannot separate. This reaction is called *cross-linking of the DNA chains.* It disrupts the function of DNA because the chains must separate for duplication of the DNA chains and for synthesis of RNA. Alkylating agents also disturb cell function by altering the structure of the DNA chains. In contrast to most anticancer drugs, these agents are effective against nondividing ("resting") cells as well as actively growing cells.

Another large group of anticancer drugs is called **antimetabolites.** They resemble essential compounds required for cell growth and multiplication, but they cannot be utilized by the cell. Therefore, they disrupt the cell's metabolic processes. (Some antimicrobial agents inhibit bacterial growth in this way, as described in the section on competitive inhibition in chapter 6.)

All anticancer drugs are quite toxic. They injure normal cells as well as cancer cells and must be administered very carefully in order to assure maximum damage to tumor cells without irreparable injury to normal cells. Lymphoid tissue is quite susceptible to the destructive effects of these potent drugs, and, consequently, one unavoidable side effect of anticancer drugs is impairment of cell-mediated and humoral immunity.

Adjuvant Chemotherapy

Sometimes, surgical resection of a cancer appears to be successful, but metastases appear several years later and eventually prove fatal. The operation fails to eradicate the tumor because small, unrecognized metastases have already spread throughout the body. Even though the main tumor has been removed, the minute metastases continue to grow until eventually they form many large, bulky deposits of metastatic tumor that kill the patient.

In order to forestall the development of late metastases, a current trend is to administer a course of anticancer drugs after surgical resection of some tumors. This is called **adjuvant chemotherapy** (*adjuvare* = to assist). The drugs destroy any small, undetected foci of metastatic tumor before they become large enough to produce clinical manifestations. In some cases, adjuvant chemotherapy combined with surgery appears to achieve better results than surgery alone. Anticancer drugs are quite toxic, however, and the potential benefits of adjuvant chemotherapy must be weighed against the harmful effects of the drugs on normal tissues.

Immunotherapy

The immune system has evolved a number of ways to deal with abnormal cells that can proliferate and form tumors, and to deal with established tumors.

1. Cytotoxic T cells recognize antigens on tumor cells that are displayed along with the cells' own MHC Class I proteins and can damage the tumor cells by secreting destructive lymphokines.
2. Natural killer lymphocytes can attack and destroy tumor cells without prior antigenic stimulation, and some killer lymphocytes specialize in attacking antibody-coated tumor cells.
3. Activated macrophages can destroy tumor cells by phagocytosis, and by secreting tumor necrosis factor along with other cytokines that stimulate lymphocytes to attack tumor cells.
4. Antibodies formed against tumor cell antigens can affix to tumor cells and activate complement; products of complement activation attract lymphocytes and macrophages and form destructive attack complexes that damage the cell membranes of the tumor cells.

Despite the array of immunologic defenses, many tumors circumvent or overwhelm the body's immune defenses and so they become ineffective and no longer retard the growth of the tumor. Some tumor cells produce little or no MHC Class I protein. Because cytotoxic T cells can recognize tumor cell antigens only if they are displayed along with MHC Class I proteins, the lymphocytes cannot attack the tumor cells because they cannot recognize the tumor antigens without the associated MHC Class I proteins. Some tumor cells thwart the immune system because the tumor cells release large amounts of soluble tumor-specific antigens that saturate the body to such an extent that the lymphocytes are no longer capable of responding to the tumor-specific antigens on the surface of the tumor cells. In addition, the chemotherapy and irradiation used to treat tumors also suppress the body's immune responses. When the patient's immune capacity is impaired for any reason, the growth of the tumor is no longer inhibited, indicating a poor prognosis. Various attempts have been made to stimulate the body's immune system so that it can deal more effectively with the tumor, in order to improve the patient's prognosis. Treatment of tumors by stimulating the body's immune defenses is called **immunotherapy.** Nonspecific immunotherapy is directed toward bolstering the patient's own immune defenses so that the patient can deal more effectively with the tumor. Specific immunotherapy directs the immune system against the specific antigens present in the patient's own tumor.

Nonspecific Immunotherapy

Initially, attempts were made to stimulate the immune system nonspecifically by immunizing the patient with vaccines prepared from various types of bacteria or bacterial products, but this approach had very limited success and was associated with serious complications. Sometimes the therapy actually accelerated rather than retarded tumor growth because antitumor antibodies were produced that coated the surface of the tumor cells, protecting them from the cytotoxic T cells and activated macrophages that were trying to destroy them.

More recent approaches have consisted of the administration of various cytokines that either stimulate cells of the immune system or act against the tumor cells. The two cytokines that have been used with greatest success against tumors are *interferon* and *interleukin-2.*

Interferon   Interferon is the name given to a group of carbohydrate-containing, "broad spectrum" antiviral protein substances produced by cells in response to viral infection (described in chapter 6), but interferon has other functions. It regulates the functions of the immune system and regulates cell growth, inhibiting the growth of rapidly dividing cells. These latter properties have led to the use of interferon for treating tumors as well as viral infections. After methods for producing interferon commercially were developed, large quantities of interferon became available for clinical use, and studies were undertaken in patients with various tumors in order to evaluate the usefulness of this material. To date, the best results have been obtained in patients with a relatively rare type of leukemia called "hairy cell" leukemia (so named because the hairlike processes projecting from the cytoplasm of the tumor cell). Interferon has also produced responses in some patients with other types of leukemia, multiple myeloma (described later in this chapter), some lymphomas, and some widely disseminated carcinomas that had not responded to other methods of treatment. Interferon has the advantage of being much less toxic than many anticancer drugs, and treatment by intramuscular injection several times per week is usually well tolerated.

Interleukin-2   Interleukin-2 is a lymphokine produced by T cells. It stimulates the production of natural killer cells and cytotoxic T cells that can destroy tumor cells, but it has no direct effects against the tumor cells. Interleukin-2 is administered in multiple courses and has produced beneficial effects in the treatment of metastatic melanoma and renal cell carcinoma. High doses of interleukin-2 produce a variety of toxic effects that limit its use to some extent.

Interleukin-2 has also been administered along with lymphocytes obtained from the patient, an approach called *cell transfer immunotherapy*. One method is to collect blood from the patient and incubate the blood with interleukin-2 in the laboratory, which stimulates the lymphocytes to proliferate and generates a large population of natural killer lymphocytes. Then the lymphocytes (which are called *lymphokine-activated killer cells*) are infused into the patient to seek out and destroy the tumor.

Other Cytokines   Various other cytokines have been produced by genetic engineering and are undergoing clinical evaluation. They include *tumor necrosis factor* and a cytokine produced by macrophages called *interleukin-1,* which has antitumor activity.

Specific Immunotherapy

Specific immunotherapy targets the patient's own tumor cells for attack. Three different approaches appear promising: (1) administration of cytotoxic T lymphocytes directed against the tumor, which are called *tumor-infiltrating lymphocytes;* (2) administration of tumor vaccines; and (3) administration of antitumor antibodies.

Tumor-Infiltrating Lymphocyte Therapy   This is a specific type of cell transfer immunotherapy in which the lymphocytes infused back into the patient are obtained from the patient's own tumor. These lymphocytes are actually infiltrating the tumor and are trying to destroy it, and they are obtained when the tumor is biopsied or excised. The tumor-infiltrating lymphocytes contain a large concentration of cytotoxic T lymphocytes specifically targeted against the antigens in the patient's own tumor, as well as numbers of natural killer lymphocytes that also can destroy tumor cells. The lymphocytes from the tumor are grown in the laboratory with interleukin-2, to stimulate their growth, and then infused back into the patient to attack and destroy the tumor. This approach has been used with some success to treat metastatic malignant melanoma.

Tumor Vaccines   Tumor vaccines prepared from the patient's own tumor also have been used to immunize the patient against the tumor, in an effort to reduce the likelihood that the tumor will recur or metastasize after it has been resected. Tumor cells are obtained from the resected tumor, grown in the laboratory, and then killed so that they cannot proliferate in the patient but can still generate an immune response. They are then used to prepare a vaccine that will stimulate an immune response to the resected tumor.

Tumor vaccines have been used as an additional treatment after resection of a malignant melanoma or a colon carcinoma when the patient is considered at high risk of recurrence.

Tumor Antibody Therapy In this approach, antibodies are prepared against tumor cell antigens and then the antibodies are linked to some anti-tumor drug or toxin that can kill tumor cells. The antibodies with attached drug or toxin are then infused back into the patient to seek out and destroy the tumor cells without damaging normal cells.

Results of Immunotherapy

Results of immunotherapy have been mixed. There have been some notable successes, as in the use of interferon therapy for one type of leukemia called hairy cell leukemia. Some types of immunotherapy have produced gratifying results in persons with specific types of widespread tumors when no other methods of treatment were available to control the tumor. No single method works against all types of tumors, and ongoing clinical trials continue to assess the applications and limitations of these various methods. Unfortunately, most patients treated with immunotherapy have advanced diseases, and often the body's immune defenses are incapable of dealing with such large amounts of tumor even when stimulated by immunotherapy.

Leukemia

The term **leukemia** refers to a neoplasm of hematopoietic tissue. In contrast to solid tumors, which form nodular deposits, leukemic cells diffusely infiltrate the bone marrow and lymphoid tissues, spill over into the bloodstream, and infiltrate throughout the various organs of the body. The leukemic cells may be mostly mature or they may be extremely primitive. The overproduction of white cells in leukemia may be revealed in the peripheral blood by a very high white blood count. In some cases of leukemia, however, the proliferation of the white cells is largely confined to the bone marrow, and there is no significant increase in the number of white cells in the bloodstream.

Classification of Leukemia

Leukemia is classified on the basis of both the cell type and the maturity of the proliferating cells. Any type of hematopoietic cells can give rise to leukemia, but the most common types are granulocytic, monocytic, and lymphocytic. Leukemia developing from stem cells that would normally give rise to the leukocytes containing specific granules (neutrophils, eosinophils, and basophils) is called *granulocytic leukemia. Monocytic leukemia* develops from precursor cells that give rise to monocytes. *Lymphocytic leukemia* is derived from lymphoid precursor cells. Various subclassifications have been established within these major groups on the basis of the characteristics of the cell membranes and the enzymes present within the leukemic cells, as determined by highly specialized techniques. Another type of leukemia also arises from lymphoid cells and has some unusual features. Cytoplasmic processes projecting from the cells give the cells a distinctive appearance, which is responsible for the descriptive term *hairy cell leukemia.*

If the leukemia cells are mostly primitive forms, the leukemia is classified as *acute leukemia* (figure 10–25). In *chronic leukemia,* the abnormal cells are mostly mature (figures 10–26 and 10–27).

In most instances, the total number of white blood cells in the peripheral blood is significantly above normal. Occasionally, however, the marrow may be crowded with abnormal cells, but the number of white blood cells

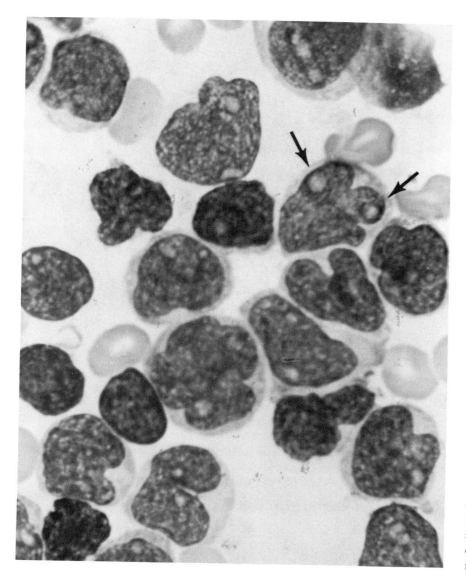

FIGURE 10–25

Photomicrograph of blood smear from patient with acute leukemia. The nuclei of the white cells have a fine chromatin structure and contain nucleoli indicating immaturity (*arrows*). Nuclei are irregular in size and configuration. (Original magnification × 1000.)

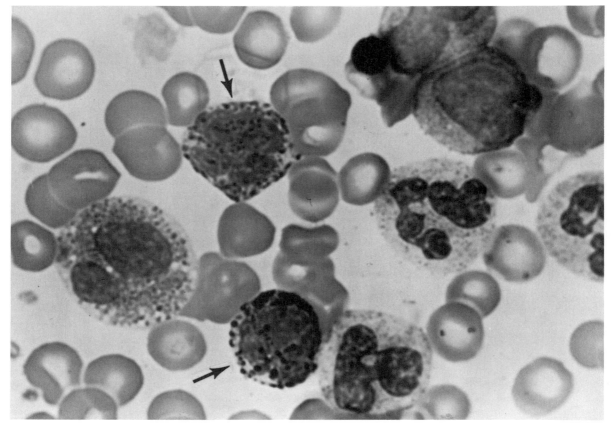

FIGURE 10–26

Chronic granulocytic leukemia. Most of the cells in the photomicrograph are mature. Note basophils (*arrows*), eosinophils (left of *arrows*), and three neutrophils (right of *arrows*). (Original magnification × 1000.)

in the blood is normal or decreased. This variety of leukemia is sometimes called *aleukemic leukemia.* The term is merely descriptive and does not denote a type of leukemia with any special clinical features or any difference in prognosis.

Generally, the classifications by cell type and maturity are used together. Thus, one may speak of chronic granulocytic leukemia, acute lymphocytic leukemia, or acute monocytic leukemia. The term *aleukemic* is often added if the number of white cells in the circulating blood is reduced.

Clinical Features and Principles of Treatment

The clinical features of leukemia are of two kinds: those caused by impairment of bone marrow function and those caused by infiltration of the viscera by leukemic cells. The overgrowth of leukemic cells in the bone marrow often

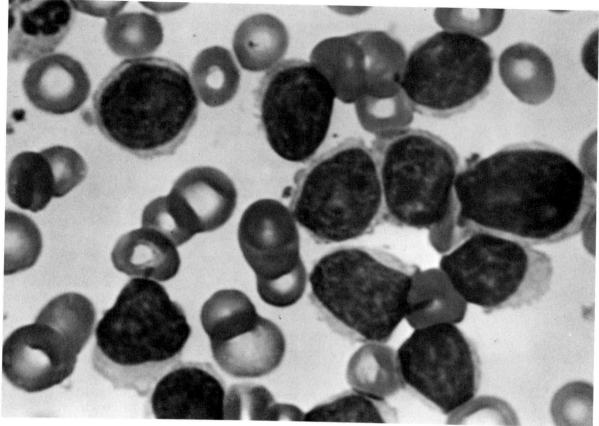

FIGURE 10–27

Chronic lymphocytic leukemia. The dense nuclear chromatin structure indicates that the lymphocytes are mature (compare with figure 10–25). Total white count is elevated. (Original magnification × 1000.)

crowds out normal bone marrow cells. This leads to anemia as a result of inadequate red cell production, bleeding caused by thrombocytopenia, and infection resulting from inadequate numbers of normal white blood cells, which are an important part of the body's defenses against pathogenic organisms.

The leukemic cells not only infiltrate the bone marrow, but also spread into the spleen, liver, lymph nodes, and other tissues. In chronic leukemia, the evolution of the disease proceeds at a relatively slow pace and often can be well controlled by treatment for long periods of time. Therefore, the patient with chronic leukemia may survive for many years in relatively good health. In contrast, acute leukemia is often a rapidly progressive disease. Symptoms of bone marrow infiltration and visceral infiltration make their appearance early and are quite conspicuous. In some patients with acute leukemia, the abnormal proliferation of the leukemic cells can be stopped for a variable period of time by various anticancer drugs, and the patient appears to have completely recovered. An arrest of the disease induced by therapy is called a *remission*. In many cases, however, the patient undergoes a relapse and the disease ultimately proves fatal. Acute leukemia in children responds better to anticancer chemotherapy than acute leukemia in adults, and some children have been completely cured by intensive therapy.

Some patients with acute leukemia and chronic granulocytic leukemia can be treated successfully by *bone marrow transplantation* from a compatible donor. Marrow transplantation has also been used successfully to treat patients with multiple myeloma, widespread lymphoma affecting the bone marrow, and Hodgkin's disease when the bone marrow is infiltrated by the neoplasm. In this treatment, the patient's own marrow is destroyed first by large doses of anticancer drugs and radiation. Then several hundred milliliters of bone marrow are aspirated from multiple sites in the pelvic bones of a suitable donor, filtered to break up the clusters of marrow cells and form a homogeneous suspension of individual cells, and injected into the patient. The marrow cells circulate in the patient's blood but become established and grow only in the marrow, producing within a few weeks a new population of leukemia-free marrow cells derived from the donor. The marrow transplant is a foreign tissue, however, and the patient's own immunologic defenses must be suppressed (described in chapter 5) in order for the transplanted marrow to survive.

The transplant patient also faces another problem related to immunologic differences between the cells of the donor and those of the patient, which is called a *graft-versus-host reaction*. The donor lymphocytes in the transplanted marrow recognize the patient's cells as antigenically different and attempt to destroy them, leading to various clinical manifestations including skin rash, liver injury, and gastrointestinal symptoms. This is the reverse of the usual situation in which the patient tries to reject the transplant. Here, the transplant tries to reject the patient!

Although marrow transplantation is an important advance, it is not always successful. Patients may develop life-threatening infections related to the immunosuppression required to maintain the transplant, and in some patients the leukemia recurs, arising from the patient's surviving leukemic cells that were not destroyed by the prior chemotherapy and radiation.

Newer transplantation methods are being developed in which the patient's own marrow is used for transplantation, which is called an *autologous bone marrow transplant* (*auto* = self). One approach comprises collecting the patient's own marrow while the patient is in remission, treating the marrow to destroy any surviving leukemic cells, and storing the marrow in liquid nitrogen for later use should the patient develop recurrent leukemia. If this occurs, the patient's leukemic marrow is destroyed by anticancer drugs and radiation, and the stored leukemic-free marrow is reinfused into the patient as a transplant. Because the transplant is the patient's own marrow, immunosuppression is not required and complications related to immunosuppression are avoided. Autologous bone marrow transplants have also been used to treat patients with acute leukemia when no compatible marrow transplant donor is available. In this situation, the leukemic patient's marrow is collected in the same way as marrow is from a donor. Then the patient is treated with chemotherapy and radiation to destroy the diseased marrow. Meanwhile, the patient's previously collected marrow is treated with specific antibodies that destroy the leukemic cells without affecting the normal marrow cells. Then the treated marrow is returned to the patient, and, if all goes well, the leukemia-free marrow becomes reestablished and functions normally.

Precursors of Leukemia: The Myelodysplastic Syndromes

For many years it has been recognized that acute leukemia in older patients may not have an abrupt onset but is preceded by a period lasting from several months to several years in which the affected patients have only a moderate anemia, sometimes associated with reduced white cells (leukopenia) and low blood platelets (*thrombocytopenia*). Examination of the bone marrow of these patients reveals variable degrees of disturbed growth and maturation of red cells, white cell precursors, and megakaryocytes but not leukemia. This condition has been called *preleukemia,* although it was realized that not all patients with bone marrow maturation disturbances of this type develop leukemia, and one could not reliably predict which patients would eventually become leukemic. Recently these conditions have been grouped together under the general term **myelodysplastic syndromes** (*myelo* = marrow + *dysplasia* = disturbed growth). Several different types have been described that differ somewhat in their clinical and hematologic manifestations. In general, the more severe the maturation disturbance in the bone marrow, the greater the likelihood that leukemia would eventually occur. Unfortunately, there is no specific treatment available for most patients with these conditions, although some patients with severe "preleukemic" changes in their bone marrow have been treated successfully by bone marrow transplantation.

Multiple myeloma is a neoplasm arising from plasma cells within the bone marrow (figure 10–28). In many ways, it resembles leukemia, but the neoplastic plasma cell proliferation is generally confined to the bone marrow. Infiltration of the viscera by the abnormal plasma cells is unusual; outpouring of large numbers of plasma cells into the peripheral blood also is uncommon. The abnormal plasma cells either may infiltrate the bone marrow diffusely or may form discrete tumors that weaken the bone, leading to spontaneous fractures, pain, and disability (figure 10–29).

Multiple Myeloma

Normal plasma cells produce antibody proteins (*immunoglobulins*), as described in chapter 5. In myeloma, the neoplastic cells also often produce large amounts of protein. This greatly increases blood proteins and, correspondingly, blood viscosity. The protein produced by the myeloma cells is generally a single type of immunoglobulin, usually IgG. In some patients, the

FIGURE 10–28

Photomicrograph illustrating
aspirated bone marrow
from patient with multiple
myeloma. Almost all cells
are immature plasma cells
containing large eccentric
nuclei and abundant cyto-
plasm. (Original magnification × 400.)

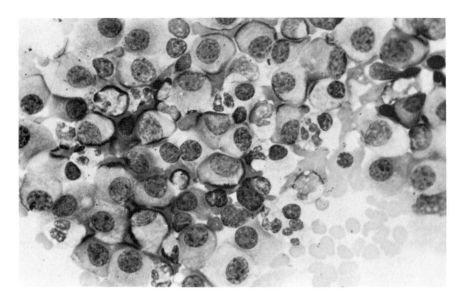

FIGURE 10–29

Skull x-ray from patient with
multiple myeloma. Multiple
punched-out areas in skull
bones (*arrow*) result from
bone destruction caused by
nodular masses of neoplastic
plasma cells growing in
bone marrow.

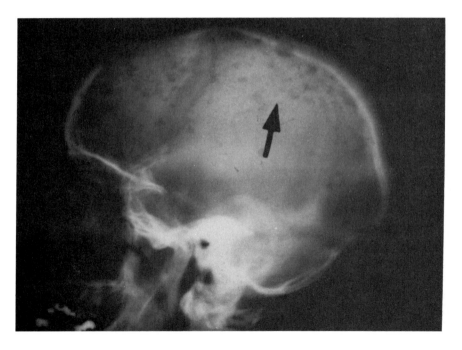

production of immunoglobulins also is abnormal, and an excess of light chains
is produced. Any light chains that are not incorporated into the immunoglobulin molecules are excreted in the urine. The myeloma protein can be identified in the blood (figure 10–30), and the free light chains can be identified in
the urine by special laboratory tests.

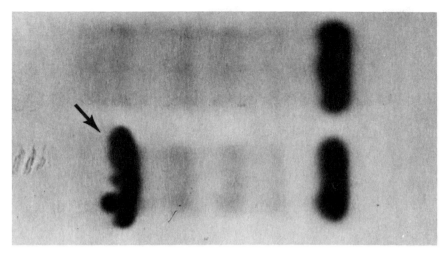

FIGURE 10–30

Examination of serum proteins by special technique (*electrophoresis*) that separates serum proteins into various fractions. The upper pattern is a fraction of a normal serum, with the dense albumin band at the *far right* in the photograph. The lower pattern is from a patient with multiple myeloma. *Arrow* indicates homogeneous band representing protein produced by the abnormal plasma cells.

Masses of coagulated myeloma protein may accumulate within the patient's own tissues, and so the function of the affected tissues is severely impaired. Some patients with myeloma die of kidney failure because masses of protein produced by the plasma cells infiltrate the kidneys and block the renal tubules.

Malignant neoplasms are a leading cause of disability and death. Cancer is second only to heart disease as a cause of death in the United States, accounting for almost 17 percent of all deaths in this country. It has been estimated that one in every four persons will eventually develop cancer. Of the cancers affecting major organs, lung carcinoma is the most common malignant tumor in men, and breast carcinoma is the most frequent in women. Carcinoma of the intestine is quite common in both sexes. The survival rate for patients with malignant tumors depends on whether the disease has been diagnosed and treated early, before it has spread. The chances for survival are significantly reduced if the tumor has metastasized to regional lymph nodes or to distant sites.

The curability of the various types of cancer can be assessed in terms of five-year survival rates, which range from more than 80 percent for patients with thyroid cancer to a discouraging 1 percent for those with pancreatic carcinoma (table 10–5). Attempts are being made continually to improve survival rates by means of earlier diagnosis and more effective therapy. Unfortunately, five-year survival does not necessarily indicate that the patient is cured, because some types of malignant tumors may recur and prove fatal many years after initial treatment. Breast carcinoma and malignant melanomas are two such tumors that are prone to late recurrence. For breast carcinoma, for example, the overall five-year survival rate in this group of patients is approximately 65 percent (although more recent five-year survival data reveal

Survival Rates in Neoplastic Disease

TABLE 10–5

Malignant neoplasms: five-year survival rates

| | Five-year survival (%) | | | Five-year survival (%) | |
Type of neoplasm	White	Black	Type of neoplasm	White	Black
Thyroid	95	91	Kidney	59	54
Melanoma	87	70	Non-Hodgkins lymphoma	52	45
Uterus, cervix	71	56	Ovary	44	38
Uterus, body	85	56	Multiple myeloma	28	29
Breast	84	69	Leukemia	41	32
Bladder	82	59	Stomach	19	20
Larynx	68	52	Lung	14	11
Prostate	87	71	Esophagus	11	7
Hodgkin's disease	81	70	Pancreas	3	5
Colon-rectum	61	52			

Note: Cases diagnosed 1986–1991. Survival for all stages with survival of blacks and whites listed separately. Average survival for both sexes used when neoplasm occurs in both sexes.
SOURCE: *CA: A Cancer Journal for Clinicians,* January/February 1996.

FIGURE 10–31

Continuing mortality from breast carcinoma after mastectomy, as a result of late recurrences of carcinoma as described in text. (Data from J. Berg and G. Robbins, *Surg. Gynec. Obst.,* June 1966.)

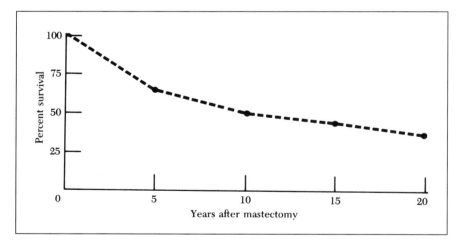

higher survival rates). The ten-year rate in this group is only 50 percent, owing to late recurrences and metastases. Even after ten years, a small proportion of patients eventually die of their original tumor (figure 10–31). In such cases, the tumor had already spread by the time it was first recognized and treated, but the metastatic deposits were held in check by the body's immune defense mechanisms. The recurrence was caused by an eventual failure of the body's defenses, which allowed the tumor to become reactivated.

Review Questions

1. What are the major differences between a benign and a malignant tumor? (See table 10–1.)

2. How are tumors named? What are the common prefixes used in naming tumors? How would you name the following tumors: a benign tumor of fat, a malignant tumor of muscle, a malignant tumor of squamous epithelium, a benign tumor of glandular epithelium arising from the surface of the colon and projecting into the lumen, a malignant tumor of cartilage?

3. How does the body defend itself against abnormal cells that arise spontaneously in the course of cell division? What is the consequence of failure of these defense mechanisms? (See figure 10–20.)

4. What is a lymphoma? What is the difference between a nevus and a melanoma? What is a teratoma?

5. What is a Pap smear? How is it used in the early diagnosis of tumors? What is the significance of a Pap smear containing atypical cells?

6. What is a frozen section? How is it used in the diagnosis of tumors? How are neoplasms treated?

7. What is leukemia? What are its major clinical manifestations? How is leukemia classified? What is the difference between multiple myeloma and leukemia?

Supplementary Readings

Blattner, W. A., et al. 1983. Human T-cell leukemia-lymphoma virus and adult T-cell leukemia. *Journal of the American Medical Association* 250:1074–80. Reviews the isolation and characterization of a virus that causes leukemia and lymphoma in human beings and the diseases caused by the virus.

Breo, D. L. 1994. The cancer revolution: From "black box" to "genetic disease." *Journal of the American Medical Association* 271:1452–54. Reviews recent advances that may affect future treatment.

Cavenee, W. K. 1991. Recessive mutations in the causation of human cancer. *Cancer* 67:1431–35. A review of the inheritance of retinoblastoma.

Chabner, B. A. 1977. Second neoplasm: A complication of cancer chemotherapy. *New England Journal of Medicine* 297:213–14. Anticancer chemotherapy is carcinogenic, and risk-benefit ratio should be considered when contemplating use of this type of treatment.

Cooper, G. M. 1990. *Oncogenes.* Boston: Jones and Bartlett Publishers. A comprehensive in-depth treatment of oncogenes and how they function.

Cooper, G. M. 1992. *Elements of human cancer.* Boston: Jones and Bartlett Publishers. A well-written, easy-to-understand textbook dealing with various aspects of cancer biology, genetics, prevention, and treatment. Good sections on oncogenes and tumor suppressor genes.

Gordon, H. 1985. Oncogenes. *Mayo Clinic Proceedings* 60:697–713. A discussion of genes controlling processes of cell division. Derangement or mutation of these genes leads to disorderly cell division leading to cancer. Describes the role of RNA viruses in converting a benign host cell into a malignant one.

Gutterman, J. U., et al. 1980. Leukocyte interferon-induced tumor regression in human metastatic breast cancer, multiple myeloma, and malignant lymphoma. *Annals of Internal Medicine* 93:399–406. Interferon can induce tumor regression in patients with advanced cancer.

Hellman, S. 1994. Immunotherapy for metastatic cancer (Editorial). *Journal of the American Medical Association* 271:945. Interleukin-2 treatment activates killer lymphocytes and stimulates production of cytotoxic T cells.

Hoagland, H. C. 1995. Myelodysplastic (preleukemia) syndromes: The bone marrow factory failure problem. *Mayo Clinic Proceedings* 70:673–77. A review of classification, clinical features, cytogenetic abnormalities, diagnosis, and management.

Jacobs, A. D., et al. 1985. Recombinant α-2 interferon for hairy cell leukemia. *Blood* 65:1017–20. Interferon is a highly effective therapy for hairy cell leukemia.

Klee, G. G., et al. 1982. Serum tumor markers. *Mayo Clinic Proceedings* 57:129–32. Reviews major tumor markers, their applications and limitations.

Sandberg, A. A. 1994. Cancer cytogenetics for clinicians. *CA: A Cancer Journal for Clinicians* 44:136–59. An overview of the chromosomal changes associated with human cancer and their clinical consequences.

Weinberg, R. A. 1994. Oncogenes and tumor suppressor genes *CA: A Cancer Journal for Clinicians* 44:160–70. Reviews the role of these mutant genes in pathogenesis of cancer.

Chapter 10 ■ Outline Summary

Classification and Nomenclature / 225
Benign Tumors

Descriptive: polyp, papilloma.

Tissue of origin + *oma*.

Malignant Tumors

Cancer: general term.

Carcinoma: arising from surface, glandular, or parenchymal epithelium.

Sarcoma: solid tumor arising from other primary tissues.

Leukemia: neoplasm of blood-forming tissues.

Comparison of Benign and Malignant Tumors / 225
Benign Tumors

Grow slowly.

Grow by expansion.

Remain localized.

Cells well differentiated.

Malignant Tumors

Grow more rapidly.

Grow by infiltration.

Metastasize.

Cells not well differentiated.

Variations in Terminology / 233
Lymphoid Tumors

Lymphoma: a malignant lymphoid tumor.

Classification:

Hodgkin's disease: characteristic Reed-Sternberg cells.

Non-Hodgkin's lymphoma: well-differentiated and poorly differentiated.

Skin Tumors

From melanocytes:

Benign: nevus.

Malignant: melanoma.

From keratinocytes:

Benign: keratoses.

Malignant: basal cell carcinoma, squamous cell carcinoma.

Sun exposure damages skin and predisposes to development of tumors.

Tumors of Mixed Components (Teratomas)

Frequently occur in reproductive tract.

Must specify as either benign or malignant.

Embryonic (Embryonal) Tumors

Arise from persisting groups of embryonic cells.

Named from tissue of origin + *blastoma*.

Necrosis in Tumors / 238
Pathogenesis

Tumor outgrows blood supply.

Necrosis occurs in center of deeply placed tumor.

Necrosis occurs on the surface of tumors growing from epithelial surface.

Noninfiltrating (in Situ) Carcinoma / 239
Characteristics

Remains localized for many years.

Frequently occurs in cervix, but encountered in other locations as well.

Most favorable stage for cure.

Precancerous Conditions

Characteristics:

Nonmalignant conditions with tendency to eventually become malignant.

Treatment prevents progression.

Common precancerous conditions:

Actinic keratosis: arises in sun-damaged skin and may form skin cancers.

Lentigo maligna: arises in sun-damaged skin and may lead to melanoma.

Leukoplakia: affects oral mucosa, usually caused by exposure to tobacco tars. May affect vulva (described in chapter 17).

Some colon polyps.

Etiologic Factors in Neoplastic Disease / 243
Viruses

Some animal tumors are caused by viruses.

Some human tumors also may be virus induced.

Gene and Chromosome Abnormalities

Activation of oncogenes and inactivation of tumor suppressor genes deregulates cell, which proliferates to form tumor.

Translocation or deletion may change relation of genes on chromosome, disturbing cell regulation and growth functions.

Philadelphia chromosome is best-known abnormality.

Reciprocal translocation of ends of chromosomes 9 and 22.

Oncogene on translocated piece of chromosome 9 exhibits increased activity.

Failure of Immunologic Defenses

Body produces abnormal cells periodically.

Immune defenses eliminate abnormal cells.

Failure of elimination may allow overgrowth, forming malignant tumors.

Heredity and Tumors

No strong hereditary predisposition to most tumors.

Slightly increased susceptibility in relatives of cancer patients may be caused by multifactorial inheritance pattern.

Some breast carcinomas have strong hereditary background, owing to inheritance of mutant gene.

Rare tumors:

Autosomal dominant inheritance:

Some retinoblastomas.

Multiple polyposis of colon.

Neurofibromatosis.

Multiple endocrine adenomas.

Only small fraction of all tumors affecting humans.

Diagnosis of Tumors / 250
Early Recognition

An abnormality of form or function requires evaluation by physician.

If abnormality discovered, perform biopsy or excise.

Excision of benign tumor is curative; malignant tumor may require further treatment.

Cytologic Diagnosis

Tumor cells shed from surface or can be scraped from epithelial surface.

Abnormal smear indicates need for further studies but not diagnostic of neoplasm.

Frozen-Section Diagnosis

Means of rapid evaluation of abnormal tissue obtained at surgery.

Permits immediate decision about proper course of treatment.

Tumor-Associated Antigen Tests

Carbohydrate-protein complexes secreted by tumor cells.

Can be detected in the blood.

Used to monitor response to treatment.

Treatment of Tumors / 255
Surgery

Extensive resection of tumor with draining lymph nodes.

Not curative if tumor has already metastasized to distant sites.

Radiotherapy

Lymphomas and some epithelial tumors treated primarily by radiotherapy.

May be used in conjunction with surgery.

Useful for pain relief.

Hormones

Hormone-dependent tumors undergo temporary regression when deprived of required hormones.

Some tumors inhibited by hormones, corticosteroids, estrogens.

Anticancer Drugs

Impede processes concerned with cell growth and cell division.

Most effective against rapidly growing tumors.

Alkylating agents.

Antimetabolites.

Adjuvant Chemotherapy

Used after surgical resection of tumor.

Attempts to eradicate small metastases before they become apparent clinically.

Immunotherapy

Nonspecific immunotherapy:

Interferon:

Interferon regulates cell growth and functions of immune system in addition to antiviral activity.

Large quantities available from commercial production.

Best results in hairy cell leukemia, but useful for causing regression of some other neoplasms.

Low toxicity.

Interleukin-2:

Stimulates production of natural killer cells that attack tumor.

Best results in metastatic melanoma and renal cell carcinoma.

Other cytokines under investigation.

Specific immunotherapy:

Tumor infiltrating lymphocytes:

Cytotoxic T cells attack patient's own tumor.

Some success in treating metastatic melanoma.

Tumor vaccines:

Vaccine prepared from patient's own tumor induces immune response.

Used as additional treatment after melanoma or colon cancer if patient at high risk of recurrence.

Tumor antibody therapy:

Antibodies prepared against tumor antigens and coupled with antitumor drug or toxin.

Antibody infused into patient and damages tumor cells without injuring normal cells.

Leukemia / 260
Classification

By cell type: granulocytic, lymphocytic, or monocytic.

By maturity of cells: acute (primitive cells) or chronic (mature cells).

By number of circulating white cells: descriptive term *aleukemic* indicates low white count in peripheral blood.

Clinical Features/Principles of Treatment

As a result of impaired bone marrow function: anemia, thrombocytopenia, and infections caused by reduced numbers of mature functional leukocytes.

As a result of infiltration of organs: splenomegaly, hepatomegaly, lymphadenopathy.

Chronic leukemia well controlled by treatment; relatively long survival.

Acute leukemia difficult to treat and has poor prognosis in many cases; childhood leukemia has better prognosis and may be cured by treatment.

Bone marrow transplant available in selected patients.

Preleukemia/Myelodysplasia / 265
Manifestations

Disturbed growth and maturation of marrow cells.

Anemia, leukopenia, thrombocytopenia.

May be precursor of leukemia in some patients.

Multiple Myeloma / 265
Characteristics

A neoplasm of plasma cells.

Differs somewhat from leukemia.

Nodular deposits of plasma cells in bone.

Plasma cells produce protein.

Usually no visceral infiltration.

Survival Rates in Neoplastic Disease / 267
Nature of Problem

Cancer is leading cause of disability and mortality.

Survival rates vary from 1 percent to more than 80 percent, depending on tumor.

Early diagnosis and treatment may enhance survival.

Some tumors may recur many years after treatment.

Abnormalities of Blood Coagulation

Learning Objectives

1. Describe the functions of blood vessels and platelets in controlling bleeding.
2. Explain the three phases of coagulation and list the coagulation factors involved.
3. Describe the laboratory tests used to evaluate hemostasis.
4. List the most common clinically significant disturbances of hemostasis and describe their clinical manifestations.

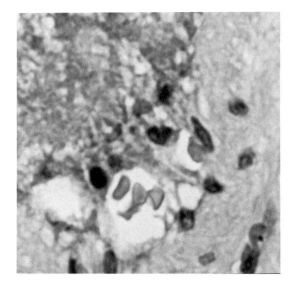

Chapter 11 ▪ Contents

If one cuts a finger with a knife, the cut bleeds, but the bleeding soon stops and healing ensues. The body has a complex mechanism for causing blood to clot when and where it is necessary, while keeping the blood fluid within the capillaries and larger blood vessels.

The proper functioning of the hemostatic mechanism depends on the proper integrated functioning of the five major factors that affect hemostasis:

Factors Concerned with Hemostasis

1. Integrity of the small blood vessels
2. Adequate numbers of structurally and functionally normal platelets
3. Normal amounts of coagulation factors (proteins present in small quantities in the blood plasma)
4. Normal amounts of coagulation inhibitors
5. Adequate amounts of calcium ions in the blood

Blood Vessels and Platelets

The small blood vessels and blood platelets function together to prevent bleeding. The small blood vessels are the body's first line of defense. If a blood vessel is injured, it automatically contracts (*reflex vasoconstriction*), narrowing its caliber and facilitating closure of the vessel by a blood clot. Injury to the vessel also leads to disruption of the endothelium, exposing the underlying connective tissue. Platelets accumulate and adhere to the site of injury, where they perform three important functions:

1. They plug the defect in the vessel wall
2. They liberate chemical compounds (*vasoconstrictors*) that cause the vessel to contract
3. They release substances (*phospholipids*) that initiate the process of blood coagulation

Platelets play a very important part in preventing bleeding from capillaries. Small breaks in the walls of capillaries occur frequently, but the defects are promptly sealed by platelets, and bleeding does not occur. However, if the quantity of platelets in the blood is seriously reduced, as occurs in some diseases, the "platelet sealing mechanism" is impaired. As a result, the affected individual develops multiple small pinpoint areas of bleeding (called **petechiae** or *petechial hemorrhages*) in the skin and deeper tissues owing to leakage of blood through minute defects in the capillary endothelium.

Plasma Coagulation Factors

The blood plasma contains several different proteins called *coagulation factors,* which are designated both by name and by roman numerals. When these factors are activated, they interact to produce a blood clot. The process of blood coagulation is a chain reaction in which each component of the chain is formed from an inactive precursor in the blood, and each activated component in turn activates the next member of the chain. The process has been compared to what happens when the first in a long chain of dominoes is knocked over. Tipping the first domino represents the initiation of the clotting mechanism, and the fall of the last domino represents the formation of a firm blood clot.

The process of blood coagulation is a highly complex and bewildering sequence of interactions involving plasma and tissue components, platelets, and calcium. At the risk of oversimplifying its complexities, however, it is convenient to divide it into three phases for descriptive purposes (figure 11–1).

Phase 1 leads to the formation of *thromboplastin,* which may be produced by either of two different mechanisms. One mechanism depends on the interaction of platelets and plasma coagulation factors. If the wall of a blood vessel is injured, platelets accumulate at the site and release a phospholipid that interacts with plasma components to form thromboplastin. This is called the *intrinsic system* because the thromboplastin is produced from substances present in the bloodstream. Tissues also have thromboplastic

FIGURE 11–1

A simplified concept of the blood coagulation mechanisms. In the intrinsic system, plasma factors (XII, XI, and IX) are activated, and they interact with factor VIII and platelets to yield intrinsic thromboplastin. In the extrinsic system, tissue injury yields extrinsic thromboplastin that reacts with a plasma factor (VII). Then the thromboplastin interacts with additional components (factors V, X, and platelet phospholipid) to form the complex (prothrombin activator) that converts prothrombin into thrombin in the second phase. Thrombin converts fibrinogen into fibrin in the third phase.

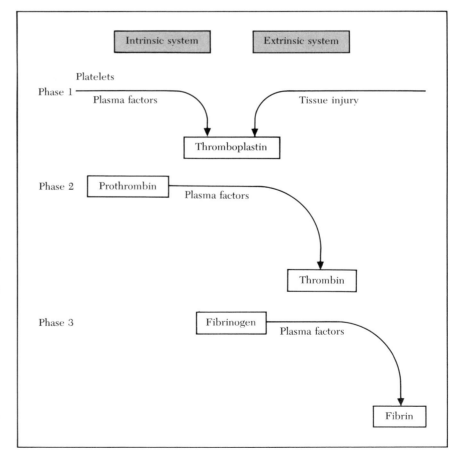

activity, and thromboplastin is also liberated from injured tissues. This is called the *extrinsic system* because the thromboplastin is not derived from the blood but from tissue outside the vascular compartment.

Actually, the intrinsic and extrinsic pathways may not be completely independent. Recent evidence suggests that both pathways may be activated at the same time when tissues are injured, and both pathways may interact to initiate the blood-clotting process.

The conversion of *prothrombin* into *thrombin* takes place in phase 2. The thromboplastin formed in either the intrinsic or the extrinsic system interacts with additional plasma factors and platelet phospholipid to form a complex (called prothrombin activator) that converts the prothrombin into thrombin. Prothrombin is a protein manufactured in the liver. It is split into several fragments by thromboplastin. One of these is the active component **thrombin,** an enzyme capable of digesting protein. The formation of thrombin from prothrombin requires other plasma coagulation factors (called *accessory factors*) that function by speeding the rate of the conversion.

Phase 3 leads to the conversion of *fibrinogen* into *fibrin* by thrombin. Fibrinogen is a high molecular weight protein produced by the liver. Thrombin splits off a part of the fibrinogen molecule, forming a smaller molecule called **fibrin monomer.** The fibrin monomer molecules then become joined end to end (*polymerized*) to form long strands of fibrin, and the fibrin strands also become linked together side to side. Another plasma factor (*fibrin stabilizing factor*) acts by strengthening the bonds between the fibrin molecules and increasing the strength of the fibrin clot. The blood clot is the end stage in the clotting process. It consists of an interlacing meshwork of fibrin threads containing entrapped plasma, red cells, white cells, and platelets.

Table 11–1 summarizes the coagulation factors and their role in the clotting process.

Coagulation Inhibitors and Fibrinolysins

Coagulation factors are counterbalanced by various coagulation inhibitors that restrict the clotting process to a limited area. An important member of this group is *antithrombin III,* which inhibits not only thrombin, but also other activated coagulation factors generated in the clotting process.

An equally important control system is one that dissolves fibrin after it has formed. A precursor compound in blood plasma called *plasminogen* (profibrinolysin) is activated to form *plasmin* (fibrinolysin), which dissolves fibrin in blood clots. The fibrinolytic system is activated at the same time that the coagulation process is initiated, and thrombin produced in the coagulation process also activates this system. Another important plasminogen activator is a substance called *tissue plasminogen activator,* which is released from endothelial cells in the region where the clot is forming. As described in chapter 13, tissue plasminogen activator or another plasminogen activator, called *streptokinase,* produced by streptococci is administered intravenously to dissolve blood clots in the coronary arteries of patients who have had a recent heart attack. Prompt administration of one of these plasminogen acti-

TABLE 11–1 Coagulation factors	Factor number	Name	Functions
	I	Fibrinogen	Protein synthesized in liver; converted into fibrin in Stage 3
	II	Prothrombin	Protein synthesized in liver (requires Vitamin K); converted into thrombin in Stage 2
	III	Tissue thromboplastin	Released from damaged tissue; required in extrinsic Stage 1
	IV	Calcium ions	Required throughout entire clotting sequence
	V	Proaccelerin (labile factor)	Protein synthesized in liver; required to form prothrombin activator in both intrinsic and extrinsic Stage 1
	VII	Serum prothrombin conversion accelerator (stable factor, proconvertin)	Protein synthesized in liver (requires vitamin K); functions in extrinsic Stage 1
	VIII	Antihemophilic factor (antihemophilic globulin)	Protein synthesized in liver; required for intrinsic Stage 1
	IX	Plasma thromboplastin component	Protein synthesized in liver (requires vitamin K); required for intrinsic Stage 1
	X	Stuart factor (Stuart-Prower factor)	Protein synthesized in liver (requires vitamin K); required to form prothrombin activator in both intrinsic and extrinsic Stage 1
	XI	Plasma thromboplastin antecedent	Protein synthesized in liver; required for intrinsic Stage 1
	XII	Hageman factor	Protein required for intrinsic Stage 1
	XIII	Fibrin-stabilizing factor	Protein required to stabilize the fibrin strands in Stage 3

vators within a few hours after onset of symptoms dissolves the clot and restores flow through the artery, which minimizes heart muscle damage resulting from the blockage.

Calcium and Blood Coagulation

Adequate amounts of calcium ions (Ca^{2+}) are required in all phases of blood coagulation, and blood will not clot in the absence of calcium. However, there are no diseases in which a disturbance of blood coagulation results from an abnormally low level of blood calcium, because calcium levels sufficiently low to affect blood coagulation would be incompatible with life.

Disturbances of blood coagulation may be classified as one of four major categories:

Clinical Disturbances of Blood Coagulation

1. Abnormalities of small blood vessels
2. Abnormalities of platelet function
3. Deficiency of one or more of the plasma coagulation factors
4. Liberation of thromboplastic material into the circulation

Abnormalities of Small Blood Vessels

Some rare diseases characterized by abnormal bleeding have been found to be a result of abnormal function of the small blood vessels. Normally, small blood vessels contract after injury, helping to seal the defect by a blood clot. Sometimes this function is defective, leading to excessive bleeding. There are a few other rare diseases in which the small blood vessels are abnormally formed and cannot function properly.

Abnormalities of Platelet Numbers or Function

A decrease in platelets is called **thrombocytopenia** (*thrombus* = clot + *cyte* = cell + *penia* = deficiency). This decrease may be a result of injury or disease of the bone marrow, which damages the *megakaryocytes* in the marrow, the precursor cells of the platelets. In other cases, thrombocytopenia occurs because the bone marrow has been infiltrated by leukemic cells or by cancer cells that have spread to the skeletal system, and the megakaryocytes have been crowded out by the abnormal cells. Thrombocytopenia may also occur if antiplatelet autoantibodies destroy the platelets in the peripheral blood (as seen in some autoimmune diseases). Sometimes platelets are normal in quantity but abnormal in function, and so they are ineffective in initiating the clotting process.

Bleeding associated with defective or inadequate platelets is generally manifested by small petechial hemorrhages rather than by large areas of hemorrhage (figure 11–2A).

Deficiency of Plasma Coagulation Factors

Deficiencies of plasma coagulation factors often lead to large areas of hemorrhage called **hematomas** (*heme* = blood + *oma* = swelling) (figure 11–2B). Deficiencies of factors concerned with the first phase of coagulation are usually hereditary and are relatively rare. Only three hereditary bleeding diseases occur with any frequency. Hemophilia, an X-linked hereditary disease affect-

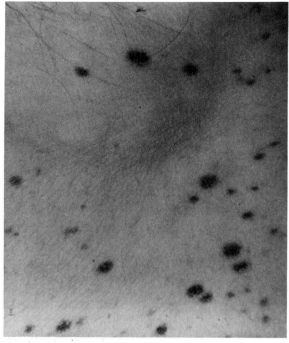 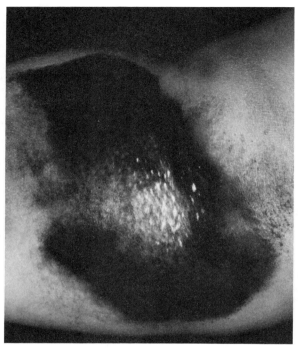

A   **B**

FIGURE 11–2

Characteristics of bleeding in patients with disturbed hemostatic function. **A,** Petechial hemorrhages indicative of thrombocytopenia or defective platelet function. **B,** Large hemorrhage (*hematoma*) associated with deficiency of plasma coagulation factors.

ing males, is the most common and best known. Clinically, the disease is characterized by episodes of hemorrhage in joints and internal organs after minor injury. There are two forms of hemophilia. Both have the same clinical manifestations and X-linked method of transmission. The most common type, which is called *hemophilia A* or *classic hemophilia,* is characterized by a decrease in coagulation factor VIII, which is also called *antihemophiliac globulin.* Its method of inheritance was considered in chapter 9. The less-common form of hemophilia is called *hemophilia B* or *Christmas disease.* It is caused by a deficiency of coagulation factor IX, which is also called *Christmas factor* (named after an affected patient, not the holiday). Both factors VIII and IX, which are produced in the liver, are required in the first phase of coagulation.

A third hereditary bleeding disease is called *von Willebrand's disease* and is usually transmitted as a Mendelian dominant trait. This disease also is characterized by excessive bleeding after minor injury, but usually the bleeding is not in the joints, as is so characteristic of hemophilia. The manifestations of von Willebrand's disease result from a deficiency of a large protein molecule that is produced primarily by the endothelial cells lining blood vessels. This factor is required in order for platelets to adhere to the vessel wall at the site of injury. The protein is also released into the bloodstream, where it forms a complex in the circulation with factor VIII, and it is needed in order to maintain a normal level of factor VIII in the blood.

Von Willebrand's factor functions by adhering to the vessel wall where the endothelium is disrupted, forming a latticelike framework that allows platelets and coagulation factors to adhere, interact, and form a blood clot.

The level of factor VIII is low in patients with von Willebrand's disease, as it is in hemophilia A, but for a different reason. Patients with von Willebrand's disease can synthesize factor VIII, but an adequate level of von Willebrand's factor is required to form a complex with factor VIII and maintain a normal amount of factor VIII in the circulation. The factor VIII deficiency in von Willebrand's disease occurs because the affected persons lack adequate amounts of circulating von Willebrand's factor with which the factor VIII can combine.

Because von Willebrand's factor is also required in order for platelets to adhere at the site of vascular injury, some platelet functions also are disturbed in persons with this disease, which can be identified by special laboratory tests.

Patients with hemophilia A, hemophilia B, and von Willebrand's disease who have bleeding episodes can be treated by administration of factor concentrates prepared from human blood plasma. A factor VIII concentrate prepared by recombinant DNA technology also has become available and can be used to treat patients with classic hemophilia.

Disturbances affecting the second phase of blood coagulation result from a deficiency of prothrombin or various accessory coagulation factors that are required for the conversion of prothrombin into thrombin. These factors are produced in the liver, and vitamin K is required for the synthesis of most of these factors (called *vitamin-K–dependent factors*). Vitamin K is synthesized by intestinal bacteria. It is a fat-soluble vitamin, and bile is required for its absorption.

A disturbance of blood coagulation caused by a deficiency of prothrombin or related factors suggests four possibilities:

1. Administration of anticoagulant drugs
2. Inadequate synthesis of vitamin K
3. Inadequate absorption of vitamin K
4. Severe liver disease

Anticoagulant drugs such as coumadin and similar compounds are sometimes used to treat patients who have shown an increased tendency to develop blood clots in their leg veins. These drugs are also sometimes given to patients with some types of heart disease. Anticoagulant drugs act by inhibiting the synthesis of biochemically active vitamin K-dependent factors. Inadequate synthesis of vitamin K also occurs if the intestinal bacteria have been eradicated by prolonged antibiotic therapy, as sometimes occurs in seriously ill, hospitalized patients. The usual cause of inadequate uptake of vitamin K is blockage of the common bile duct by a gallstone or tumor, preventing bile from entering the intestine to promote absorption of the vitamin. Patients with severe liver diseases have deficiencies of prothrombin and accessory factors because the liver is so badly damaged that it can no longer synthesize adequate amounts of coagulation factors.

Intramuscular administration of vitamin K corrects coagulation disturbances resulting from coumadin anticoagulants, inadequate synthesis of vitamin K, or insufficient absorption of the vitamin. The coagulation disturbance associated with severe liver disease does not respond, because the diseased liver is no longer capable of synthesizing sufficient coagulation factors to provide efficient hemostasis.

Liberation of Thromboplastic Material into the Circulation

In a number of diseases associated with shock, overwhelming bacterial infection, or extensive necrosis of tissue, products of tissue necrosis and other substances with thromboplastic activity are liberated into the circulation, leading to widespread intravascular coagulation of the blood (figure 11–3). In the process of clotting, platelets and the various plasma coagulation factors are utilized, and the levels of these components in the blood drop precipitously.

In order to defend itself against widespread intravascular clotting, the body activates the fibrinolysin system; this dissolves clots and prevents potentially lethal obstruction of the circulatory system by massive intravascular coagulation. The breakdown products produced during degradation of the fibrin act as additional inhibitors of the clotting process.

The net effect of these various events is a bleeding disturbance, sometimes in a patient already seriously ill because of an underlying disease that caused the blood-clotting mechanism to be activated. This abnormal bleeding state is called *disseminated intravascular coagulation* or *consumption coagulopathy*. The latter term alludes to consumption of the clotting factors as a result of the pathogenic coagulation process. Figure 11–4 summarizes the pathogenesis of this bleeding syndrome.

Relative Frequency of the Various Coagulation Disturbances

In one group of 350 hospitalized patients with bleeding problems that I studied, most of the disorders were caused by inadequate numbers of platelets or abnormal platelet function. Next in frequency were coagulation disturbances caused by deficient formation of coagulation factors in patients with liver disease. In acutely ill patients, the majority of acquired coagulation disturbances are the result of disseminated intravascular coagulation, with depletion of both platelets and plasma coagulation factors.

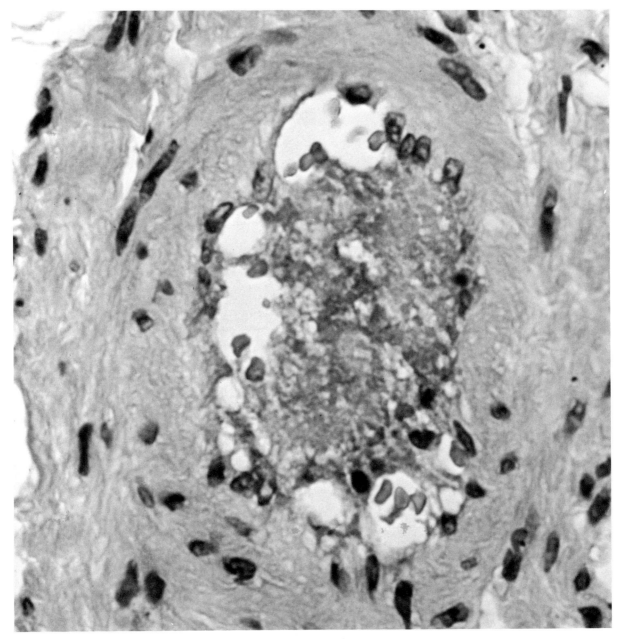

FIGURE 11–3

Fibrin thrombus in small blood vessel of patient with disseminated intravascular coagulation syndrome. (Original magnification × 400.)

FIGURE 11–4

Pathogenesis of disseminated intravascular coagulation syndrome.

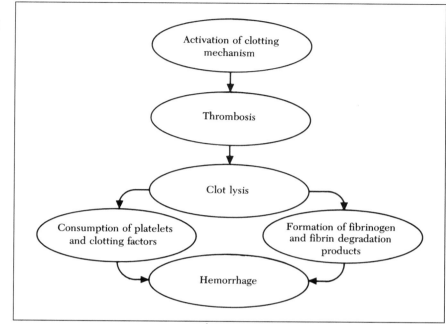

FIGURE 11–5

Common laboratory tests used to measure hemostatic function, indicating the phases of the clotting mechanism measured by the various tests.

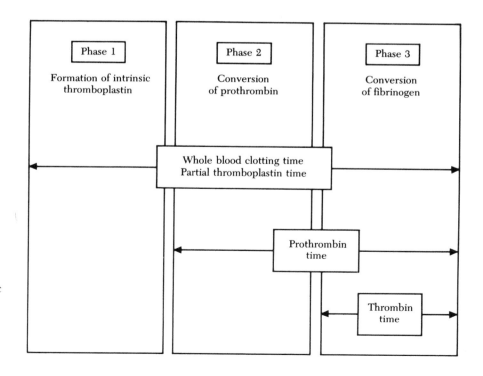

Several laboratory tests can evaluate the overall efficiency of the coagulation process, detect the presence of inhibitors of coagulation, and estimate the number and function of the platelets (figure 11–5).

The number of platelets in the blood can be estimated by examining the blood smear, and more precise data can be obtained by a numerical platelet count. Special tests also are available to evaluate platelet function. The function of the capillaries in the hemostatic process is evaluated by the *bleeding time,* which reflects the time it takes for a small, standardized skin incision to stop bleeding.

The time that it takes for blood to clot in a test tube under standard conditions is a crude test that measures the overall efficiency of the clotting process. A much more sensitive test is called the **partial thromboplastin time.** This test measures the time that it takes for blood plasma to clot after a lipid substance is added to the plasma sample. This lipid is similar to the lipid material released from platelets to initiate the clotting process in the intrinsic system. If any of the plasma factors concerned with blood coagulation is deficient, the clotting process is slowed, and the partial thromboplastin time is prolonged.

The test commonly used to measure the combined second and third phases of blood coagulation is called the **prothrombin time.** In this test, the first stage of the coagulation process is bypassed. One measures the clotting time of blood plasma after adding a tissue thromboplastin that is normally generated in the first stage of coagulation. The thromboplastin is usually prepared from rabbit brain. A normal prothrombin time indicates that the second and third phases of blood coagulation are normal. If the test is prolonged, an abnormality of either the second or the third stage is indicated. The abnormality cannot be in the first stage of clotting, because this stage includes the formation of thromboplastin, and thromboplastin has already been supplied in the test. The prothrombin time test is commonly used to monitor the effect of coumadin anticoagulants administered to patients in order to reduce the coagulability of the blood.

The third stage of coagulation can be evaluated by bypassing the first and second stages. One determines the clotting time of plasma after addition of thrombin (which is normally generated in the second phase of the clotting process). Therefore, the test primarily measures the level of fibrinogen, which may be deficient in some conditions. The level of fibrinogen can also be measured directly by other tests, and one can also test for fibrinogen and fibrin degradation products, which are increased if fibrinolysis is excessive.

In the event that abnormalities are detected in any phase of coagulation, it is necessary to determine whether they have occurred because a coagulation factor is deficient or because an inhibitor is impairing the action of the factor. If necessary, one can also determine the concentrations of the various factors.

The following cases illustrate the spectrum of coagulation abnormalities encountered in clinical medicine. The cases also illustrate how laboratory

Laboratory Tests to Evaluate Hemostasis

Case Studies

tests can help to determine the nature of the abnormality and suggest a proper course of treatment.

CASE 11–1

Factor VIII Deficiency

A ten-month-old child was admitted to the hospital through the emergency room because he was bleeding profusely from a cut under the lip that he received when falling. The history revealed easy bruising since birth but no episodes of bleeding into the joints, and the child was considered by the parents to be in good health.

Physical examination revealed ecchymoses over the left chest and a small bruise on the abdomen. Small bruises were noted on both lower extremities. Laboratory studies revealed moderate anemia and normal platelets. Coagulation studies revealed a normal plasma prothrombin time, but the partial thromboplastin time was significantly prolonged.

The bleeding was controlled by applying pressure for about 10 minutes. The next day, the child has a tarry stool, apparently owing to swallowed blood. After this, the stools became normal in color, and no further bleeding was noted.

In this case, the abnormal partial thromboplastin time indicated an abnormality of blood coagulation, but the normal prothrombin time indicated that the abnormality was not in the second or third stages of coagulation. Therefore, the defect must have been in the first phase, which suggests either hemophilia or von Willebrand's disease as diagnostic possibilities. Further tests showed a very low level of factor VIII (antihemophiliac globulin), and additional diagnostic tests established the diagnosis of von Willebrand's disease.

CASE 11–2

Vitamin K Deficiency

A fifty-five-year-old woman was admitted to the hospital with a severe staphylococcal pneumonia that was complicated by an accumulation of pus in the left pleural cavity. She received intensive antibiotic therapy. She was unable to take food or fluid orally because of severe nausea and vomiting and was maintained almost entirely on intravenous fluids. It was difficult to maintain satisfactory fluid balance and nutrition. After several weeks in the hospital, she developed bleeding from her urinary tract and rectal bleeding.

Coagulation studies revealed a prolonged partial thromboplastin time, and prolonged plasma prothrombin time (27 seconds, control 13 seconds). The patient was given a vitamin K preparation. Both the partial thromboplastin time and the prothrombin time returned to normal, and she had no further bleeding.

In this case, the coagulation data indicate an acquired depression of vitamin-K–dependent coagulation factors primarily caused by deficient synthesis of vitamin K by intestinal bacteria, which were eliminated by the intensive antibiotic treatment. The excellent response to vitamin K confirmed the diagnosis.

Chronic Liver Disease

A fifty-seven-year-old man was admitted to the hospital because of bleeding from his urinary tract. Blood coagulation studies revealed a prolonged partial thromboplastin time and prothrombin time. The plasma prothrombin time was 18 seconds (control 13 seconds). Other studies revealed that his liver function was very abnormal. The prothrombin time did not return to normal after administration of a vitamin K preparation. A needle biopsy of the liver revealed a type of chronic liver disease called *portal cirrhosis* (described in chapter 21).

Here the abnormality was localized to the second stage of blood coagulation. Failure to respond to vitamin K suggested chronic liver disease rather than vitamin K deficiency or a decrease in coagulation factors caused by anticoagulant therapy. The needle biopsy confirmed the presence of chronic liver disease.

Disseminated Intravascular Coagulation Syndrome as a Result of Retained Dead Fetus

A thirty-six-year-old pregnant woman was admitted to the hospital at thirty-eight weeks gestation. She had not felt fetal movement for the previous month, and no fetal heart tones were detected by her physician. Coagulation studies revealed prolonged partial thromboplastin time and prothrombin time. Fibrinogen was markedly reduced. The patient's blood contained high levels of fibrinogen and fibrin degradation products. Labor was induced, and delivery was accomplished with very little loss of blood. The next day, the fibrinogen returned to normal and all coagulation studies were within normal limits.

In this case, all the coagulation factors were decreased because they had been used up in the coagulation process induced by release of thromboplastic material into the maternal circulation from the retained dead fetus. The high levels of fibrinogen and fibrin degradation products were the result of activation of the fibrinolytic system—the body's defense against a potentially lethal intravascular coagulation process.

Questions for Review

1. How does blood clot?

2. What are some of the common disturbances of blood coagulation?

3. What is thrombocytopenia? What type of bleeding is produced when platelets are markedly reduced? What types of diseases are associated with thrombocytopenia?

4. What types of diseases produce abnormalities in the first phase of blood coagulation?

5. What is the consequence of liberation of thromboplastic material into the circulation?

6. What laboratory tests are used to evaluate the coagulation of blood?

7. A patient with a bleeding tendency has a prolonged partial thromboplastin time with a normal prothrombin time. In what phase of the clotting process is the disturbance located? Name one possible disease that could produce these findings.

8. What are the effects of coumadin anticoagulants on the clotting mechanism? How do they work? What laboratory test can be used to monitor the effect of the anticoagulant?

Supplementary Readings

Crowley, L. V. 1968. Diagnosis of blood clotting disorders in a community hospital. *Lancet* 88:295–302. Thrombocytopenia, chronic liver disease, and disseminated intravascular coagulation syndrome are common problems.

Rapaport, S. I. 1992. Hemorrhagic disorders. In *The Merck manual of diagnosis and therapy*. 16th ed. Ed. R. Berkow, pp. 1195–1225. Rahway, N.J.: Merck and Co. An excellent comprehensive review.

Vander, A. J., Sherman, J. H., and Luciano, D. S. 1994. *Human physiology*. 6th ed. New York: McGraw-Hill. A review of the interaction of coagulation factors, emphasizing the interrelation of the intrinsic and extrinsic systems.

Vansell, J. E., et al. 1977. The spectrum of vitamin K deficiency. *Journal of the American Medical Association* 238:40–42. A common problem, especially in postoperative patients and those with cancer or renal failure. Treatment with parenteral vitamin K confirms the diagnosis and stops bleeding.

Weiss, H. J. 1975. Platelet physiology and abnormalities of platelet function. *New England Journal of Medicine* 293:531–40; 580–88. A comprehensive review article.

Chapter 11 ■ Outline Summary

Factors Concerned with Hemostasis / 275
Blood Vessels and Platelets

Reflex contraction of blood vessels after injury.

Platelets adhere to site of injury: plug vessel, liberate vasoconstrictors, release phospholipids to initiate clotting.

Small breaks in capillaries are sealed by platelets as they occur.

Plasma Coagulation Factors

Phase 1: generation of prothrombin activator:

Intrinsic system: components derived from blood.

Extrinsic system: tissue injury yields tissue thromboplastin.

Phase 2: formation of thrombin.

Phase 3: formation of fibrin.

Coagulation Inhibitors
Calcium

Required for all phases of coagulation.

No clinical disturbances of coagulation caused by low calcium.

Clinical Disturbances of Blood Coagulation / 279
Abnormalities of Small Blood Vessels

Abnormal function of small blood vessels.

Abnormal form of small blood vessels.

Abnormalities of Platelet Numbers and Functions

Thrombocytopenia:

As a result of bone marrow infiltration.

As a result of autoantibodies.

Defective platelet function.

Deficiency of Plasma Coagulation Factors

First phase:

Usually congenital.

Hemophilia is best-known defect.

Second phase:

Administration of anticoagulant drugs.

Inadequate synthesis of vitamin K.

Inadequate absorption of vitamin K.

Severe liver disease.

Liberation of thromboplastic materials into circulation:

Activation of coagulation mechanism by products of tissue injury.

Intravascular coagulation.

Activation of fibrinolysin.

Consumption of coagulation factors and platelets.

Products of fibrin breakdown have anticoagulant activity.

Frequency of Coagulation Disturbances

Frequently a result of inadequate platelets or defective platelet function.

Chronic liver disease.

Disseminated intravascular coagulation syndrome.

Laboratory Tests to Evaluate Hemostasis / 285
Platelets

Platelet count.

Examination of blood smear for platelet numbers.

Overall Evaluation of Coagulation Mechanism

Clotting time of whole blood.

Partial thromboplastin time.

Second and Third Stages

Evaluation by prothrombin time.

Test bypasses first stage of blood coagulation.

Third Stage

Thrombin time.

Determine fibrinogen and fibrin degradation products.

12

Circulatory Disturbances

Learning Objectives

1. Describe the causes and effects of venous thrombosis.
2. Explain the pathogenesis of pulmonary embolism. Describe the clinical manifestations and compare the techniques of diagnosis.
3. Describe the causes and effects of arterial thrombosis.
4. List the four factors regulating the circulation of fluid between capillaries and interstitial tissue. Explain the major clinical disturbances leading to edema.
5. Describe the pathogenesis of the hypercoagulable state sometimes seen in patients with carcinoma.

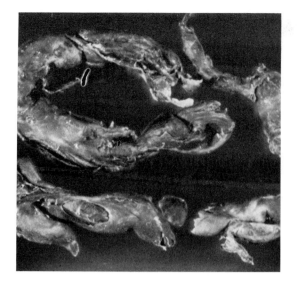

Chapter 12 ▪ Contents

Normally, blood does not clot within the vascular system. Under unusual circumstances, however, intravascular clotting may occur, owing to one or more of the following factors:

1. Slowing or stasis of the blood flow
2. Damage to the walls of the blood vessel
3. Increase in the coagulability of the blood

An intravascular clot is called a *thrombus;* the condition is termed **thrombosis.** Intravascular thrombi may form within veins or arteries and occasionally within the heart itself. A clot in the vascular system may become detached and may be carried in the circulation. Such a clot is termed an *embolus* (*embolus* = plug or stopper); the condition is termed **embolism.** Depending on where the blood clot was formed initially, the embolus may be carried into either the pulmonary circulation or the systemic arterial circulation. Eventually, it is arrested in an artery of smaller caliber than the diameter of the clot. When the embolus plugs the vessel, it blocks the blood flow to the tissue beyond (*distal to*) the obstruction, and the damaged tissue may undergo necrosis if the collateral blood supply is inadequate. The area of tissue breakdown is called an infarct or *infarction.*

Venous Thrombosis and Pulmonary Embolism

Formation of blood clots within leg veins is primarily a result of slowing or stasis of the blood in the veins. This is likely to occur during periods of prolonged bed rest or after a cramped position has been maintained for a long period of time. Under these circumstances, the "milking action" of the leg musculature, which normally promotes venous return, is impaired, leading to stasis of the blood. Varicose veins or any condition preventing normal emptying of veins predisposes an individual to thrombosis by causing venous stasis.

Postoperative thrombosis in leg veins is a common problem. The surgical patient is susceptible to venous thrombosis owing to the combined effects of venous stasis resulting from inactivity and increased blood coagulability resulting from an increased concentration of coagulation factors. (Blood coagulation factors usually increase as a result of tissue injury or necrosis from any cause.)

A venous thrombosis may partially block venous return in the leg, making the leg swell. However, the major complication of venous thrombosis is related to detachment of the clot from the wall of the vein. The thrombus often is not firmly attached to the vein wall. It may break loose, forming an embolus that is carried rapidly up the inferior vena cava into the right side of the heart. From there it is ejected into the pulmonary artery, where it may become lodged in either the main pulmonary artery or one of its branches. The clinical manifestations of a pulmonary embolism depend on the size of the embolus and where it lodges in the pulmonary artery.

Large Pulmonary Emboli

A large embolus that completely blocks the main pulmonary artery or its two major branches obstructs the flow of blood through the lungs (figure 12–1). The right side of the heart becomes overdistended with blood because blood cannot be expelled into the lungs. The pulmonary artery leading to

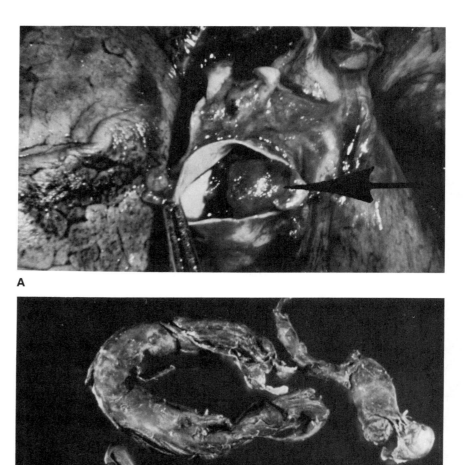

A

B

FIGURE 12–1

Massive pulmonary embolism. **A,** Main pulmonary artery occluded by embolus. **B,** Several emboli filled both pulmonary arteries and obstructed blood flow to lungs.

(*proximal to*) the obstructing embolus also becomes overdistended with blood, and the pressure in the pulmonary artery rises. Because less blood flows through the lungs into the left side of the heart, the left ventricle is unable to pump an adequate volume of blood to the brain and other vital organs. The systemic blood pressure falls, and the patient may go into shock. Blood still flows into the lungs from the bronchial arteries, which arise from the descending aorta and interconnect with the pulmonary arteries by means of collateral channels. This flow normally prevents infarction of the lung (figure 12–2).

Clinically, the patient becomes very short of breath and the skin and mucous membranes assume a bluish coloration (*cyanosis*) because of inadequate oxygenation of the blood. If the massive embolism is not immediately fatal, some blood may be able to flow around the embolus and circulate through the lungs, because the caliber of the pulmonary artery is increased by overdistention, and the high arterial pressure forces blood around the site of obstruction. In favorable circumstances, the embolus is eventually dissolved by the body's normal clot-dissolving mechanisms, and blood flow through the pulmonary artery is restored. In unfavorable cases, however, thrombus material builds up on the surface of the obstructing embolus and enlarges it. The sluggishly flowing blood in the branches of the pulmonary artery distal to the obstructing embolus may also become thrombosed. These events further impair pulmonary blood flow and may ultimately cause death several days after the initial embolization.

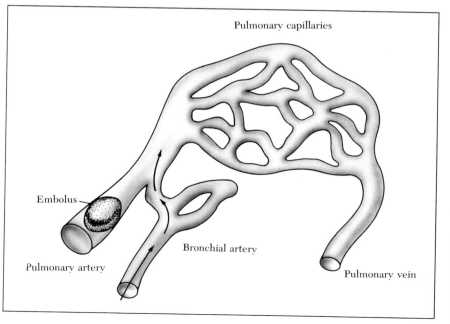

FIGURE 12–2

Anastomoses between bronchial and pulmonary arteries. The presence of an alternative pathway for blood flow often prevents infarction of the lung when the pulmonary artery is blocked by an embolus.

Small Pulmonary Emboli

If emboli are small, they may pass through the main pulmonary arteries and become impacted in the peripheral branches, usually in the arteries supplying the lower lobes of the lungs. Smaller emboli impede the flow of blood through the lungs and raise pulmonary artery pressure, but they have a less-devastating effect than large emboli. Frequently, the segment of lung supplied by the obstructed pulmonary artery undergoes necrosis, resulting in a pulmonary infarct. The alveolar septa break down, and blood flows from the ruptured capillaries into the pulmonary alveoli, which become distended with blood. The typical infarct is a wedge-shaped hemorrhagic area that extends to the pleural surface (figure 12–3). Infarction does not always follow a pulmonary embolism because anastomoses between the bronchial artery and pulmonary artery distal to the obstruction provide an alternative pathway for blood flow. If the pulmonary venous pressure is elevated, however, as occurs in heart failure or when the lungs are poorly expanded, an adequate collateral circulation often does not develop and the lung becomes infarcted.

The clinical manifestations of smaller pulmonary emboli are quite variable and are frequently minimal if the lung does not become infarcted. Common symptoms of pulmonary infarction are difficulty in breathing (*dyspnea*), pleuritic chest pain, cough, and expectoration of bloody sputum. The chest pain occurs because the pleura overlying the infarct become inflamed and rub against the overlying parietal pleura as the lung expands and contracts

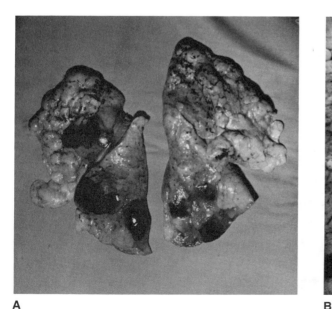

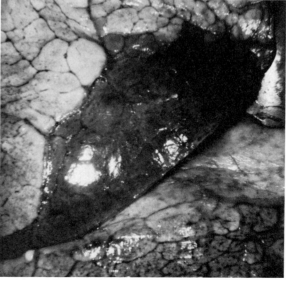

A   **B**

FIGURE 12–3

A, Multiple hemorrhagic pulmonary infarcts in both lungs. **B,** Closer view of infarct illustrating typical wedge-shaped hemorrhagic area that extends to pleural surface.

during respiration. The cough is caused by irritation of the bronchi in the injured area. The bloody sputum appears because blood escapes from the infarcted segment of lung into the bronchi and is subsequently coughed up.

Septic Pulmonary Emboli

Sometimes thrombi form in pelvic veins as a result of a bacterial infection in adjacent pelvic organs, as may occur following a uterine infection, and the bacteria may spread to infect the venous thrombi as well. If an infected thrombus breaks loose and causes a pulmonary infarct, the bacteria transported to the lung in the embolus invade the infarcted tissue, which breaks down to form a lung abscess. An infected embolus is called a *septic embolus*. If a patient sustains a pulmonary infarct owing to a septic embolus, the usual manifestations of pulmonary infarction are overshadowed by those of the systemic infection and the pulmonary abscess.

Diagnosis of Pulmonary Embolism

Diagnosis of pulmonary embolism requires a high index of suspicion. Unexplained dyspnea, cough, or pleuritic chest pain in a predisposed patient may be the only manifestations of a pulmonary embolism. These symptoms should alert the physician to undertake further diagnostic studies. Some of the more useful studies are chest x-ray, radioisotope lung scans, and pulmonary angiography.

Chest X-ray

If the embolus has caused pulmonary infarction, a routine chest x-ray will often demonstrate the infarct, which appears as a wedge-shaped area of increased density in the lung (figure 12–4). Because emboli cannot be visualized on x-ray films, the lung will appear normal if it is not infarcted.

Radioisotope Lung Scan

To perform a radioisotope lung scan, one first injects a peripheral vein with a solution of specially prepared albumin labeled with a radioisotope. The injected material flows through the lung and is filtered out in the pulmonary capillaries. The radioactivity in the lungs, which is related to pulmonary blood flow, is then recorded by special instruments. If pulmonary blood flow is normal, the isotope is uniformly distributed throughout both lungs, and a uniform pattern of radioactivity appears on the lung scan. When blood flow to a part of the lung is blocked by an embolism, however, the isotope does not flow into the portion of lung supplied by the blocked artery, and no radioactivity is detected in the affected part of the lung. The isotope study does not actually demonstrate the embolus; it indicates only that a part of the lung has a reduced blood supply. Nevertheless, the isotope study does detect the abnormal pulmonary blood flow caused by the embolus (figure 12–5). Consequently, the lung scan will be abnormal even when the lung is not infarcted and the routine chest x-ray appears normal.

FIGURE 12–4

Chest roentgenograph illustrating pulmonary infarct in lower part of right lung (*left side of photograph*), which appears as area of increased density (*arrow*). Opposite lung appears normal.

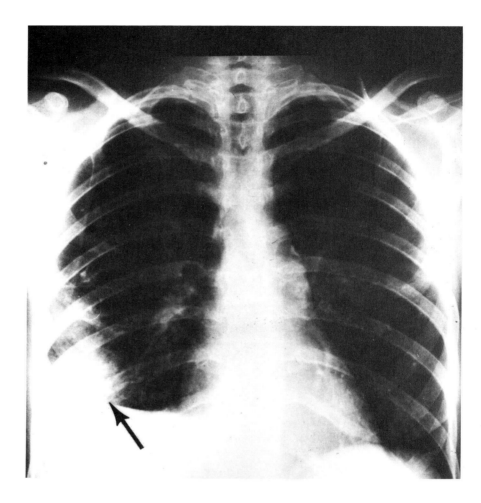

Pulmonary Angiography

A definitive diagnosis of pulmonary embolism requires *pulmonary angiography,* a procedure that directly visualizes the pulmonary artery and its branches. A catheter is inserted into a vein in the arm and advanced up the vein through the superior vena cava, into the right side of the heart, and out the pulmonary artery. A radiopaque material is then injected into the artery through the catheter, and the flow of the material through the pulmonary arteries is visualized by means of serial x-ray films. If the pulmonary artery or one of its branches is completely obstructed by an embolus, no contrast material flows into the blocked vessel (figure 12–6). If the embolus does not completely obstruct the artery, some contrast medium flows around the embolus, which appears as a filling defect in the column of contrast material within the partially occluded vessel.

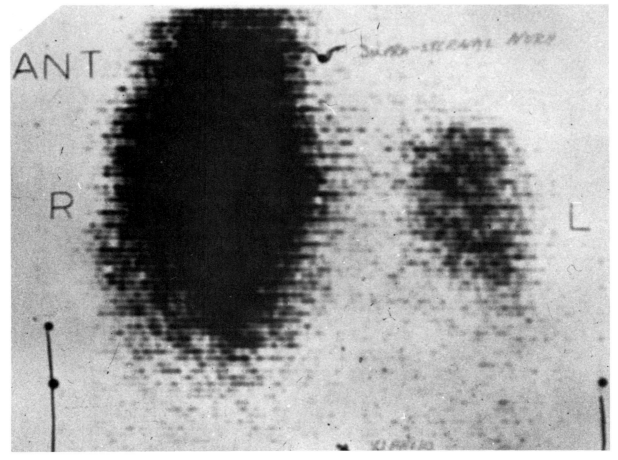

FIGURE 12–5

Lung scan illustrating impaired blood flow to left lung (*right side of photograph*), represented by decreased radioactivity. Radioactivity of opposite lung is normal (uniform dark appearance), indicating normal pulmonary blood flow.

Treatment of Pulmonary Embolism

Treatment of patients with pulmonary embolism includes general supportive care and administration of anticoagulants. Heparin, which has an immediate effect, is generally used initially, followed by administration of coumadin-type anticoagulants, which act by depressing hepatic synthesis of coagulation factors. The purpose of anticoagulant therapy is twofold: (1) to prevent recurrent pulmonary emboli by preventing the formation of more thrombi in leg and pelvic veins and (2) to prevent thrombus formation in branches of the pulmonary artery distal to the embolism. If adequate therapy is given, further thromboembolism is prevented, and the embolus will slowly dissolve.

FIGURE 12–6

Angiogram used to identify pulmonary embolism illustrated by view of left lung and pulmonary artery. Catheter has been inserted into the pulmonary artery and radiopaque contrast material injected. Flow of contrast material is almost completely blocked (*upper arrow*) by a large pulmonary embolus obstructing the left main pulmonary artery. Only a thin trickle of contrast material flows around the embolus (*middle arrow*) to fill the pulmonary artery branches supplying part of the lower lobe (*lower arrow*).

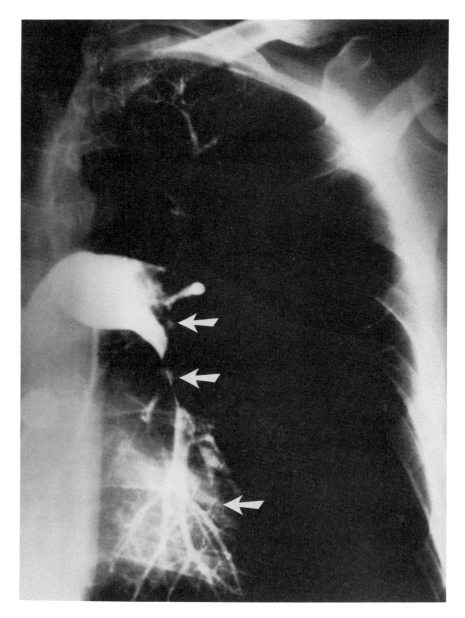

Rarely, if the patient has sustained a massive embolus and is in critical condition, it is necessary to remove the embolus surgically.

If the patient continues to have pulmonary emboli despite adequate anticoagulant therapy, it may be necessary to perform surgery on the inferior vena cava to interrupt the passage of clots from the peripheral veins to the lungs. Generally, the operative procedure consists of either complete or partial interruption of the vena cava below the level of the renal veins. Complete interruption is accomplished by surgical ligation of the vein. Partial interruption has been performed by various methods in such a way as to allow normal blood flow and yet trap emboli.

The following case illustrates the clinical features of a large pulmonary embolism treated successfully by anticoagulant therapy.

A twenty-six-year-old woman consulted her physician because of cough and marked shortness of breath. Physical examination revealed that she was in severe respiratory distress with a dry, hacking cough. Her lips and fingernails were slightly cyanotic, indicating poor oxygenation of the blood. Chest x-ray revealed prominent pulmonary arteries but no evidence of pulmonary consolidation suggesting an infarct. The oxygen saturation of the arterial blood was reduced, which was compatible with a pulmonary embolus. An angiographic study revealed that the left main pulmonary artery was occluded by a pulmonary embolus. The patient received anticoagulant therapy and supplementary oxygen. Her condition gradually improved. Past medical history was significant in that the patient was taking a relatively high estrogen contraceptive pill for control of a menstrual irregularity. The pill apparently predisposed her to thrombosis of a leg vein, which was followed by a pulmonary embolus.

CASE 12–1

Arterial Thrombosis

Blood flow in arteries is rapid, and intravascular pressure is high; so stasis of blood is not a factor in arterial thrombosis. The main cause of arterial thrombosis is injury to the wall of the vessel, usually secondary to arteriosclerosis. The arteriosclerotic deposits cause ulceration and roughening of the lining to the artery, and thrombi form on the roughened area. The effects of arterial thrombus formation depend on the location and size of the artery that has become obstructed. Blockage of a coronary artery frequently causes infarction of the heart muscle and consequent "heart attack." If a major artery supplying the leg is occluded, the extremity undergoes necrosis, usually called **gangrene** (figure 12–7). (This differs from gas gangrene, which is caused by a species of *Clostridium.*) Occlusion of an artery to the brain leads to infarction of a portion of the brain, commonly called a "stroke."

Intracardiac Thrombosis

Occasionally, blood clots may form within the heart itself. Thrombi may form within the atrial appendages when heart function is abnormal, as in heart failure, or when the atria are not contracting normally. Thrombi may also form on the surfaces of heart valves that have been damaged as a result of disease. Occasionally, thrombi may form on the internal lining of the ventricle adjacent to an area where the heart muscle is infarcted. Intracardiac thrombi may become dislodged and may be carried into the systemic circulation, resulting in infarction of the spleen, kidneys, brain, or other organs. The symptoms produced depend on the size and location of the infarction.

FIGURE 12–7

Gangrene of right foot as a result of arterial obstruction.

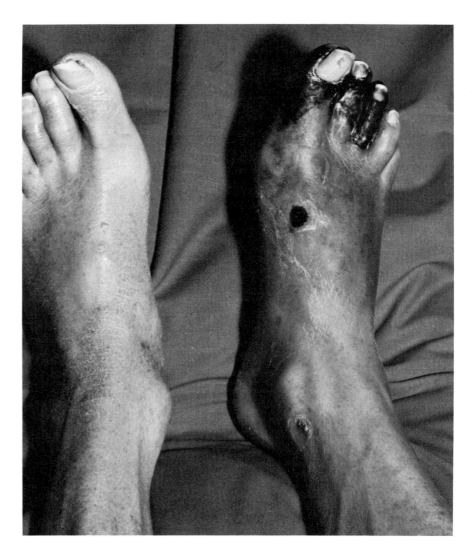

Thrombosis Caused by Increased Blood Coagulability

In some conditions, the concentration of various blood coagulation factors is elevated, increasing the coagulability of the blood and predisposing the individual to intravascular clotting. After injury or operation, products of tissue necrosis with thromboplastic activity stimulate the synthesis of many clotting factors. This increases the likelihood of postoperative thrombosis in leg veins.

The estrogen in contraceptive pills has been found to stimulate synthesis of coagulation factors, raising their concentration and predisposing the women who use the pills to both venous and arterial thrombosis. This observation has led to concern about the safety of "the Pill" when used for long periods of time.

Men with prostatic carcinoma are sometimes treated with estrogen to cause regression of the tumor. Sometimes this treatment is complicated by intravascular thrombosis because large doses of estrogen increase the concentration of the plasma coagulation factors.

Thrombosis in Patients with Cancer

Many patients with advanced cancer have elevated platelets and increased concentrations of coagulation factors in their blood, and they are predisposed to both venous and arterial thromboses. This tendency results from the release of thromboplastic materials into the circulation from deposits of tumor. The same basic mechanism induces hemorrhage in patients with a disseminated intravascular coagulation syndrome (chapter 11). The variations in clinical manifestations result from differences in the rate at which the thromboplastic material enters the circulation. In the acute process, a large quantity of thromboplastic material is rapidly released into the circulation. Platelets and coagulation factors are consumed faster than they can be replenished, and bleeding results. In patients with widespread cancer, the thromboplastic material is liberated slowly but continuously from the tumor. The blood coagulation mechanism is activated, and clot lysis occurs. Production of coagulation factors and platelets increases in response to increased demand, but the body overcompensates. Production exceeds destruction, which leads to a hypercoagulable state. Figure 12–8 compares these two processes.

Most emboli are caused by blood clots, but other materials occasionally gain access to the circulation. Fat, air, and foreign particles within the vascular system may sometimes cause serious difficulties.

Embolism as a Result of Foreign Material

Fat Embolism
After a severe bone fracture, fatty bone marrow and surrounding adipose tissue may be disrupted. The emulsified fat globules may be sucked into the veins and carried into the lungs, leading to widespread obstruction of the pulmonary capillaries. Some of the fat may be carried through the pulmonary capillaries and may reach the systemic circulation, eventually blocking small blood vessels in the brain and other organs.

Air Embolism
Sometimes a large amount of air is sucked into the venous circulation after a chest wound with injury to the lung. Air may also be accidentally injected into the circulation in attempts at abortion by persons without medical training. The air is carried to the heart and accumulates in the right heart chambers, preventing filling of the heart by returning venous blood. As a result, the heart is unable to pump blood, and the individual dies rapidly of circulatory failure.

FIGURE 12–8

Pathogenesis of hypercoagulable state that occurs in patients with cancer, contrasted with pathogenesis of disseminated intravascular coagulation syndrome. Different clinical manifestations reflect differing rates of fibrinolysis and compensatory regeneration of hemostatic components.

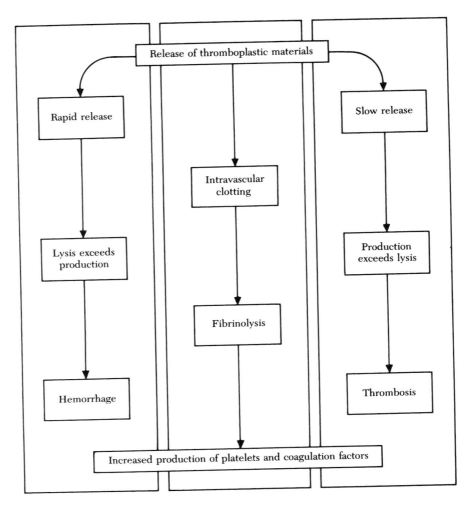

Embolism of Particulate Foreign Material

Various types of particulate material may be injected into veins by drug abusers, who crush and dissolve tablets intended for oral use and inject the material intravenously. The material is usually trapped within the small pulmonary blood vessels, producing symptoms of severe respiratory distress caused by obstruction of the pulmonary capillaries by the foreign material.

Edema

The term **edema** refers to accumulation of fluid in the interstitial tissues. Edema is most conspicuous in the skin and subcutaneous tissues of the dependent parts of the body and is usually noted first in the legs and ankles. When the edematous tissue is compressed by indenting the tissue with the fingertips, the fluid is pushed aside, leaving a pit or indentation that gradually refills with fluid. This characteristic is responsible for the common term *pitting edema.* Fluid may also accumulate in the pleural cavity (**hydrothorax**) or in the peritoneal cavity (**ascites**).

Edema may result from any condition in which the circulation of extracellular fluid between the capillaries and the interstitial tissues becomes disturbed.

Factors Regulating Fluid Flow between Capillaries and Interstitial Tissue

The flow of fluid through the interstitial space depends on four factors:

1. The *capillary hydrostatic pressure,* which tends to filter fluid from the blood through the capillary endothelium.
2. The *permeability of the capillaries,* which determines the ease with which the fluid can pass through the capillary endothelium.
3. The *osmotic pressure* exerted by the proteins in the blood plasma (called *colloid osmotic pressure*), which tends to attract fluid from the interstitial space back into the vascular compartment. Osmotic pressure, which was considered in chapter 2, may be defined as the property causing fluid to migrate in the direction of a higher concentration of molecules. The osmotic pressure of the plasma depends primarily on the concentration of the plasma proteins. Because the capillaries are impermeable to protein, the protein tends to draw water from the interstitial fluid into the capillaries and to hold it there.
4. The presence of open *lymphatic channels,* which collect some of the fluid forced out of the capillaries by the hydrostatic pressure of the blood and return the fluid to the circulation.

Figure 12–9 illustrates the mechanism by which fluid flow is regulated through interstitial tissues.

Flow of Fluid into and out of Capillaries

The pressure of the blood at the arterial end of the capillary is higher than the colloid osmotic pressure, which causes fluid to be filtered through the endothelium of the capillaries into the interstitial space. The capillary endothelium acts as a semipermeable membrane and limits the rate at which fluid is filtered from the blood. At the venous end of the capillary, the hydrostatic pressure is lower than the colloid osmotic pressure, and fluid tends to diffuse back into the capillaries. In this way, the fluid containing dissolved nutrients is carried from the blood into the interstitial tissues to nourish the cells, and waste products are returned to the circulation for excretion.

FIGURE 12–9

Factors regulating flow of fluid through the interstitial tissues, as described in text. HP_A, hydrostatic pressure at arterial end of capillary. HP_V, hydrostatic pressure at venous end of capillary. OP, osmotic pressure. Fluid is forced from the arterial end of the capillary because hydrostatic pressure exceeds osmotic pressure. At the venous end of the capillary, hydrostatic pressure is lower than osmotic pressure and fluid returns. Lymphatic channels also collect some of the fluid forced from the capillaries by the hydrostatic pressure.

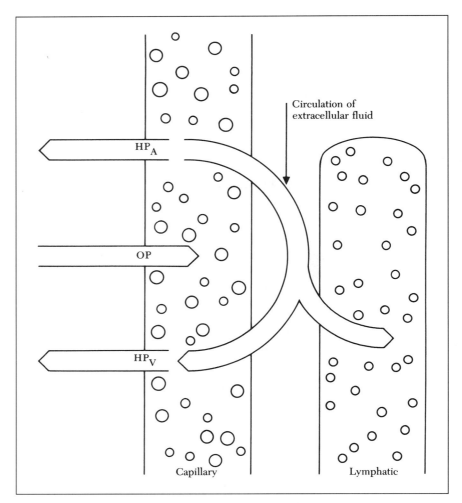

Pathogenesis and Classification of Edema

Increased Capillary Permeability

Normally, the endothelium of the capillaries limits the amount of fluid filtered from the blood. If the capillaries are excessively permeable, filtration of fluid into the interstitial space is greater than normal. Increased capillary permeability is responsible for the swelling of the tissues associated with an acute inflammation such as a boil or a severe sunburn. Some systemic diseases also cause a generalized increase in capillary permeability, which leads to widespread edema of the subcutaneous tissues (figure 12–10).

Low Plasma Proteins

If the concentration of plasma proteins is decreased, the colloid osmotic pressure is reduced correspondingly. Consequently, less fluid is attracted

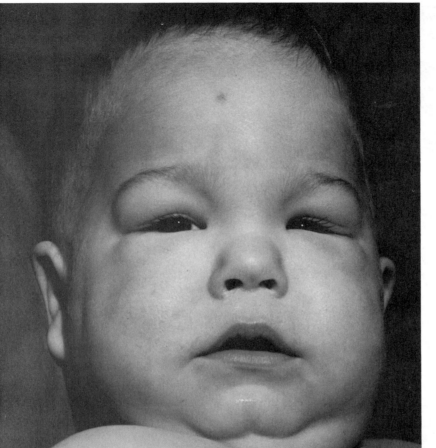

FIGURE 12–10
Edema as a result of
increased capillary
permeability. Note
swelling of eyelids
and face.

back into the capillaries, and the fluid accumulates in the tissues. A low concentration of plasma proteins may result from excessive loss of plasma proteins in the urine, as occurs in patients with some types of kidney disease, or from inadequate synthesis of plasma proteins as a result of malnutrition or starvation (figure 12–11). Hypoproteinemia caused by inadequate protein intake may be encountered in patients with chronic debilitating diseases who are unable to eat an adequate amount of food and in patients with intestinal diseases in whom assimilation of food is impaired.

Increased Hydrostatic Pressure

Increased pressure in the veins draining the capillaries is reflected as a higher-than-normal pressure at the venous end of the capillaries. As a result,

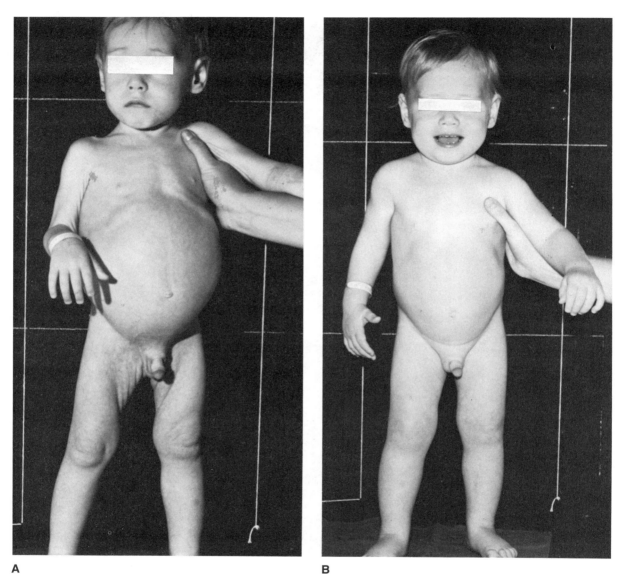

A   **B**

FIGURE 12–11

Edema resulting from low plasma proteins as a result of malnutrition. **A,** Child prior to treatment, illustrating emaciation, abdominal distention caused by an accumulation of fluid in peritoneal cavity, and edema of legs. **B,** Same child after treatment by nutritious high-protein diet.

more fluid is filtered from the capillaries, causing it to accumulate in the tissues. A localized increase in venous pressure may be encountered if the veins draining a part of the body become compressed, twisted, or obstructed by a blood clot that fills the lumen (figure 12–12). More commonly, the increased venous pressure is a manifestation of heart failure, and the pressure is elevated in all the systemic veins.

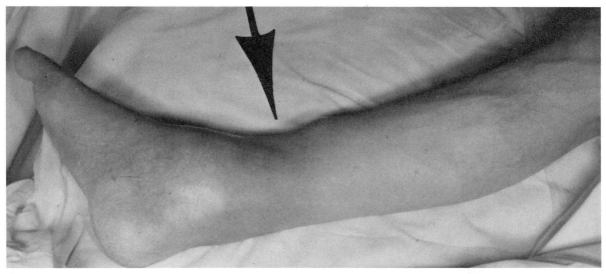

A

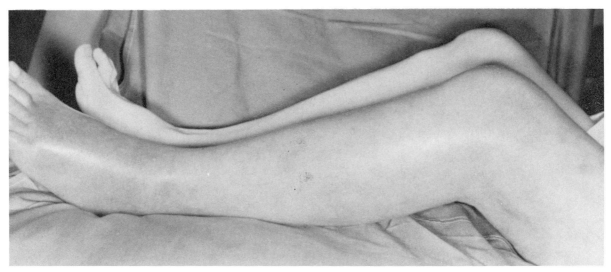

B

FIGURE 12–12

A, Noticeable pitting edema of leg (*arrow*) as a result of chronic heart failure. **B,** Localized edema of left leg caused by a venous obstruction. Right leg appears normal.

Lymphatic Obstruction

Sometimes lymphatic channels draining a part of the body become obstructed owing to disease. The obstruction blocks a pathway by which fluid is returned from the interstitial space into the circulation and leads to edema in the region that is normally drained by the obstructed lymphatic vessels (figure 12–13).

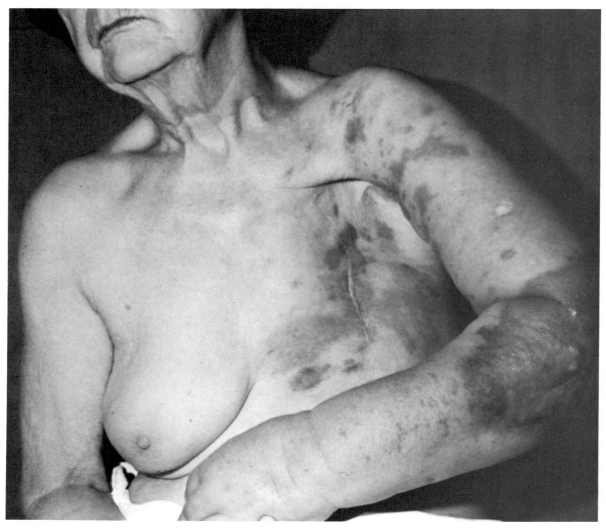

FIGURE 12–13

Severe edema of left arm as a result of lymphatic obstruction. Patient had a radical operation for breast cancer. Scarring in the axilla blocked lymphatic drainage from arm, leading to chronic edema.

Questions for Review

1. What is the difference between a thrombus and an embolus? What is an infarct?

2. What factors predispose to venous thrombosis? What is the major complication of a thrombus in a leg vein?

3. What factors predispose to arterial thrombosis?

4. What are the causes and effects of intracardiac thrombi?

5. What conditions predispose to thrombosis by increasing the coagulability of the blood?

6. What factors regulate the flow of fluid between capillaries and interstitial tissue? What are the major causes of edema?

7. What coagulation disturbances may be encountered in patients with tumors?

8. What is the difference between a pulmonary embolus and a pulmonary infarct? What are the clinical manifestations of a pulmonary infarct?

Supplementary Readings

Alperin, J. B. 1987. Coagulopathy caused by vitamin K deficiency in critically ill hospitalized patients. *Journal of the American Medical Association* 258:1916–19. Vitamin K deficiency in hospitalized patients is common and can be misdiagnosed as disseminated intravascular coagulation syndrome. It can be prevented by prophylactic vitamin K in seriously ill patients receiving antibiotics.

Consensus Conference. 1986. Prevention of venous thrombosis and pulmonary embolism. *Journal of the American Medical Association* 256:744–49. A current summary of the magnitude of thromboembolism, groups at high risk, and measures to prevent thromboembolic complications.

Dalen, J. E., and Alpert, J. S. 1975. The natural history of pulmonary embolism. *Progress in Cardiovascular Disease* 17:259–69. A good review of the problem.

Litin, S. C., and Gastineau, D. A. 1995. Current concepts in anticoagulant therapy. *Mayo Clinic Proceedings* 70:266–272. Discusses various anticoagulation strategies for treating venous thromboembolic disease and methods for monitoring anticoagulant therapy.

Miller, G. H., and Feied, C. F. 1995. Suspected pulmonary embolism: The difficulties of diagnostic evaluation. *Postgraduate Medicine* 97:51–58. Discusses the use of various diagnostic procedures in the diagnosis of pulmonary embolism.

Moser, K. M. 1994. Frequent asymptomatic pulmonary embolism in patients with deep venous thrombosis. *Journal of the American Medical Association* 271:223–25. Pulmonary embolism is a frequent complication of deep venous thrombosis and is asymptomatic in many patients.

Senior, R. M. 1992. Pulmonary embolism. In *Cecil textbook of medicine*. 19th ed. Ed. J. B. Wyngaarden, et al. pp. 421–29. Philadelphia: Saunders. A summary of current concepts.

Stein, P. D., et al. 1992. Complications and validity of pulmonary angiography in acute pulmonary embolism. *Circulation* 85:462–68. Small pulmonary emboli may be missed by angiography.

Chapter 12 ▪ Outline Summary

Thrombosis and Embolism / 293
Pathogenesis
  Slowing or stasis of blood flow.
  Damage to wall of blood vessel.
  Increased coagulability of blood.
Terminology
  Thrombosis: intravascular clot.
  Embolus: detached clot carried in circulation.
  Infarct: tissue necrosis caused by interruption of blood supply.

Venous Thrombosis / 293
Predisposing Factors
  Stasis of blood in veins.
  Varicose veins.
  Increased blood coagulability.
Pulmonary Embolism / 294
Large Pulmonary Emboli
  Obstructs main pulmonary artery or major branches.
  Obstructs blood flow to lungs.
  Causes severe dyspnea and cyanosis.

May cause shock and sudden death.

Usually lung is not infarcted, because adequate collateral blood flow is provided by bronchial arteries.

Small Pulmonary Emboli

Become impacted in peripheral branches of pulmonary artery.

Collateral circulation may be inadequate, and lung infarct develops.

Causes chest pain, cough, and bloody sputum secondary to infarct.

Diagnosis

Chest x-ray: detects infarct, not embolus.

Lung scan: detects impaired lung perfusion secondary to embolus.

Pulmonary angiography: detects blocked pulmonary artery.

Treatment

Anticoagulants.

Operation on inferior vena cava to prevent passage of clots if anticoagulants ineffective.

Septic Pulmonary Emboli

Thrombi form in pelvic veins after pelvic infection.

Bacteria invade thrombi.

Infected thrombus is transported to lungs and causes pulmonary infarct.

Bacteria in clot invade infarct, which becomes infected and forms lung abscess.

Arterial Thrombosis / 301

Pathogenesis

Roughening of arterial wall owing to arteriosclerosis.

Thrombus forms on roughened surface.

Clinical Manifestations Depend on Vessel Affected

Heart attack.

Stroke.

Gangrene of extremity.

Intracardiac Thrombosis / 301

Location

Atrial appendage: in heart failure.

Heart valves: secondary to valve injury.

Left ventricle: secondary to infarct of heart muscle.

Thrombosis Caused by Increased Blood Coagulability / 302

Predisposing Factors

Postoperative increase in coagulation factors.

Estrogens in contraceptive pills.

Malignant tumors: induce hypercoagulable state.

Embolism as a Result of Foreign Material / 303

Sources

Fat embolism: after fracture.

Air embolism: after chest injury.

Particulate material: associated with illicit drug use.

Edema / 304

Factors Regulating Flow of Fluid between Capillaries and Interstitial Tissue

Hydrostatic pressure.

Capillary permeability.

Osmotic pressure.

Open lymphatic channel.

Pathogenesis and Classification

Increased capillary permeability.

Low plasma proteins:

Excess protein loss: kidney disease.

Inadequate synthesis: malnutrition.

Increased hydrostatic pressure:

Heart failure.

Localized venous obstruction.

Lymphatic obstruction.

13

The Cardiovascular System

Learning Objectives

1. Explain the basic anatomy and physiology of the heart as they relate to the common types of heart disease.

2. Describe the common causes of valvular heart disease. Explain its effects. Outline the methods of treating valvular heart disease.

3. Describe the pathogenesis of coronary heart disease. List the four most important risk factors. Describe the clinical manifestations of coronary heart disease. Explain the methods of treatment and their rationales.

4. List the major complications of myocardial infarction and describe their clinical manifestations.

5. Explain the general principles applied to the diagnosis and treatment of coronary heart disease and myocardial infarction.

6. Explain the current concepts regarding the effect of diet on coronary heart disease. Describe how cholesterol is transported by lipoproteins. Distinguish between "good" and "bad" cholesterol.

7. Describe the adverse effects of hypertension on the cardiovascular system and the kidneys.

8. Differentiate between pathogenesis of acute and chronic heart failure. Describe the pathogenesis of each and list the principles of treatment.

9. Differentiate between the pathogenesis and clinical manifestations of arteriosclerotic and dissecting aneurysms of the aorta. Explain the principles of treatment.

10. List the common diseases affecting veins, their clinical manifestations, and methods of treatment.

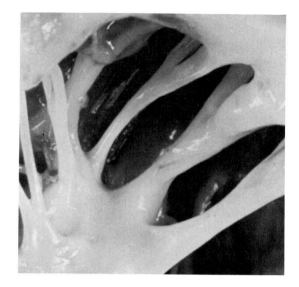

Chapter 13 ▪ Contents

The heart is a muscular pump that propels blood through the lungs and to the peripheral tissues. Heart disease is caused by a disturbance in the function of the cardiac pump. A working knowledge of the normal structure and function of the heart is essential to an understanding of the various types of heart disease.

Cardiac Chambers

The heart is divided by partitions into four chambers, the right and left atria and the right and left ventricles. No direct communication exists between the right and left halves of the heart, and it is convenient clinically to consider each half of the heart as an independent structure. The "right heart" circulates blood into the pulmonary artery and through the lungs (the *pulmonary circulation*); the "left heart" pumps blood into the aorta for distribution to the various organs and tissues of the body (the *systemic circulation*).

Cardiac Valves

The flow of blood into and out of the cardiac chambers is controlled by a system of valves that normally permits flow in only one direction. The **atrioventricular (AV) valves** are flaplike valves surrounding the orifices between atria and ventricles. The free margins of the valves are connected to the papillary muscles of the ventricular walls by narrow, stringlike bands of fibrous tissue called the *chordae tendineae* (figure 13–1). These bands

Normal Cardiac Function

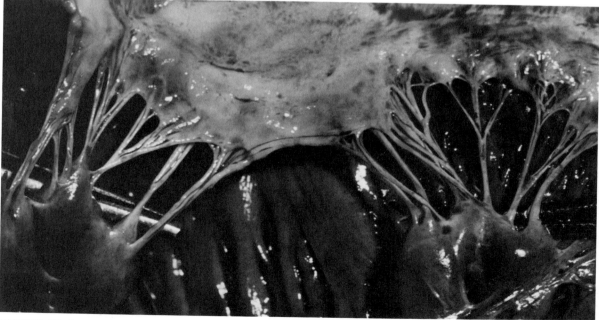

FIGURE 13–1

Normal mitral valve, illustrating thin chordae extending from valve leaflets to papillary muscles.

prevent the valves from prolapsing into the atria during ventricular systole. The **semilunar valves** surrounding the orifices of the aorta and pulmonary artery are positioned so that the free margins of the valves face upward. This structural arrangement defines cuplike pockets between the free margins of the valves and the roots of the blood vessels to which the valves are attached (figure 13–2).

When the heart relaxes in diastole, the chordae produce tension on the valves and pull the atrioventricular valves apart. When the ventricles contract, the chordae are no longer under tension, and the force of the blood flow pushes the valves together so that no blood flows from the ventricles into the atria. During ventricular contraction, the semilunar valves are forced apart by the jets of blood leaving the ventricles. When ventricular contraction ceases, the weight of the column of ejected blood forces the valves back into position, preventing reflux of blood into the ventricles during diastole. The atrioventricular and semilunar valves function reciprocally. Ventricular

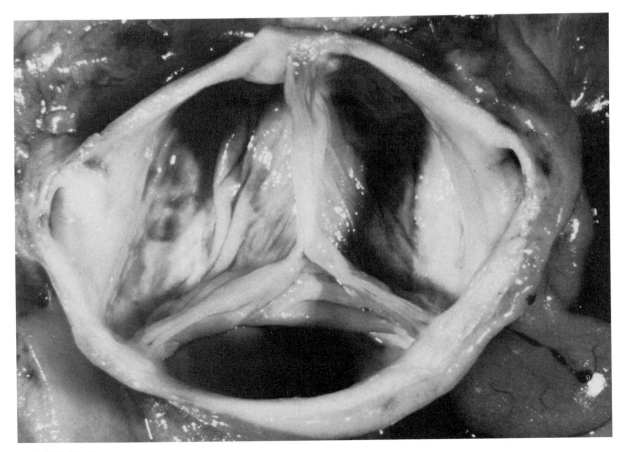

FIGURE 13–2

Aortic valve viewed from above, illustrating cup-shaped configuration of valve leaflets.

contraction relaxes tension on the chordae, causing the atrioventricular valves to close at the same time that the jets of blood open the semilunar valves. Closure of the semilunar valves in diastole is also associated with opening of the atrioventricular valves. Figure 13–3 illustrates the reciprocal action of the two sets of valves which is responsible for the unidirectional flow required for normal cardiac function.

Blood Supply to the Heart

The Left and Right Coronary Arteries

The heart is supplied by two large **coronary arteries** that arise from the aortic sinuses at the root of the aorta (figure 13–4). The *left coronary artery*

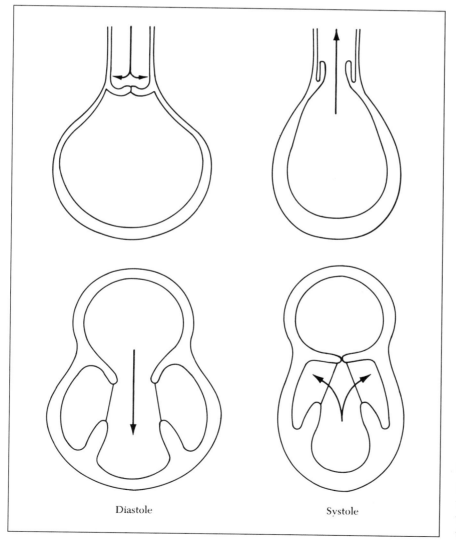

Diastole   Systole

FIGURE 13–3

Reciprocal action of atrioventricular and semilunar valves, resulting in unidirectional blood flow.

FIGURE 13–4

Distribution of coronary arteries.

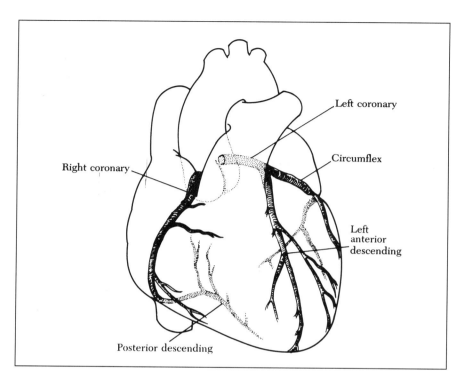

is a short vessel that soon divides into two major branches. The *left anterior descending artery* descends to supply the front of the heart and the anterior part of the interventricular septum. The *circumflex artery* swings to the left (*circum* = around + *flex* = bend) to supply the left side of the heart. The *right coronary artery* swings to the right, supplying the right side of the heart, and then descends to supply the back of the heart and the posterior part of the interventricular septum. Each coronary artery gives off many branches that supply the heart muscle. The terminal branches of the coronary arteries frequently communicate with each other by means of connections called **anastomoses.** Because of these connections, obstruction of one of the arteries does not necessarily completely interrupt the blood flow to the tissues supplied by the blocked vessel. There may be enough blood flow through anastomoses with other arteries to supply the heart muscle. This is called a **collateral circulation.**

Conduction System of the Heart

The impulses that cause the heart to beat are initiated and propagated by groups of specialized muscle cells called the *conduction system of the heart* (figure 13–5). Impulses are normally initiated in the *sinoatrial* (SA) *node,* which is located in the right atrium near the opening of the superior vena cava. The SA node is connected to the *atrioventricular* (AV) *node* by small

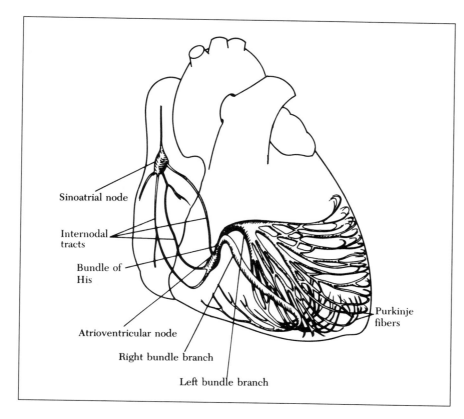

Sinoatrial node

Internodal tracts

Bundle of His

Atrioventricular node

Right bundle branch

Left bundle branch

Purkinje fibers

FIGURE 13–5

Diagram of the cardiac conduction system. The cardiac impulse originates in the SA node and is conducted to the ventricles via the internodal tracts, the AV node, the bundle of His, and the right and left bundle branches, which terminate in the network of Purkinje fibers.

bundles of fibers called the *internodal tracts.* The *atrioventricular bundle* (bundle of His) is a continuation of the AV node, which divides into *right and left branches* in the upper part of the interventricular septum. The branches extend downward on either side of the interventricular septum and break into a fine meshwork of terminal fibers called *Purkinje fibers,* which relay the impulses to the muscle fibers.

Blood Pressure

The flow of blood in the arteries is a result of the force of ventricular contraction. The pressure within the arteries varies rhythmically with the beating of the heart. The highest pressure is reached during the ventricular contraction (*systolic pressure*); the pressure is lowest when the ventricles are relaxed (*diastolic pressure*). The peripheral arterioles regulate the rate of blood flow into the capillaries by varying the degree of arteriolar construction. In many respects, the effect is analogous to the resistance to outflow of water from a garden hose, which can be varied by tightening or loosening the nozzle on the hose. Because of the resistance offered by the arterioles, the blood pressure during cardiac diastole does not fall to zero but declines slowly as blood leaves the large arteries through the arterioles into the capillaries.

In summary, the systolic blood pressure is a measure of the force of ventricular contraction as blood is ejected into the large arteries. The diastolic pressure is a measure of the rate of "run off" of blood into the capillaries, which is governed by the peripheral resistance caused by the small arterioles throughout the body. The mean (average) pressure of blood in the large arteries is midway between systolic and diastolic pressure.

Heart Disease as a Disturbance of Pump Function

For a pump to function properly, several conditions are required:

1. The pump must be properly constructed so that it is free of mechanical defects.
2. The pump must have a system of valves to permit unidirectional flow. If valves do not function properly, the force of the pump stroke is dissipated and effective pumping is impaired.
3. The pump must have an adequate fuel supply. It will not run properly if the fuel line is dirty or plugged.
4. The pump must be used within its rated capacity. One must not use a pump rated at 3 horsepower to perform a job requiring a 10-horsepower pump. Either the pump will not function at all or it will wear out very rapidly.
5. The pump motor must function smoothly and efficiently. If the motor functions erratically, the efficiency of the pump is reduced greatly.

The heart is a muscular pump that is subject to the same requirements as any mechanical pump. Each type of heart disease can be roughly compared to one of the derangements that would impair the function of a mechanical pump (table 13–1).

Congenital heart disease corresponds to faulty pump construction. The term *valvular heart disease* indicates that heart valves have been damaged by rheumatic fever or other diseases and so they fail to open and close properly. It is comparable to a malfunction in the unidirectional valve system of a mechanical pump. *Coronary heart disease* is a result of deposits of fatty material in the arterial walls that narrow their lumens and eventually may completely block the flow of blood through the arteries. This type of heart disease corresponds to failure of a mechanical pump caused by a dirty or plugged fuel

TABLE 13–1

Heart disease compared with mechanical pump dysfunctions

Mechanical abnormality	Comparable heart disease
Faulty pump construction	Congenital heart disease
Faulty unidirectional valves	Valvular heart disease
Dirty or plugged fuel line	Coronary heart disease
Overloaded pump	Hypertensive heart disease
Malfunctioning pump	Primary myocardial disease

line. *Hypertensive heart disease* results when the heart is forced to pump blood at high pressure against an excessively high resistance in the peripheral arterioles and corresponds to overloading a mechanical pump. *Primary myocardial disease* corresponds to malfunction of the pump motor.

The heart undergoes a complicated developmental sequence. It is formed by fusion of paired tubes. The fused cardiac tube undergoes segmental dilatations and constrictions along with considerable growth and change in configuration. Eventually, the individual chambers, valves, and large arteries develop, leading to the final structural configuration of the normal heart.

Congenital Heart Disease

Sometimes the heart fails to develop normally, and so communication between cardiac chambers is defective (figure 13–6). The cardiac valves or septa are malformed (figure 13–7), or the large vessels entering and leaving the cardiac chambers are malformed. Some viral infections, especially German measles in the mother in the early phases of fetal development, may

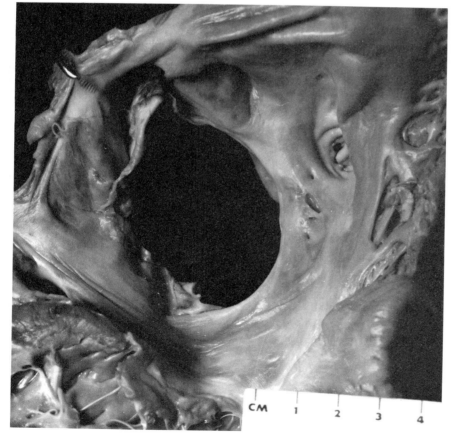

CM 1 2 3 4

FIGURE 13–6

Large congenital atrial septal defect.

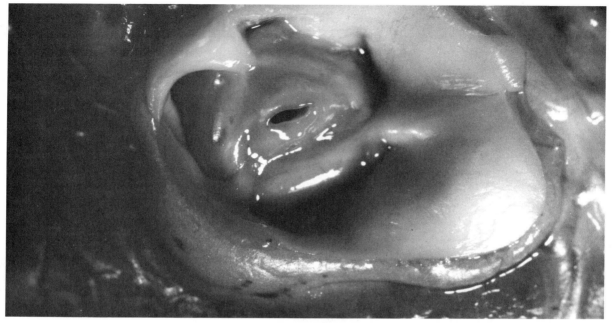

FIGURE 13–7

Congenital pulmonary stenosis. Valve orifice is reduced to a narrow slit, obstructing outflow from right ventricle.

cause improper development of the heart as well as other organs. Some chromosomal abnormalities, such as Down syndrome, also are frequently associated with abnormal cardiac development. In many instances, the reason for congenital heart abnormalities cannot be determined.

The effect of a structural abnormality depends on the nature of the defect. Some congenital abnormalities can be corrected relatively easily by various types of surgical operations. Some cannot be corrected by surgery but may be compatible with a relatively normal life. Still others cause serious malfunction of the heart and are rapidly fatal in the neonatal period.

Prevention of Congenital Heart Disease

The only way to prevent congenital heart disease is to attempt to protect the developing fetus from intrauterine injury during the early phases of pregnancy when it is extremely vulnerable. The factors that may cause intrauterine fetal injury are discussed in chapter 9.

Valvular Heart Disease

Rheumatic fever is much less frequent now than formerly. As a result, rheumatic valvular heart disease has also declined, and other conditions that cause valve malfunction have assumed greater importance. These include various degenerative conditions of the aortic valve and an abnormality of the mitral valve that causes it to prolapse into the atrium during ventricular systole.

Rheumatic Fever and Rheumatic Heart Disease

Rheumatic fever is a complication of infection by the group A beta hemolytic streptococcus, the organism responsible for streptococcal sore throat and scarlet fever. This disease, encountered most commonly in children, is a febrile illness associated with inflammation of connective tissue throughout the body, especially in the heart and joints. Clinically, the affected individual has an acute arthritis affecting multiple joints (which is why the disease is called "rheumatic" fever) and evidence of inflammation of the heart.

Rheumatic fever is not a bacterial infection but a type of hypersensitivity reaction induced by various antigens present in the streptococcus. This reaction develops several weeks after the initial streptococcal infection. It is uncertain exactly how the streptococcus induces the development of rheumatic fever. Apparently, some persons form antibody against antigens present in the streptococcus, and the antistreptococcal antibody cross-reacts with similar antigens in the individual's own tissues. The antigen-antibody reaction injures connective tissue and is responsible for the febrile illness. Fortunately, rheumatic fever develops only in a small proportion of persons with group A beta streptococcal infections.

Some patients with acute rheumatic fever die as a result of severe inflammation of the heart and consequent acute heart failure. In most instances, however, the fever and signs of inflammation eventually subside. Healing is often associated with some degree of scarring. In the joints and in many other tissues, scarring causes no difficulties, but scarring of heart valves may produce various deformities that impair function.

Unfortunately, rheumatic fever is likely to recur when the patient develops another streptococcal infection, because any subsequent contact with the streptococcus reestablishes the sequence of hypersensitivity and connective-tissue damage.

Rheumatic heart disease, a complication of rheumatic fever, is caused by scarring of the heart valves subsequent to the healing of a rheumatic inflammation. This complication is relatively common and primarily affects the valves of the left side of the heart, the mitral and aortic valves (figure 13–8). If the valve does not close properly, blood refluxes back through it (called *regurgitation*). Frequently, the damaged valve also does not open properly, and the valve orifice is narrowed. This is called a valve *stenosis*. Valve lesions impair cardiac function. When valvular stenosis is present, the heart must exert more effort than normal to force blood through the narrowed orifice. In regurgitation, a portion of the ventricular output is not expelled normally and leaks through the incompetent valve. This is a serious disadvantage, because the heart must repump the volume of regurgitated blood to deliver the same amount of blood to the peripheral tissues.

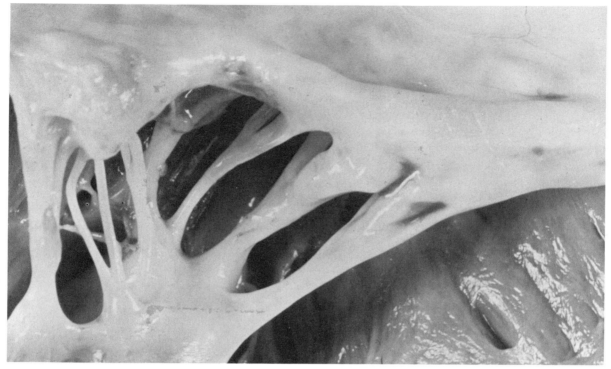

FIGURE 13–8

Scarring of mitral valve leaflet and chordae as a result of earlier rheumatic fever. Compare with figure 13–1.

An individual with a mild rheumatic valvular deformity that does not seriously interfere with cardiac function may experience little or no disability. However, a severe valve deformity may place a serious strain on the heart, eventually causing heart failure many years after the initial attack of rheumatic fever. When a person is seriously disabled by a rheumatic valvular deformity, it is possible to excise the abnormal, scarred heart valve surgically and replace it with an artificial valve.

Prevention of Rheumatic Heart Disease

Rheumatic heart disease can be largely prevented by treating beta streptococcal infection promptly, thereby forestalling the hypersensitivity state that causes rheumatic fever. Because a person who has once had rheumatic fever is susceptible to recurrent attacks after beta streptococcal infections, many physicians recommend that persons who have had rheumatic fever receive prophylactic penicillin therapy throughout childhood and young adulthood. Penicillin treatment prevents streptococcal infections and reduces the risk of recurrent rheumatic fever and further heart valve damage.

Nonrheumatic Aortic Stenosis

In about 2 percent of all people, the aortic valve has two rather than the usual three cusps. This abnormality is called a *congenital bicuspid aortic valve*. The valve functions satisfactorily for a time but is subjected to unusual stress during opening and closing because of its bicuspid configuration. As a result, the valve gradually becomes thickened and may eventually become calcified after many years, leading to marked rigidity of the valve when a person reaches middle age (figure 13–9). This condition is called *aortic stenosis secondary to bicuspid aortic valve*.

Fibrosis and calcification of the aortic valve leaflets also may occur as a degenerative change in elderly persons, and sometimes the valve becomes so rigid that is unable to open properly. This entity is called *calcific aortic stenosis* (figure 13–10).

Mild degrees of aortic stenosis may not greatly compromise cardiac function, but severe aortic stenosis places a great strain on the left ventricle, which must expel blood through the greatly narrowed and rigid valve orifice. This leads to marked left ventricular hypertrophy and eventual heart failure. Treatment of severe aortic stenosis consists of surgically replacing the stenotic valve with an artificial heart valve.

Mitral Valve Prolapse ("Floppy Mitral Valve")

Sometimes the dense connective-tissue framework of one or both mitral valve leaflets undergoes an unusual degenerative change that causes it to become transformed into loose, spongy tissue. The cause is unknown. The affected valve leaflets gradually stretch as a result of degeneration of their fibrous framework. Eventually one or both leaflets may become enlarged and redundant, tending to prolapse into the left atrium during ventricular systole. As a result of the prolapse, the free margins of the valve may fail to

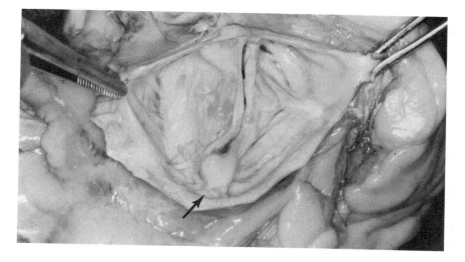

FIGURE 13–9

Congenital bicuspid aortic valve viewed from above. Beginning scarring is seen at lower margin of valve (*arrow*).

FIGURE 13–10

Aortic valve viewed from above, illustrating marked thickening and nodularity of valve leaflets. **A,** Partial fusion of valve cusps (*left side of photograph*). Normal coronary artery is seen in cross-section at right of aortic valve. **B,** Severe calcific stenosis with fusion of adjacent cusps (*upper part of photograph*).

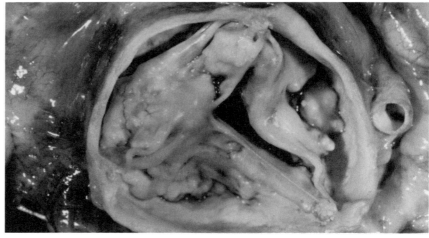

A

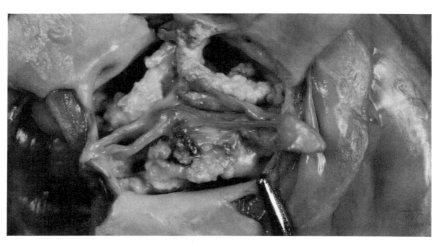

B

come together normally during systole, and some blood may reflux into the left atrium, causing a mild degree of mitral insufficiency (figure 13–11). The prolapsing valve also tends to produce excessive strain of the chordae and papillary muscles, which may provoke bouts of cardiac arrhythmia. Rarely, the excessive stress causes one of the chordae to rupture. The stretched prolapsing mitral valve, held at its free margin by the chordae, somewhat resembles an open parachute (figure 13–12).

Infective Endocarditis

Infective endocarditis is an infection of a heart valve, usually caused by bacteria but occasionally caused by other pathogens. In most cases, the infec-

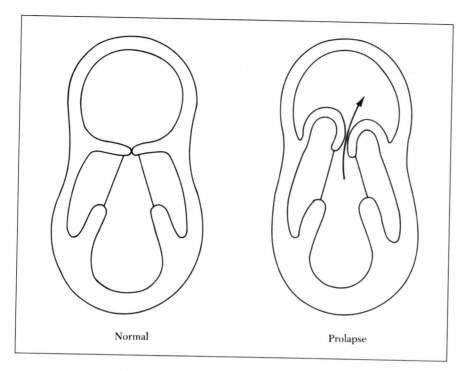

Normal   Prolapse

FIGURE 13–11

Normal mitral valve leaflets (*left*) compared with prolapsing valve leaflets associated with mild mitral insufficiency (*right*).

tion is in the valves in the left side of the heart. It is customary to classify infective endocarditis into two groups: (1) *subacute infective endocarditis,* which is caused by organisms of low virulence, may be a complication of any type of valvular heart disease and is associated with relatively mild symptoms of infection; and (2) *acute infective endocarditis,* caused by highly virulent organisms that infect previously normal heart valves, is associated with symptoms of a severe systemic infection.

Subacute Infective Endocarditis

An abnormal or damaged valve is susceptible to infection because small deposits of agglutinated platelets and fibrin may accumulate on the roughened surface of the valve, serving as a site for implantation of bacteria. Transient bacteremias occasionally develop from superficial skin infections, after tooth extractions, and in association with various minor infections. In normal persons, transient bacteremia causes no problems, because the organisms are normally destroyed by the body's defenses. However, an individual with a damaged valve runs the risk that bacteria may become implanted on the valve and incite an inflammation (figure 13–13). Frequently, thrombi form at the site of the valve infection, and bits of thrombus may be dislodged and carried as emboli to other parts of the body, producing infarcts in various organs. Because of the hazards of bacterial endocarditis in persons with damaged heart valves, prophylactic antibiotic therapy is commonly given to susceptible individuals about to undergo a tooth extraction or an elective sur-

Large prolapsing mitral valve leaflet (*arrow*) that was associated with rupture of a chorda and mitral insufficiency.

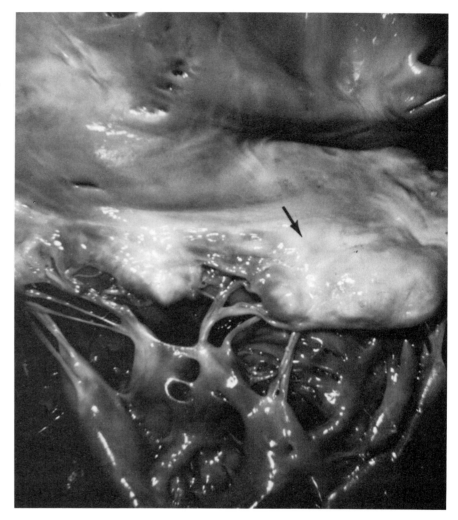

gical procedure. Febrile illnesses in such persons also are treated promptly with appropriate antibiotics. Prophylactic antibiotic therapy given to prevent streptococcal infection in persons who have had rheumatic fever also provides some protection against bacterial endocarditis.

Acute Infective Endocarditis

Acute infective endocarditis results when highly pathogenic organisms spread into the bloodstream from an infection elsewhere in the body and infect a previously normal heart valve. Virulent staphylococci are a common cause of acute endocarditis and may cause considerable destruction of the affected valve (figure 13–14).

Another group at high risk are intravenous drug abusers; in this group, the infection is usually in the tricuspid valve rather than the valves on the

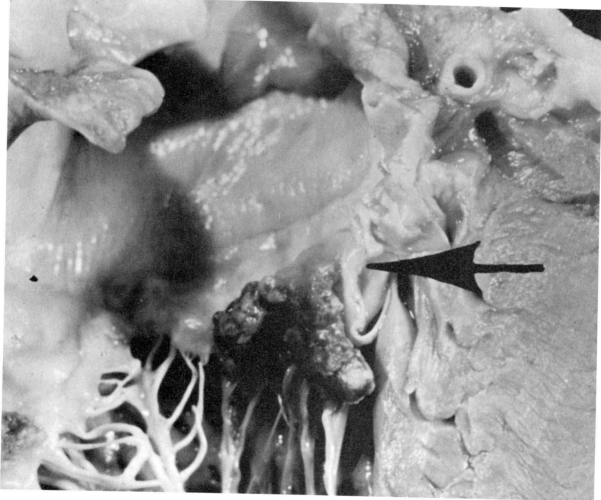

FIGURE 13–13

Bacterial endocarditis illustrating vegetations on mitral valve (*arrow*). Normal coronary artery is seen in cross-section at *upper right.*

left side of the heart. Infection is a result of the use of unsterile materials to dissolve and inject the drug. In addition to bacterial contamination, undissolved particles and other debris contaminate the injected material. Intravenous injection carries the contaminated solution directly to the right side of the heart, where the particles and debris abrade the surface of the tricuspid valve. Platelets adhere to the site of injury and form thrombi, providing a favorable site for the injected microorganisms to implant and start an infection. Often, large bacteria-laden vegetations form on the valve. Pieces often break loose and are swept into the pulmonary arteries where they lodge in

FIGURE 13–14

Severe bacterial endocarditis caused by staphylococcal infection of normal mitral valve. Infection has caused extensive destruction of valve leaflet.

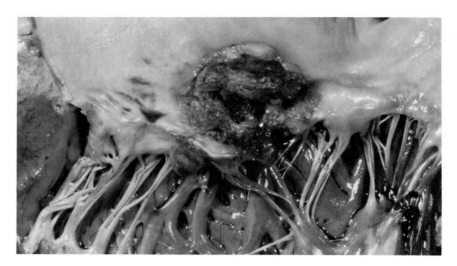

the lungs, causing multiple infected pulmonary infarcts and lung abscesses. Case 13–1 illustrates some of the clinical features of an acute endocarditis in a drug abuser.

CASE 13–1

A thirty-two-year-old hospital employee was admitted to the hospital because of chills and fever of about two weeks duration. She was an intravenous cocaine user. Physical examination revealed numerous needle marks on the extremities and neck. Laboratory studies revealed increased numbers of polymorphonuclear leukocytes in the blood, suggesting an infection, and blood culture revealed Staphylococcus aureus. Special cardiac studies (echocardiograms) demonstrated a large vegetation on the tricuspid valve, and chest x-ray revealed multiple densities throughout both lungs, suggesting pulmonary infarcts secondary to emboli from the infected tricuspid valve. She eventually required surgical removal of the tricuspid valve and entered a drug treatment program.

Coronary Heart Disease

Coronary heart disease results from arteriosclerosis of the large coronary arteries. The arteries narrow owing to accumulation of fatty materials within the vessel walls. The lipid deposits, consisting of neutral fat and cholesterol, accumulate in the arteries by diffusion from the bloodstream. The initial event may be an injury to the endothelium of the vessel, which is followed by proliferation of cells within the inner layer of the arterial wall (called the *intima*) and accumulation of cholesterol and other lipids within their cytoplasm (figure 13–15). Some of the cells accumulate so much cholesterol that it precipitates as crystals within the cytoplasm, disrupting the cells and causing cell necrosis. Cholesterol crystals, debris, and enzymes escape from the disrupted cells, inducing secondary fibrosis, calcification, and other degenerative changes in the arterial wall. The end result is an irregular mass of yellow, mushy debris that encroaches on the lumen of the artery and extends

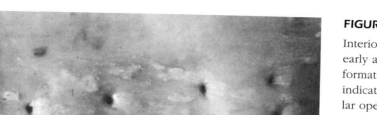

FIGURE 13–15

Interior of aorta, illustrating early atheromatous plaque formation. Two plaques are indicated by *arrows*. Circular openings are orifices of intercostal arteries.

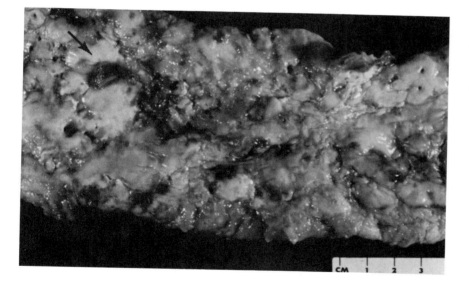

FIGURE 13–16

Advanced atherosclerosis of aorta. Many plaques are ulcerated and covered by thrombus material (*arrow*).

more deeply into the muscular and elastic tissue of the arterial wall. Often the smooth internal lining of the vessel becomes ulcerated over the surface of the fatty deposits, leaving a roughened surface that predisposes to thrombus formation. The plaquelike deposit of material is called an *atheromatous plaque* or **atheroma** (*athere* = mush); the term for this type of arteriosclerosis is **atherosclerosis** (figure 13–16).

The initial stage in the development of atherosclerosis is reversible. The later stages, characterized by crystallization of cholesterol and secondary degenerative changes, are irreversible, and the vessel becomes permanently narrowed.

Risk Factors

A number of factors are known to increase the risk of developing coronary heart disease and its associated complications. The four most important of these are (1) elevated blood lipids, (2) high blood pressure, (3) cigarette smoking, and (4) diabetes. If one risk factor is present, the likelihood of coronary heart disease and heart attacks is twice that in an individual lacking risk factors. If two risk factors are present, the risk increases fourfold, and if three factors are present, the risk of heart attack is seven times that for an individual with none.

Other factors also may increase risk but play a less-important role. Obesity increases risk, but probably because an obese person usually has high blood lipids and elevated blood pressure. The personality of the individual may also play a role. One investigator has classified individuals on the basis of personality traits into two large groups. The *type A* person is aggressive, hard driving, and competitive and is thought to have a greater risk of coronary heart disease than the *type B* person who is less aggressive and more easygoing.

Manifestations and Complications

If atherosclerotic plaques narrow the coronary arteries by 50 percent or more, the arteries may still be able to supply enough blood to the heart muscle if the individual is not very active and no excessive demands are placed on the heart (figure 13–17). However, blood supply may become inadequate if the subject exerts himself and the heart requires more blood to satisfy the increased demands. *Myocardial ischemia* is the term commonly used to describe a reduced blood supply to the heart muscle caused by narrowing or obstruction of the coronary arteries, and the term **ischemic heart disease** is frequently used interchangeably with *coronary heart disease.* Although flow rate through a tube falls as the tube narrows, the decrease is related not directly to the tube diameter but to the fourth power of the diameter. Consequently, a moderate decrease in the caliber of a coronary artery causes a disproportionately large reduction in its flow rate (figure 13–18).

The clinical manifestations of coronary heart disease are quite variable (figure 13–19). Although many individuals are free of symptoms, some experience bouts of oppressive chest pain that may radiate into the neck or arms. The pain, which is caused by myocardial ischemia, is called *angina pectoris,* which means literally "pain of the chest." The usual type of angina is a midsternal pressure discomfort that occurs on exertion and subsides when the person rests or takes a nitroglycerine tablet, which dilates the coronary arteries and increases blood flow to the heart muscle. This kind of angina is often called *stable angina* to distinguish it from *unstable angina,* which is a manifestation of more severe and progressive narrowing of the coronary arteries. Unstable angina is characterized by episodes of pain that occur more frequently, last longer, and are less completely relieved by nitroglycerine.

A few patients exhibit another type of angina that characteristically occurs at rest rather than on exertion and is caused by coronary artery spasm. This

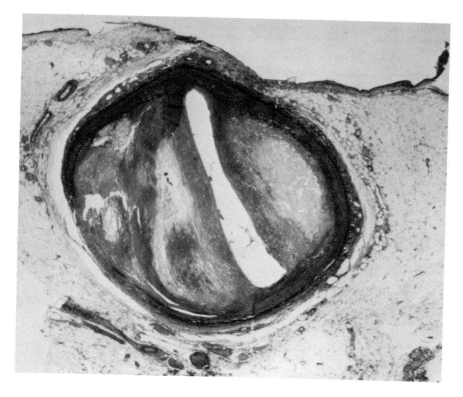

FIGURE 13–17

Low-magnification photomicrograph of coronary artery in cross-section. Atheromatous deposits reduce lumen of artery to a narrow slit. (Original magnification × 40.)

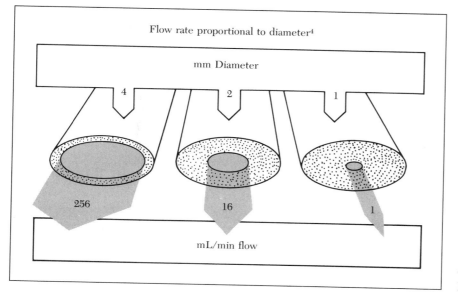

FIGURE 13–18

Relation of caliber of artery to flow rate, illustrating how a small reduction in diameter causes a disproportionately large drop in flow rate.

FIGURE 13–19

Causes and effects of severe myocardial ischemia, as described in text.

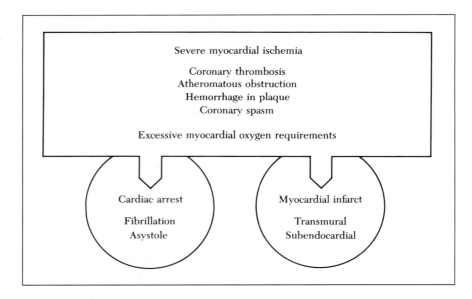

type of angina is usually called *Prinzmetal's angina,* named after the physician who first described it. Although angina is a common manifestation of coronary artery disease, it is not invariably present even though the coronary arteries are severely narrowed.

More severe and prolonged myocardial ischemia may precipitate an acute episode called a "heart attack." This event may be manifested as either cessation of normal cardiac contractions, called a **cardiac arrest,** or an actual necrosis of heart muscle, which is termed a **myocardial infarction.** Any one of four basic mechanisms may trigger a heart attack in a patient with coronary artery disease.

1. *Sudden blockage of a coronary artery.* Usually this is the result of a blood clot that forms on the roughened surface of an ulcerated atheromatous plaque. This is called a *coronary thrombosis.* A less-common cause of blockage is an obstruction of the lumen by atheromatous debris. This sometimes occurs if a break develops in the endothelium and fibrous tissue covering a plaque, allowing the contents of the plaque to be extruded and block the lumen (figure 13–20).

2. *Hemorrhage into an atheromatous plaque.* Bleeding into a plaque usually results from rupture of a small blood vessel in the arterial wall adjacent to the plaque. The blood seeping into the plaque causes it to enlarge, which further narrows or obstructs the lumen of the coronary artery.

3. *Arterial spasm.* Spasm of coronary arteries has been shown to occur adjacent to atheromatous plaques. This may be the mechanism that precipitates arterial obstruction in some patients with heart attacks.

4. *Sudden greatly increased myocardial oxygen requirements.* Vigorous activity such as running, snow shoveling, or tennis abruptly increases

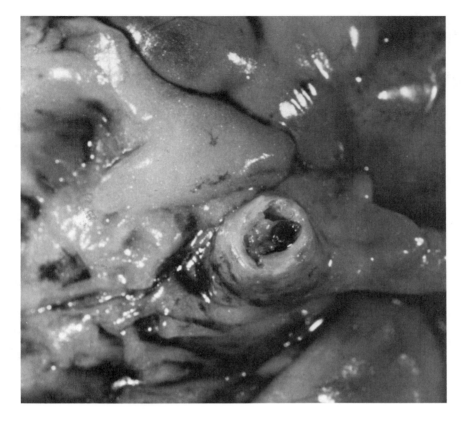

FIGURE 13–20
Severely sclerotic coronary artery in cross-section. Lumen is almost completely blocked.

cardiac output, which in turn raises myocardial oxygen consumption. But the sclerotic coronary arteries are incapable of delivering an adequate blood supply to the heart muscle, and severe myocardial ischemia develops.

Cardiac Arrest

Myocardial ischemia increases myocardial irritability, which may lead to disturbances of cardiac rhythm called cardiac **arrhythmias.** A cardiac arrest occurs when an arrhythmia induced by prolonged or severe myocardial ischemia disrupts the pumping of the ventricles. The most devastating arrhythmia is an uncoordinated quivering of the ventricles that is called *ventricular fibrillation.* It is the most common cause of cardiac arrest and sudden death in patients with coronary heart disease. Ventricular fibrillation is rapidly fatal, because the normal pumping action of the ventricles ceases. If the condition is recognized promptly, it is often possible to stop the fibrillation by delivering an electric shock to the heart by means of electrodes applied to the chest. This procedure frequently causes the ventricles to resume normal contractions, but in many cases ventricular fibrillation occurs without warning and the patient dies before medical attention can be obtained. A less-common cause of cardiac arrest is complete cessation of cardiac contractions, which is called an *asystole* (*a* = without + *systole*).

Myocardial Infarction

A *myocardial infarct* is a necrosis of heart muscle resulting from severe ischemia (figure 13–21). It occurs when blood flow through one of the coronary arteries is insufficient to sustain the heart muscle and when collateral blood flow into the ischemic muscle from other coronary arteries is inadequate. The infarction is associated with severe chest pain and often with shock and collapse.

An infarct may involve the full thickness of the muscular wall or only part of the wall. A full-thickness infarct extending from endocardium to epicardium is called a *transmural infarct* (*trans* = across + *muris* = wall) and is usually the result of thrombosis of a major coronary artery. If only a part of the wall undergoes necrosis, the term *subendocardial infarct* is used.

Location of Myocardial Infarcts

Myocardial infarcts involve the muscle of the left ventricle and septum almost exclusively. Only rarely are the walls of the atria or right ventricle involved. This is because the left ventricle is much more vulnerable to interruption of its blood supply than are other parts of the heart. The left ventricular wall is much thicker than the walls of the other chambers, and it works much harder because it must pump blood at high pressure into the systemic circulation. Consequently, it requires a very rich blood supply. In contrast, the other chambers have much thinner walls, pump blood under much lower pressures, need a less-abundant blood supply, and can usually "get by" by means of collateral blood flow if a major coronary artery is blocked.

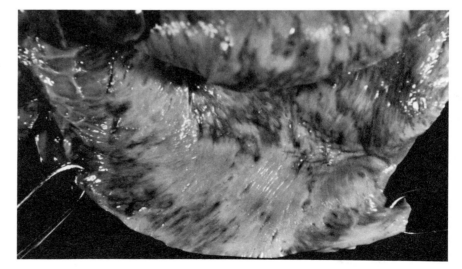

FIGURE 13–21

Longitudinal section through infarcted heart muscle, illustrating pale zone of necrotic muscle that has been infiltrated by inflammatory cells.

The size and location of myocardial infarcts are determined both by the location of the obstructions in the coronary arteries and by the amount of collateral blood flow. Generally, an obstruction of the *left anterior descending artery* leads to an infarct of the anterior wall and often of the adjacent anterior part of the interventricular septum as well. If the *circumflex artery* is blocked, it is usually the lateral wall that is damaged. Occlusion of the *right coronary artery* generally causes an infarction of the back wall of the left ventricle and adjacent posterior part of the interventricular septum. A block of the *main left coronary artery,* which fortunately is quite uncommon, causes an extensive infarction of both the anterior and the lateral walls of the left ventricle and is frequently fatal.

Complications of Myocardial Infarcts

Patients who sustain a myocardial infarction are subject to complications that fall into seven categories (figure 13–22):

1. Disturbances of cardiac rhythm (arrhythmias)
2. Heart failure
3. Cardiac rupture
4. Intracardial thrombi
5. Pericarditis
6. Papillary muscle dysfunction
7. Ventricular aneurysm

Arrhythmias
Disturbances of cardiac rhythm are common subsequent to a myocardial infarct. The arrhythmias result from the extreme irritability of the ischemic heart muscle adjacent to the infarct and can frequently be controlled by drugs that reduce myocardial irritability. The most serious arrhythmia is ventricular fibrillation, which leads to cessation of the circulation. Another type of disturbance of cardiac rhythm occurs if the conduction system of the heart is damaged by the infarct. Conduction of impulses from the atria to the ventricles may be disturbed, which is called a **heart block.** The conduction disturbance may subside spontaneously as the infarct heals, but sometimes it is necessary to insert various types of electrodes directly into the heart in order to stimulate the ventricles to contract properly. A device of this type is called a *cardiac pacemaker.* Usually the electrode is passed into a large vein in the upper arm, near the shoulder, and threaded downward into the heart until it makes contact with the wall of the right ventricle. Then the electrode is connected to a small battery. The electrode stimulates the ventricles at a predetermined rate and causes them to contract at a faster, more normal rate.

Heart Failure
The ventricle may be so badly damaged that it is unable to maintain normal cardiac function, and the heart fails. Heart failure may develop abruptly

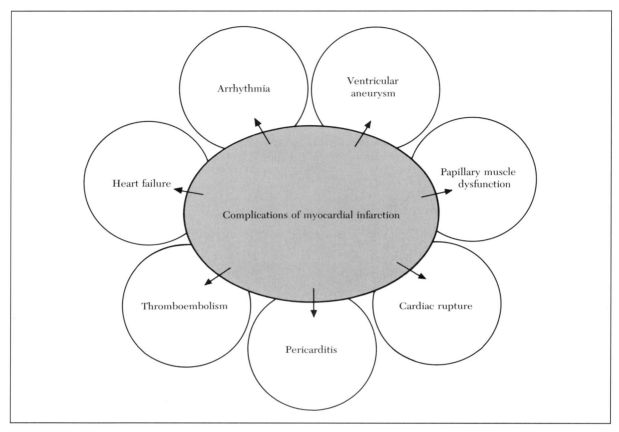

FIGURE 13–22

Possible complications of a myocardial infarction, as described in text.

(*acute heart failure*) or more slowly (*chronic heart failure*), as described in a subsequent section, and may be difficult to treat.

Intracardial Thrombi
If the infarct extends to involve the endocardium, thrombi may form on the interior of the ventricular wall and cover the damaged endocardial surface. This is called a *mural thrombus* (figure 13–23). Bits of the thrombus may break loose and be carried as emboli into the systemic circulation, causing infarctions in the brain, kidneys, spleen, or other organs. Some physicians attempt to forestall this complication by administering anticoagulants when a patient has sustained a severe infarction.

Pericarditis
If an infarct extends to involve the epicardial surface, the inflammatory process resulting from myocardial necrosis may spread to include the overlying epicardium and lead to accumulation of fluid and inflammatory cells

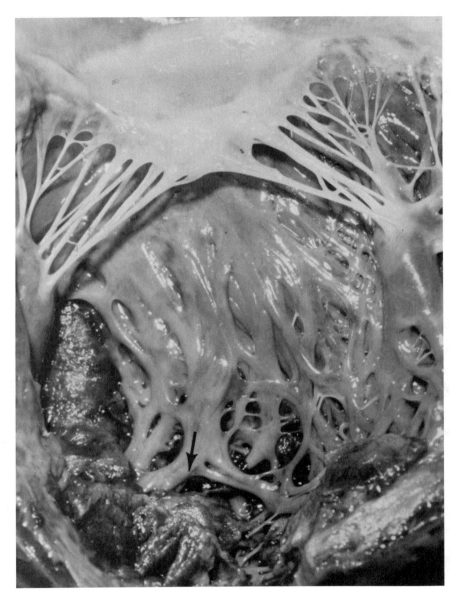

FIGURE 13–23
Interior of left ventricle, illustrating mural thrombus (*arrow*) adherent to endocardium adjacent to myocardial infarct. Normal mitral valve leaflet and chordae are seen at *top* of photograph.

in the pericardial sac (figure 13–24). This condition is called *pericarditis* (not epicarditis). Pericarditis may cause chest pain but usually does not cause other serious problems.

Cardiac Rupture

If a patient sustains a transmural infarct, a perforation may occur through the necrotic muscle (figure 13–25). This permits blood to leak through the rupture into the pericardial sac and, as the blood accumulates, it compresses the

FIGURE 13–24

Acute pericarditis secondary to transmural myocardial infarct. Normal epicardium appears at *upper left* of photograph (*arrow*). The rest of the epicardial surface exhibits fibrinous inflammation.

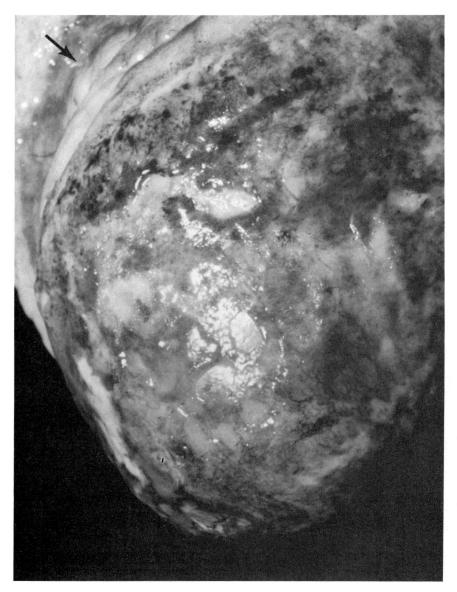

heart, so the ventricles cannot fill in diastole. This event is called a *cardiac tamponade*. Eventually the circulation ceases because the heart is no longer able to pump blood (figure 13–26). Less commonly, rupture occurs through the ventricular septum or papillary muscle. Full-thickness infarction of the ventricular septum may lead to septal perforation, which allows blood to leak from the left ventricle into the right ventricle during ventricular contractions instead of being ejected normally. As a result, the output of blood from the left ventricle is reduced greatly, which often leads to severe heart

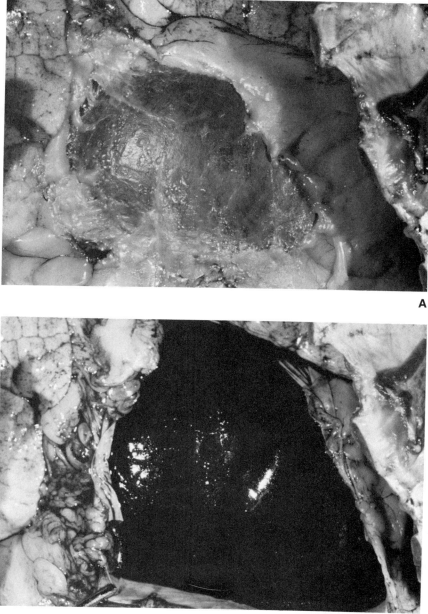

A

B

FIGURE 13–25
Cardiac tamponade
secondary to myocardial
rupture. **A,** Distended pericardial sac. **B,** Pericardium
opened, showing clotted
blood surrounding heart
which prevented the filling
of ventricles in diastole.

failure. An infarcted papillary muscle may tear loose from its attachment to the ventricular wall. This leads to loss of "guy wire" support for the mitral valve leaflet to which it is attached and permits the leaflet to prolapse into the left atrium during systole. This complication results in severe mitral insufficiency, which often leads to heart failure.

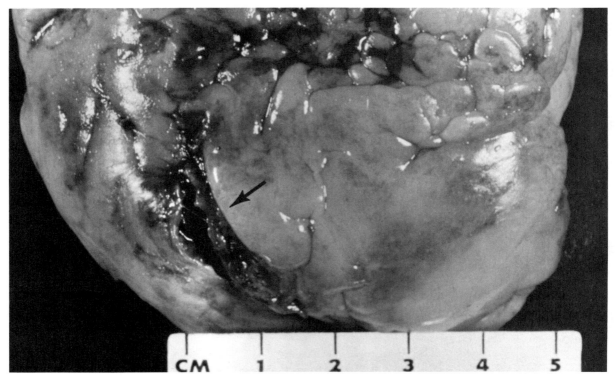

FIGURE 13–26

Rupture of heart muscle (*arrow*) through large transmural myocardial infarct.

Papillary Muscle Dysfunction

Normally, the papillary muscles contract during ventricular systole along with the rest of the ventricle, exerting tension on the chordae to prevent prolapse of the mitral valve leaflets into the left atrium during systole. If a papillary muscle becomes infarcted, it is unable to contract normally and is less able to control the movement of the attached mitral valve leaflet. So, even if the papillary muscle does not rupture, its malfunction often allows the mitral valve to prolapse slightly into the left atrium, and a mild degree of mitral insufficiency develops (figure 13–27).

Ventricular Aneurysm

A **ventricular aneurysm** is usually a late complication of myocardial infarction. It is an outward bulging of the healing infarct during ventricular systole (figure 13–28). There are two adverse effects on ventricular function. The damaged area is unable to contract; so the overall efficiency of left ventricular function is reduced. Moreover, as the ventricle contracts and the intraventricular pressure rises during systole, the aneurysm fills with blood and balloons out. Consequently, part of the volume of blood within the ven-

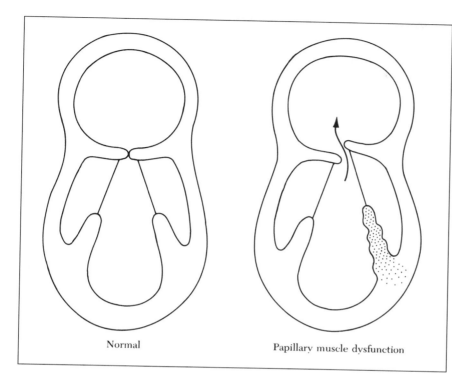

FIGURE 13-27

Pathogenesis of papillary muscle dysfunction. *Left,* Normal mitral valve function in systole. Papillary muscle contraction exerts tension on chordae to prevent prolapse of mitral valve into atrium. *Right,* Papillary muscle infarcted and unable to contract normally. Attached mitral leaflet prolapses into atrium, leading to mitral insufficiency.

Normal — Papillary muscle dysfunction

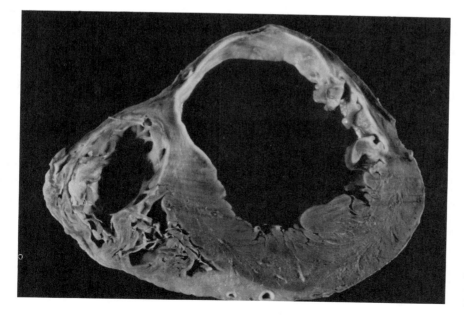

FIGURE 13-28

Cross-section of heart through ventricles illustrating large ventricular aneurysm protruding from posterior wall of left ventricle (*upper part of photograph*). Heart muscle of anterior wall is of normal thickness.

tricle is "wasted" because it fills the aneurysm rather than being ejected into the aorta, and the cardiac output is reduced correspondingly (figure 13–29).

Survival After Myocardial Infarction

The survival rate of patients who have had a myocardial infarct depends on many factors, the more important being (1) the size of the infarct, (2) the patient's age, (3) the development of complications, and (4) the presence of other diseases that would adversely affect the patient's survival. Mortality rates vary from about 6 percent in patients who have had small infarcts and who do not develop heart failure to more than 50 percent in patients with large infarcts who develop severe heart failure. Major causes of death following myocardial infarction are fatal arrhythmia, heart failure, and cardiac rupture with cardiac tamponade. Coronary care units staffed by specially trained personnel have reduced the mortality from cardiac arrhythmias, which are prone to occur in the first several days after myocardial infarction, but these facilities have not had any significant effect on the rates of death from heart failure or cardiac rupture.

FIGURE 13–29

Hemodynamic derangements associated with large ventricular aneurysm (*right*), as described in text, compared with normal ventricular function (*left*).

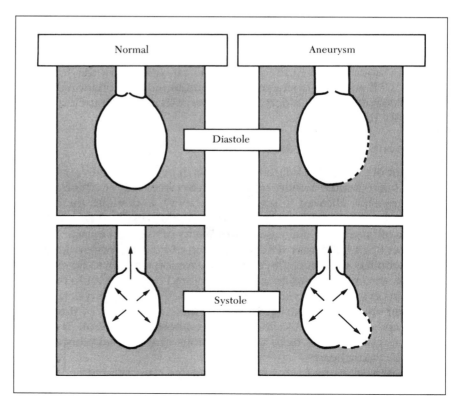

If we consider all hospitalized patients as a group, about 90 percent survive and are able to leave the hospital. The data on survival, however, relate only to patients with myocardial infarction who are admitted to the hospital. They do not include patients with severe heart attacks who die suddenly or within a few hours. This is a significant number of patients, because it is estimated that one-third of all deaths from heart attacks occur outside the hospital. On the other hand, the survival data also do not include patients with small infarcts that may not be detected clinically. Many small myocardial infarcts cause relatively mild symptoms and heal without complications. The patients may ascribe the chest discomfort associated with the infarction to indigestion or other causes and never seek medical attention. Some studies indicate that as many as 25 percent of all patients with myocardial infarcts have very few symptoms and do not consult a physician.

Diagnosis of Myocardial Infarction

Diagnosis of myocardial infarction rests on evaluation and interpretation of the medical history, physical examination, and laboratory data. The clinical history may at times be inconclusive, because severe angina may be quite similar to the pain of a myocardial infarction. Conversely, many patients who develop subendocardial myocardial infarcts may have minimal symptoms. Physical examination will usually not be abnormal unless the subject exhibits evidence of shock, heart failure, or a heart murmur as a result of papillary muscle dysfunction. Consequently, the physician must rely on specialized diagnostic studies to demonstrate infarction of heart muscle. The most helpful diagnostic aids are the electrocardiogram and determination of blood levels of various enzymes that leak from damaged heart muscle.

The Electrocardiogram

The **electrocardiogram** (ECG or EKG), which measures the transmission of electrical impulses associated with cardiac contraction, reveals rather characteristic abnormalities when heart muscle becomes infarcted. By means of the electrocardiogram, the physician can often determine the location and approximate size of the infarct. The process of healing can be followed by means of serial cardiograms. The electrocardiogram can also detect arrhythmias and various disturbances in the transmission of impulses through the cardiac conduction system.

Enzyme Tests

Heart muscle is rich in various enzymes that regulate the metabolic activities of the cells. If heart muscle becomes infarcted, the enzymes leak from the necrotic cells into the circulation. Enzyme levels begin to rise soon after the infarction, reach a peak within a few days, and then gradually return to normal. In general, the larger the infarct, the greater the elevation of enzyme activity and the longer it takes for the elevated level to fall to normal. The pattern of rapid rise of enzyme activity followed by a fall over the succeeding several days is characteristic of a myocardial infarct. The following three enzymes are most widely used to monitor the course of a myocardial infarction:

1. *Aspartate aminotransferase* (AST), which some physicians still designate by its older name, *glutamic-oxalacetic transaminase* (GOT)
2. *Creatine phosphokinase* (CPK)
3. *Lactic dehydrogenase* (LDH)

These enzymes are found not only in heart muscle, but in other tissues as well. There are several different varieties (*isoenzymes*) of CPK and LDH, which can be distinguished by specialized tests. The isoenzymes of CPK and LDH found in heart muscle differ slightly from the isoenzymes present in other organs. Consequently, one can analyze for the "cardiac specific" CPK and LDH isoenzymes as an additional confirmation that the elevated enzyme activity is derived from necrosis of heart muscle and not from injury to other tissues.

Thrombolytic (Clot-Dissolving) Treatment of Coronary Thrombosis

Most myocardial infarctions are caused by thrombi that form on a roughened atheromatous plaque within a coronary artery, and in many cases it is possible to unblock the artery by dissolving the clot. Clot dissolution reestablishes the flow through the artery and salvages at least some of the heart muscle supplied by the blocked artery before the muscle becomes completely necrotic. Initially, clot-dissolving agents were introduced directly into the occluded coronary artery. Cardiac catheterization was performed; the obstructing thrombus was located by means of a coronary arteriogram, and the clot-dissolving drug was injected directly into the blocked artery by means of a catheter inserted into the coronary artery. Later, it was found that coronary artery thrombi could be dissolved just as well by administering thrombolytic (*thrombus* = clot + *lysis* = dissolving) drugs intravenously, and cardiac catheterization was no longer required.

In order for thrombolysis to be successful, the thrombus must be dissolved very soon after the vessel has become occluded and before the myocardium has sustained extensive and irreparable damage. The sooner the clot is dissolved, the better the results. Excellent results are obtained and mortality is reduced greatly if the clot can be dissolved within one hour after the patient experiences the first symptoms of a heart attack. The benefit of thrombolytic therapy decreases progressively as the time interval between coronary thrombosis and clot lysis lengthens. After about six hours, administration of a thrombolytic drug is of no benefit because by this time the heart muscle has progressed from ischemia to complete infarction, and it can no longer be salvaged by restoring blood flow through the occluded vessel.

Three different thrombolytic drugs are available for intravenous administration: streptokinase, a chemically modified more slowly acting streptokinase preparation, and tissue plasminogen activator. All act by converting plasminogen into plasmin, which is the fibrinolytic agent that dissolves the clot. (The coagulation and fibrinolytic mechanisms are described in chapter 11). Each agent has advantages and disadvantages, and each is quite effective.

Streptokinase is a fibrinolytic enzyme derived from beta streptococci; its chemically modified derivative is similar but has a slower and more prolonged duration of action. Streptokinase preparations not only activate plasminogen, but also attack other blood coagulation components, which greatly reduces the coagulability of the blood as well as dissolving fibrin clots. Tissue plasminogen activator (TPA), which is produced commercially by recombinant DNA technology, is the same material that is normally produced by the endothelial cells of blood vessels to dissolve clots. It binds to the fibrin within the clot in the coronary artery, where it converts plasminogen into plasmin within the clot and dissolves the clot without producing generalized effects on the coagulation mechanism. Unfortunately, the preparation is much more expensive than other thrombolytic agents.

Aspirin and heparin are often used along with thrombolytic agents. Aspirin reduces the tendency of platelets to aggregate and initiate the coagulation process at the site where the clot was dissolved. Heparin reduces the coagulability of the blood and decreases the likelihood that the clot will reform.

Although thrombolytic therapy improves survival and salvages myocardium, it also tampers with the body's coagulation mechanisms, and treatment may be complicated by serious bleeding episodes, including brain hemorrhage (hemorrhagic stroke) that can severely disable the patient or may even be fatal. Consequently, patients who are at greater-than-normal risk of hemorrhagic complications are not suitable candidates for thrombolytic therapy. In this group are: (1) patients who have had a stroke or have any other disease affecting the cerebral blood vessels, because they are at greater risk of a hemorrhagic stroke; (2) patients with severe hypertension, which increases the risk of a cerebral hemorrhage; (3) patients who have had a recent operation, because the site of the operation may not be completely healed and may bleed if the clotting mechanism is disturbed; and (4) patients with any type of bleeding disorder or with any condition (such as a gastric or duodenal ulcer) in which thrombolytic therapy may precipitate bleeding. Patients who are not suitable candidates for thrombolytic therapy can be treated by immediate coronary angioplasty to unblock the occluded artery.

Many studies have confirmed that thrombolytic therapy is effective. A large international study called *the global utilization of streptokinase and TPA in occluded coronary arteries study* (usually referred to by the acronym "the GUSTO study") included more than forty thousand patients from more than a thousand different institutions. The study reached several conclusions: Thrombolytic therapy is effective, and the sooner it is administered, the better the results will be. All available thrombolytic agents are effective. Tissue plasminogen activator seems to have a slight advantage over other thrombolytic agents but is much more expensive and is associated with a slightly higher risk of hemorrhagic strokes.

Treatment of Myocardial Infarction

After as much myocardium as possible has been salvaged by restoring flow through the occluded artery, further treatment of myocardial infarction consists of bed rest initially, gradually progressing to limited activity and then to full activity. Sometimes the injured heart is quite irritable and prone to abnormal rhythms. Therefore, various drugs are often given to decrease the irritability of the heart muscle. Development of heart block may require insertion of a cardiac pacemaker. The patient who has sustained a myocardial infarction may develop intracardiac thrombi if the endocardium is injured or may develop thrombi in leg veins as a result of reduced activity. Therefore, some physicians also administer anticoagulant drugs to reduce the coagulability of the blood and thereby decrease the likelihood of thromboses and emboli. If the patient shows evidence of heart failure, various drugs are administered to sustain the failing heart.

Patients recovering from a myocardial infarct are at increased risk of sudden death from a fatal arrhythmia of another infarct, and the risk is greatest within the first six months after the infarct. Many physicians treat postinfarct patients for at least two years with drugs that reduce myocardial irritability (called beta-blockers), because this seems to reduce the incidence of these postinfarct complications and improves survival. Ingestion of a small amount of aspirin daily also is beneficial. As mentioned earlier, aspirin inhibits platelet function, making them less likely to adhere to roughened atheromatous plaques and initiate a thrombosis in the coronary artery.

Case Studies

The following three cases illustrate some of the clinical features and complications of myocardial infarctions. At the time that these patients were admitted to the hospital, thrombolytic therapy was not being used routinely.

CASE 13–2

A seventy-four-year-old man was admitted to the emergency room because of severe oppressive chest pain of about five hours' duration. For the previous two weeks, he had also experienced episodes of less-severe chest pain when he walked rapidly, but the pain soon subsided when he rested.

Physical examination revealed an elderly man in no acute distress. Heart sounds were normal. Lungs were clear. Blood pressure was 190/110 (normal about 120/80) Electrocardiogram showed the pattern of acute myocardial infarction involving the anterior wall of the left ventricle.

Laboratory studies obtained soon after admission revealed elevated levels of cardiac enzymes aspartate aminotransferase (glutamic oxalacetic transaminase), creatine phosphokinase, and lactic dehydrogenase. Repeat studies the following morning revealed a further elevation of these enzymes.

He received the usual treatment for acute myocardial infarction. His condition stabilized, and he appeared to be progressing well. About 6:10 P.M. on the second hospital day, the cardiac monitor showed a drop in heart rate to 60, soon followed by ventricular fibrillation. The patient failed to respond to resuscitative measures and was pronounced dead at 6:30 p.m.

An autopsy revealed severe arteriosclerosis of all coronary arteries. The left anterior descending coronary artery was occluded by a thrombus, and there was a large transmural anterolateral myocardial infarction. A myocardial perforation at the apex had permitted blood to leak into the pericardial sac and caused death by cardiac tamponade.

A fifty-seven-year-old man was admitted to the hospital from his place of employment. While at work he complained of a sweaty feeling and then lost consciousness. When he regained consciousness, he noted a constant, oppressive substernal pain. In the preceding month, he had experienced similar episodes of substernal pain that would last for several minutes and disappear spontaneously. The pain was associated with a feeling of numbness in the arms. The patient had sustained a myocardial infarction two years earlier.

CASE 13–3

Physical examination was normal and blood pressure was normal. An electrocardiogram showed changes of acute myocardial infarction involving the anterior wall and interventricular septum.

At 3:40 P.M. on the day of admission, the patient complained of more chest pain. At about 5:30 P.M., his blood pressure fell to shock levels and could not be restored to normal. He was considered to be in shock caused by severe myocardial damage. At approximately 6:00 P.M., the cardiac monitor recorded ventricular fibrillation. Resuscitative measures were instituted but were unsuccessful, and the patient was pronounced dead at 6:35 P.M.

The autopsy revealed old scarring in the posterior wall and the posterior portion of the interventricular septum in the distribution of the right coronary artery. There was a recent area of infarction in the anterior and lateral wall and in the anterior portion of the interventricular septum in the distribution of the anterior descending left coronary artery. The coronary arteries showed a variable degree of arteriosclerosis. The main left and circumflex arteries showed from 35 to 50 percent narrowing. The anterior descending left artery was 85 to 90 percent narrowed but was not occluded. The right coronary artery was occluded by old thrombus material that extended within the vessel for a distance of 7 to 8 cm. Lungs exhibited marked pulmonary edema.

A fifty-two-year-old man experienced an episode of severe precordial pain associated with nausea and vomiting. He attributed this to indigestion and did not consult a physician. He remained at home on restricted activity but felt quite weak and experienced periodic episodes of sweating and chest pain. Eventually he was able to be up and about around the house and felt somewhat better. While eating supper two weeks later, he experienced sudden onset of weakness in the right arm and difficulty with speech. When he attempted to get up from the table, his right leg did not support him and he fell to floor.

CASE 13–4

On admission to the hospital, he exhibited a paralysis of the right side of the body. His blood pressure was elevated (210/110). The remainder of the physical examination was normal.

The electrocardiogram showed the pattern of a recent anterior-wall myocardial infarction. Serum cardiac enzyme studies on admission, at twenty-four hours, and at forty-eight hours were all within normal limits, because the myocardial infarct had occurred two weeks earlier. The elevated levels of enzyme activity had returned to normal by the time the patient entered the hospital.

The patient's disorder was treated as a recent myocardial infarction. A mural thrombus had apparently formed in the left ventricle at the site of the infarct. A piece of the clot had broken loose and had been carried as an embolus to the brain, where it had obstructed a cerebral artery and caused the paralysis. He made a satisfactory recovery but was left with some residual weakness and speech difficulty.

Coronary Artery Disease

Diagnosis of Coronary Artery Disease

Physicians can now evaluate the extent of coronary artery disease as well as the exact sites where the main coronary arteries are obstructed. This is accomplished by passing a catheter into the aorta and injecting a radiopaque dye directly into the orifices of the coronary arteries. The filling of the coronary arteries can be observed, along with the location and degree of arterial obstruction (figure 13–30). This procedure is called a *coronary angiogram* (described in chapter 1).

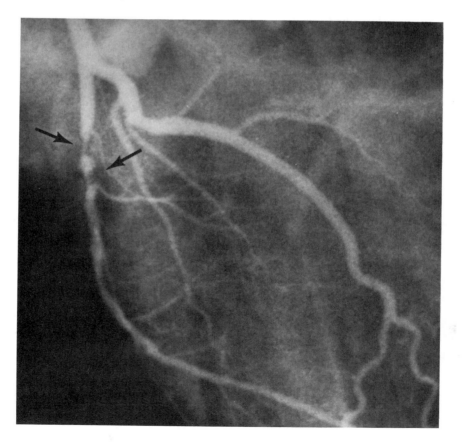

FIGURE 13–30

Coronary arteriogram illustrating segmental narrowing (*arrows*).

Treatment of Coronary Artery Disease

Medical Treatment

Medical treatment of coronary heart disease consists of administering drugs that reduce myocardial oxygen consumption and improve coronary circulation (*antianginal drugs*). If the patient exhibits cardiac irregularities, drugs that reduce myocardial irritability also are prescribed (*antiarrhythmial drugs*). Factors that potentiate coronary artery disease also are controlled or eliminated as follows whenever possible (figure 13–31):

1. Cessation of smoking, which has an adverse effect on the coronary circulation
2. Control of hypertension, which increases myocardial work and accelerates development of atherosclerosis
3. An "anticoronary diet," which lowers levels of cholesterol and fat in the blood
4. Weight reduction
5. A program of graduated exercises, which seems to improve myocardial performance

Surgical Treatment

Several surgical approaches, called *myocardial revascularization procedures,* have been devised to improve blood supply to the heart muscle. Surgery is often recommended for patients who do not respond satisfactorily to medical treatment. The usual surgical method is to bypass the obstructions in the coronary arteries by means of segments of saphenous vein

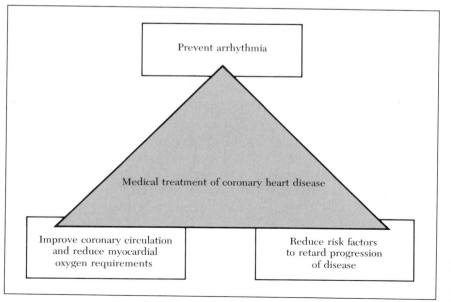

FIGURE 13–31

Principles of medical treatment of coronary heart disease.

obtained from the patient's legs. The proximal ends of the grafts are sutured to small openings made in the aorta above the normal openings of the coronary arteries, and the distal ends are sutured into the coronary arteries beyond the areas of narrowing (figure 13–32). Sometimes the vein grafts are combined with procedures that "ream out" parts of the arteriosclerotic lining of the narrowed arteries (figure 13–33). Myocardial revascularization operations are generally reserved for patients with severe sclerosis of all three major coronary arteries, and usually grafts are used to bypass all three arteries. The operation alleviates or greatly improves symptoms of angina and may also improve survival in some groups of patients. Unfortunately, the high arterial pressure carried by the vein grafts sometimes causes the grafts to undergo progressive intimal thickening, which may lead to complete occlusion of the grafts. Many of the grafts eventually also develop the same type of atherosclerosis that occurred in the coronary arteries.

The internal mammary arteries also can be used to bypass obstructed coronary arteries. The internal mammary arteries are paired arteries that arise from the aorta and descend along the undersurface of the thoracic cavity just lateral to the sternum. They can be dissected from their normal location and connected to the coronary arteries, thereby delivering blood directly from the aorta to the coronary arteries beyond the narrowed or blocked areas. Because the arteries are able to carry blood under much higher pressure than veins, artery grafts are less likely to become narrowed or obstructed. In some patients, both vein grafts and internal mammary arteries are used to restore adequate blood flow to the myocardium.

Coronary Angioplasty

In some patients, it is possible to dilate areas of narrowing within coronary arteries instead of bypassing them, thereby avoiding major surgery. The procedure is called *coronary angioplasty* (*angio* = vessel + *plasty* = molding) and is illustrated in figure 13–34. By means of a technique similar to that

FIGURE 13–32

Principle of surgical treatment of coronary heart disease by means of saphenous vein grafts that bypass obstructions in coronary arteries.

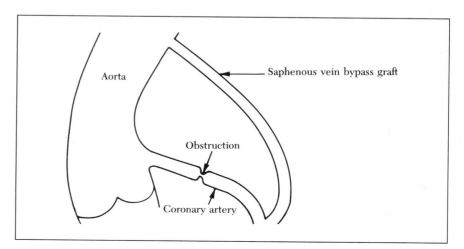

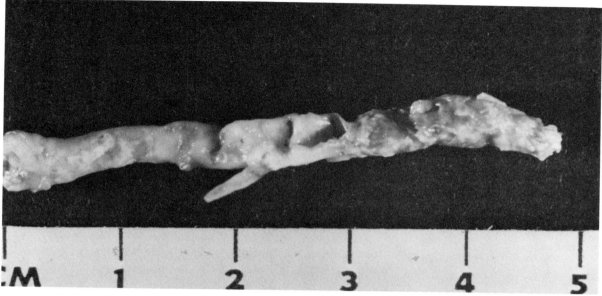

FIGURE 13–33

Tubular mass of atheromatous plaque material dissected from coronary artery (*endarterectomy*) to increase the caliber of the artery.

used to perform a coronary arteriogram (described in chapter 1), a guiding catheter is introduced through the skin and into a large artery in the arm or leg, threaded under fluoroscopic control into the narrowed coronary artery, and positioned at the site of narrowing. Then, the balloon catheter is threaded through the guide catheter until the balloon lies within the narrowed area. After the balloon is properly positioned, it is inflated briefly under very high pressure, which smashes the plaque and pushes it into the arterial wall, enlarging the lumen of the artery and improving blood flow to the myocardium. At first, the procedure was used to treat patients who had only a single narrowed artery, but it is now used to treat patients who have multiple obstructing plaques in their coronary arteries and can also be used to dilate saphenous vein grafts that have become narrowed or obstructed.

Successful dilatation of a narrowed artery promptly restores normal flow through the artery, as illustrated in figure 13–35. Unfortunately, in about 25 percent of successfully treated patients, the stenosis eventually recurs and may require redilatation.

Dilatation is not always successful and may be complicated by thrombosis of the artery being dilated, which may cause a myocardial infarction. If complications arise in attempts to dilate an artery, then emergency coronary artery bypass graft surgery is required in order to restore myocardial blood flow.

New techniques to restore blood flow through narrowed coronary arteries are being evaluated continually, including vaporization of plaque mate-

FIGURE 13–34

Principle of coronary angioplasty. **A,** Overview illustrating positioning of guide catheter and balloon catheter within narrowed coronary artery. **B,** Details of catheter placement. Guide catheter positioned at site of narrowing. **C,** Balloon catheter passed through guide catheter and positioned within narrowed segment of artery. **D,** Balloon inflated, smashing plaque and relieving obstruction.

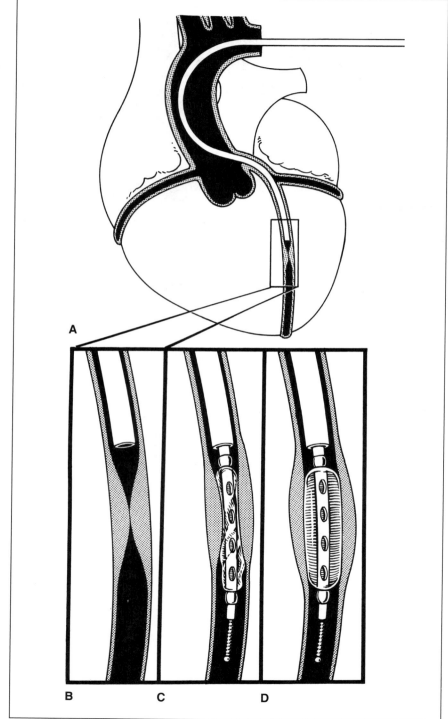

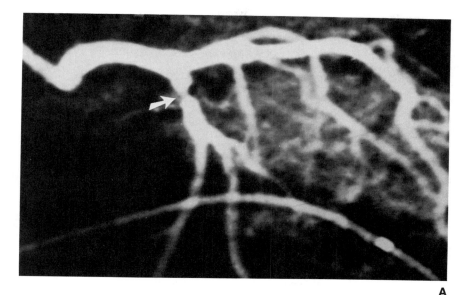

A

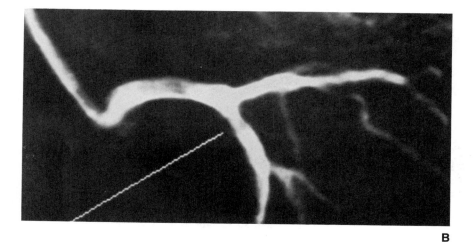

B

FIGURE 13–35

Coronary angioplasty. **A,** Severely narrowed coronary artery (*arrow*) shown by arteriogram. **B,** Same artery after successful dilatation by angioplasty.

rial by means of lasar light energy. Other procedures to enlarge narrowed coronary arteries involve fragmentation of plaque material. One technique inserts a rapidly rotating cutting blade contained in a rigid sheath through an endarterectomy-type cardiac catheter into the narrowed coronary artery. Then the cutting instrument is advanced into the narrowed area, where it cuts the plaque material into fragments. Another method uses a more slowly rotating blade to excise fragments that are removed by a vacuum suction device used with the cutting instrument. Still another variation of these procedures employs a drill with an abrasive tip to cut the plaque material into fragments. In an attempt to solve the problem of restenosis of a coronary artery after angioplasty, some investigators have inserted tubular coiled springs into the segment dilated by angioplasty to keep the dilated lumen open.

Cocaine-Induced Arrhythmias and Myocardial Infarcts

Cocaine has very powerful effects on the cardiovascular system and, as the recreational use of cocaine has increased in recent years, so has the number of cocaine-related cardiac deaths.

The drug prolongs and intensifies the effects of sympathetic nerve impulses that regulate the heart and blood vessels. As a result, the heart beats faster and more forcefully, thereby increasing myocardial oxygen requirements. The heart muscle becomes more irritable, which predisposes to arrhythmias, and the peripheral arterioles constrict, which raises the blood pressure. Cocaine also constricts the coronary arteries and may induce coronary artery spasm, which leads to severe myocardial ischemia and may be followed by a myocardial infarction. Cocaine-related fatal arrhythmias and myocardial infarcts may occur in persons with normal coronary arteries, and cocaine users who already have some degree of coronary atherosclerosis are at even greater risk.

Blood Lipids and Coronary Artery Disease

The level of lipids in the blood has been shown to be an important factor in the pathogenesis of coronary atherosclerosis. The lipids of clinical importance are neutral fat (*triglyceride*) and cholesterol.

Neutral Fat

Chemically, fat is composed of three molecules of fatty acid combined with one molecule of glycerol. Glycerol is a three-carbon alcohol containing a hydroxyl group (OH) attached to each carbon atom. A fatty acid is a long, straight-chain carbon compound containing a terminal carboxyl group (COOH); this constitutes the acid group of organic molecules. The carboxyl groups of the fatty acids are linked to the hydroxyl groups of glycerol, with loss of a molecule of water, in a linkage called an *ester*.

A neutral fat may be classified as saturated or unsaturated. In unsaturated fats, the fatty acids linked to glycerol contain one or more double bonds between adjacent carbon atoms in the molecule. A *polyunsaturated fat* is one in which the fatty acids contain several double bonds. A *saturated fat* is one in which there are no double bonds in the fatty acid molecules. At room temperature, saturated fats are solid, whereas unsaturated fats are liquid. In general, fats of animal origin are saturated. Most vegetable oils and fats found in fish and poultry are unsaturated.

High levels of neutral fat (along with cholesterol) in the blood promote atherosclerosis. Carbohydrate is converted readily into fat in the body, and much of the blood triglyceride is derived not from ingested fat but from ingested carbohydrate. In clinical medicine, most examples of high blood triglycerides can be traced to diets excessively high in carbohydrate. Sugar has been found to be more potent in elevating blood triglycerides than the more complex carbohydrates derived from cereals and other starches.

Cholesterol

Cholesterol is a complex carbon compound containing several ring structures and is classified as a *sterol*. Most cholesterol is present in the body in combination with fatty acids as cholesterol esters. Cholesterol is synthesized in the body and is also present in many foods. Normally, cholesterol is excreted in the bile into the gastrointestinal tract.

Much evidence indicates that a high dietary intake of cholesterol leads to high levels of blood cholesterol and premature atherosclerosis. Americans subsist on a diet relatively high in cholesterol; they also have one of the highest rates of death from coronary heart disease. In contrast, other populations whose diet is much lower in cholesterol have much lower rates of death from coronary heart disease.

The level of blood cholesterol is influenced not only by the amount of cholesterol in the diet, but also by the type of dietary fat. *Saturated fats,* the type found in meats and dairy products, tend to raise blood cholesterol, whereas *unsaturated fats,* which are found in fish, poultry, and most vegetable oils, tend to lower blood cholesterol. Cholesterol and saturated fat are found together in many foods. In general, foods high in cholesterol also have a high content of saturated fats, whereas foods low in cholesterol contain polyunsaturated fats rather than saturated fats.

Transport of Cholesterol by Lipoproteins

Cholesterol is carried in the blood plasma combined with proteins and other lipids as complexes called **lipoproteins.** There are two different cholesterol-carrying lipoproteins. They have different functions and are classified by their weight (density) into *low-density lipoprotein* (**LDL**) and *high-density lipoprotein* (**HDL**). About 80 percent of the circulating cholesterol is carried bound to LDL, and the remaining 20 percent is transported by HDL.

The function of LDL is to transport cholesterol from the bloodstream into the cells, whereas the HDL apparently removes cholesterol from the cells and carries it to the liver for excretion in the bile. High-density lipoprotein may also "tie up" cholesterol so that it cannot infiltrate the arterial wall (figure 13–36). This has led to the belief that there is a "bad cholesterol" and a "good cholesterol." The "bad cholesterol" is the fraction bound to LDL, which can infiltrate the arterial wall and is correlated with atherosclerosis. The "good cholesterol" is the cholesterol fraction carried attached to HDL, and elevations of this cholesterol fraction actually protect against coronary heart disease. Several factors are known to raise HDL cholesterol and thereby reduce risk of coronary heart disease. These factors include regular exercise, cessation of cigarette smoking, and (surprisingly) a modest regular intake of alcoholic beverages.

FIGURE 13–36

Role of lipoproteins in transport of cholesterol. Low-density lipoprotein (L) promotes atherosclerosis by transporting cholesterol into arterial wall. High-density lipoprotein (H) protects against atherosclerosis by transporting cholesterol to the liver for excretion.

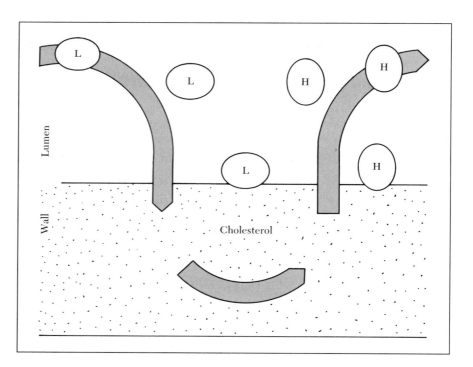

Alteration of Blood Lipids by Change in Diet

Various studies have demonstrated that the levels of both cholesterol and triglycerides in the blood can be lowered by dietary change. These studies have also demonstrated that individuals maintained on a modified diet have a lower incidence of coronary artery disease than a comparable group subsisting on an average American diet. The diet (often called an "anticoronary" diet) is modified by decreasing the amount of cholesterol and saturated fat and substituting foods containing polyunsaturated fats. This involves restricting the intake of animal fat and substituting fish and poultry. Carbohydrates are derived primarily from starches and cereals. The consumption of sugar and foods rich in sugar (pies, cakes, candies) is reduced. Alcohol consumption is restricted but not forbidden because of its favorable effect on HDL levels, which seems to protect against coronary heart disease. In addition to raising HDL, modest alcohol intake also helps protect against heart attacks by raising the level of circulating tissue plasminogen activator. This substance, which is one of the body's physiologic clot-dissolving components, is produced by the endothelial cells of blood vessels and diffuses into the circulation. Blood containing a higher concentration of tissue plasminogen activator has increased fibrinolytic activity. Consequently, any small clots that begin to form over atheromatous plaques in coronary arteries would be dissolved by the body's own tissue plasminogen activator before the clots become large enough to occlude the vessel.

Modifying the typical American diet is difficult, because it requires breaking old dietary habits. However, some change in diet is desirable because it will significantly reduce the incidence of coronary artery disease in the U.S. population. An "anticoronary" diet is essential for individuals who have high levels of blood lipids, because they run a greatly increased risk of death or disability from coronary artery disease.

It should be emphasized that the factors influencing the development of atherosclerosis are complex; an elevated level of blood lipids is only one of many factors concerned with atherogenesis. A number of other conditions, among them obesity, hypertension, cigarette smoking, and genetic factors, also predispose individuals to atherosclerosis.

Hypertension results from excessive vasoconstriction of the small arterioles throughout the body; this, in turn, raises the diastolic blood pressure. Because of the high peripheral resistance, the heart is required to increase the force of ventricular contraction in order to supply blood to the tissues, which produces a compensatory increase in the systolic blood pressure. Severe hypertension exerts injurious effects not only on the heart, but also on the blood vessels and kidneys.

Hypertension and Hypertensive Cardiovascular Disease

Cardiac Effects

The heart responds to the increased workload resulting from the high peripheral resistance by becoming enlarged. Although the enlarged heart may be able to function effectively for many years, the cardiac pump is being forced to work beyond its "rated capacity." Eventually, the heart can no longer maintain adequate blood flow, and the patient develops symptoms of cardiac failure.

Vascular Effects

Because the blood vessels are not designed to carry blood at such a high pressure, the vessels wear out prematurely. Hypertension accelerates the development of atherosclerosis in the larger arteries. The arterioles also are injured; they thicken and undergo degenerative changes, and their lumens become narrowed. This process is termed **arteriolosclerosis.** Sometimes the walls of the small arterioles become completely necrotic owing to the effects of the sustained high blood pressure. Weakened arterioles may rupture, leading to hemorrhage. The brain is particularly vulnerable, cerebral hemorrhage being a relatively common complication of severe hypertension.

Renal Effects

The narrowing of the renal arterioles decreases the blood supply to the kidneys, which, in turn, leads to injury and degenerative changes in the glomeruli and renal tubules. Severe hypertension may cause severe derangement of renal function and eventually lead to renal failure.

Cause and Treatment of Hypertension

Occasionally, hypertension is the result of an adrenal tumor secreting hormones that elevate the blood pressure. Certain uncommon types of renal disease also may occasionally cause hypertension. In most instances, however, the reason for excessive vasoconstriction in the peripheral arterioles is unknown.

Although the reason for the hypertension cannot be determined in most instances, the blood pressure can be reduced to more normal levels, thereby lowering risk of complications of high blood pressure. This is accomplished by administering various drugs that lower the blood pressure by lessening the vasoconstriction of the peripheral blood vessels.

Primary Myocardial Disease

In a small number of patients, heart disease results not from valvular or coronary disease or hypertension but from primary disease of the heart muscle itself. There are two major types of primary myocardial disease. One type results from inflammation of heart muscle and is called *myocarditis*. The second type, in which there is no evidence of inflammation, is designated by the noncommittal term *cardiomyopathy* (*cardio* = heart + *myo* = muscle + *pathy* = disease).

Myocarditis

Myocarditis is characterized by an active inflammation in the heart muscle associated with injury and necrosis of individual muscle fibers. In the United States, most cases are caused by viruses. A few are caused by parasites, such as *Trichinella* (described in chapter 7) that lodge in the myocardium and cause an inflammation. Occasionally other pathogens such as *Histoplasma* are responsible, especially in immunocompromised patients. Some cases are the result of a hypersensitivity reaction, such as the myocarditis occurring in acute rheumatic fever.

The onset of myocarditis is usually abrupt and may lead to acute heart failure. Fortunately, in most cases, the inflammation subsides completely and the patient recovers without any permanent heart damage. There is no specific treatment other than treating the underlying condition that caused the myocarditis and decreasing cardiac work by bed rest and limited activity while the inflammation subsides.

Cardiomyopathy

The general term cardiomyopathy encompasses two different conditions: *dilated cardiomyopathy* and *hypertrophic cardiomyopathy*. Dilated cardiomyopathy is characterized by enlargement of the heart and dilatation of its chambers. The pumping action of the ventricles is greatly impaired, which leads to chronic heart failure. Its cause is uncertain, and there is no specific treatment.

Hypertrophic cardiomyopathy is hereditary and transmitted as a dominant trait. The condition is characterized by disarray of muscle fibers that intersect at odd angles with no apparent organized pattern and marked hypertrophy of heart muscle to such an extent that the thick-walled chambers become greatly reduced in size and do not dilate readily in diastole. Frequently, the muscle of the septum is hypertrophied to a greater extent than the rest of the myocardium and hinders outflow of the blood from the ventricle into the aorta. At times, the thick septum may actually impinge on the anterior mitral valve leaflet, intermittently completely blocking the outflow of blood from the left ventricle (figure 13–37). This type of cardiomyopathy is often called *idiopathic hypertrophic subaortic stenosis,* usually abbreviated IHSS. The term indicates that the obstruction (stenosis) is located below the aortic valve (subaortic), resulting from myocardial hypertrophy (hypertrophic) of unknown cause (idiopathic).

Patients with IHSS frequently exhibit manifestations related to inadequate cardiac output, such as episodes of excessive fatigue and lightheadedness

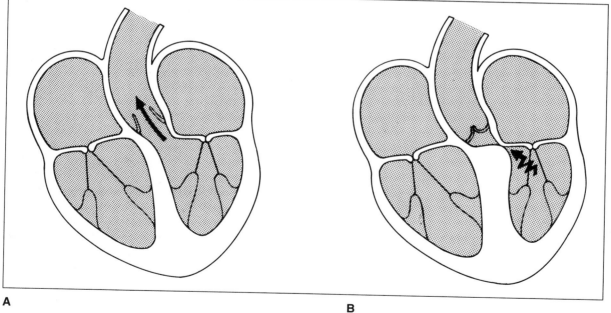

A   **B**

FIGURE 13–37

Comparison of normal cardiac function with malfunction characteristic of hypertrophic cardiomyopathy. **A,** Normal heart, illustrating unobstructed flow of blood from left ventricle into the aorta during ventricular systole. **B,** Hypertrophic cardiomyopathy, illustrating obstruction to outflow of blood from left ventricle by hypertrophied septum, which impinges on anterior leaflet of mitral valve.

related to exertion. The characteristic myocardial hypertrophy with greatly thickened septum can be identified by echocardiography (described in chapter 1). Treatment consists of administering drugs that slow the heart (allowing more time for ventricular filling) and reduce the force of ventricular contraction (which tends to reduce the degree of obstruction caused by the hypertrophied septum). Commonly used drugs are those that block the sympathetic nerve impulses that normally increase heart rate and the force of contraction (beta blockers) and those that decrease myocardial contractility by impeding the flow of calcium into myocardial cells (called calcium channel blocking agents). Persons who do not respond to medical treatment may require surgical resection of part of the thickened septum.

Heart Failure

Heart failure exists whenever the heart is no longer able to pump adequate amounts of blood to the tissues. It may result from any type of heart disease. Rapid failing of the heart, as when a large portion of muscle undergoes infarction, is called *acute heart failure*. In most cases, however, cardiac failure develops slowly and insidiously; this is called *chronic heart failure*. Because the most prominent feature in chronic heart failure is congestion of the tissues as a result of engorgement by blood, the physician often uses the term *congestive heart failure* when referring to chronic heart failure and its attendant clinical manifestations.

Sometimes the terms "forward failure" and "backward failure" are used to describe the mechanisms leading to the development of heart failure. In *forward failure,* the initial effect of inadequate cardiac output is considered to be insufficient blood flow to the tissues. The inadequate renal blood flow results in retention of salt and water by the kidneys. (This effect is mediated indirectly through the adrenal glands.) Fluid retention, in turn, leads to an increased blood volume, and this is soon followed by a rise in venous pressure. The high venous pressure and high capillary pressure cause excessive transudation of fluid from the capillaries, leading to edema of the tissues. In *backward failure,* the inadequate output of blood is considered to cause "back up" of blood within the veins draining back to the heart, leading to increased venous pressure, congestion of the viscera, and edema. Figure 13–38 illustrates the interrelation of the various factors concerned in the development of cardiac failure. Probably both forward failure and backward failure are present to some degree in every patient with heart failure. Treatment consists of diuretic drugs, which promote excretion of excess salt and water by the kidneys, thereby lowering blood volume. In addition, digitalis preparations are sometimes administered. They act to increase the efficiency of ventricular contractions.

Acute Pulmonary Edema

Acute pulmonary edema is a manifestation of acute heart failure. It is caused by a temporary disproportion in the output of blood from the ventricles. If the output of blood from the left ventricle is temporarily reduced more than

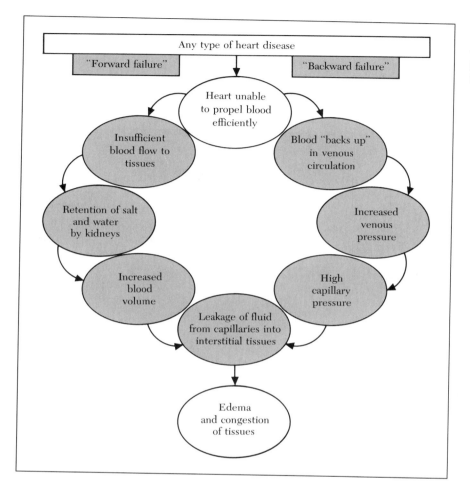

FIGURE 13–38

Mechanisms in the pathogenesis of congestive heart failure.

Any type of heart disease

"Forward failure" "Backward failure"

Heart unable to propel blood efficiently

Insufficient blood flow to tissues

Blood "backs up" in venous circulation

Retention of salt and water by kidneys

Increased venous pressure

Increased blood volume

High capillary pressure

Leakage of fluid from capillaries into interstitial tissues

Edema and congestion of tissues

the output from the right ventricle, the "right heart" will pump blood into the lungs faster than the "left heart" can deliver the blood to the peripheral tissues. This rapidly engorges the lungs with blood, raises the pulmonary capillary pressure, and produces transudation of fluid into the pulmonary alveoli. The patient becomes extremely short of breath because fluid accumulates within the alveoli, and oxygenation of the blood circulating through the lungs is impaired. The edema fluid becomes mixed with inspired air, forming a frothy mixture that "overflows" into the bronchi and trachea, filling the patient's upper respiratory passages.

An aneurysm is a dilatation of the wall of an artery or an outpouching of a portion of the wall. Most aneurysms are acquired as a result of arteriosclerosis, which causes weakening of the vessel wall. One type of aneurysm involv-

Aneurysms

ing the cerebral arteries is the result of a congenital abnormality of the vessel wall and is considered in conjunction with the nervous system (chapter 26).

Arteriosclerotic Aneurysm

A small artery that undergoes arteriosclerotic change becomes narrowed and may eventually become thrombosed. A large artery such as the aorta has a diameter so large that complete obstruction is uncommon. However, atheromatous deposits tend to damage the wall of the aorta, reducing its elasticity and weakening the wall (figure 13–39). The aortic wall tends to balloon out under the stress of the high pressure within the vessel. Aortic aneurysms usually develop in the distal part of the abdominal aorta, where the pressure is highest and the atheromatous change is most severe (figures 13–40 and 13–41). Usually the interior of the aneurysm becomes covered with a layer of thrombus material, and the wall often becomes partially calcified. Aortic aneurysms are dangerous because they may rupture, leading to massive and often fatal hemorrhage. In general, the larger the aneurysm, the greater the likelihood of rupture (figure 13–42). The treatment of aneurysm is surgical excision of the dilated portion and replacement of the diseased segment by

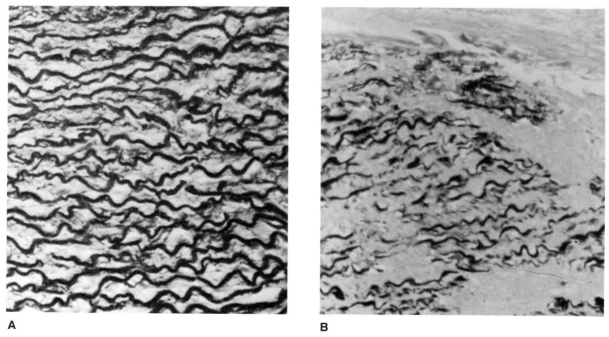

A   B

FIGURE 13–39

A, Photomicrograph of normal arterial wall stained for elastic tissue. Elastic fibers appear as dark wavy bands. **B,** Aortic wall from patient with severe aortic arteriosclerosis, illustrating marked fragmentation and destruction of elastic fibers, which weakens wall and predisposes to aneurysm. (Original magnification × 400.)

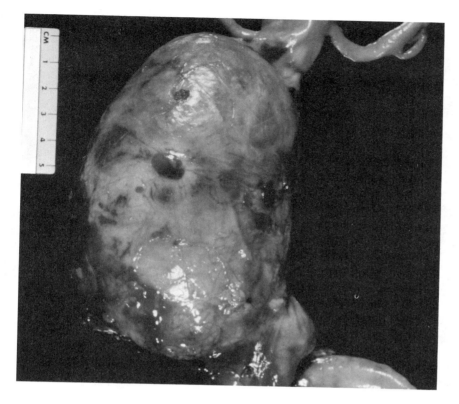

FIGURE 13–40

Large arteriosclerotic aneurysm of aorta extending from renal arteries (*above*) to iliac arteries (*below*).

nylon or Dacron grafts (figure 13–43). Occasionally, arteriosclerotic aneurysms develop in other large arteries.

Dissecting Aneurysm of the Aorta

The thick middle layer of the aorta is called the *media*. It is composed of multiple layers of elastic tissue and muscle bonded together by fibrous connective tissue. Degenerative changes sometimes occur in the media, causing the layers to lose their cohesiveness and separate. Then the pulsatile force of the blood flowing through the aorta may cause the inner half of the aortic wall to pull away from the outer half in the region where the media has degenerated, and sometimes the inner lining (*intima*) tears as the media separates. This complication is especially likely to occur in persons with high blood pressure.

Once an intimal tear has developed, blood is forced into the aortic wall. The area of medial degeneration forms a cleavage plane that permits the blood to dissect within the media for a variable distance. This event, a **dissecting aneurysm of the aorta,** is associated with severe chest and back pain. The term *dissecting* refers to the splitting (dissection) of the media by the blood, and the somewhat misleading term *aneurysm* was applied

FIGURE 13–41

Aortic aneurysm demonstrated on x-ray by injection of contrast material into aorta.

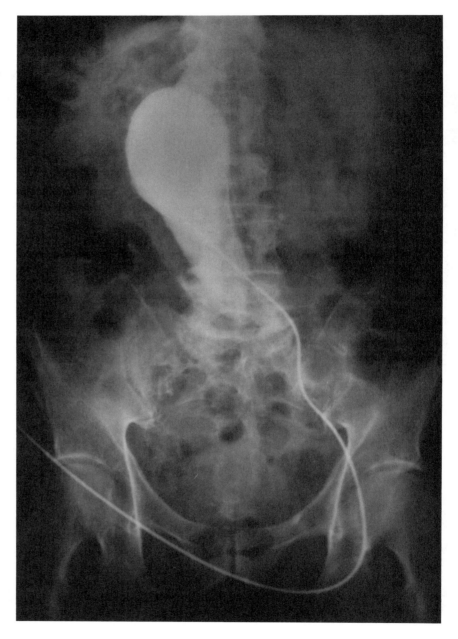

because the affected part of the aorta appears wider than normal. The widening results from the hemorrhage within the aortic wall, but the lumen of the aorta is not dilated.

The intimal tear that starts the dissection is usually either in the ascending aorta just above the aortic valve or in the descending aorta just beyond the origin of the large arteries that arise from the aortic arch (figure 13–44).

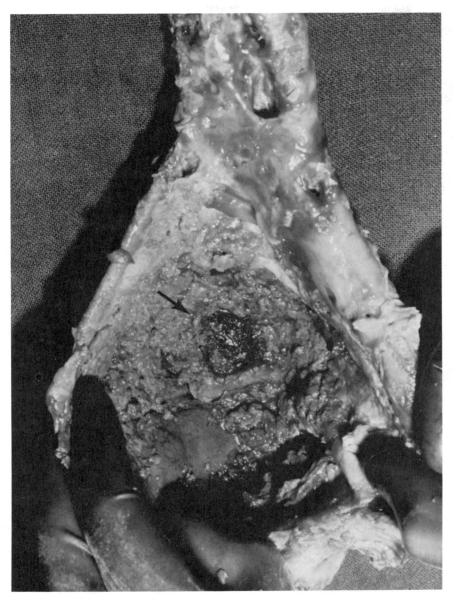

FIGURE 13–42

Interior of arteriosclerotic aneurysm, illustrating marked degenerative change in wall. Extremely thin area in wall (*arrow*) predisposes to rupture.

If the tear is in the ascending aorta, the blood often dissects proximally as well as distally within the aortic wall, extending into the base of the aorta where the aortic valve attaches and the coronary arteries arise. The dissection may separate the aortic valve from its attachment to the deeper aortic wall so that it no longer functions properly, and severe aortic regurgitation develops. The origins of the coronary arteries may also be compressed by the hemorrhage in the wall, which compromises the blood supply to the

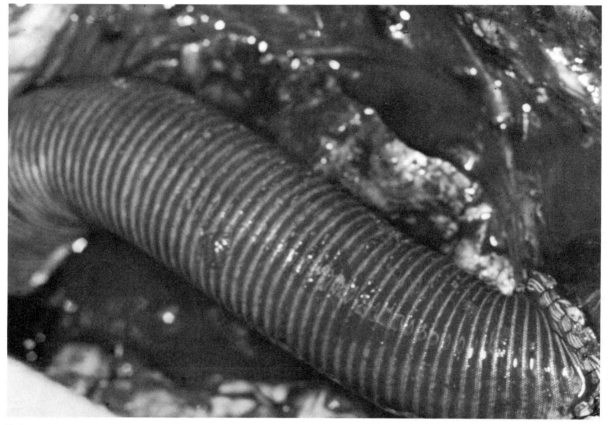

FIGURE 13–43

Repair of aortic aneurysm by means of tubular Dacron graft.

heart muscle. A dissection in the ascending aorta is often fatal because the blood frequently ruptures through the outer wall of the aorta at the base of the heart, leading to extensive hemorrhage into the mediastinum or pericardial sac.

If the intimal tear is in the descending aorta, the blood dissects distally and may extend the entire length of the aorta. The blood in the aortic wall may also compress the origins of the large arteries that arise from the aorta, leading to impairment of blood flow to the kidneys, the intestines, or other vital organs. Sometimes the dissection may rupture back into the lumen of the aorta. If this occurs, blood flows not only through the lumen of the aorta, but also through the channel in the aortic wall created by the dissection, which communicates with the lumen of the aorta both proximally and distally (figure 13–45).

Various surgical procedures have been devised to correct this condition.

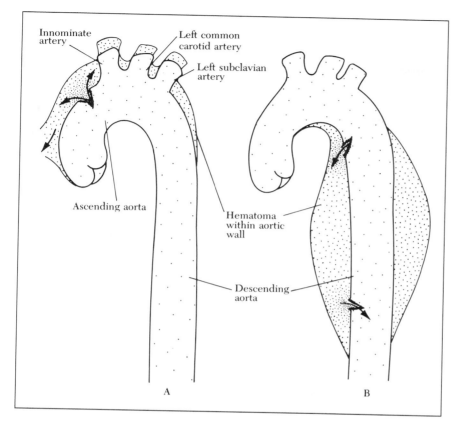

FIGURE 13–44

Sites of aortic dissection. **A,** Tear in ascending aorta causes both proximal and distal dissection and may rupture externally. **B,** Tear in descending aorta may cause extensive distal dissection and may rupture back into lumen of aorta.

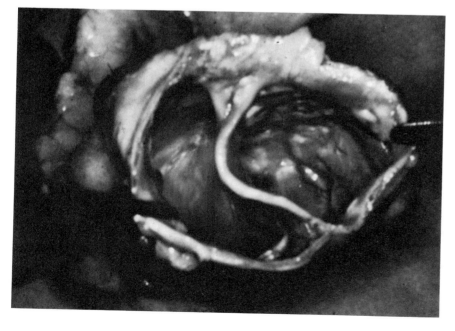

FIGURE 13–45

Cross-section of aorta illustrating two channels ("double-barreled aorta") caused by dissecting aneurysm. Channel on *right* of photograph is true lumen of aorta. Channel on *left* is the channel in the aortic wall created by the dissection.

Diseases of the Veins

The main diseases of veins are (1) venous thrombosis, (2) inflammation of veins, and (3) excessive dilatation and tortuosity of veins.

Venous thromboses occur most commonly in leg veins, but sometimes clots form within veins elsewhere in the body. Inflammation of a vein is called *phlebitis* (*phleb* = vein + *itis* = inflammation). If there is an associated thrombosis of the affected vein, the term *thrombophlebitis* is used. Dilated tortuous veins are called *varices* or *varicose veins.* (*Varix* is a Latin word meaning *dilated vessel;* the plural term is *varices.*) Varicosities occur most often in leg veins but may occur in other veins as well.

Venous Thrombosis and Thrombophlebitis

Thrombus formation in deep leg veins is a frequent problem in postoperative patients and in those confined to bed, and it may be complicated by a pulmonary embolism, as described in chapter 12. The risk of leg vein thromboses in susceptible patients can be minimized by encouraging active leg exercises to improve venous blood flow and prevent venous stasis and by early ambulation.

Venous thrombosis and thrombophlebitis are treated by elevation of the leg, heat, and anticoagulant drugs. The anticoagulation stops the progression of the intravascular clotting process while the body's normal protective mechanisms remove the clot. The clot is dissolved by activation of the fibrinolytic mechanism and by ingrowth of connective tissue from the vein wall at the site where the clot adheres to the vein wall. Damage to the vein wall and its valves after thrombophlebitis may disturb venous return and predispose to later development of varicose veins.

Varicose Veins of the Lower Extremities

Two main groups of veins return blood from the lower limbs: the deep veins and the superficial veins. The *deep veins* carry most of the venous return. They accompany the major arteries and drain into the iliac veins, which in turn empty into the inferior vena cava. The *superficial veins* form a network of intercommunicating channels that travel just beneath the skin in the subcutaneous tissue and eventually drain into the deep veins. The largest superficial vein is the *great saphenous vein,* which extends up the medial surface of the leg from the ankle to the groin and drains into the more deeply placed femoral vein just below the groin. A second large superficial vein called the *small saphenous vein* ascends the back of the leg and drains into the deep venous system at the back of the knee. Both the superficial and deep veins contain cup-shaped valves, fashioned somewhat like the semilunar valves in the heart, which are interposed along the course of the veins. The arrangement of the valves is such that blood can flow upward in the veins but cannot flow in the reverse direction. The superficial and deep venous systems are also interconnected by short communicating branches that contain valves arranged so that blood normally flows only from superficial to deep veins and not in the reverse direction.

Blood is propelled upward within the deep veins by contraction of the leg and thigh muscles, which intermittently compress the veins and force the blood upward within the veins against gravity. The valves within the veins prevent retrograde flow. In contrast, the superficial veins are relatively unsupported, and venous return is much less efficient. Nevertheless, venous return through the superficial veins is normal provided that the veins do no become excessively dilated and the valves function properly to prevent retrograde flow and venous stasis.

Varicose veins result if the saphenous veins become dilated and their valves become incompetent. As a result, the blood tends to stagnate in the veins instead of flowing back normally to the heart, causing the veins to become elongated and tortuous. The condition tends to run in families, suggesting that the basic cause is a congenital weakness of the vein wall or its valves, which predisposes to the varicosities.

Varicose veins of the saphenous system may also develop if the deeper veins become blocked or if their valves become damaged by previous thrombophlebitis. As a result of damage to the deep veins, more of the venous return is shifted to the unsupported superficial veins, which are unable to cope with the increased flow and become varicose.

Complications of Varicose Veins

Complications result from stasis of blood in the veins, with poor nutrition of the tissues owing to chronic venous engorgement. The skin of the distal leg and ankle becomes thin and atrophic and quite susceptible to infection. Skin ulcers may develop and heal poorly. The dilated veins are easily injured and may rupture, leading to extravasation of blood and chronic discoloration of the skin. Stasis of blood in the veins also predisposes to repeated bouts of thrombophlebitis.

Treatment of Varicose Veins

Varicosities of the saphenous veins are treated by elastic stockings to support the veins and elevation of the legs whenever possible to promote more efficient venous return. Sometimes surgical removal of the varicose veins may be required. This is usually performed in conjunction with ligation of the communicating veins that interconnect the superficial and deep venous systems.

Varicose Veins in Other Locations

Dilated veins around the rectum are called **hemorrhoids** and are described in chapter 23 in conjunction with disorders of the gastrointestinal tract. Varicose veins of the esophagus often occur in patients with a disease called *cirrhosis of the liver. Esophageal varices* may rupture and cause profuse life-threatening hemorrhage. Their pathogenesis and treatment are considered in chapter 21. Varicose veins of the spermatic cord appear as a mass of vessels in the scrotum above the testicle. The condition is called a *varico-*

cele (*varix* = vein + *cele* = swelling). The varicosities usually do not cause symptoms but at times may cause mild scrotal discomfort. Rarely, they may impair fertility in some men. Usually no treatment is required.

Questions for Review

1. How do the heart valves function to provide unidirectional blood flow? What factors determine the level of the systolic and diastolic blood pressure?

2. What are the major causes of heart disease? What is the difference between rheumatic fever and rheumatic heart disease?

3. What is bacterial endocarditis? How does it arise? How is it prevented?

4. What is coronary heart disease? What are its manifestations? What is the difference between angina pectoris and myocardial infarction?

5. What is the effect of high blood pressure on the heart and on the blood vessels?

6. What is heart failure? What is meant by the following terms: *forward failure, backward failure, acute heart failure, chronic heart failure, acute pulmonary edema?*

7. What is the usual cause of an aortic aneurysm? How is an aneurysm treated?

8. What is the difference between an arteriosclerotic aneurysm of the aorta and a dissecting aneurysm of the aorta?

9. What are the possible complications of a large myocardial infarction?

10. What is meant by the following terms: *mitral valve prolapse, calcific aortic stenosis, ventricular aneurysm, ventricular fibrillation?*

11. What factors predispose to thrombus formation in leg veins? What are the major complications of venous thrombi?

12. What are varicose veins? What veins are commonly affected? What are the clinical manifestations?

Supplementary Readings

Baker, D. W., Konstam, M. A., Bottorff, M., et al. 1994. Management of heart failure: Pharmacologic treatment. *Journal of the American Medical Association* 272: 1361–66. ACE inhibitors should be given to all patients. Diuretics should be used judiciously. Digoxin should be reserved for patients who do not respond to other measures.

Bigger, J. T., 1987. Why patients with congestive heart failure die: Arrhythmias and sudden cardiac death. *Circulation* 75 (Suppl):28–35. Patients with advanced heart disease are at high risk of death from cardiac arrhythmia. Correction of factors predisposing to arrhythmia may improve survival. See also other articles in this issue dealing with various aspects of cardiovascular disease.

Bourassa, M. G., et al. 1982. Changes in grafts and coronary arteries after saphenous vein aortocoronary bypass surgery: Results at repeat angiography. *Circulation* (Suppl II):90–97. Rate of vein graft occlusion was about 2 percent per year after first year. Patency at end of one year was about 80 percent. Late graft occlusion was the result of atherosclerosis.

Cregler, L. L., et al. 1986. Cardiovascular dangers of cocaine abuse. *American Journal of Cardiology* 57:1185–86. A review article. Cocaine predisposes to acute myocardial infarctions and cerebrovascular accidents. Headache after cocaine use may indicate cerebral hemorrhage.

DeBakey, M., et al. 1974. Aneurysm of abdominal aorta. *Annals of Surgery* 160:622–39. One of the classic articles on this subject. Outlines natural history of untreated aneurysm, methods of treatment, and results.

Furster, V., et al. 1987. Platelet-inhibitor drugs' role in coronary artery disease. *Progress in Cardiovascular Disease* 29:325–46. Reviews the role of platelet aggregation in producing coronary thrombosis and the role of antiplatelet drugs.

Hennekins, C. H. 1979. Effects of beer, wine, and liquor in coronary death. *Journal of the American Medical Association* 242:1973–74. Daily consumption of small to moderate amounts of alcohol protects against coronary heart disease.

Holmes, D. R., Jr., et al. 1990. Advances in interventional cardiology. *Mayo Clinic Proceedings* 65:565–83. Discusses percutaneous coronary angioplasty applications and limitations and newer approaches including laser-light vaporization of intimal plaque material within coronary arteries.

Howard, R. E., Hueter, D. C., and Davis, G. 1985. Acute myocardial infarction following cocaine abuse in a young woman with normal coronary arteries. *Journal of the American Medical Association* 254:95–96. Describes cardiovascular hazards of cocaine documented by a myocardial infarction in a young woman.

Jeresaty, R. M. 1985. Mitral valve prolapse: An update. *Journal of the American Medical Association* 254:793–95. Mitral valve prolapse affects about 5 percent of the population and is the most common cause of pure mitral insufficiency. Complications include ruptured chordae, strokes, and infective endocarditis.

Lavie, C. J., and Gersh, B. J. 1990. Acute myocardial infarction: Initial manifestations, management, and prognosis. *Mayo Clinic Proceedings* 65:531–48. A comprehensive review article.

Lavie, C. J., and Gersh, B. J. 1990. Mechanical and electrical complications of acute myocardial infarction. *Mayo Clinic Proceedings* 65:709–30. A survey of major complications.

Lavie, C. J., et al. 1990. Reperfusion in acute myocardial infarction. *Mayo Clinic Proceedings* 65:549–64. Systemic thrombolytic therapy administered early after onset of symptoms of acute myocardial infarction can restore artery patency, salvage myocardium, and reduce mortality.

Lewis, H. D., et al. 1983. Protective effects of aspirin against acute myocardial infarction and death in men with unstable angina: Results of the Veterans Administration Cooperative Study. *New England Journal of Medicine* 309:396–403. Aspirin therapy greatly reduced the mortality and risk of infarction.

McIntosh, H. D. 1978. Benefits from aortocoronary bypass graft. *Journal of the American Medical Association* 239:1197–99. Procedure provided relief of pain. A significant proportion of vein grafts eventually become occluded. Survival is improved in selected patients.

Mooney, M. R. 1994. Interventional cardiology: Update on devices and procedures for mechanical revascularization. *The Medical Journal of Healthspan* 3:17–21. Reviews new techniques and devices for treating coronary artery disease.

Reeder, G. S. 1994. Thrombolysis for acute myocardial infarction: t-PA for everyone? *Mayo Clinic Proceedings* 69:796–99. Thrombolysis saves lives. The time interval is critical. t-PA costs seven times as much as streptokinase. Some trials have found no difference between t-PA and streptokinase.

Reeder, G. S., Bailey, K. R., Gersh, B. J., et al. 1994. Cost comparison of immediate angioplasty versus thrombolysis followed by conservative therapy for acute myocardial infarction: A randomized prospective trial. *Mayo Clinic Proceedings* 69:5–12. There is no difference in cost between these two methods of treatment, and results are comparable.

Ridker, P. M., Vaughan, D. E., Stampfer, M. J., et al. 1994. Association of moderate alcohol consumption and plasma concentration of endogenous tissue-type plasminogen activator. *Journal of the American Medical Association* 272:929–33. The elevated t-PA associated with moderate alcohol consumption decreases risk of coronary heart disease and is independent of changes in HDL cholesterol.

Ross, J., Jr., et al. 1987. Guidelines for coronary angiography. *Journal of the American College of Cardiology* 10:935–50. Indications and procedures.

Ryan, J. S. 1988. Guidelines for percutaneous transluminal coronary angioplasty. *Circulation* 78:486–502. Describes indications, techniques, and results of the procedure.

Seides, S. F., et al. 1978. Long-term anatomic fate of coronary artery bypass grafts and functional status of patients five years after operation. *New England Journal of Medicine* 298:1213–17. Most grafts that remain patent several months after operation will remain patent for several years, but arteriosclerosis will continue to progress in ungrafted vessels and symptoms will recur in many patients.

Simari, R. D., Berger, P. B., Bell, M. R., et al. 1994. Coronary angioplasty in acute myocardial infarction: Primary, immediate adjunctive, rescue, or deferred adjunctive approach? *Mayo Clinic Proceedings* 69:346–58. Primary coronary angioplasty without prior thrombolytic therapy is as effective as thrombolytic therapy for salvaging myocardium.

Slone, D., et al. 1978. Relation of cigarette smoking to myocardial infarction in young women. *New England Journal of Medicine* 298:1273–76. Cigarette smoking is a risk factor for myocardial infarction in young women who are otherwise apparently healthy.

Turi, Z., and Braunwald, E. 1983. The use of β-blockers after myocardial infarction. *Journal of the American Medical Association* 249:2512–16. Beta-blocking drugs reduce late mortality after myocardial infarcts. Treatment should be started between one and four weeks after infarction and continued for at least two years.

Veterans Administration Cooperative Study Group on Anti-Hypertensive Agents. 1967. Effects of treatment on morbidity in hypertension: Results in patients with diastolic blood pressures averaging 129 through 155 mm Hg. *Journal of the American Medical Association* 202:1028–34. Treatment of severe hypertension reduces morbidity.

Veterans Administration Cooperative Study Group on Anti-Hypertensive Agents. 1970. Effects of treatment on morbidity in hypertension: II. Results in patients with diastolic blood pressures averaging 90 through 114 mm Hg. *Journal of the American Medical Association* 213:1143–52. Treatment reduces morbidity and mortality.

Walker, W. J. 1977. Changing United States life-style and declining vascular mortality: Cause or coincidence. (Editorial.) *New England Journal of Medicine* 297:163–65. There has been a decline in coronary mortality since 1963 that may be the result of a more healthy life style. About 60 percent of coronary deaths continue to occur before the subjects reach any medical facility.

Willet, W., et al. 1980. Alcohol consumption and high density lipoprotein cholesterol in marathon runners. *New England Journal of Medicine* 303:1159–61. Alcohol consumption raises high-density lipoprotein cholesterol beyond the increase related to physical activity.

Chapter 13 ■ Outline Summary

Normal Cardiac Function / 315
Cardiac Chambers

Right heart circulates blood to lung.

Left heart circulates blood to peripheral tissues.

Cardiac Valves

AV valves attached to papillary muscles by chordae.

Cup-shaped semilunar valves.

Blood Supply to Heart

Left coronary artery:

Anterior descending: supplies anterior wall.

Circumflex: supplies lateral wall.

Right coronary artery: supplies posterior wall.

Conduction System

SA node.

AV node.

AV bundle, branches, and Purkinje fibers.

Blood Pressure

Systolic pressure: reflects force of ventricular contraction.

Diastolic pressure: measure of peripheral resistance.

Heart Disease as a Disturbance of Cardiac Function / 320
Congenital Heart Disease

Manifestations:

Defective communication between cardiac chambers.

Malformation of valves.

Malformation of septa.

Prevention: protect fetus from intrauterine injury.

Valvular Heart Disease

Rheumatic fever and rheumatic heart disease:

Rheumatic fever is complication of beta-streptococcal infection and causes valvular damage.

Healing leads to valve scarring. Prevented by prompt treatment of beta-streptococcal infection.

Nonrheumatic aortic stenosis:

Bicuspid aortic valve: congenital malformation eventually leads to valve thickening and scarring.

Calcific aortic stenosis: degenerative change in elderly individuals.

Mitral valve prolapse.

Valve stretches owing to degeneration of connective tissue and prolapses into left atrium.

Chordae may rupture owing to stress.

Predisposes to arrhythmia.

Infective Endocarditis

Subacute: organisms of low virulence implant on damaged valves.

Acute: virulent organisms implant on normal valves and may destroy valve. Intravenous drug abusers at high risk.

Coronary Heart Disease / 330
Pathogenesis of Atherosclerosis

Endothelial injury.

Lipids accumulate and precipitate.

Secondary fibrosis and calcification.

Major Risk Factors

High blood lipids.

High blood pressure.

Cigarette smoking.

Diabetes.

Manifestations and Complications

Angina pectoris.

Classification:

Stable angina: pain on exertion, subsides with rest or medication.

Unstable angina: more frequent episodes, last longer, poor response to rest or medications.

Prinzmetal's angina: occurs at rest, caused by coronary artery spasm.

Heart attack.

Pathogenesis:

Blockage of coronary artery.

Hemorrhage in plaque.

Arterial spasm adjacent to plaque.

Significant increase in myocardial oxygen requirements (severe exertion).

Manifestations:

Cardiac arrest.

Myocardial infarction.

Myocardial Infarction / 336
Location: Almost Always Left Ventricle
Anterior wall: left anterior descending artery distribution.

Lateral wall: circumflex artery distribution.

Posterior wall: right coronary distribution.

Massive anterior and lateral wall: main left coronary distribution.

Complications
Arrhythmias

Heart failure.

Intracardiac thrombi.

Pericarditis.

Cardiac rupture: a complication of transmural infarct.

Papillary muscle dysfunction.

Ventricular aneurysm.

Survival After Myocardial Infarction
Depends on patient's age, size of infarct, presence of complications.

Average survival: 90 percent of hospitalized patients.

Survival frequency does not reflect patients who die before entering hospital or patients with small infarcts who do not consult physician.

Diagnosis
History and physical: often inconclusive.

Electrocardiogram: can detect location and size of infarct.

Enzyme tests: enzymes leak from infarcted muscle.

Treatment of Coronary Thrombosis
Thrombolytic therapy (clot-dissolving) improves survival and salvages myocardium

Bed rest advancing to graded activity.

Antiarrhythmia drugs: to reduce myocardial irritability.

Treatment of complications.

Heart block: requires pacemaker.

Heart failure: digitalis and diuretics.

Long-term treatment with antiarrhythmia drugs (beta blockers) and aspirin improves prognosis.

Diagnosis and Treatment of Coronary Heart Disease / 350
Diagnosis
Angiography: detects extent of disease and localizes sites of obstruction.

Treatment
Medical treatment:

Drugs to reduce myocardial oxygen consumption and improve coronary circulation.

Drugs to reduce myocardial irritability.

Reduction of risk factors:

Cessation of smoking.

Control of hypertension.

Anticoronary diet.

Weight reduction where appropriate.

Graduated exercises.

Surgical treatment: myocardial revascularization.

Coronary angioplasty: balloon catheter smashes atheromatous plaque and dilates artery.

Cocaine-Induced Arrhythmias/Infarcts
Drug intensifies effects of sympathetic nerve impulses.

Rapid heart rate: increases oxygen requirements.

Myocardial irritability: predisposes to arrhythmias.

Constricts blood vessels: raises blood pressure.

Drug may induce coronary artery spasm/severe ischemia/myocardial infarcts.

Fatal arrhythmias/myocardial infarcts may occur in persons with normal coronary arteries. Persons with coronary atherosclerosis are at even greater risk.

Blood Lipids and Coronary Heart Disease / 356
Neutral Fat: Triglyceride
Composed of fatty acid combined with glycerol.

Fatty acids may be saturated, unsaturated, or polyunsaturated.

Cholesterol
High levels associated with increased incidence of coronary heart disease.

Transport of cholesterol by lipoprotein.

LDL cholesterol is atherogenic: "bad cholesterol."

HDL cholesterol is protective: "good cholesterol."

Alteration of Blood Lipids by Change in Diet
Decrease cholesterol intake.

Decrease intake of saturated fats.

Derive carbohydrates from complex carbohydrates.

Reduce alcohol intake.

Hypertension and Hypertensive Cardiovascular Disease / 359

Increased Peripheral Resistance Increases Work of Heart

Vascular effects:

Vessels wear out prematurely.

Weakened arteries may rupture in brain causing cerebral hemorrhage.

Renal effects: narrowing of arterioles damages kidneys.

Causes and Treatment

In most cases cause unknown.

Treatment by drugs that lower blood pressure.

Primary Myocardial Disease / 360

Myocarditis

Usually viral; occasionally, other pathogens or hypersensitivity state.

Onset usually abrupt, with eventual complete recovery.

Cardiomyopathy

Dilated cardiomyopathy:

Heart enlarged and dilated.

Cause uncertain, no specific treatment available.

Hypertrophic cardiomyopathy:

Hereditary dominant transmission.

Disorganized muscle fibers and greatly hypertrophied heart.

Thick septum impinging on mitral valve leaflet may block outflow of blood from ventricle (idiopathic hypertrophic subaortic stenosis).

Treated by drugs that slow heart and reduce force of contraction.

Surgical resection of part of septum if medical management fails.

Heart Failure / 362

Definition

Heart no longer able to function efficiently:

Acute heart failure: rapid progression.

Chronic heart failure: slow onset and progression.

Pathogenesis:

Forward failure: inadequate cardiac output leads to salt and water retention by kidneys.

Backward failure: blood backs up in venous circulation.

Treatment:

Diuretics: promote salt and water excretion.

Digitalis: increases efficiency of cardiac contraction.

Acute Pulmonary Edema / 362

Pathogenesis

Temporary disproportion in output of blood from left and right ventricles.

Blood accumulates in lung.

Extravasation of fluid in alveoli.

Aneurysms / 363

Arteriosclerotic Aneurysm

Arteriosclerosis damages wall, which dilates owing to high intraluminal pressure.

Aneurysm may rupture and cause profuse hemorrhage.

Treatment by replacement with nylon or Dacron graft.

Dissecting Aneurysm of the Aorta

Splitting of layers of wall.

Blood dissects through intimal tear and may rupture back into lumen or externally.

Can be treated surgically.

Diseases of the Veins / 370

Venous Thrombosis and Thrombophlebitis

Deep veins of lower extremities most commonly affected.

Postoperative and bed patients predisposed.

Predisposing factors, pathogenesis, manifestations, and treatment covered in chapter 12.

Varicose Veins of Lower Extremities

Usually a result of congenital weakness of vein wall or valves predisposing to varicosities.

May occur if deeper veins blocked or valves damaged by thrombophlebitis, diverting more blood flow to superficial veins.

Complications:

Stasis ulcers.

Rupture with bleeding.

Thrombophlebitis.

Treatment:

Medical: elastic stockings, elevation of limb.

Surgical: ligation and excision of varicosities.

Varicose Veins in Other Locations

Hemorrhoids: varicose veins of rectum. See chapter 23.

Esophageal varices: in patients with cirrhosis of liver. See chapter 21.

Varicocele: veins of spermatic cord. Usually asymptomatic, requiring no treatment.

14

The Hematopoietic and Lymphatic Systems

Learning Objectives

1. Describe the composition of the blood and enumerate its functions. Explain the functions of the lymphatic system.
2. Explain the principles by which anemias are classified and treated.
3. List and describe the usual causes of hypochromic microcytic anemia and macrocytic anemia. Explain how these anemias are treated.
4. List the usual causes of anemia as a result of bone marrow damage and anemia caused by accelerated blood destruction. Explain their treatment.
5. Describe the causes and effects of polycythemia and thrombocytopenia.
6. Describe the cause and clinical manifestations of infectious mononucleosis.
7. List the common causes of lymph node enlargement.
8. Explain the role of the spleen in protecting the body against infection. Describe the effects of a splenectomy on the body's defenses and relate them to the management of the patient who has had a splenectomy.

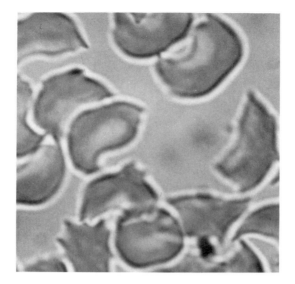

Chapter 14 ▪ Contents

Composition and Function of Human Blood

Blood is essential to transporting oxygen and nutrients to the tissues; carbon dioxide and other waste products of cell metabolism to the excretory organs; and leukocytes, hormones, and antibodies to various locations in the body. The volume of blood, which varies with the size of the individual, is about 5 quarts in the average man. Almost half of the blood consists of cellular elements: red cells, white cells (leukocytes), and platelets suspended in a viscous fluid called blood plasma (figure 14–1). The numbers of circulating red cells, white cells, and platelets are so great that their numbers are expressed as the number per microliter (μL) of blood (1 ml = 1000 μL). This same quantity can also be expressed as the number per cubic millimeter (mm^3) of blood. The terms are equivalent because 1 microliter is the same as 1 cubic millimeter.

Red cells, which are concerned primarily with oxygen transport, are the most numerous cells, averaging about 5 million per microliter of blood. Red cells normally survive about four months in the circulation.

Leukocytes are much less numerous, averaging about 7000 per microliter. The following types of leukocytes are recognized:

1. Neutrophils
2. Eosinophils
3. Basophils
4. Monocytes
5. Lymphocytes

Although *lymphocytes* are produced chiefly in the lymph nodes and spleen, they are also manufactured in the bone marrow and elsewhere throughout the body where lymphoid tissue is present. Under normal circumstances, production of the other types of white cells is confined to the bone marrow. In contrast with the relatively long survival of red cells, most white cells have a short survival time within the circulation, varying from several hours to several days, and they must be replenished continually. Lymphocytes are an exception. Two populations of lymphocytes are present in the circulation, one surviving about the same length of time as most of the other leukocytes and another surviving for several years.

The proportions of the various leukocytes vary with the age of the individual. The most numerous in the adult are the **neutrophils,** constituting about 70 percent of the total circulating white cells. Neutrophils are actively phagocytic and predominate in acute inflammatory reactions. **Lymphocytes** are the next most common type of white cells in adults and are the predominant leukocytes in the blood of children. The lymphocytes in the peripheral blood constitute only a small fraction of the total lymphocytes, most being located in the lymph nodes, spleen, and other lymphoid tissues. Lymphocytes continually recirculate from the bloodstream into lymphoid tissues. Eventually, they leave the lymphoid tissue through the lymphatic channels and the thoracic duct, returning to the circulation and later becoming reestablished for a time in a different site of lymphoid tissue. Lymphocytes take part in cell-mediated and humoral defense reactions.

FIGURE 14–1

Normal blood. Red cells appear as biconcave disks. A neutrophil appears near *center* of photograph. Small, dark structures are platelets. (Original magnification × 400.)

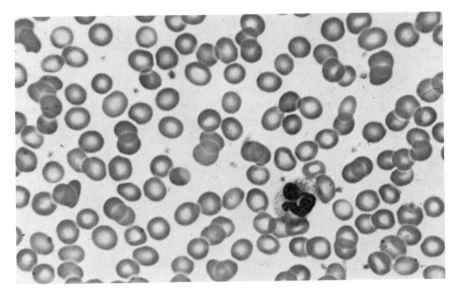

Small numbers of eosinophils, basophils, and monocytes also are normally present in the blood. **Eosinophils** are related in some manner to allergy. One of their functions appears to be phagocytosis and digestion of antigen-antibody complexes. Eosinophils increase in allergic diseases, in the presence of worm or other animal-parasite infestations, and in a few other conditions. **Basophils** are similar to mast cells. Their granules contain histamine and an anticoagulant called **heparin. Monocytes** are actively phagocytic and increase in certain types of chronic infections. Monocyte-lymphocyte interaction is necessary in the initial phase of response to a foreign antigen; it also plays a role in the cell-mediated immune reaction.

Blood **platelets,** which are essential for normal blood coagulation, are much smaller than leukocytes. They represent bits of the cytoplasm of *megakaryocytes,* large precursor cells present in the bone marrow. Platelets have a short survival, comparable to that of most leukocytes.

Normal Hematopoiesis

The *bone marrow* can be compared to a large manufacturing plant. It replenishes the blood cells that are continually being worn out and removed from the circulation. As with any manufacturing process, adequate quantities of raw materials are required. Moreover, the factory must be able to process these raw materials efficiently into finished products (the blood cells). The major raw materials necessary for hematopoiesis are protein, vitamin B_{12}, folic acid (one of the vitamin B group), and iron. Inadequate supplies of these substances will handicap the production of blood cells.

Development, Maturation, and Survival of Red Cells

Red cells develop from large precursor cells in the bone marrow called **erythroblasts** (*erythro* = red + *blast* = a primitive cell). **Hemoglobin,** the oxygen-carrying protein that is formed by the developing red cells, is composed of four separate pieces called *subunits,* which in turn fit together to form a much larger aggregate called a *tetramer* (*tetra* = four). Each subunit consists of two parts: *heme* and *globin.*

Heme is a complex nitrogen-containing ring structure (called a *porphyrin ring*) containing an iron atom. Globin, which forms the largest part of each hemoglobin subunit, is a short, coiled protein (*polypeptide*) chain. Several types of globin chains, differing in their amino acid composition, are formed at varying times and in differing proportions in the fetus and in the adult. The chains are designated by Greek letters: alpha (α), beta (β), gamma (γ), delta (δ), and epsilon (ϵ).

Two different types of hemoglobin are found in the red cells of the normal adult. About 98 percent is called *hemoglobin A* or *adult hemoglobin,* in which two subunits of the tetramer contain alpha chains and two contain beta chains. The hemoglobin can also be designated by the shorthand notation $\alpha_2\beta_2$. (The chain is designated by the Greek letter and the number of subunits by the subscript.) The remaining 2 percent is called *hemoglobin A_2,* a tetramer composed of two alpha and two delta chains ($\alpha_2\delta_2$).

The heme and globin are synthesized separately in different locations within the erythroblast. The porphyrin ring is produced by the mitochondria. Then the iron, brought to the cell by a transport protein called *transferrin,* is inserted into the porphyrin ring to form heme. The globin chains are synthesized by groups of ribosomes (*polyribosomes*) in the cytoplasm and are joined to heme to form a hemoglobin subunit. Finally, the four subunits aggregate to form the complete hemoglobin tetramer.

The developing red cell accumulates increasing amounts of hemoglobin as it matures. When about 80 percent of its total hemoglobin has been synthesized, the nucleus is extruded. The cell is then discharged from the bone marrow into the circulation, where it completes its maturation and hemoglobin synthesis over the succeeding 24 hours. A newly formed red cell, which lacks a nucleus but still retains is mitochondria and other organelles for a short time, is called a **reticulocyte.** The name comes from its special staining characteristics. Certain stains precipitate the organelles within the cell cytoplasm, causing them to appear as a network (*reticulum*) of dark blue strands and granules. A reticulocyte is slightly larger than a mature red cell, and it also has a faint blue color because it contains less red-staining hemoglobin than a mature cell. These distinguishing features, which differentiate a reticulocyte from a mature red cell, are soon lost as the cell matures within the circulation.

The red cell, which derives its energy from the enzymatic breakdown of glucose, possesses enzyme systems that permit the cell to perform the diverse metabolic functions necessary for survival. Because the cell lacks a nucleus, it cannot synthesize new enzyme molecules to replace those that gradually wear out. As the cell ages, its enzyme systems gradually become depleted until eventually, after about four months, the cell is no longer able to function. The worn-out red cell is then removed by the *mononuclear phagocyte system (reticuloendothelial system)*, primarily in the spleen, and its hemoglobin is degraded. The globin chains are broken down, and their component amino acids are used to make other proteins. The iron is extracted and saved to make new hemoglobin. The porphyrin ring, however, cannot be salvaged. It is degraded and is excreted by the liver as bile pigment.

Regulation of Hematopoiesis

Red cell production is regulated by the oxygen content of the arterial blood. Decreased oxygen supply to the tissues stimulates erythropoiesis. However, low oxygen tension does not act directly on the bone marrow. The effect is mediated by the kidneys. Certain specialized cells in the kidneys elaborate a hormonelike material that interacts with certain factors in the plasma, leading to the production of an erythrocyte-stimulating material called **erythropoietin.**

The factors regulating the production of white blood cells and their delivery into the circulation are not well understood. Products of cell necrosis may cause the number of white blood cells in the peripheral blood to increase. Hormone secretion by the adrenals and some other endocrine glands also influences white cell production.

Anemia

Anemia literally means "without blood." Specifically, the term is used to refer to a decrease in red cells or to subnormal hemoglobin levels. Many classifications of anemia have been proposed, and two different methods of classification are widely used. One system, based on the factor responsible for the anemia, is an etiologic classification. A second system, based on the shape and appearance of the red blood cells (as determined by microscopic examination of a stained blood smear), is a morphologic classification.

Etiologic Classification of Anemia

One simple classification of the anemias is based on the "bone marrow factory" concept (figure 14–2). Anemia is classified as being caused by either inadequate production of red cells or excessive loss of cells. Inadequate production, in turn, may result from an insufficiency of raw materials or from factors that render the factory inoperative and no longer able to deliver enough finished products into the circulation. Examples of the latter would be marrow damage or replacement of marrow by abnormal cells. Excessive loss of red cells may be caused either by external blood loss or by accelerated destruction of the cells (and hence shortened survival) in the circulation. Table 14–1 presents a classification of the various causes of anemia.

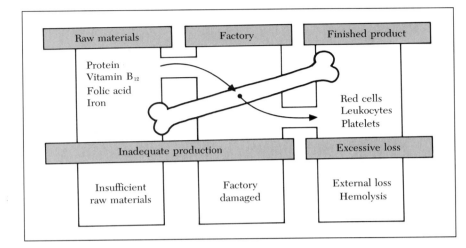

FIGURE 14–2

Classification of anemia based on "bone marrow factory" concept.

Morphologic Classification of Anemia

An anemia in which the cells are normal in size and appearance is called a *normocytic anemia*. If the cells are larger than normal, the anemia is called a *macrocytic anemia*. If the cells are smaller than normal, the anemia is called a *microcytic anemia*. Many times, microcytic cells also have a reduced

TABLE 14–1

Etiologic classification of anemia

As a result of inadequate production of red cells

Inadequate "raw materials"

Iron-deficiency anemia
Vitamin B$_{12}$ deficiency
Folic acid deficiency

Bone marrow factory function impaired, damaged, or inoperative

Anemia of chronic disease
Bone marrow depressed or destroyed (aplastic anemia)
Bone marrow replaced by foreign or abnormal cells

As a result of excessive loss of red cells

As a result of external blood loss

As a result of shortened survival of red cells in the circulation (hemolytic anemia)

Caused by defective red cells (hereditary hemolytic anemia)
    Abnormal shape
    Abnormal hemoglobin
    Defective hemoglobin synthesis
    Deficient enzymes
Caused by "hostile environment" (acquired hemolytic anemia)
    Antibodies present
    Mechanical trauma to red cells

hemoglobin content, appearing quite pale when examined under the microscope; here, the term *hypochromic anemia* is used. Often the latter two terms are combined, and the anemia is called a *hypochromic microcytic anemia.* Classification of anemia on the basis of red cell appearance is useful, because the appearance of the cells provides a clue to the etiology. Iron-deficiency anemia is a hypochromic microcytic anemia. Anemia caused by vitamin B_{12} or folic acid deficiency is a macrocytic anemia. Most other types of anemia are normocytic.

Iron-Deficiency Anemia

The body contains about four grams of iron, of which about 75 percent is contained in hemoglobin. Most of the rest is a reserve supply that is stored in the bone marrow, liver, and spleen. The usual diet of an adult contains from about 10 to 20 mg of iron, but men absorb merely 1 mg per day, and only slightly more iron is absorbed by women and children. Women need more iron to make up for menstrual blood losses, because 1 mL of blood contains about 0.5 mg of iron. Additional iron is also required during pregnancy to supply the needs of the developing fetus. Children require greater amounts of iron in order to synthesize more hemoglobin during periods of growth when the blood volume is increasing. Iron is absorbed with difficulty from the gastrointestinal tract, and the iron stores within the body are carefully conserved.

Iron-deficiency anemia is the most common anemia encountered in clinical practice. Iron forms an essential part of the hemoglobin molecule, and normal synthesis of hemoglobin requires adequate supplies of iron.

When red blood cells, which have a normal life-span of about four months, become "senile," they are removed from the circulation. The iron from the destroyed cells is transported back to the bone marrow and is reused by the bone marrow to be incorporated into newly formed red cells. Iron-deficiency anemia may result from either insufficient intake of iron in the diet or inadequate reutilization of the iron present in red cells.

Iron deficiency caused by inadequate dietary intake may occur in infants during periods of rapid growth. A normal, full-term infant has been provided with a reserve supply of iron that was transferred to the fetus from the mother during the last part of pregnancy. Consequently, the newborn infant generally has an adequate short-term supply of iron available for hematopoiesis during the neonatal period when the production of red cells accelerates to supply the needs of an increasing blood volume. A premature infant, however, may not get its full component of iron stores and may not have enough reserve to supply its postnatal needs. Even in full-term infants, the reserve supply of iron for hematopoiesis is limited and must be supplemented by iron from the diet. Breast milk contains very little iron, although the amount available is well absorbed. If the diet is not supplemented by cereals, fruits, vegetables, other foods containing iron, or some type of iron supplement, iron stores will become rapidly exhausted and iron-deficiency anemia will develop in the first year of life. For this reason, many physicians gradually add supplementary foods containing additional sources of iron to infants' diets. Occasionally, adolescents subsisting on an inadequate or poorly balanced diet develop iron deficiency anemia.

Most cases of iron-deficiency anemia in adults results from failure to recapture the iron present in red cells for hemoglobin synthesis. This failure is a result of chronic blood loss. The iron contained in red cells that is lost from the circulation by bleeding is no longer available to the body for the production of new red cells. Because each milliliter of blood contains 0.5 mg of iron, loss of 500 mL of blood represents loss of 250 mg of iron, which is equivalent to one-fourth of the body's entire iron reserves. Unless dietary intake of iron is extremely liberal, iron stores soon become exhausted, and iron-deficiency anemia develops (figure 14–3).

Iron-deficiency anemia is a hypochromic microcytic anemia (figure 14–4). The cells are pale because they contain less hemoglobin than normal. The cells are also abnormally small, because the body apparently attempts to "scale down" the size of the cell to conform to the reduced hemoglobin content.

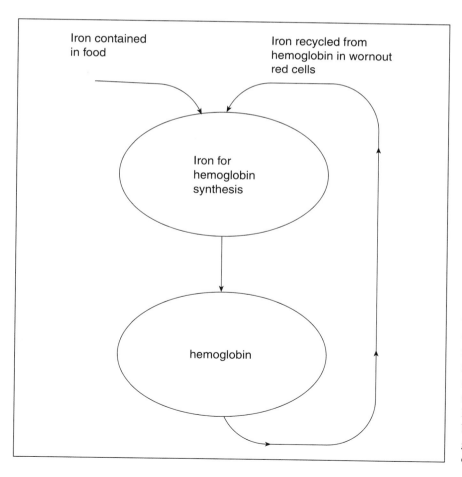

FIGURE 14–3

Sources of iron for hemoglobin synthesis, and role of chronic blood loss in pathogenesis of iron-deficiency anemia. Dietary iron contributes to hemoglobin synthesis but is absorbed with difficulty. Most of the iron used for hemoglobin synthesis is recycled from worn-out red cells. Chronic blood loss removes iron-containing red cells from the circulation, and the iron contained in the lost red cells can no longer be recycled to make hemoglobin, which leads to iron-deficiency anemia.

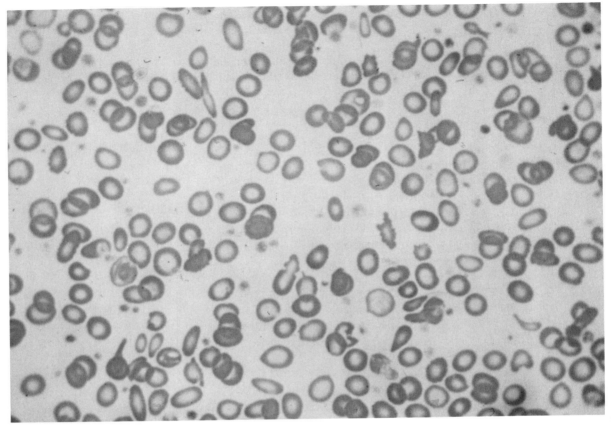

FIGURE 14–4

Hypochromic microcytic anemia caused by chronic iron deficiency. (Original magnification × 400.)

A physician treating a patient with iron-deficiency anemia is primarily concerned with learning the cause of the anemia and then directing therapy toward the cause rather than the symptoms. In an infant with a history of a very poor diet, the cause may be obvious. In an adult, the anemia is usually a result of blood loss, and the physician must always investigate to determine the source of the bleeding. Blood loss may be caused by a bleeding ulcer or an ulcerated carcinoma of the colon. In women, excessive menstrual bleeding is a common cause of iron-deficiency anemia. Another sometimes overlooked cause of iron-deficiency anemia in otherwise healthy young adults is too-frequent blood donations. Once the cause of the blood loss has been determined, proper treatment of the underlying cause can be instituted. In addition, the patient is given supplementary iron to replenish the body's depleted iron stores.

Vitamin B$_{12}$ and Folic Acid Deficiency

Vitamin B$_{12}$ is found in meat, liver, and other foods rich in animal protein. Folic acid is widely distributed in nature, being found in abundance in green leafy vegetables as well as many foods of animal origin.

Vitamin B$_{12}$ and folic acid are required not only for normal hematopoiesis, but for normal maturation of many other types of cells. In the absence of either vitamin B$_{12}$ or folic acid, DNA synthesis is impaired and the developing red cells in the bone marrow exhibit a characteristic disturbance of cell maturation. The developing red cells, which are larger than normal, are called **megaloblasts** (*megalos* = large). The abnormal red cell maturation is called *megaloblastic erythropoiesis.* The mature red cells derived from the abnormal maturation also are larger than normal. Therefore, the anemia is classified morphologically as a macrocytic anemia. The development of white cell precursors and megakaryocytes is also abnormal. Consequently, patients with megaloblastic anemia usually also have **leukopenia** and **thrombocytopenia** as well as a macrocytic anemia. Vitamin B$_{12}$, but not folic acid, is required to maintain the structural and functional integrity of the nervous system; thus, a deficiency of this vitamin is often associated with pronounced neurologic disturbances.

Anemia As a Result of Folic Acid Deficiency

The body has very limited stores of folic acid, which rapidly become depleted if not replenished continually. As a result, folic-acid–deficiency anemia is relatively common and may result from reduced dietary intake, impaired absorption, or increased folic acid requirements.

Deficiency caused by inadequate dietary intake is found in persons subsisting on inadequate diets and is encountered frequently in chronic alcoholics because of their typically deficient diet and, possibly, impaired absorption of folic acid, compared with nondrinkers. Persons with chronic intestinal diseases may become folic acid deficient because of impaired ability to absorb the vitamin. Pregnant women also are at risk because pregnancy greatly increases folic acid requirements. Folic-acid–deficiency anemia in pregnancy is uncommon because physicians routinely prescribe folic acid supplements to pregnant women.

Anemia As a Result of Vitamin B$_{12}$ Deficiency

Efficient absorption of vitamin B$_{12}$ ingested in food requires a substance called *intrinsic factor,* secreted by gastric mucosal cells along with hydrocholoric acid and digestive enzymes. The intrinsic factor combines with the vitamin B$_{12}$, and the B$_{12}$–intrinsic-factor complex is absorbed from the distal small intestine. The absorbed vitamin is stored in the liver and made available to the bone marrow and other tissues as required for cell growth and maturation.

A common cause of vitamin B$_{12}$ deficiency is **pernicious anemia.** The basic defect in pernicious anemia is atrophy of the gastric mucosa, which sometimes develops in middle-aged and elderly individuals and is often associated with autoantibodies directed against gastric mucosal cells and intrinsic factor. The atrophic mucosa fails to secrete intrinsic factor, acid, and digestive enzymes, and consequently vitamin B_{12} is not absorbed. The vitamin B_{12} deficiency causes impaired hematopoiesis as well as various neurologic disturbances.

Pernicious anemia is not the only cause of vitamin B_{12} deficiency. Persons who have had most of their stomach surgically removed because of ulcer or gastric cancer or who have had a gastric bypass procedure to control obesity (described in chapter 25) may not be able to secrete enough intrinsic factor. Persons who have had a small bowel resection of the distal ilium, where the vitamin B_{12}-intrinsic factor complex is absorbed, may not be able to absorb enough vitamin to supply their needs, and an individual with chronic intestinal disease affecting the vitamin B_{12}-absorbing area (such as regional enteritis, described in chapter 23) also may be unable to absorb the vitamin adequately.

Pernicious anemia and other vitamin B_{12} deficiencies are treated with intramuscular administration of vitamin B_{12}. Parenteral administration avoids the problem of poor absorption of the vitamin.

Bone Marrow Suppression, Damage, or Infiltration

Many conditions can depress bone marrow function. Chronic diseases of all types may impair hematopoiesis and lead to mild or moderate anemia, which is called the *anemia of chronic disease*. In this condition, iron and other "raw materials" supplied to the bone marrow are adequate, but they are not utilized efficiently to make red cells. White blood cell and platelet production are usually not disturbed. The most common cause of this type of anemia is chronic infection, but other chronic diseases and some malignant tumors also may be responsible.

The anemia of chronic disease improves when the disease that caused it is identified and treated. Chronic infections may respond to treatment, but unfortunately it is often not possible to "cure" many of the other chronic diseases that lead to this type of anemia.

The anemia of chronic disease usually causes only a relatively mild suppression of bone marrow function. In contrast, much more serious and sometimes irreversible damage to the bone marrow factory is caused by many different drugs and chemicals and by excessive radiation. These agents damage or destroy hematopoietic cells. In some cases, the cause of the marrow injury cannot be determined. Anemia that is a result of bone marrow failure is called *aplastic anemia* (*a* = without + *plasia* = growth). The term is not strictly accurate, because all hematopoietic precursors are damaged, and leukopenia and thrombocytopenia are present as well as anemia. In aplastic anemia, the red cells are normal in size and shape but inadequate in number. Therefore, aplastic anemia is classified as a normocytic anemia.

A similar type of anemia is produced if marrow cells are crowded out and replaced by such abnormal cells as leukemic cells or metastatic tumor. As a consequence, production of all blood cells is inadequate. The anemia is normocytic, and leukopenia and thrombocytopenia also tend to be present. The term *bone marrow replacement anemia* is sometimes used to denote any type of anemia caused by infiltration of the bone marrow and consequent displacement of normal marrow cells.

Anemias of this kind are treated by administering blood transfusions to maintain an adequate volume of circulating blood cells while the disease that caused the marrow failure is being treated. Unfortunately, in many cases, there is no specific treatment to restore marrow function to normal. In some highly selected patients with aplastic anemia, it is possible to perform a *bone marrow transplantation,* using methods similar to those used to treat patients with leukemia (described in chapter 10). A large volume of bone marrow is aspirated from the pelvic bones of a suitable donor and injected intravenously into the circulation of the recipient. Sometimes the donor cells become established in the recipient's marrow and begin to produce blood cells. A marrow transplant is foreign tissue, however, and the recipient's own immune defenses must be suppressed (described in chapter 5) in order to permit the transplanted bone marrow to survive.

Acute Blood Loss

A normocytic anemia may result from an episode of acute blood loss, as from a massive hemorrhage from the uterus or gastrointestinal tract. Provided that iron stores are adequate, the lost blood is rapidly replaced by the bone marrow and the newly formed red cells are normal. This is in contrast with the anemia of chronic blood loss, in which the red cells are hypochromic and microcytic because prolonged bleeding has depleted the body's iron stores.

Accelerated Blood Destruction

Normal red cells survive for about four months. Sometimes, however, their survival is considerably shortened, and anemia results because the regenerative capacity of the marrow is not sufficient to keep up with the accelerated destruction. This type of anemia is called a *hemolytic anemia* and may be a result of either defective red cells or a "hostile environment." Hemolytic anemias caused by defective red cells are called *hereditary hemolytic anemias.* Those resulting from damage to normal red cells by antibodies or other injurious agents are called *acquired hemolytic anemias.*

Hereditary Hemolytic Anemias
The genetically determined abnormalities of red cells that may shorten their survival fall into four major groups (table 14–2):

1. Abnormally shaped cells
2. Abnormal hemoglobins
3. Defective hemoglobin synthesis
4. Enzyme deficiencies

TABLE 14–2

Inheritance and manifestations of some hereditary hemolytic anemias

Anemia	Inheritance	Characteristics of red cells	Manifestations
Hereditary spherocytosis	Dominant or recessive	Spherocytic	Mild to moderate chronic hemolytic anemia
Hereditary ovalocytosis	Dominant	Oval	Usually asymptomatic; may have mild anemia
Sickle cell anemia	Codominant	Normocytic; cells sickle under reduced oxygen tension	Marked anemia
Hemoglobin C disease	Codominant	Normocytic	Mild to moderate anemia
Sickle cell–hemoglobin C disease	Codominant	Normocytic; cells sickle under reduced oxygen tension	Moderate anemia
Thalassemia minor	Dominant (heterozygous)	Hypochromic-microcytic; total number of red cells usually increased	Mild anemia
Thalassemia major	Dominant (homozygous)	Hypochromic-microcytic	Severe anemia; usually fatal in childhood
Glucose-6-phosphate dehydrogenase deficiency	X-linked recessive	Normocytic; enzyme-deficient cells	Episodes of acute hemolytic anemia precipitated by drugs or infections

Shape Abnormalities   The most common abnormality of shape is called *hereditary spherocytosis.* There appear to be two distinct genetic forms. Most are transmitted as a Mendelian-dominant trait, but some follow a recessive-inherited pattern. The basic red cell defect is a deficiency of a structural protein called *spectrin,* which enters into the formation of the basic framework of the red cell. As a result of the deficiency, the red cells are unable to retain the normal biconcave disk configuration characteristic of normal red cells and tend to adopt a progressively more spherical shape within the circulation. Because of their abnormal shape, the spherocytic cells tend to become trapped within the spleen, where they are destroyed at an accelerated rate by the phagocytic cells within the splenic pulp. This results in a chronic hemolytic anemia. Splenectomy cures the anemia by removing the main site of red cell destruction, but it has no effect on the basic red cell defect.

A somewhat similar condition, which is also transmitted as a Mendelian-dominant trait, is called *hereditary ovalocytosis.* As the name indicates, the red cells are oval rather than round. Most affected persons are not inconvenienced by the abnormality, but some have a mild hemolytic anemia that can be cured by splenectomy.

Abnormal Hemoglobins   The arrangement of amino acids in the globin chains of hemoglobin is controlled by genes. If the gene is abnormal, the amino acids forming the globin chains will be altered, leading to the formation of an abnormal hemoglobin. Genes directing the synthesis of the various types of hemoglobin are codominant. If an abnormal gene is present, the abnormal hemoglobin appears in the red cells. Many different abnormal hemoglobins can be identified and characterized by various laboratory tests. Some of the abnormal hemoglobins function normally, but others have unusual properties that impair their function. *Hemoglobin S* (sickle hemoglobin) is one of the more important abnormal hemoglobins. Its formation results from a change in only a single amino acid in the beta chains of hemoglobin. Hemoglobin S crystallizes when the oxygen tension is reduced and causes the erythrocytes to become distorted into bizarre sickle and holly-leaf shapes (figure 14–5). The crystallization is largely reversible, and the hemo-

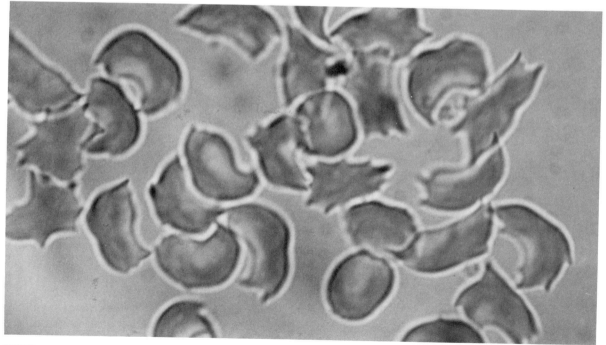

FIGURE 14–5

Unstained red cells containing sickle hemoglobin incubated under reduced oxygen tension. Sickle hemoglobin crystallizes, causing cells to adopt sickle and holly-leaf configurations. (Original magnification × 1000.)

globin becomes soluble again when the oxygen tension is raised. About 10 percent of the Black population are heterozygous carriers of the sickle cell gene. Their erythrocytes contain both hemoglobin S and hemoglobin A. This condition, which is called *sickle cell trait,* does not usually cause symptoms unless the red cells are exposed to extremely low oxygen concentrations, a situation that is unlikely to occur under normal circumstances. The homozygous state is called *sickle cell anemia* and is a serious disease. The cells of the affected individual contain no hemoglobin A and become sickled within the capillaries, where the oxygen tension is lower than in arterial blood. The clumps of sickled red cells obstruct blood flow and cause progressive damage to the heart, kidneys, and other organs, owing to impaired circulation. Anemia develops because the abnormal cells have a shortened survival.

Another common abnormal hemoglobin, called *hemoglobin C,* also is found predominantly in Blacks. Heterozygous individuals, whose cells contain both hemoglobin A and hemoglobin C, are normal clinically. Persons homozygous for the hemoglobin C gene have a mild hemolytic anemia.

Some persons possess genes for two abnormal hemoglobins. This may occur, for example, if one parent carries the hemoglobin S gene and the other carries the hemoglobin C gene, and each parent transmits the abnormal gene. In this case, the red cells of the affected person contain both abnormal hemoglobins in approximately equal amounts, and a hemolytic anemia results.

Defective Hemoglobin Synthesis   Sometimes the globin chains of hemoglobin are normal, but their synthesis is defective. This genetically determined condition is called *thalassemia* and is transmitted as a Mendelian-dominant trait. The defective synthesis may be of either the alpha chains (*alpha thalassemia*) or the beta chains (*beta thalassemia*), but the latter defect is the more common and the more important clinically. This genetic abnormality is relatively common in persons of Greek and Italian ancestry. (The term *thalassemia* comes from the Greek word *thalassa,* meaning sea, and derives from the high incidence of the condition in persons who live in the regions surrounding the Mediterranean Sea.)

In the more common beta thalassemia, the production of beta chains is reduced but alpha chain production is not, and synthesis of the two types of chains is unbalanced. An excess of alpha chains accumulates and precipitates within the red cells, which shortens their survival. Because hemoglobin synthesis is reduced, the red cells appear hypochromic and microcytic, somewhat like the appearance of the cells in iron-deficiency anemia. In thalassemia, however, the hypochromia is the result of deficient hemoglobin production because of inadequate beta chain synthesis, rather than deficient production caused by iron deficiency. Usually, the cells also contain an increased amount of hemoglobin A_2, which does not contain beta chains, to compensate in part for the reduced synthesis of hemoglobin A.

If a person is heterozygous for the thalassemia gene, the anemia is mild and the condition is called *thalassemia minor.* The red cells are hypochromic and microcytic, and usually there is a compensatory overproduction of red cells and so their numbers are greater than normal. The homozygous condi-

tion, which is called *thalassemia major,* occurs if both parents have thalassemia minor and each transmits the abnormal gene. The affected individual has a severe chronic hemolytic anemia that is usually fatal in childhood.

Red Cell Enzyme Deficiencies   Red cells derive energy by metabolizing
glucose by a series of chemical reactions that are catalyzed by various
enzyme systems. These same energy-producing reactions also indirectly
help prevent oxidation of the hemoglobin, thereby protecting the hemoglobin from the potentially harmful effects of oxidizing drugs or other agents
that can damage it. This protective function is compromised if certain red cell
enzymes are deficient. Under such circumstances, exposure of the red cells
to an oxidizing agent causes denaturation and precipitation of the protein
chains of hemoglobin, as well as the cell-membrane proteins.

One of the more common red cell enzyme defects is a deficiency of the
enzyme *glucose-6-phosphate dehydrogenase,* which is transmitted as an X-
linked recessive trait. (X-linked inheritance is considered in chapter 3.)
About 10 percent of Black men are affected, and 30 percent of Black
women carry the abnormal gene on one of their X chromosomes. The
abnormal gene occurs with high frequency in some White populations as
well. The enzyme-deficient cells are highly susceptible to injury by drugs that
do not affect normal red cells, and to various bacterial and viral infections.
More than forty drugs are known to induce an acute hemolytic anemia in
susceptible subjects, including such commonly used drugs as sulfonamides,
aspirin, some diuretics, some antibiotics, and some vitamins. Hemolysis
begins soon after exposure to the drug or infectious agent and continues for
about a week. Considerable red cell destruction results, followed by red cell
regeneration and return of red cell levels to normal in about four or five
weeks.

Acquired Hemolytic Anemia

Sometimes the red cells are normally formed but are unable to survive normally because they are released into a "hostile environment." For example,
antibodies that attack and destroy the red cells may be present in the circulation. Some of the autoimmune diseases, such as lupus erythematosus
(described in chapter 5), and some diseases of the lymphatic system may be
associated with a hemolytic anemia caused by autoantibodies.

Some drugs also cause a hemolytic anemia by inducing formation of antibodies that damage red cells. Three different immunologic mechanisms have
been identified. The most common mechanism results from the effect of the
drug on the body's immune system. Certain drugs disrupt the immune system
in some way, leading to the formation of an autoantibody directed against the
red cell membrane. The autoantibody may persist for some time after the drug
has been discontinued. Other mechanisms include formation of drug-protein
complexes. In some cases, the drug combines with a plasma protein, forming
a drug-protein complex that is antigenic and induces antibody formation. The
antigen and antibody interact within the circulation, forming complexes that
attach to the red cells and cause their destruction. In other cases, the drug

binds to the red cell membrane, forming an antigenic drug-membrane complex. An antibody against the complex then forms, attacks the cell membrane, and damages the red cells.

In another type of acquired hemolytic anemia, red cells may be destroyed by mechanical trauma. Some diseases are characterized by significant enlargement of the spleen. Red cells passing through a greatly enlarged spleen may be subject to considerable mechanical trauma, accelerating their destruction. Occasionally, a hemolytic anemia may follow the insertion of an artificial heart valve. The red cells are injured by contact against some part of the artificial valve.

Diagnostic Evaluation of Anemia

Once it is determined that a patient is anemic, the physician's function is to determine the cause so that proper, effective treatment can be instituted. A careful medical history and physical examination may provide important clues to the most likely cause. A complete blood count is essential in order to assess the degree of anemia and to determine whether leukopenia and thrombocytopenia also are present. Careful microscopic examination of a blood smear allows the physician to determine whether the anemia is hypochromic microcytic, normocytic, or macrocytic. This information is helpful in identifying the probable cause of the anemia. The rate of production of new red cells can be estimated by determining the percentage of reticulocytes in the circulation. This is called a *reticulocyte count.* An increased percentage of reticulocytes indicates rapid regeneration of red cells, as would be encountered after acute blood loss or hemolysis. Many times, an examination of the bone marrow also is desirable. In this procedure, a small amount of bone marrow is removed from the pelvic bone, sternum, or other site and examined microscopically. Characteristic abnormalities in the maturation of the marrow cells are seen in pernicious anemia and in anemia caused by folic acid deficiency. Bone marrow examination also detects interference with bone marrow functions secondary to infiltration by leukemic cells or metastatic tumor. Aplastic anemia can generally be recognized by studying the bone marrow. Certain other tests are used when chronic blood loss from the gastrointestinal tract is suspected. Stools are examined for blood, and x-ray studies of the gastrointestinal tract are frequently performed to localize a site of bleeding. Other diagnostic procedures are performed in special circumstances.

Polycythemia

An increase of red cells and hemoglobin above normal levels is called **polycythemia.** Polycythemia may be secondary to an underlying disease that produces decreased arterial oxygen saturation (*secondary polycythemia*). Or, it may represent a manifestation of a leukemia-like overproduction of red cells for no apparent reason (*primary polycythemia*).

Secondary Polycythemia

Any condition associated with decreased arterial oxygen tension leads to increased erythropoietin production and hence to increased levels of red cells. The condition may accompany pulmonary emphysema, pulmonary fibrosis, or some other type of chronic lung disease that lowers the oxygenation of the blood. Some types of congenital heart disease associated with shunting of unsaturated venous blood into the systemic circulation lead to low arterial oxygen tension and may cause secondary polycythemia. Rarely, polycythemia may be the result of a renal tumor. Apparently, such polycythemia is caused by excess erythropoietin production by the tumor; it subsides after removal of the neoplasm.

Primary Polycythemia

Primary polycythemia, also called *polycythemia vera* (true polycythemia), is a manifestation of a diffuse hyperplasia of the bone marrow of unknown etiology. It is characterized by overproduction not only of red cells, but also of white blood cells and platelets. The disease has many features of a neoplastic process, and some patients with polycythemia vera eventually develop granulocytic leukemia.

Complications and Treatment of Polycythemia

The symptoms of polycythemia are related to the increased blood volume and increased blood viscosity. Many patients with polycythemia develop thromboses owing to the increased blood viscosity and elevated platelet levels. Polycythemia vera is usually treated by drugs that suppress the bone marrow overactivity. Secondary polycythemia is sometimes treated by periodic removal of excess blood.

Thrombocytopenia

Blood platelets are fragments of the cytoplasm of megakaryocytes that are released into the bloodstream. These small structures serve a hemostatic function, sealing small breaks in capillaries and interacting with plasma factors in the initial stages of blood clotting. A significant reduction in the numbers of platelets in the blood leads to numerous small, pinpoint hemorrhages from capillaries in the skin and mucous membranes, called *petechiae,* and to larger areas of hemorrhage, called *ecchymoses.* This type of skin and mucous membrane bleeding is called *purpura,* and the disease entity is called *thrombocytopenic purpura.* The number of platelets may be reduced by bone marrow disease, which impairs platelet production, or by accelerated destruction of platelets in the circulation.

Many cases of thrombocytopenic purpura develop when drugs, chemicals, or other substances damage the bone marrow. Others develop when the bone marrow is infiltrated by leukemic cells or metastic carcinoma. These conditions are called *secondary thrombocytopenic purpura,* because the purpura results from an underlying disease of the bone marrow.

Sometimes the bone marrow produces platelets normally, but the platelets are rapidly destroyed in the circulation. Autoantibodies directed against platelets can often be detected in the blood of affected individuals. Cases of this type, in which no underlying disease can be detected, are called *primary thrombocytopenic purpura.* Primary thrombocytopenic purpura is often encountered in children and subsides spontaneously within a short time. When the disease develops in adults, it tends to be more chronic.

The Lymphatic System

The lymphatic system consists of the lymph nodes and spleen, together with various organized masses of lymphoid tissue elsewhere throughout the body; these include the tonsils, the adenoids, the thymus, and lymphoid aggregates in the intestinal mucosa, respiratory tract, and bone marrow. The primary function of the lymphatic system is to provide immunologic defenses against foreign material by means of cell-mediated and humoral defense mechanisms. The lymph nodes, which constitute a major part of the system, form an interconnected network linked by lymphatic channels.

Lymph nodes are small, bean-shaped structures that vary from a few millimeters to as much as 2 centimeters in diameter. They are interspersed along the course of lymphatic channels, where they act somewhat like filters. Frequently, they form groups at locations where many lymphatic channels converge, such as around the aorta and inferior vena cava, in the mesentery of the intestine, in the axillae (armpits) and groin, and at the base of the neck. Each node consists of a mass of lymphocytes supported by a meshwork of reticular fibers in which are scattered phagocytic cells of the mononuclear phagocyte system (reticuloendothelial system). As the lymph flows through the nodes, the phagocytic cells filter out and destroy any microorganisms or other foreign materials that have gotten into the lymphatic channels. The lymphocytes and mononuclear phagocytes within the node also interact with the foreign material and initiate an immune response, as described in chapter 5.

The spleen is specialized to filter blood rather than lymph. Much larger than lymph nodes, it is about the size of a man's fist and is located under the ribs in the left upper part of the abdomen. It consists of compact masses of lymphocytes and a network of *sinusoids* (capillaries having wide lumens of variable width) within a supporting framework composed of reticular fibers and numerous phagocytic cells. As the blood flows through the spleen, worn-out red cells are removed from the circulation by the phagocytic cells, and the iron that they contain is salvaged for reuse. Abnormal red cells—such as those that are damaged by disease, are abnormal in shape, or contain a large amount of an abnormal hemoglobin—also are destroyed by the splenic phagocytes, which accounts for their shortened survival in the circulation.

The thymus is a bilobed lymphoid organ overlying the base of the heart. It is a large structure during infancy and childhood but gradually undergoes atrophy in adolescence. Only a remnant persists in the adult. The thymus plays an essential role in the prenatal development of the lymphoid system and in the formation of the body's immunologic defense mechanisms.

Development of the Lymphatic System

The precursor cells of the lymphocytes are formed initially from stem cells in the bone marrow. In the fetus, some of these precursor cells migrate from the marrow into the thymus, where they undergo further maturation and develop into cells that are destined to form a specific type of lymphocyte called **T** (*thymus-dependent*) **lymphocytes.** Other lymphoid cells remain within the bone marrow, where they differentiate and develop into cells destined to form a second specific type of lymphocyte called **B** (*bone-marrow*) **lymphocytes.** Before birth, the precursor cells of both T and B lymphocytes migrate into the spleen, lymph nodes, and other sites. Here they proliferate to form the masses of mature lymphocytes that populate the various lymphoid organs. Lymphocytes do not remain localized within the various lymphoid organs. They continually recirculate between the bloodstream and the various lymphoid organs. The functions of the various lymphoid cells and their role in immunity are considered in chapter 5.

The principal diseases affecting the lymphatic system are infections and neoplasms.

Diseases of the Lymphatic System

Inflammation of Lymph Nodes (Lymphadenitis)

Lymph nodes draining an area of infection may become enlarged and tender, owing to spread of infection through the lymphatic channels and acute inflammation in the node. This is called *lymphadenitis.*

Infectious Mononucleosis

Infectious mononucleosis is a relatively common viral disease. The virus belongs to the same family as the herpes virus that causes fever blisters. The virus has been named the **Epstein-Barr virus** (usually simply called *EB virus*). The disease is encountered most frequently in young adults and is transmitted by close contact, often by kissing. The virus causes an acute, debilitating, febrile illness associated with a diffuse hyperplasia of lymphoid tissue throughout the body. The lymphoid hyperplasia is manifested clinically by enlargement and tenderness of lymph nodes, some degree of splenic enlargement, and a moderate increase of lymphocytes in the peripheral blood. The lymphocytes show rather distinctive morphologic abnormalities, and the diagnosis can generally be made by the pathologist from a careful examination of the blood smear. The lymphocytes are larger than normal, with abundant deep blue cytoplasm and an irregularly shaped nucleus (figure 14–6). Enlargement and ulceration of lymphoid tissue in the throat is responsible for the sore throat often accompanying the disease.

The EB virus infects B lymphocytes, which proliferate actively during the first week of the infection. Then the T lymphocytes and antibodies produced by plasma cells against the EB virus destroy the virus-infected cells. The atypical lymphocytes seen in the blood of an infected individual are activated T lymphocytes attacking the virus-infected cells. Most persons infected with EB virus never develop clinical manifestations of infectious mononucleosis, because the body's defenses destroy the virus-infected cells. Only a small proportion of infected persons develop the characteristic elevated temperature, sore throat, and enlarged lymph nodes.

The blood of patients with infectious mononucleosis frequently contains antibodies capable of clumping red cells taken from sheep. These are called *heterophile antibodies*. Antibodies against the EB virus can also be detected in the blood. The diagnosis of infectious mononucleosis can be established on the basis of the clinical features of the febrile illness in a young adult with lymphadenopathy, the characteristic appearance of the blood smear, and the presence of heterophile and EB virus antibodies in the patient's blood. The disease is self-limited, and no specific treatment is available.

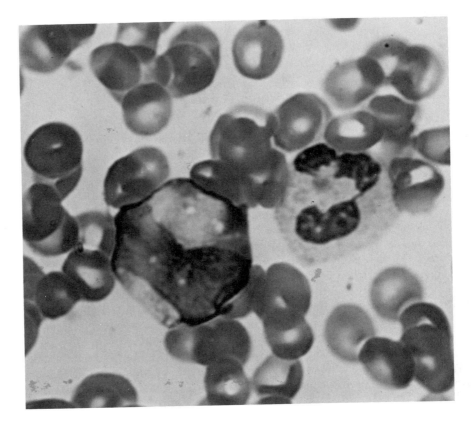

FIGURE 14–6

Large lymphocyte from subject with infectious mononucleosis, illustrating characteristic morphologic abnormalities, as described in text. Normal neutrophil appears to the right of the lymphocyte. (Original magnification × 1000.)

Neoplasms Affecting Lymph Nodes

Metastatic Tumors

Lymph nodes may be affected by the spread of metastatic tumor from malignant tumors arising in the breast, lung, colon, or other sites. The nodes first affected lie in the immediate drainage area of the tumor. The tumor may then spread to other, more distant lymph nodes through lymphatic channels and may eventually gain access to the circulatory system through the thoracic duct (figure 14–7).

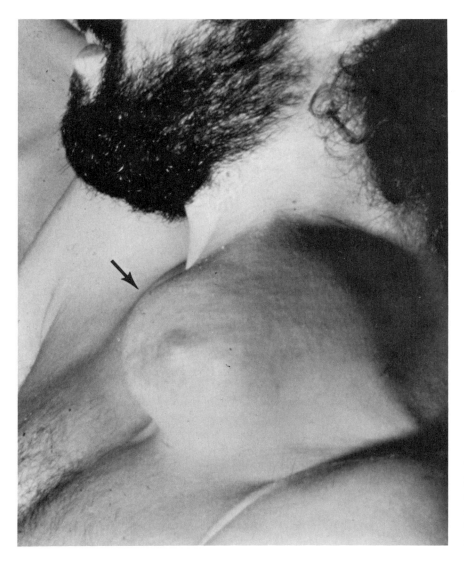

FIGURE 14–7

Large deposit of metastatic carcinoma (*arrow*) in supraclavicular lymph nodes of young man with carcinoma of testicle.

Malignant Lymphoma

A *lymphoma* is a primary malignant neoplasm of lymphoid tissue. The two main types of lymphoma are *Hodgkin's disease* and *non-Hodgkin's lymphoma* (described in chapter 10). A lymphoma usually begins in a single lymph node or a small group of nodes but often spreads to other nodes; frequently, the disease becomes widespread. The spread of lymphoma to multiple groups of nodes is probably a consequence of the recirculation of lymphocytes within the lymphatic system.

Lymphocytic Leukemia

Leukemia may develop from lymphoid cells in the bone marrow or from lymphoid tissue elsewhere in the body. Leukemia is covered in chapter 10.

Alteration of Immune Reactions in Diseases of the Lymphatic System

Because of the central role of the lymphatic system in immune reactions, many diseases affecting the lymphatic system diffusely, such as leukemias and lymphomas, are frequently associated with abnormal immune responses. These responses may be manifested either by production of autoantibodies directed against the red cells, white cells, or platelets of the affected individual or by loss of normal cell-mediated and humoral defenses, leading to an increased susceptibility to infection.

The Enlarged Lymph Node as a Diagnostic Problem

The patient who visits a physician because one or more lymph nodes are enlarged may present a difficult diagnostic problem. Lymph node enlargement may be a manifestation of a localized infection in the area drained by the node; it may be caused by a systemic infection with initial manifestations in the node; it may be caused by metastatic tumor in the node; or it may be caused by metastatic tumor in the node; or it may be an early manifestation of leukemia or malignant lymphoma. Often the cause of the lymphadenopathy can be determined by the physician from the clinical evaluation of the patient in conjunction with laboratory studies, including an examination of the peripheral blood. Sometimes the cause cannot be established, however, and the physician must perform a lymph node biopsy to determine the reason for the enlargement. The enlarged lymph node is surgically excised and submitted to the pathologist for microscopic examination and microbiologic studies. In difficult cases, more elaborate and sophisticated studies may be required. It is possible, for example, to determine whether a lymphocyte proliferation within a lymph node arose from a single abnormal lymphocyte that formed a clone of identical cells (a monoclonal proliferation), indicating a lymphoid neoplasm, or from many different lymphocytes that formed multiple clones of cells (a polyclonal proliferation), which is characteristic of a benign lymphocyte proliferation. Generally, the pathologist can make a specific diagnosis on the basis of such studies.

The Role of the Spleen in Protection against Systemic Infection

The spleen is an efficient blood-filtration system. Any bacteria or other foreign material that gain access to the bloodstream are promptly removed by the splenic phagocytes as the blood flows through the spleen. In addition, the spleen manufactures antibodies that facilitate prompt elimination of pathogenic organisms.

Sometimes it is necessary to remove the spleen. Splenectomy is often required to prevent fatal hemorrhage if the spleen has been lacerated in an automobile accident or other injury. Splenectomy is also frequently performed on patients with blood diseases characterized by excessive destruction of blood cells within the spleen, such as thrombocytopenic purpura and some types of hereditary hemolytic anemia. Splenectomy is sometimes performed on patients with Hodgkin's disease before treatment is started, to determine whether the spleen is affected by the disease. Splenic involvement may influence the type of treatment the patient receives.

Splenectomized persons are less able to eliminate bacteria that gain access to the bloodstream and do not produce antibodies as well as before removal of the spleen. Consequently, they are likely to develop serious bloodstream infections caused by pathogenic bacteria. These infections respond poorly to antibiotics. To reduce this risk, splenectomized patients are often immunized with bacterial vaccines, because high levels of antibacterial antibodies facilitate removal of bacteria from the circulation, and this can substitute for splenic function to some extent. Many physicians also recommend that a splenectomized individual either take antibiotics continuously or begin taking antibiotics at the first sign of a respiratory infection or other febrile illness.

Questions for Review

1. What types of cells are found in the circulating blood and what are their major functions?

2. What is anemia? What is the difference between an etiologic and a morphologic classification of anemia? Outline a simple etiologic classification of anemia.

3. What is an iron-deficiency anemia? How does it arise? How is it treated? What is the morphologic appearance of the red cells?

4. What is the effect of vitamin B_{12} and folic acid on blood cell maturation? What type of anemia results from deficiency of these vitamins?

5. What is the difference between an aplastic anemia and a hemolytic anemia? What is the difference between polycythemia and thrombocytopenia?

6. What is the lymphatic system? How is it organized? What are the major cells of the lymphatic system? What are the major functions of the lymphatic system?

7. What is the EB virus? What is its relation to infectious mononucleosis? What are the clinical manifestations of infectious mononucleosis? How is the disease treated?

8. A patient has an enlarged lymph node. What types of diseases could produce lymph node enlargement? How does the physician arrive at a diagnosis when the patient presents with enlarged lymph nodes?

9. What types of altered immune reaction are sometimes encountered in diseases of the lymphatic system?

10. What are the functions of the spleen? What are the adverse effects of splenectomy?

Supplementary Readings

Agre, P. 1990. Hereditary spherocytosis. *Journal of the American Medical Association* 262:2887–90. Reviews the genetics, pathophysiology, and clinical manifestations.

Allison, A. C., and Ferluga, J. 1976. How lymphocytes kill tumor cells. *New England Journal of Medicine* 295: 165–67. An interesting review article.

Berlin, N. I. 1975. Diagnosis and classification of the polycythemias. *Seminars in Hematology* 12:339–52. A good review article.

Beutler, E., Lichtman, M. A., Coller, B. S., and Kipps, T. J. (eds.). 1995. *Hematology.* 5th ed. New York: McGraw-Hill. A standard textbook.

Evans, A. S. 1972. Infectious mononucleosis and other mono-like syndromes. (Editorial.) *New England Journal of Medicine* 286:836–37. The clinical syndrome of infectious mononucleosis can be caused by EB virus, cytomegalovirus, and several other pathogenic organisms.

Likhite, V. V. 1976. Immunologic impairment and susceptibility to infection after splenectomy. *Journal of the American Medical Association* 236:1376–77. Describes the adverse effects of splenectomy on phagocytosis of bacteria and on antibody formation.

Marieb, E. N. 1992. *Human anatomy and physiology.* 2nd ed. Redwood City, Calif.: Benjamin/Cummings. Basic anatomy and physiology of the hematopoietic system.

Simon, T. L., and Garry, P. J. 1981. Iron stores in blood donors. *Journal of the American Medical Association* 245:2038–43. Frequent blood donations deplete iron stores.

Stites, D. P., Terr, A. I., and Parslow, T. G. 1994. *Basic and clinical immunology.* 8th ed. Norwalk, Conn.: Appleton & Lange. Deals with immunologic aspects of hematologic problems.

Chapter 14 ■ Outline Summary

Composition and Function of Human Blood / 379
Composition

Five quarts of blood in adult male.

Contains formed elements suspended in plasma.

Normal Hematopoiesis

Marrow comparable to manufacturing plant.

Requires raw materials: iron, vitamin B_{12}, and folic acid, protein.

Erythropoiesis regulated by erythropoietin.

Anemia / 382
Etiologic Classification

Inadequate raw materials.

"Factory" damaged or inoperative.

Excessive loss of red cells.

Morphologic Classification

Normocytic anemia: normal-sized cells.

Macrocytic anemia: larger than normal cells.

Hypochromic microcytic anemia: small cells with reduced hemoglobin content.

Iron-Deficiency Anemia / 384
Pathogenesis

Inadequate iron intake.

Depletion of iron stores: external blood loss.

Treatment

Establish cause and correct.

Supply supplementary iron.

Folic Acid Deficiency / 387
Pathogenesis

As a result of inadequate diet or poor absorption caused by intestinal disease.

Occasionally occurs in pregnancy.

Treatment

Establish cause and correct.

Supply supplementary folic acid.

Vitamin B_{12} Deficiency / 387
Mechanism of Vitamin B_{12} Absorption

Vitamin B_{12} in food combines with intrinsic factor in gastric juice.

Vitamin B_{12}-intrinsic factor complex absorbed in ilium.

Pernicious anemia: lack of intrinsic factor.

Gastric resection/bypass: lack of intrinsic factor.

Distal small bowel resection or disease: impaired absorption of B_{12}-intrinsic factor complex.

Treatment

Supply vitamin B_{12} intramuscularly.

Bone Marrow Suppression, Damage, or Infiltration / 388
Pathogenesis

Anemia of chronic disease.

Marrow injured by drugs or chemicals.

Marrow infiltrated by tumor.

Marrow replaced by fibrous tissue.

Treatment

Blood transfusions.

No specific treatment in most cases.

Bone marrow transplant in highly selected cases.

Acute Blood Loss or Accelerated Blood Destruction / 389
Acute Blood Loss

Usually the result of massive bleeding from gastrointestinal tract or uterus.

Lost blood regenerated if iron stores adequate.

Hemolytic Anemia

Hereditary hemolytic anemia: genetic abnormality in red cells prevents normal survival.

Shape abnormalities: hereditary spherocytosis and ovalocytosis.

Abnormal hemoglobins: sickle cell anemia.

Defective hemoglobin synthesis: thalassemia.

Enzyme defects: glucose-6-phosphate dehydrogenase deficiency predisposes to episodes of acute hemolysis.

Acquired hemolytic anemia.

Caused by antibodies.

As a result of mechanical trauma: associated with marked splenomegaly or artificial heart valves.

Diagnostic Evaluation of Anemia / 394
Approach

History and physical examination.

Complete blood count.

Morphologic classification of anemia: clue to etiology.

Reticulocyte count: measures red cell regeneration.

Bone marrow study: may be required to evaluate hematopoiesis.

Evaluation of blood loss from gastrointestinal tract:

Stool examination.

X-ray studies of gastrointestinal tract.

Other diagnostic procedures as indicated.

Polycythemia / 394
Secondary Polycythemia

Decreased arterial oxygen saturation leads to compensatory increase in red cells:

Chronic lung disease.

Some types of congenital heart disease.

Increased erythropoietin production by renal tumor.

Primary Polycythemia

Diffuse marrow hyperplasia of unknown cause.

Overproduction of white cells, platelets, and red cells.

Some cases evolve into granulocytic leukemia.

Complications

As a result of increased blood viscosity.

Increased tendency to thromboses.

Treatment

Primary polycythemia treated by drugs that suppress marrow function.

Secondary polycythemia treated by periodic removal of excess blood.

Thrombocytopenia / 395
Classification

Secondary: as a result of marrow damage or infiltration.

Primary: usually associated with antiplatelet autoantibodies.

Structure and Function of the Lymphatic System / 396
Lymph Nodes

Function as filters.

Grouped where lymph channels converge.

Clear foreign material from lymph.

Spleen

Specialized to filter blood.

Phagocytosis of worn-out red cells.

Thymus

Located at base of heart.

Concerned with prenatal development of the lymphatic system.

Development of the Lymphatic System

T and B lymphocytes formed from precursors in bone marrow.

T lymphocyte precursors processed by thymus.

T and B lymphocytes populate spleen, lymph nodes, and other lymphoid tissues.

Diseases of the Lymphatic System / 397
Lymphadenitis

Infection spreads to regional lymph nodes.

Nodes become enlarged and tender.

Infectious Mononucleosis

Caused by EB virus.

Causes enlargement and tenderness of nodes.

Virus infects B lymphocytes; T lymphocytes and antibodies destroy virus.

Neoplasms

Metastatic carcinoma: tumor spreads from primary sites to regional nodes.

Malignant lymphoma: see chapter 10.

Lymphatic leukemia: see chapter 10.

Alteration of Immune Reactions in Diseases of the Lymphatic System / 400

Abnormal Immune Response

Autoantibodies formed against red cells, white cells, and platelets.

Loss of cell-mediated or humoral immunity or both.

The Enlarged Lymph Node as a Diagnostic Problem / 400

Diagnostic Possibilities

Localized infection.

Systemic infection.

Lymphoma.

Metastatic tumor.

Investigation

Clinical evaluation.

Laboratory studies.

Lymph node biopsy.

Role of the Spleen in Protection against Systemic Infection / 401

Functions of the Spleen

Phagocytosis.

Antibody formation.

Reasons for Splenectomy

Traumatic injury.

Patients with Hodgkin's disease prior to treatment.

Effects of Splenectomy

Less-efficient elimination of bacteria from bloodstream.

Impaired production of antibodies.

Predisposition to systemic bloodstream infection.

Treatment of Splenectomized Patients

Immunize with antibacterial vaccines.

Antibiotic prophylaxis.

15

The Respiratory System

Learning Objectives

1. Explain the basic anatomic and physiologic principles of ventilation and gas exchange.
2. Describe the causes, clinical effects, complications, and treatment of pneumothorax and atelectasis.
3. Describe the histologic characteristics of a tuberculous infection. Explain the possible outcome of an infection. Describe methods of diagnosis and treatment.
4. Differentiate between bronchitis and bronchiectasis.
5. List the anatomic and physiologic derangements in chronic obstructive lung disease. Explain its pathogenesis. Describe the clinical manifestations and methods of treatment.
6. Describe the pathogenesis and manifestations of bronchial asthma and the respiratory distress syndrome.
7. Explain the causes and effects of pulmonary fibrosis. Describe the special problems associated with asbestosis.
8. List the major types of lung carcinoma. Describe the clinical manifestations of lung carcinoma and explain the principles of treatment.

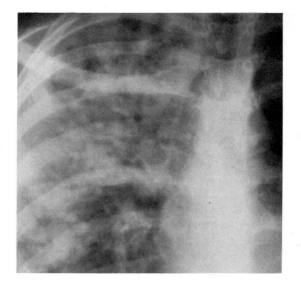

Chapter 15 ▪ Contents

Normal life processes require that an adequate supply of oxygen be delivered to the tissues and that the waste products of cell metabolism be removed. These functions are carried out by a cooperative effort of the respiratory and circulatory systems. The respiratory system oxygenates the blood and removes carbon dioxide. The circulatory system transports these gases in the bloodstream.

The lungs consist of two distinct components: a system of tubes whose chief function is to conduct air into and out of the lungs and the **alveoli** (singular, *alveolus*), where oxygen and carbon dioxide are exchanged between air and the pulmonary capillaries. Just as a tree branches progressively and ends in a foliage of leaves, so the conducting tubes branch repeatedly and terminate in clusters of pulmonary alveoli.

Structure and Function of the Lungs

Bronchi, Bronchioles, and Alveoli

The largest conducting tubes are called **bronchi** (singular, *bronchus*). Tubes less than about 1 mm in diameter are called **bronchioles** (little bronchi), and the smallest bronchioles, which function only for conduction of air, are called *terminal bronchioles*. The tubes distal to the terminal bronchioles are called *respiratory bronchioles* because they have alveoli in their walls and not only transport air, but also participate in gas exchange. Each terminal bronchiole gives rise to several *respiratory bronchioles,* which branch to form *alveolar ducts.* The alveolar ducts in turn subdivide and give rise to *pulmonary alveoli* (figure 15–1).

Each alveolus is a small air space surrounded by a thin wall, the *alveolar septum,* which is composed of a network of capillaries supported by a few connective-tissue fibers and lined by a layer of epithelial cells (figure 15–2). Each alveolus contains a relatively small volume of air surrounded by a large network of capillaries, conditions that promote rapid diffusion of oxygen and carbon dioxide between alveolar air and pulmonary capillaries as the blood flows through the lung. Any condition that enlarges the pulmonary alveoli or reduces the number of pulmonary capillaries impedes the efficiency of pulmonary ventilation.

Two types of cells line the alveoli. Most are flat squamous cells. A few are larger secretory cells that produce a lipid material called **surfactant,** which reduces surface tension. *Surface tension* is the attraction between molecules of a fluid that causes the fluid to aggregate into droplets instead of spreading as a thin film. The surface tension of the molecules in the fluid lining the alveoli would normally tend to pull the alveolar walls together. This effect would hinder expansion of the lungs during inspiration and would cause the alveoli to collapse during expiration owing to the cohesive force of the water molecules. Surfactant acts somewhat like a detergent by lowering the surface tension of the fluid and thereby facilitating respiration.

FIGURE 15–1

Structure of terminal air passages. The interior of one alveolar duct is illustrated in cut-away view.

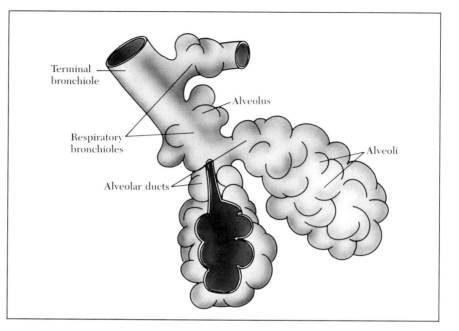

FIGURE 15–2

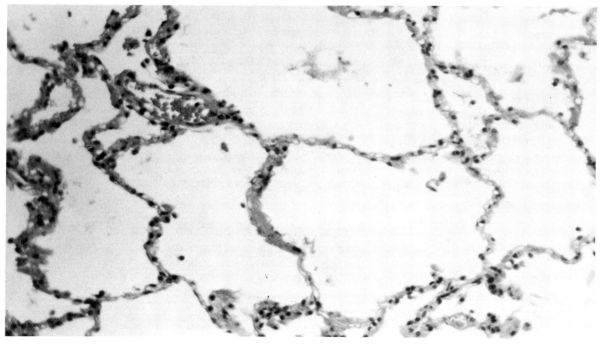

Histologic structure of the lung, illustrating alveoli and thin alveolar septa containing pulmonary capillaries. (Original magnification × 100.)

The functional unit of the lung is called an **acinus.** It is formed by the cluster of respiratory bronchioles, alveolar ducts, and alveoli derived from a single terminal bronchiole. A *lung lobule* is a small group of terminal bronchioles and the acini that arise from them. Lobules are partially circumscribed by connective-tissue septa and are easiest to identify just beneath the pleura, where the connective-tissue septa defining the lobules can be easily seen.

Respiration has two functions, corresponding to the two structural components of the lungs:

1. *Ventilation,* which concerns the movement of air into and out of the lungs.
2. *Gas exchange* between alveolar air and pulmonary capillaries.

Both ventilation and gas exchange must function normally if respiration is to be effective.

Ventilation

Air is moved into and out of the lungs by the bellows action of the *thoracic cage.* During inspiration, the ribs become more horizontal, owing to the action of the intercostal muscles, and the diaphragm descends. Consequently, the volume of the thoracic cage increases. The lungs expand to fill the larger intrathoracic space, and air is drawn into the lungs through the trachea and bronchi. During expiration, the ribs become more vertical and the diaphragm rises. The volume of the thoracic cage is reduced. The lungs, which conform to the size of the thorax, also decrease in volume, and air is expelled.

Normal respiratory movements require that respiratory muscles, innervation of the muscles, and mobility of the thoracic cage be normal. Ventilation is impaired if the nerve supply to the respiratory muscles is damaged by disease, as in poliomyelitis, or if the respiratory muscles undergo atrophy and degeneration, as in some uncommon types of muscle disease. Ventilation is also impaired if the thoracic cage is immobile. For example, a person buried in sand up to his neck will suffocate because he is unable to move his thoracic cage and therefore cannot move air into and out of his lungs.

Gas Exchange

Oxygen and carbon dioxide, along with nitrogen and water vapor, are in the atmospheric air that we breathe, in the air within the pulmonary alveoli, and in the blood. At sea level, the atmospheric pressure exerted by the mixture of all the gases is 760 mm Hg. Each gas exerts a proportionate part of the total atmospheric pressure, depending on its concentration in the mixture of gases. For example, the concentration of oxygen in atmospheric air is 20 percent. Therefore, the pressure exerted by oxygen is 20 percent of the total pressure exerted by all the gases ($0.20 \times 760 = 152$ mm Hg). The part of the total atmospheric pressure exerted by a gas is called the *partial pressure* of the gas. Partial pressure is usually expressed by the letter "P" preceding the chemical symbol for the gas, as for example PO_2 152 mm Hg.

Gases diffuse between blood, tissues, and pulmonary alveoli because of differences in their partial pressures. Venous blood returning from the tissues is low in oxygen (PO_2 40 mm Hg) and high in carbon dioxide (PCO_2 47 mm Hg). This blood is pumped through the pulmonary capillaries, where it comes into contact with the air in the pulmonary alveoli. Alveolar air has a much higher concentration of oxygen (PO_2 105 mm Hg) but a lower concentration of carbon dioxide (PCO_2 35 mm Hg). Therefore, oxygen diffuses from alveolar air into pulmonary capillaries, and carbon dioxide diffuses from pulmonary capillaries into the aveoli. The situation is reversed in the tissues. The tissue oxygen concentration is much lower (PO_2 about 20 mm Hg), and the carbon dioxide concentration is much higher (PCO_2 about 60 mm Hg); so oxygen diffuses into the tissues from the blood, and carbon dioxide diffuses in the opposite direction.

Exchange of gases between alveolar air and pulmonary capillaries is accomplished by diffusion across the alveolar membrane. Efficient gas exchange requires (1) a large capillary surface area in contact with alveolar air, (2) unimpeded diffusion of gases across the alveolar membrane, (3) normal pulmonary blood flow, and (4) normal pulmonary alveoli. The spongy structure of the lungs, in which each tiny air sac is surrounded by a large network of capillaries, provides the large surface area required for efficient gas exchange (figure 15–3A). Destruction of alveolar septa leads to coalescence of alveoli and reduction in size of the capillary network surrounding the alveoli, resulting in less-efficient gas exchange (figure 15–3B).

If the alveolar septa are thickened and scarred, the diffusion of gases across the thickened alveolar membranes is impeded (figure 15–3C). Gas exchange is also impaired if pulmonary blood flow to a portion of the lung is obstructed, as might be caused by a pulmonary embolus obstructing a large pulmonary artery or by blockage of pulmonary capillaries by fat emboli or foreign material (figure 15–3D). If the pulmonary alveoli become filled with fluid or inflammatory exudate, inspired air cannot enter the diseased alveoli, and pulmonary gas exchange is impeded (figure 15–3E).

Pulmonary Function Tests

Pulmonary function tests can be used to evaluate the efficiency of pulmonary ventilation and pulmonary gas exchange. Pulmonary ventilation is usually tested by measuring the volume of air that can be moved into and out of the lung under standard conditions. Two commonly used measurements are **vital capacity,** which measures the maximum volume of air that can be expelled after a deep inspiration, and the **one-second forced expiratory volume** (FEV_1), which measures the maximum volume of air that can be expelled in one second. If the bronchioles are narrowed by inflammation or spasm, impeding the movement of air out of the lungs, FEV_1 is often reduced. Specialized tests can measure the total volume of air in the lungs and the volume of air remaining in the lungs after a maximum expiration.

One can also measure the concentrations of oxygen and carbon dioxide (O_2 and CO_2) in the patient's arterial blood in order to determine the effi-

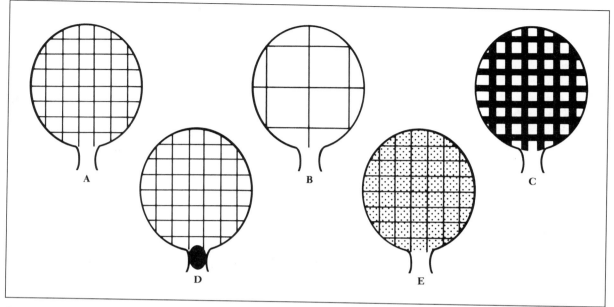

FIGURE 15–3

Types of structural and functional abnormalities that adversely affect pulmonary gas exchange. **A,** Normal alveoli and pulmonary blood flow. **B,** Destruction of alveolar septa, leading to coarsening of alveolar structure with corresponding reduction in size of the pulmonary capillary bed. **C,** Fibrous thickening and scarring of alveolar septa, impeding diffusion of gases across alveolar membrane. **D,** Obstruction of pulmonary blood flow to a portion of the lung. **E,** Alveoli filled with fluid or inflammatory exudate.

ciency of gas exchange in the lungs. In chronic pulmonary disease, oxygenation of the blood is inefficient. Oxygen concentration is reduced and arterial oxygen saturation is decreased correspondingly. Often the arterial PCO_2 also is higher than normal because carbon dioxide is inefficiently eliminated by the lungs. Arterial blood for analysis is usually collected by inserting a small needle into the radial artery in the wrist and withdrawing a small amount of blood.

The Pleural Cavity

The lungs are covered by a thin membrane called the **pleura,** which also extends over the internal surface of the chest wall. Because the lungs fill the thoracic cavity, the two pleural surfaces are in contact. The potential space between the lung and chest wall is the *pleural cavity.* Normally, the apposing pleural surfaces move smoothly over one another. In disease, however, the pleural surfaces may become roughened owing to inflammation and may become adherent. Inflammatory exudate may accumulate in the pleural cavity and separate the two pleural surfaces.

Intrapleural and Intrapulmonary Pressures

The lungs are held in an expanded position within the pleural cavity because the pressure within the pleural cavity (the *intrapleural pressure*) is less than the pressure of the air within the lungs (*intrapulmonary pressure*). The pressure differences develop when the thoracic cavity enlarges after birth. When respirations are initiated, the size of the thoracic cavity increases. The lungs become filled with air at atmospheric pressure and expand to fill the enlarged thoracic cavity, stretching the elastic tissue within the lungs. The tendency of the stretched lung to pull away from the chest wall and return to its original contracted state creates a slight vacuum within the pleural cavity. Because the intrapleural pressure is slightly less than atmospheric pressure, it is often called "negative pressure."

Pneumothorax

Because the intrapleural pressure is subatmospheric, air flows into the pleural space if the lung or chest wall is punctured. When this occurs, the subatmospheric ("negative") pressure that holds the lung in the expanded position is lost, and the lung collapses because the elastic tissue within the lung contracts. This condition, which is called **pneumothorax** (*pneumo =* air), may follow any type of lung injury or pulmonary disease that allows air to escape from the lungs into the pleural space. It may also result from a stab wound or some other penetrating injury to the chest wall that permits atmospheric air to enter the pleural space (figure 15–4).

Occasionally, a pneumothorax occurs without apparent cause. This is called *spontaneous pneumothorax.* Most cases occur in young healthy men, usually as a result of rupture of a small, air-filled, subpleural bleb at the apex of the lung.

The sudden escape of air into the pleural cavity that is associated with any type of pneumothorax usually causes *chest pain* and often some *shortness of breath.* The breath sounds, which normally can be heard with a stethoscope when the air moves in and out of the lung during respiration, are diminished on the affected side. A chest x-ray reveals partial or complete collapse of the lung and the presence of air in the pleural cavity (figure 15–5).

The development of a positive (higher than atmospheric) pressure in the pleural cavity, called *tension pneumothorax,* may accompany any type of pneumothorax. This dangerous complication may occur if the lung has been perforated in such a way that the pleural tear acts as a one-way valve (figure 15–6). In this circumstance, air flows through the perforation into the pleural cavity as the pleural pressure falls on inspiration. On expiration, however, the intrapleural pressure rises and forces the edges of the pleural tear together, trapping the air within the pleural space. With each inspiration, more air enters the pleural cavity but cannot escape. Eventually the pleural cavity becomes overdistended with air under pressure, and the affected lung collapses completely. As the pressure builds up in the pleural cavity, the heart and mediastinal structures are displaced away from the side of the pneumothorax and encroach on the opposite pleural cavity, impairing the expan-

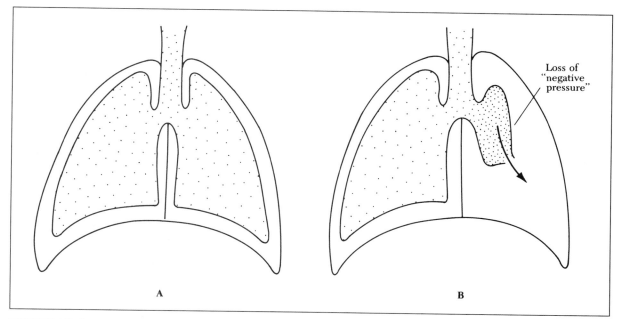

FIGURE 15–4

A, Normal relation of lung to chest wall. Pleural space is exaggerated, and surfaces are normally in contact. "Negative pressure" is a result of the tendency of the stretched lung to pull away from the chest wall. **B,** Pneumothorax caused by a perforating injury of lung.

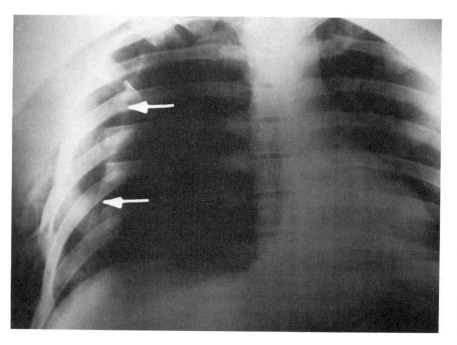

FIGURE 15–5

X-ray illustrating pneumothorax secondary to multiple rib fractures in which fractured ribs have torn underlying lung. *Arrows* indicate surface of lung that is no longer in contact with chest wall.

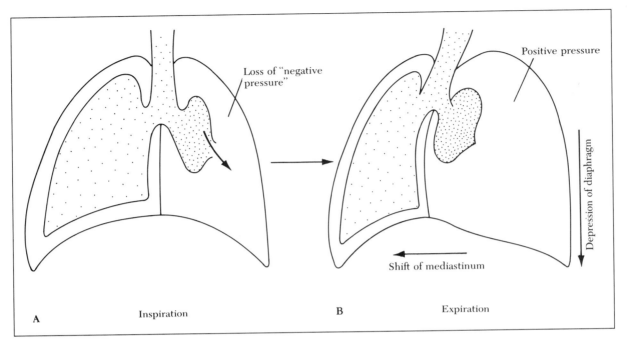

FIGURE 15–6

Pathogenesis of tension pneumothorax. **A,** Air enters pleural cavity during inspiration as intrapleural pressure falls. **B,** Rising intrapleural pressure on expiration closes the pleural tear, trapping air within the pleural space. Diaphragm on affected side is displaced downward. Trachea and mediastinal structures are shifted away from side of pneumothorax and encroach on opposite pleural cavity.

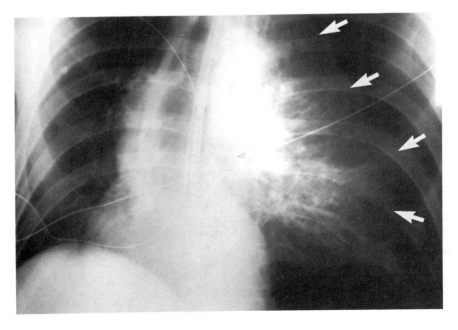

FIGURE 15–7

X-ray of tension pneumothorax. *Arrows* indicate surface of collapsed lung. Note low diaphragm on affected side and displacement of mediastinal structures.

sion of the opposite lung (figure 15–7). A tension pneumothorax can be fatal if it is not recognized and treated promptly by evacuating the trapped air to relieve the pressure.

A pneumothorax is usually treated by inserting a tube into the pleural cavity through an incision in the chest wall. The tube prevents accumulation of air in the pleural cavity and aids reexpansion of the lung. The tube is connected to an apparatus that permits the air to be expelled from the pleural cavity during expiration but prevents the air from being sucked back into the pleural cavity during inspiration. The tube is left in place until the tear in the lung heals and no more air escapes. Any air remaining in the pleural cavity is gradually reabsorbed into the bloodstream, and the lung reexpands as the air is absorbed. Sometimes a slight vacuum is applied to the tube in order to evacuate the air more rapidly and hasten reexpansion of the lung.

Atelectasis literally means incomplete expansion of the lung (*ateles* = incomplete + *ectasia* = expansion). It refers to a collapse of parts of the lung. There are two types:

Atelectasis

1. *Obstructive atelectasis,* which results from bronchial obstruction
2. *Compression atelectasis,* which is the result of external compression of the lung

Obstructive Atelectasis

Complete blockage of a bronchus by thick mucous secretions, by a tumor, or by an aspirated foreign object prevents air from entering or leaving the alveoli supplied by the blocked bronchus, and the air already present is gradually absorbed into the blood flowing through the lungs. As a result, the part of the lung supplied by the blocked bronchus gradually collapses as the air is absorbed. The volume of the affected pleural cavity also decreases correspondingly, causing the mediastinal structures to shift toward the side of the atelectasis and the diaphragm to elevate on the affected side (figure 15–8). If the bronchial obstruction is relieved promptly, the lung reexpands normally. This is illustrated by the following unusual case of obstructive atelectasis, which was initially thought to be secondary to an obstructing lung carcinoma.

A sixty-six-year-old man with a long history of heavy smoking and excessive alcohol consumption consulted his physician because of shortness of breath. He was found to have an atelectasis of the left lung (figure 15–9). An obstructing carcinoma was suspected, and a bronchoscopic examination was performed. A soft rubber stopper was found obstructing the left main bronchus. The subject apparently had been chewing the stopper while intoxicated and had accidentally inhaled it. The stopper was removed. An x-ray taken the following day revealed that the lung had reexpanded completely.

CASE 15–1

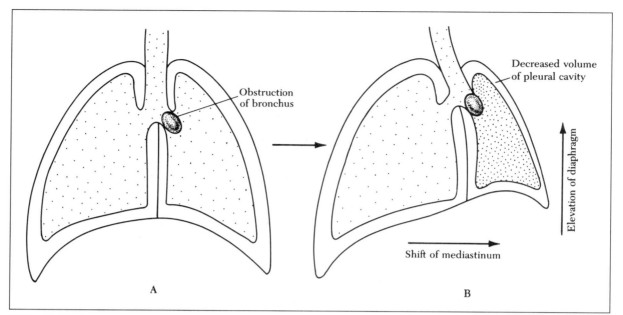

FIGURE 15–8

Atelectasis caused by bronchial obstruction. **A,** Blockage of bronchus prevents aeration of lung supplied by obstructed bronchus. **B,** Absorption of air causes collapse of lung and corresponding reduction in size of pleural cavity. Diaphragm rises and mediastinum shifts toward the affected side.

FIGURE 15–9

Complete atelectasis of left lung caused by obstruction of left main bronchus (case 15–1). **A,** Chest x-ray before development of atelectasis. **B,** Atelectasis of entire left lung. Collapsed left lung appears dense because the air has been absorbed. Left half of diaphragm is elevated. Trachea and mediastinal structures are shifted toward the side of the collapse.

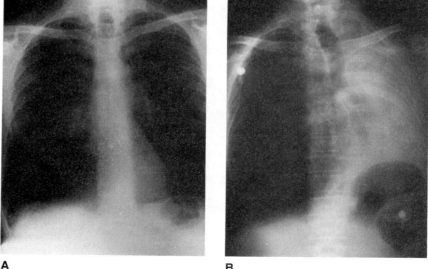

Atelectasis sometimes develops as a postoperative complication. Because of postoperative pain, the patient does not cough or breathe deeply and mucous secretions accumulate in the bronchi (figure 15–10). To prevent this problem, the physician encourages the postoperative patient to breathe deeply and cough frequently, to keep the respiratory passages clear of secretions.

Compression Atelectasis

Compression atelectasis results when fluid, blood, or air accumulates in the pleural cavity, reducing its volume and thereby preventing full expansion of the lung.

Pneumonia is an inflammation of the lung characterized by the same type of vascular changes and exudation of fluid and cells as that of inflammation in any other location. However, the inflammatory process is influenced by

Pneumonia

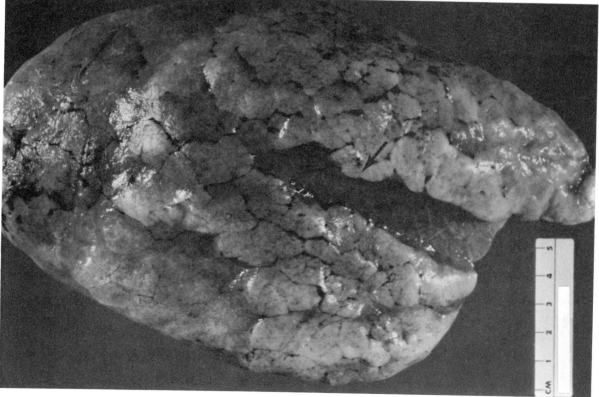

FIGURE 15–10

Atelectasis of several lung lobules caused by retained mucous secretions. Note the contrast between the pale, normally aerated lung and the atelectatic area (*arrow*), which appears dark and depressed.

the spongy character of the lungs. The inflammatory exudate spreads unimpeded through the lung, filling the alveoli, and the affected portions of lung become relatively solid (termed *consolidation*) (figure 15–11). The inflammatory exudate may reach the pleural surface in some areas, causing irritation and inflammation of the pleura; sometimes inflammatory exudate accumulates in the pleural space.

Classification of Pneumonia

Pneumonia may be classified in several ways:

1. By etiology
2. By anatomic distribution of the inflammatory process
3. By predisposing factors that led to its development

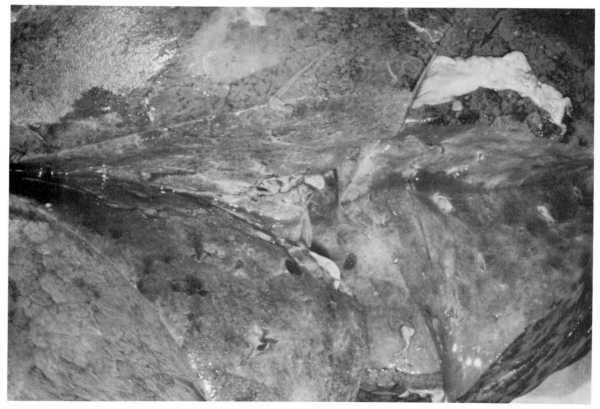

FIGURE 15–11

Consolidation of lung as a result of pneumonia. Lung has been incised and cut surfaces are exposed. *Arrow* indicates deposit of fibrin on pleura.

The etiologic classification is the most important because it serves as a guide to treatment. Pneumonia may be caused by bacteria, viruses, or fungi. Whenever possible, the pneumonia is classified in greater detail by designating the exact organism responsible for the disease, such as pneumococcus or *Staphylococcus*.

The anatomic classification describes whether an entire lobe of the lung is affected, called *lobar pneumonia,* or only the parts of one or more lobes (lung lobules) immediately adjacent to the bronchi, called *bronchopneumonia.*

Classification of pneumonia by predisposing factors is common. Any condition associated with poor lung ventilation and retention of bronchial secretions predisposes an individual to the development of pneumonia. *Postoperative pneumonia* is a pulmonary inflammation that develops in the postsurgical patient who is unable to cough or breathe deeply because of pain; the resultant poor ventilation and retention of secretions lead to pneumonia. *Aspiration pneumonia* occurs when a foreign body, food, vomit, or other irritating substance is aspirated into the lung. *Obstructive pneumonia* develops in the lung distal to an area where a bronchus is narrowed or obstructed. Blockage of a bronchus by a tumor or foreign body leads to poor aeration and to retention of bronchial secretions in the obstructed portion of lung.

Clinical Features of Pneumonia

The signs and symptoms of pneumonia are those of any systemic infection. The patient is ill and has an elevated temperature, and the number of white blood cells in the peripheral blood is frequently higher than normal. Bronchial inflammation is evident, manifested by cough and purulent sputum. If the inflammatory process involves the pleura, the patient experiences pain on respiration because the inflamed pleural surfaces rub against each other. The patient may also have symptoms related to partial loss of lung function caused by consolidation of part of the lung resulting from the accumulation of inflammatory cells within the alveoli. Oxygenation of the blood is impaired, and the patient may become quite short of breath.

Pneumonia is treated by correcting any predisposing factors that contributed to the development of the pulmonary infection and administering appropriate antibiotic therapy.

Legionnaires' disease is a type of pneumonia caused by a fastidious gram-negative organism called *Legionella pneumophila.* The infectious agent is transmitted in the air, and the infection frequently occurs in outbreaks but is not transmitted directly from person to person. The disease was first recognized in 1976 among people attending an American legion convention in Philadelphia. After the infectious agent was identified, it was determined in retrospect that this same organism had in the past caused other outbreaks of pneumonia, but the infectious agent was not identified at the time. Clinically, the disease is characterized by the usual symptoms of a pulmonary infection, and the chest x-ray reveals evidence of pneumonia. The infection responds to appropriate antibiotics.

Pneumocystis Pneumonia

Humans and many animals harbor *Pneumocystis carinii,* a protozoan parasite of low pathogenicity. The parasite does not affect normal persons but may cause serious pulmonary infections in susceptible individuals. Those at risk include adults whose immune defenses have been impaired by disease, such as by AIDS (described in chapter 8), or by administration of immunosuppressive drugs, and premature infants in whom immune defenses are poorly developed.

The life cycle of the parasite is complex. The most easily recognized form is a round or cup-shaped cyst about the size of a red blood cell that cannot be identified by routine (hematoxylin and eosin) stains but can be demonstrated by means of special stains containing silver compounds. Within the cysts are small structures called *sporozoites,* which are released from the cyst and mature to form larger structures called *trophozoites.* Some trophozoites give rise to more cysts, repeating the cycle. Others attack and injure the cells lining the pulmonary alveoli, causing a mild inflammatory reaction within the alveolar septa, which leads to exudation of large amounts of protein-rich material that accumulates within the alveoli. The parasites, intermixed in the alveolar exudate but unstained by routine stains, appear as pale areas within the brightly stained exudate, imparting a foamy, "soap bubble" appearance to the exudate. Special stains, however, demonstrate that the soap bubbles represent *Pneumocystis* cysts and may also reveal central clusters of sporozoites, which appear as dark dots within the centers of the cysts (figure 15–12).

Clinically, pneumocystis pneumonia is characterized by progressive shortness of breath and cough in a person whose immunologic defenses are impaired and who is at high risk of developing the disease. Evidence of pulmonary consolidation caused by the alveolar exudate can be demonstrated by x-ray. The diagnosis of pneumocystis pneumonia is established by biopsy of lung tissue obtained by bronchoscopy. Histologic study of the biopsy material reveals the characteristic foamy alveolar exudate containing large numbers of parasites, as demonstrated by special stains. Often the parasite also can be demonstrated in material aspirated from the bronchi by bronchoscopy. It is much more difficult to demonstrate the organisms in sputum because they are enmeshed in the alveolar exudate and do not escape from the alveoli. The infection is always very serious and is often life threatening because it affects persons whose ability to respond to infection is greatly impaired. Treatment consists of administration of drugs that inhibit the growth of the organism.

Tuberculosis

Pulmonary tuberculosis is a special type of pneumonia caused by an acid-fast bacterium, the tubercle bacillus *Mycobacterium tuberculosis*. Because the tubercle bacillus has a capsule composed of waxes and fatty substances, it is more resistant to destruction than many other organisms. The body's response to the tubercle bacillus also differs from the usual acute inflammatory reaction. Monocytes accumulate around the bacteria; many of them

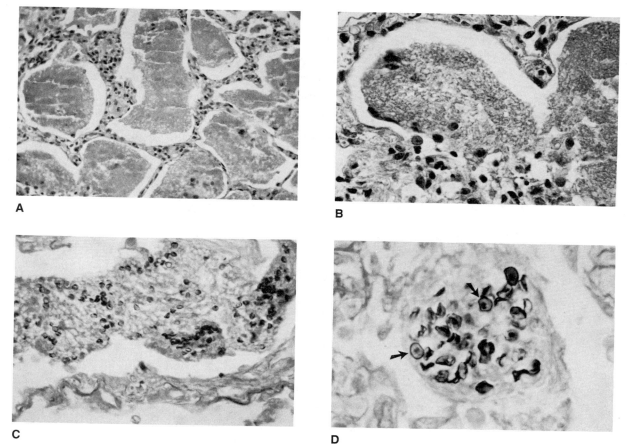

FIGURE 15–12

Pneumocystis pneumonia. **A,** Pulmonary alveoli filled with dense protein exudate (original magnification × 100). **B,** Higher magnification illustrating the foamy character of protein exudate caused by masses of pneumocystis that are not visualized by routine stains (original magnification × 400). **C,** Demonstration of *Pneumocystis carinii* cysts within exudate by means of silver-containing stains (original magnification × 400). **D,** Structure of cysts revealed by silver stains. Central dark dots within cysts (*arrow*) are clusters of sporozoites (original magnification × 1000).

fuse, forming rather characteristic large multinucleated cells called *giant cells.* Lymphocytes and plasma cells also accumulate, and fibrous tissue proliferates around the central cluster of monocytes and giant cells. The central portion of the cellular aggregation usually becomes necrotic. This characteristic nodular mass of cells with central necrosis is called *granuloma,* and the inflammatory process is called a *granulomatous inflammation* (figure 15–13). The granulomatous response to the tubercle bacillus, and the necrosis within the granulomas, indicates the development of cell-mediated immu-

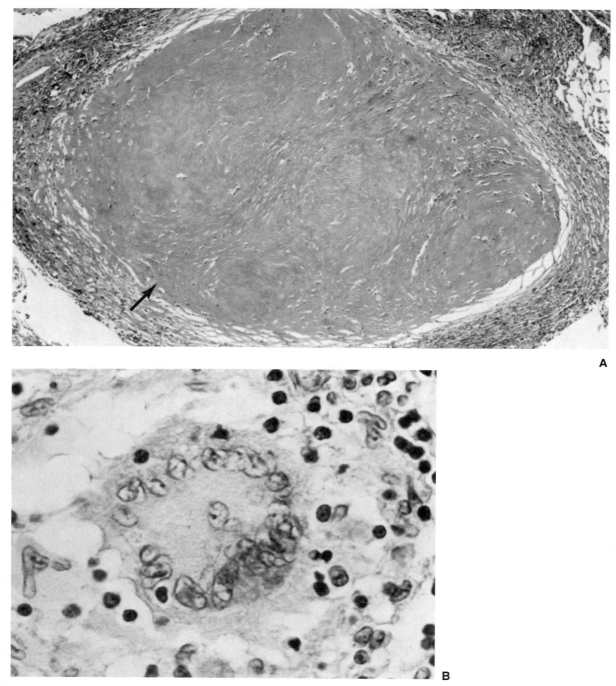

A

B

FIGURE 15–13

A, Granuloma as a result of tuberculosis. Central part (*arrow*) consists of necrotic tissue. (Original magnification ×
40.) **B,** Multinucleated giant cell characteristic of tuberculous infection. (Original magnification × 400.)

nity against the organism, which is the primary immune defense against the tubercle bacillus.

Course of a Tuberculous Infection

The initial infection is acquired from organisms inhaled in airborne droplets that have been coughed or sneezed into the air by a person with active tuberculosis who is discharging organisms into the environment. The organisms lodge within the pulmonary alveoli where they proceed to multiply. Initially, the organisms introduced into the lungs do not elicit a marked inflammatory reaction, because they do not produce any toxins or destructive enzymes that damage the tissues. Macrophages phagocytose the bacteria but are unable to destroy them; they may even carry the organisms to other parts of the lung and into the regional lymph nodes. After several weeks, however, a cell-mediated immunity develops. Sensitized lymphocytes attract and activate macrophages, which acquire a greatly enhanced phagocytic and destructive capability. The activated macrophages attack and destroy many of the organisms, forming characteristic granulomas containing areas of necrosis and surrounded by a rim of fibrous tissue. In the majority of cases, the infection is arrested; the granulomas in the lung and regional lymph nodes heal with scarring, often followed by calcification of the granulomas. In most cases, the infection does not cause any symptoms, and the person may be unaware of the infection. Sometimes the granuloma in the lung is large enough to be identified in a chest x-ray (figure 15–14), but often the area of infection is too small to be detected in an x-ray. The positive skin test (Mantoux test), which reveals a hypersensitivity to the proteins of the tubercle bacillus, may be the only evidence of recent infection.

Cell-mediated immunity generally controls the infection, and the arrested infection may never cause any further problems. The healed granulomas, however, may contain small numbers of viable organisms, and the infection may become reactivated, leading to progressive pulmonary tuberculosis if the body's cell-mediated immunity declines.

Not all primary infections respond as favorably. If a large number of organisms is inhaled or if the body's defenses are inadequate, the inflammation will progress, causing more extensive destruction of lung tissue (figure 15–15). Often the granulomatous inflammatory process makes contact with a bronchus, and the necrotic inflammatory tissue is discharged into it. A cavity then forms within the lung, surrounded by granulomatous inflammatory tissue containing masses of the tubercle bacilli. People who have active progressive tuberculosis with a tuberculous cavity can infect others because they are discharging large numbers of tubercle bacilli in their sputum.

In a tuberculous infection of the lung, organisms are often carried in lymphatic channels from the lung into the peribronchial lymph nodes, leading to a tuberculous inflammation in the regional lymph nodes.

Most cases of active progressive pulmonary tuberculosis do not result from the initial infection. They develop in persons who have been infected at some time in the past and have developed a cell-mediated immunity

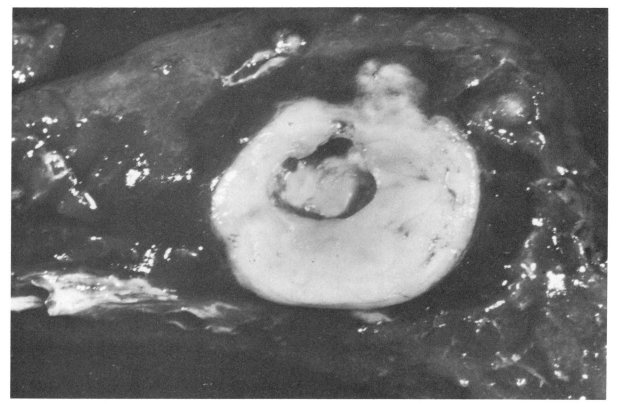

FIGURE 15–14

Old healed granuloma as a result of tuberculosis. Center of granuloma has undergone cystic degeneration.

directed against the organism. In the past, tuberculosis in previously infected persons was called reinfection tuberculosis because physicians believed that the active tuberculosis was caused by a new infection with the tubercle bacillus in a person who had been infected previously with the organism. Indeed, some cases of tuberculosis in previously infected persons are actually new infections. However, most cases of active tuberculosis in older patients result from a reactivation of an old infection rather than a new infection with the tubercle bacillus. It is well known that old tuberculous lesions that appear completely healed may harbor tubercle bacilli. If the resistance of the individual is lowered by AIDS or other debilitating disease, by treatment with adrenal corticosteroids, or by other factors, an apparently healed focus of tuberculosis may flare up and lead to active progressive tuberculosis.

Miliary Tuberculosis and Tuberculous Pneumonia

Miliary tuberculosis and tuberculous pneumonia are two uncommon but extremely serious forms of tuberculosis. *Miliary tuberculosis* develops if a

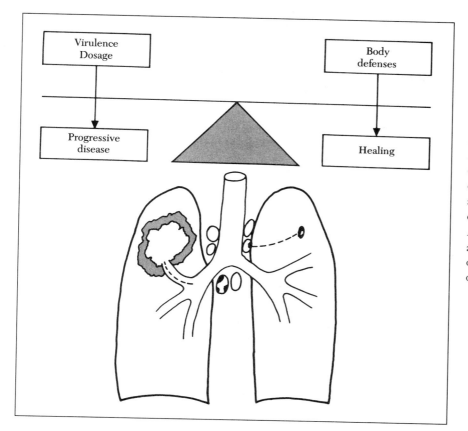

FIGURE 15–15

Possible outcome of a tuberculous infection of the lung in relation to virulence and dosage of the organism and resistance of the body. The frequent involvement of the regional lymph nodes is indicated. *Left,* Progressive disease with cavitation, caused by an infection with a large number of organisms or inadequate defenses. *Right,* Healing with scarring, as a result of a small number of organisms or high degree of resistance to infection

mass of tuberculous inflammatory tissue erodes into a large blood vessel, disseminating large numbers of organisms throughout the body through the bloodstream. The term *miliary* is derived from the resemblance of the multiple foci of disseminated tuberculosis (present in liver, spleen, kidney, and other tissues) to millet seeds. These foci are small white nodules from about 1 to 2 mm in diameter. Tuberculous pneumonia is an overwhelming infection characterized by extensive tuberculous consolidation of one or more lobes of the lung. Persons with AIDS and other immunocompromised persons are prone to this type of rapidly progressive infection.

Extrapulmonary Tuberculosis

Sometimes, tuberculosis develops in the kidneys, bone, uterus, fallopian tubes, or other extrapulmonary location. The infection results from hematogenous spread of tubercle bacilli from a focus of tuberculosis in the lung. Sometimes, the secondary focus of infection may progress even though the pulmonary infection has healed, leading to an active extrapulmonary tuberculous infection without clinically apparent pulmonary tuberculosis.

Diagnosis and Treatment of Tuberculosis

Tuberculous infection is associated with the development of hypersensitivity to proteins in the tubercle bacillus (see chapter 5). A positive skin test (*Mantoux test*) indicates the person was at one time infected with the tubercle bacillus; it does not necessarily indicate an active infection.

Tuberculosis is treated by a number of different antibiotics and chemotherapeutic agents. Drug-resistant tuberculosis is becoming a major problem, and a significant proportion of tubercle bacilli are now resistant to one or more of the drugs commonly used to treat the infection. Drug-resistant tuberculosis is more difficult to treat. The course of treatment is more prolonged, and the results of treatment are less satisfactory.

Sometimes, surgical resection of diseased lung tissue also is performed. At present, many physicians recommend that persons who develop an infection with the tubercle bacillus, as manifested by conversion of a negative into a positive skin test reaction, be treated with antituberculosis drugs. Treatment is also recommended for patients with inactive tuberculosis who have an increased risk of developing a reactivation of an old, apparently healed tuberculous infection.

Unfortunately, the frequency of tuberculosis, which declined steadily from about 1950 to 1980, has now started to increase at an alarming rate in the United States, and a number of factors appear to be responsible for the increase. A large number of persons have immigrated to the United States from Asia, Africa, and Latin American countries, where the prevalence of tuberculosis is much higher. Many of these persons have been infected, although they do not have active tuberculosis. This group serves as a reservoir of infected persons in whom active tuberculosis can develop if immunity declines, which in turn may be followed by infection of other persons with whom they are in close contact. Social problems of poverty, drug abuse, alcoholism, and homelessness create conditions favoring transmission of tuberculosis from person to person. Many of these unfortunate persons with active tuberculosis do not receive adequate ongoing medical care; they may also not be motivated to complete the full course of treatment needed to arrest the disease. Failure to complete treatment leads to treatment failure, and premature cessation of treatment also promotes the emergence of drug-resistant strains of the organism.

Tuberculosis remains a serious problem, and unrecognized cases may expose many susceptible individuals, as illustrated by the following example.

CASE 15–2

A seventeen-year-old female high school student developed a dry cough accompanied by weakness and fatigue, elevated temperature, chills, and a fifteen-pound weight loss. She had also recently noted that she became short of breath after climbing two flights of stairs. Previously, she had lived for a time with an uncle who had tuberculosis. Examination revealed extensive consolidation in the upper part of both lungs as a result of tuberculosis (figure 15–16). Smears and cultures of sputum revealed tubercle bacilli. She was hospitalized and received a course of antituberculous drug therapy. Her school was contacted, and steps were taken

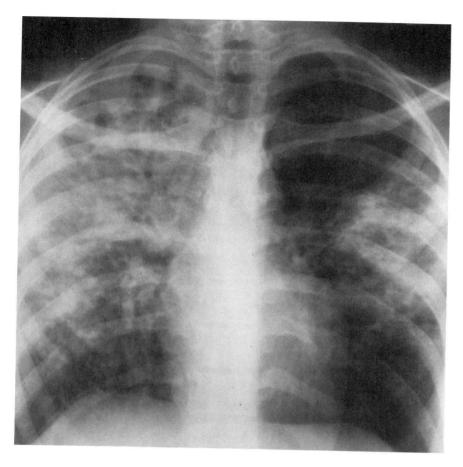

FIGURE 15–16

Chest x-ray of high school student with far-advanced pulmonary tuberculosis, illustrating extensive consolidation of both lungs (case 15–2).

to check other students with whom she had had contact for possible tuberculous infection. The infection slowly responded to therapy, and she was later released from the hospital to continue treatment as an out-patient.

Acute inflammation of the tracheobronchial mucosa is common in many upper respiratory infections. The raw throat and cough associated with many respiratory infections are a result of the associated acute bronchitis. Chronic bronchitis also is common; often it results from constant irritation of the respiratory mucosa by smoking cigarettes or breathing air containing large amounts of atmospheric pollution.

Sometimes the bronchial walls in parts of the lung become weakened as a result of severe inflammation or other factors, and the affected bronchi become markedly dilated. This condition is called **bronchiectasis** (*ectasis*

Bronchitis and Bronchiectasis

= dilation). The distended bronchi tend to retain secretions. Consequently, patients with bronchiectasis frequently have a chronic cough associated with production of large amounts of purulent sputum. Often they suffer repeated bouts of pulmonary infection. The only effective treatment of bronchiectasis is surgical resection of the affected segments of lung. Bronchiectasis can be recognized by means of a special type of radiologic examination called a *bronchogram*. The procedure consists of taking x-ray films after instilling a radiopaque oil into the trachea and bronchi. The oil covers the mucosa of the bronchi, and the abnormal bronchi can be recognized as dilated saccular or fusiform structures (figure 15–17).

Chronic Obstructive Lung Disease

Pulmonary emphysema is a disease in which the air spaces distal to the terminal bronchioles are enlarged, and their walls are destroyed. The disease is an important cause of disability and death, and its incidence is increasing

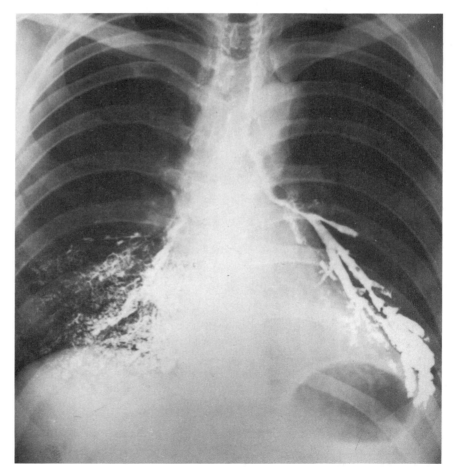

FIGURE 15–17

Chest x-ray illustrating bronchiectasis demonstrated by bronchogram. Right lower lobe bronchi (*left*) appear normal. Bronchi on opposite side exhibit saclike and fusiform dilatation, as outlined by radiopaque contrast material within the dilated bronchi.

at an alarming rate. In emphysema, the normally fine alveolar structure of the lung is destroyed, the large, cystic air spaces form throughout the lung (figure 15–18). The destructive process usually begins in the upper lobes but eventually may affect all lobes of both lungs. Usually there is an associated chronic inflammation of the terminal bronchioles. Emphysema and chronic bronchitis occur together so frequently that they are usually considered a single entity, designated *chronic obstructive pulmonary disease* (COPD). The chief clinical manifestations of any type of chronic pulmonary disease are dyspnea and cyanosis. *Dyspnea* is a sensation of shortness of breath. *Cyanosis* is a blue tinge of the skin and mucous membrane that results from an excessive amount of reduced hemoglobin in the blood. Reduced hemoglobin is dark purplish red, in contrast with normally oxygenated blood, which is bright red.

The three main anatomic derangements in chronic obstructive pulmonary disease are (1) inflammation and narrowing of the terminal bronchioles, (2) dilatation and coalescence of pulmonary air spaces, and (3) loss of lung elasticity. These derangements in turn cause severe disturbances in pulmonary function.

Derangements of Pulmonary Structure and Function

Chronic inflammation of the bronchioles probably initiates the destructive process. Chronic inflammation causes swelling of the bronchial mucosa, which reduces the caliber of the bronchi and bronchioles and stimulates increased bronchial secretions. Because a tube's resistance to air flow varies with the fourth power of its diameter, a slight reduction in the caliber of the bronchioles greatly restricts the flow of air. Normally, the bronchi and bronchioles dilate slightly during inspiration and become smaller during expiration. Consequently, air can enter the lungs more readily than it can be expelled through the narrowed bronchioles; so air tends to become trapped in the lungs during expiration. The lungs cannot empty completely, and they become chronically overinflated. As a result, the amount of additional air that can be inspired when the subject takes a deep breath is much reduced, and the subject is unable to increase his ventilation adequately in response to increased demand.

The bronchiolar obstruction also disturbs pulmonary function by causing unequal air flow to various parts of the lung. Some alveoli are overventilated; others are inadequately supplied, reducing the overall efficiency of pulmonary ventilation. The excess air supplying the overventilated alveoli is "wasted" because more is provided than is needed to completely oxygenate the blood flowing through the surrounding pulmonary capillaries. Conversely, the blood flowing to the poorly ventilated alveoli does not become fully oxygenated. When it mixes with normally oxygenated blood flowing from other parts of the lungs, the oxygen content of the blood delivered to the tissues is reduced.

The destruction of the alveolar septa leads to enlargement of the air spaces and at the same time reduces the number of pulmonary capillaries

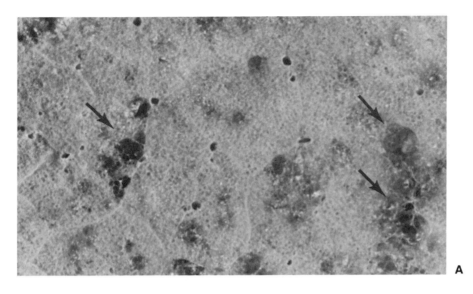

A

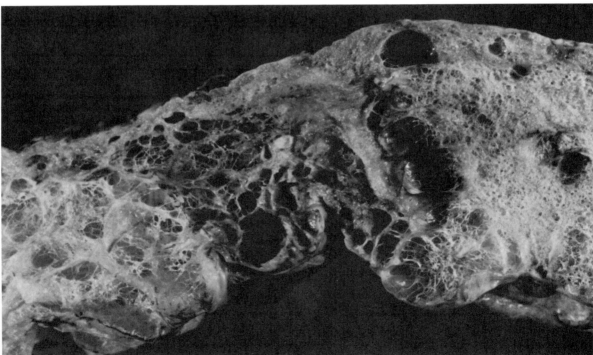

B

FIGURE 15–18

Sections of lung illustrating the gross appearance of emphysema. **A,** Mild emphysema. Beginning breakdown of lung tissue to form cystic spaces (*arrows*). Most of the alveoli appear normal. **B,** Advanced emphysema with multiple, confluent cystic spaces within the lung. Very little normal lung tissue remains. The dark color is a result of accumulation of carbon pigment in the emphysematous lung from inhaling "dirty" air.

available for gas exchange (figure 15–19). Normally, there are about 400 million alveoli in both lungs, and the surface area of the pulmonary capillaries supplying the alveoli is about thirty times as great as the surface area of the body. Each alveolus contains a relatively small volume of air surrounded by a rich network of capillaries. This arrangement promotes optimal diffusion of gases between alveolar air and pulmonary capillaries. Diffusion of gases is much less efficient from large cystic spaces because the spaces contain a much larger volume of air than does a normal alveolus and are surrounded by a relatively sparse network of capillaries. Moreover, the movement of air into and out of the enlarged spaces is impeded by the bronchiolar obstruction.

Destruction of the alveolar septa also leads to loss of the elastic tissue in the septa that forms the structural framework of the lungs, and so the lungs no longer "recoil" normally after they have been stretched during inspiration. Expiration is no longer a passive process. The air must be actively forced out of the lungs by contraction of the intercostal muscles. Breathing requires more effort that in turn requires a greater oxygen consumption. The pressure required to actively force air out of the lungs during expiration also raises the intrapleural pressure and compresses the lungs, which causes further problems with pulmonary ventilation. The bronchi and bronchioles have lost their normal structural support, owing to loss of lung elasticity, and tend to collapse during expiration, obstructing the outflow of air and trapping more air within the lungs.

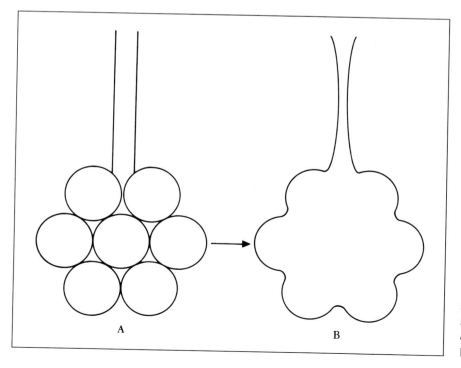

FIGURE 15–19

Derangement of pulmonary function resulting from enlargement of air spaces and reduction in pulmonary capillary bed. **A,** Normal structure, illustrating cluster of alveoli surrounded by rich capillary bed and connected to normal bronchiole. **B,** Emphysema, illustrating coalescence of air spaces to form large cystic space with greatly reduced capillary bed and narrowed bronchiole.

The chief symptom of emphysema is shortness of breath. Initially this is noted only on exertion, but later it may be present even at rest. The patient usually also has a chronic cough with purulent sputum, owing to the associated chronic bronchitis. Eventually, severely affected patients may die because they lack enough functionally normal lung tissue to sustain life or because of a superimposed pulmonary infection. Emphysema is also a frequent cause of respiratory acidosis, one of the common disturbances of acid-base balance. This will be discussed in chapter 24.

Pathogenesis of Emphysema

Cigarette smoking and atmospheric air pollution appear to be the major factors responsible for the rising incidence of emphysema. Exactly how they exert their destructive effect on the lung is not completely understood. Figure 15–20 summarizes one concept of the pathogenesis of this serious and disabling disease. Smoking and air pollution are considered to expose the bronchial mucosa to chronic irritation, eventually producing chronic bronchitis associated with a chronic cough and increased bronchial secretions.

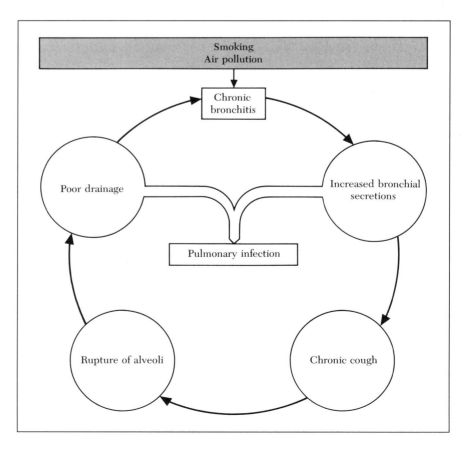

FIGURE 15–20

A concept of the pathogenesis of pulmonary emphysema.

The inflammatory swelling of the mucosa narrows the smaller bronchioles, increasing their resistance to expiration and causing air to be trapped within the lung.

Repeated bouts of coughing, with consequent extreme elevations in intra-bronchial pressure, cause the alveolar septa to rupture, gradually converting the alveoli into large, cystic air spaces. The lungs become overdistended and lose their normal elasticity. The patient cannot expel air normally from the overdistended lungs because normal lung elasticity is lost and the bronchioles are obstructed; difficulty expectorating the excessive bronchial secretions also is apparent. Retention of secretions and poor drainage of secretions from the bronchi tend to perpetuate the chronic bronchitis, and a vicious circle is created. The diseased lungs are also more susceptible to infection because of impaired pulmonary ventilation, bronchial inflammation, bronchiolar obstruction, and excessive bronchial secretions. Therefore, patients with emphysema frequently have repeated bouts of pneumonia, further damaging the lung tissue.

Prevention and Treatment of Emphysema

For the most part, emphysema can be prevented by refraining from smoking and avoiding inhalation of other substances known to be injurious to the lungs. Atmospheric air pollution contributes to the increasing incidence of emphysema, and various measures are being undertaken to control this serious public-health problem.

Once emphysema has developed, the damaged lungs cannot be restored to normal. However, several measures can be employed to promote the drainage of bronchial secretions, to improve pulmonary ventilation, and to decrease the frequency of superimposed pulmonary infections. These measures, along with cessation of smoking, will retard or arrest further progression of the disease.

The following case illustrates the clinical features of a patient with chronic pulmonary emphysema who developed severe respiratory insufficiency that was precipitated by a bout of pneumonia.

A seventy-year-old man entered the hospital because of severe, progressive shortness of breath for the previous two weeks. He had had chronic pulmonary emphysema for many years secondary to heavy cigarette smoking and had stopped smoking recently. On physical examination, he was very short of breath and there was moderate cyanosis of the lips and nailbeds. Lungs appeared overinflated and respiratory excursions were poor. Laboratory studies revealed a low arterial oxygen content (PO_2 31 mm Hg) and oxygen saturation (53 percent), with elevated carbon dioxide tension (PCO_2 53 mm Hg) and plasma bicarbonate (40 mEq/L). Blood pH was reduced to 7.29. These changes indicated severe pulmonary emphysema with respiratory acidosis. Chest x-ray revealed a pneumonia in the right lower lobe. Treatment consisted of supplementary oxygen, antibiotics, and various other measures to improve pulmonary function. The pneumonia slowly subsided, and the patient left the hospital two weeks later.

CASE 15–3

Emphysema as a Result of Alpha₁ Antitrypsin Deficiency

Blood and other body fluids contain a serum protein classified as an alpha$_1$ globulin that is capable of neutralizing trypsin and many other proteolytic (protein-digesting) enzymes such as fibrinolysins and thrombin. This specialized protein is called *alpha$_1$ antitrypsin,* and its concentration in the blood is genetically determined. Most individuals produce normal amounts of antitrypsin, others are severely deficient, and a third group have subnormal levels of this protein.

Individuals with severe antitrypsin deficiency are prone to develop an unusual type of progressive pulmonary emphysema that usually becomes manifest in adolescence or early adulthood and tends to affect chiefly the lower lobes of the lungs. It is much less common than the usual type of emphysema described. Usually there is no associated chronic bronchitis, and so cough and excessive sputum production are absent. Persons with only moderately reduced antitrypsin levels do not develop severe emphysema at an early age but are quite susceptible to lung damage from cigarette smoking, atmospheric air pollution, or respiratory infections.

Low antitrypsin levels are correlated with lung disease because alpha$_1$ antitrypsin protects the lung from injury by leukocyte enzymes. Normally, polymorphonuclear leukocytes tend to accumulate in the pulmonary capillaries, and macrophages migrate from the bloodstream into the alveolar walls and pulmonary alveoli. Some of these leukocytes degenerate and release their proteolytic enzymes, but the enzymes are normally inactivated by antitrypsin so that they do not injure the alveolar septa. However, if antitrypsin is severely deficient, the leukocyte enzymes are not inactivated and can digest the connective tissues of the alveolar septa and terminal air passages, leading to pulmonary emphysema. The individual with a subnormal level of antitrypsin manifests an increased susceptibility to chronic pulmonary disease because pulmonary irritants (such as cigarette smoke and polluted air) and pulmonary infections cause leukocytes to accumulate within the lung. The liberated leukocyte enzymes are less efficiently neutralized than in normal individuals and may injure the lungs.

Bronchial Asthma

Bronchial asthma is a spasmodic contraction of the smooth muscle in the walls of the smaller bronchi and bronchioles. It is also associated with increased secretions by the bronchial mucous glands. Asthmatic attacks cause shortness of breath, and wheezing respirations occur caused by restricted movement of air through the tightly constricted air passages. The physiologic derangements in asthma result from narrowing of the bronchioles and are similar to those in patients with emphysema. Bronchiolar spasm exerts a greater effect on expiration than on inspiration because the caliber of the bronchioles varies with the phase of respiration. Consequently, air flow is impeded more on expiration than on inspiration, which leads to trapping of air within the lungs and overinflation of the lungs.

Many cases of asthma have an allergic basis. The attacks are precipitated by inhalation of dust, pollens, animal dander, or other allergens, which interact with mast cells coated with IgE antibody. This leads to release of chemical mediators that induce the bronchospasm. Acute attacks are treated by administering drugs such as epinephrine or theophylline, which relax the bronchospasm. Often one can prevent attacks by administering drugs that block the release of mediators from mast cells. (Allergic diseases are considered in chapter 5.)

Respiratory Distress Syndrome of Newborn Infants

The condition known as respiratory distress syndrome of newborn infants is characterized by progressive respiratory distress that occurs soon after birth, leading to serious problems in oxygenation of the blood. The condition occurs most often in premature infants, infants delivered by cesarean section, and infants born to diabetic mothers. The basic cause is an inadequate quantity of surfactant in the lungs of the affected infants. As a result, the alveoli do not expand normally during inspiration and tend to collapse during expiration. The permeability of the pulmonary capillaries also is increased; so protein-rich fluid leaks from the pulmonary capillaries. The fluid, which is rich in fibrinogen, tends to clot and form adherent membranes that line the air passages. These membranes contribute to respiratory distress by impeding the diffusion of gases between the air passages and the pulmonary capillaries. There is some evidence that adrenal corticosteroid hormones administered to the mother before delivery will stimulate the maturation of the fetal lung and will also increase production of surfactant, thereby reducing the likelihood of this complication in susceptible infants.

Respiratory Distress Syndrome

Adult Respiratory Distress Syndrome

A respiratory distress syndrome similar to that encountered in newborn infants also occurs in adults, but its pathogenesis is different. The syndrome is designated *adult respiratory distress syndrome,* or simply by its initials *ARDS,* and sometimes by the term *shock lung.* The conditions causing this syndrome fall into two major groups. In the first group are many different conditions that cause shock with consequent fall in blood pressure and correspondingly reduced blood flow to the lungs. The shock may result from any type of severe injury (traumatic shock) or from a serious systemic infection (septic shock), and the pulmonary capillary and alveolar damage is an indirect result of the impaired pulmonary blood flow. In the second group are various conditions that directly damage the pulmonary capillaries and alveolar septa, such as aspiration of gastric contents or inhalation of irritants or toxic gases.

Whatever the predisposing cause of the alveolar damage, the pathophysiologic derangements are the same as in the neonatal respiratory distress syndrome: damage to alveolar capillaries and alveolar lining cells, impaired formation of surfactant, leakage of protein-rich fluid from the injured capillaries into the alveolar septa with formation of intraalveolar hyaline membranes, and impaired diffusion of oxygen across the swollen, thickened alveolar septa.

Treatment is directed toward correcting the shock, treating the underlying condition that initiated the respiratory distress, and improving the oxygenation of the blood by means of a ventilator capable of delivering an increased concentration of oxygen to the lungs under slightly increased pressure, thereby facilitating diffusion of oxygen across the swollen alveolar septa.

Pulmonary Fibrosis

The lungs are continually exposed to a number of injurious substances, such as irritant gases discharged into the atmosphere and many kinds of airborne organic and inorganic particles. Severe pulmonary injury may lead to *pulmonary fibrosis*. Fibrous thickening of alveolar septa makes the lungs increasingly rigid, restricting normal respiratory excursions. Diffusion of oxygen and carbon dioxide between alveolar air and pulmonary capillaries also is hampered because of the increased thickness of the alveolar septa. Pulmonary fibrosis causes progressive respiratory disability similar to that encountered in pulmonary emphysema.

Some types of collagen diseases, characterized by injury to connective tissue, may have as their major manifestation injury to the connective-tissue framework of the lung, leading to pulmonary fibrosis.

Certain occupational diseases are recognized as being caused by inhalation of injurious substances. The general term **pneumoconiosis** (*pneumo* = lung + *kois* = dust + *osis* = condition) is used to refer to lung injury produced by inhalation of injurious dust or other particulate material. The best known of the pneumoconioses are silicosis and asbestosis. **Silicosis** is a type of progressive nodular pulmonary fibrosis caused by inhalation of rock dust. **Asbestosis** is a diffuse pulmonary fibrosis caused by inhalation of asbestos fibers. Within the body, the fibers become coated with a protein having a high content of iron to form characteristic structures called *asbestos bodies*. Sometimes these can be identified in the sputum of patients with asbestosis (figure 15–21). Inhalation of coal dust, cotton fibers, certain types of fungus spores, and many other substances attending certain occupations also may cause pulmonary fibrosis.

Patients with asbestosis have other problems as well, because asbestos fibers appear to be carcinogenic. These patients have a higher incidence of lung carcinoma than the general population, and some develop an unusual type of malignant tumor arising from pleural mesothelial cells, called a *malignant mesothelioma*.

Lung Carcinoma

Lung carcinoma is another important disease related to cigarette smoking. Lung carcinoma was once uncommon. Now it is the most common malignant tumor in men, and the incidence in women has also increased to such

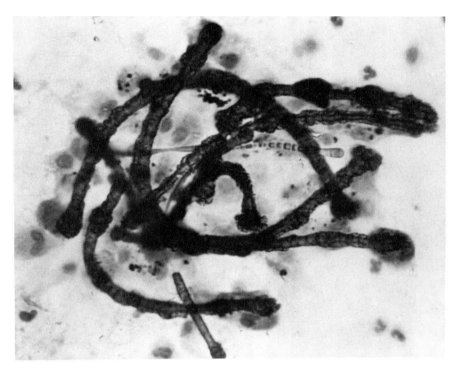

FIGURE 15–21

Cluster of asbestos bodies in sputum. (Original magnification approximately × 1000.)

an extent that the mortality from lung cancer in women now exceeds that of breast cancer. The tumor is uncommon in nonsmokers. Because the neoplasm usually arises from the bronchial mucosa, the term *bronchogenic carcinoma* is often used when referring to lung cancer. There are several different histologic types. *Squamous cell carcinoma* and *adenocarcinoma* are two of the more common (figure 5–22). A third type composed of large, bizarre epithelial cells is called by the descriptive term *large cell carcinoma*. A fourth type is composed of small, irregular dark cells with scanty cytoplasm that look somewhat like lymphocytes. This type is called a *small cell carcinoma* and carries a very poor prognosis (figure 15–23). Frequently tumor cells can be identified in the sputum of patients with lung carcinoma (figure 15–24).

Because of the rich lymphatic and vascular network in the lung, the neoplasm readily gains access to lymphatic channels and pulmonary blood vessels and soon spreads to regional lymph nodes and distant sites. Treatment usually consists of surgical resection of one or more lobes of the lung. Radiation therapy in combination with anticancer chemotherapy rather than surgery is used to treat small cell carcinoma and is also used to treat tumors that are too far advanced for surgical resection. Results of treatment are disappointing because the disease is often widespread by the time it is recognized. This tumor could largely be prevented by elimination of cigarette smoking.

FIGURE 15–22

Gross appearance of lung carcinoma. **A,** Squamous cell carcinoma partially obstructing major bronchus. **B,** Adenocarcinoma arising from smaller bronchus at periphery of lung.

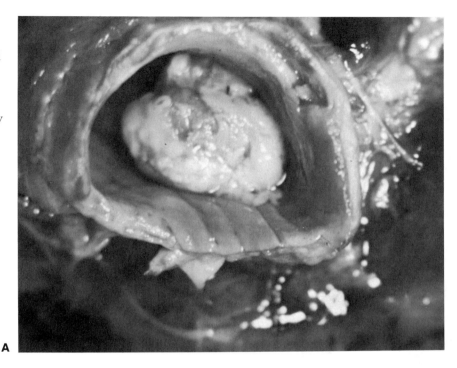

A

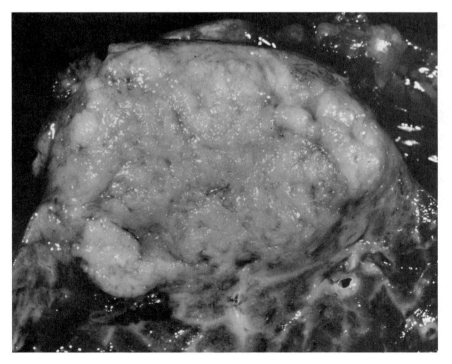

B

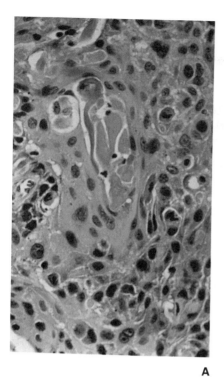
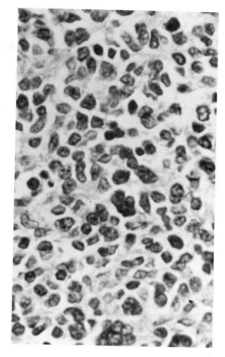

A

B

FIGURE 15–23

Histologic appearance of two common types of lung carcinoma. **A,** Moderately well differentiated squamous cell carcinoma. (Original magnification × 200.) **B,** Small cell carcinoma. (Original magnification × 200.)

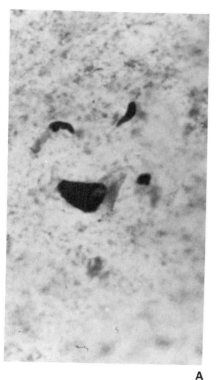
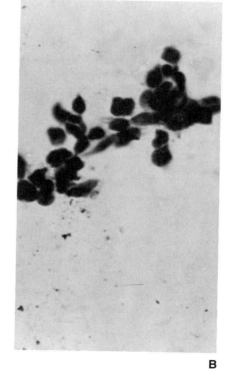

A

B

FIGURE 15–24

Tumor cells in sputum from patients with lung carcinoma. **A,** Large neoplastic squamous cell from patient with squamous cell carcinoma of lung. **B,** Cluster of small, darkly stained cells from patient with small cell carcinoma.

Review Questions

1. How do the lungs function? What is the difference between ventilation and gas exchange? How is pulmonary function disturbed if the alveolar septa are thickened and scarred?

2. What is pneumothorax? How does it develop? What is its effect on pulmonary function?

3. What is pneumonia? How is pneumonia classified? What are its major clinical features?

4. How does the tubercle bacillus differ in its staining reaction from other bacteria? What type of inflammatory reaction does it cause? What factors determine the outcome of a tuberculous infection? How does a cavity develop in lungs infected with tuberculosis? Is a person with a tuberculous cavity infectious to other persons? What is miliary tuberculosis?

5. A patient has tuberculosis of the kidney but no evidence of pulmonary tuberculosis is detected by means of a chest x-ray. How did this happen?

6. What is meant by the term "inactive tuberculosis"? Under what circumstances may an old inactive tuberculous infection become activated? What type of patients are susceptible to reactivation of a tuberculous infection?

7. What is the difference between bronchitis and bronchiectasis?

8. What is pulmonary emphysema? What factors predispose to its development? How may it be prevented? What is the difference between pulmonary emphysema and pulmonary fibrosis?

9. What is the relation between carcinoma of the lung and cigarette smoking? How is lung carcinoma treated?

Supplementary Readings

Bernard, G. R., et al. 1986. Pulmonary edema: Pathophysiologic mechanisms and new approaches to therapy. *Chest* 89:594–600. Deals with pathophysiology and principles of treatment of adult respiratory distress syndrome.

Bernard, G. R., et al. 1987. High-dose corticosteroids in patients with the adult respiratory distress syndrome. *New England Journal of Medicine* 317:1565–70. High-dose corticosteroids are not beneficial in patients with ARDS as a result of sepsis, aspiration, or mixed causes.

Cantwell, M. F., Snider, D. E., Cauthen, G. M., et al. 1994. Epidemiology of tuberculosis in the United States, 1985 through 1992. *Journal of the American Medical Association* 272:535–39. Increases in tuberculosis were concentrated among racial or ethnic minorities, persons between twenty-five and forty-four years of age, and the foreign born. Foreign-born cases accounted for 60 percent of the total increase in U.S. cases from 1986 through 1992. The number of cases among children 4 years and younger increased 36 percent, suggesting that TB transmission increased during this period as well.

Centers for Disease Control and Prevention. 1993. Initial therapy for tuberculosis in the era of multidrug resistance. *Morbidity and Mortality Weekly Report* 42:1–8. The initial treatment of tuberculosis should include four drugs.

Centers for Disease Control and Prevention. 1995. Essential components of a tuberculosis prevention and control program. Screening for tuberculosis infection in high risk populations. *Morbidity and Mortality Weekly Report* 44 (No. RR-11):1–34. Describes screening, prevention, and control procedures, emphasizing high-risk groups.

Colditz, G. A., Brewer, T. F., Berkey, C. S., et al. 1994. Efficacy of BCG vaccine in the prevention of tuberculosis. *Journal of the American Medical Association* 271:698–702. BCG vaccination reduces the risk of tuberculosis by about 50 percent.

Daley, C. L., Small, P. M., Schecter, G. F., et al. 1992. An outbreak of tuberculosis with accelerated progression among persons infected with the human immunodeficiency virus. *New England Journal of Medicine* 326:231–35. HIV infection promotes rapid progression of tuberculosis.

Driver, C. R., Valway, S. E., Morgan, W. M., et al. 1994. Transmission of *Mycobacterium tuberculosis* associated with air travel. *Journal of the American Medical Association* 272:1031–35. A flight attendant became infected after exposure to a family member who died of tuberculosis. She did not receive prophylactic treatment and developed active tuberculosis three years later. She infected other airline crew members and may also have infected passengers before her disease was diagnosed and treated.

Fraser, D. W., et al. 1977. Legionnaire's disease: Description of an epidemic of pneumonia. *New England Journal of Medicine* 297:1189–97. Describes the classic epidemic that occurred in Philadelphia in 1976.

Glantz, S. A., and Parmley, W. W. 1995. Passive smoking and heart disease: Mechanisms and risk. *Journal of the American Medical Association* 273:1047–53. Nonsmokers exposed to secondhand smoke exhibit an increased risk of cardiovascular disease.

Ranaldo, J. E., and Rogers, R. M. 1986. Adult respiratory distress syndrome. *New England Journal of Medicine*

315:578–79. An editorial with references discussing pathophysiology of the syndrome.

Selikoff, I. J., and Hammond, E. C. 1978. Asbestos-associated disease in United States shipyards. *CA: A Cancer Journal for Clinicians* 28:87–99. Asbestos exposure causes asbestosis, lung cancer, and mesotheliomas.

Talamo, R. C. 1971. The α_1-antitrypsin in man. *Journal of Allergy and Clinical Immunology* 48:240–50. Reviews the role of the substance in protecting against lung damage by leukocyte enzymes.

Weiss, S. T. 1983. The health effects of involuntary smoking. *American Review of Respiratory Diseases* 128:933–42. One of the early articles documenting the harmful effects of passive smoking on health.

White, J. R., and Froeb, H. F. 1980. Small-airways dysfunction in nonsmokers chronically exposed to tobacco smoke. *New England Journal of Medicine* 302:720–23. Nonsmokers exposed to cigarette smoke at work developed adverse effects on lung function. Chronic exposure to cigarette smoke is harmful to nonsmokers.

See also sections in standard textbooks of medicine and pathology, listed in General References.

Chapter 15 ■ Outline Summary

Structure and Function of the Lungs / 407
The Structure of Conducting Tubes and Alveoli
Bronchi: larger conducting tubes.

Bronchioles: tubes less than 1 mm in diameter.

Respiratory bronchioles: bronchioles with alveoli in their walls.

Alveoli: small air sacs where gas exchange occurs.

Ventilation
Air movement caused by movement of ribs and diaphragm.

Lungs change in volume in response to changes in size of thoracic cage.

Gas Exchange
Gases diffuse owing to differences in partial pressures.

Efficient exchange in lungs requires large capillary surface area.

Pulmonary Function Tests
Vital capacity: maximum volume of air expired after maximum inspiration.

One-second forced expiratory volume (FEV_1): maximum volume of air expelled in one second.

Arterial PO_2 and PCO_2 measure efficiency of gas exchange in lungs.

Pleural Cavity
"Negative" intrapleural pressure is caused by the tendency of stretched lung to pull away from chest wall.

Release of vacuum in pleural cavity leads to collapse of lung.

Pneumothorax / 412
Pathogenesis
Chest or lung injury permits air to escape into pleural cavity.

Spontaneous pneumothorax: no apparent cause.

Manifestations
Subjective: chest pain and dyspnea.

Objective: air in pleural cavity demonstrated by x-ray and examination.

Tension pneumothorax: complication of pneumothorax when air can enter pleural cavity but cannot escape on expiration. Air under pressure displaces mediastinum and impairs expansion of opposite lung.

Treatment
Chest tube inserted in pleural cavity; vacuum sometimes applied.

Atelectasis / 415
Classification
Obstructive: caused by bronchial obstruction.

Compression: caused by air or fluid in pleural cavity.

Treatment
Remove obstruction or material compressing lung.

Pneumonia / 417
Classification
By etiologic agent.

By anatomic distribution of inflammation in lung.

By predisposing factors.

Clinical Features
Manifestations of systemic infection.

Manifestations of lung inflammation: cough, chest pain.

Pneumocystis Pneumonia / 420
Caused by protozoan parasite of low pathogenicity.

Affects immunocompromised persons.

Organisms injure alveoli, leading to exudation of protein-rich material into alveoli.

Cysts demonstrated by special stains.

Infection characterized by dyspnea, cough, pulmonary consolidation.

Diagnosis established by lung biopsy.

Treatment available but infection has high mortality.

Tuberculosis / 420
Characteristics of Tuberculosis
A granulomatous inflammation characterized by necrosis and giant cells.

Manifestations
Depends on dosage and resistance. May heal by scarring or progress to cavitation.

Miliary tuberculosis: dissemination of organisms by bloodstream.

Extrapulmonary tuberculosis: hematogenous dissemination from lungs to distant site.

Diagnosis and Treatment
Skin test: indicates previous exposure to organism.

Chest x-ray: indicates pulmonary infiltrate.

Culture: identifies organism in sputum.

Treatment by means of antibiotic and chemotherapeutic agents.

Bronchitis and Bronchiectasis / 427
Classification
Acute bronchitis: common and self-limited.

Chronic bronchitis: secondary to chronic irritation.

Bronchiectasis: walls weakened by inflammation and dilate.

Diagnosis and Treatment
Acute bronchitis: self-limited.

Chronic bronchitis: cease irritation, as by cessation of smoking.

Bronchiectasis: bronchogram demonstrates dilation.

Diseased areas resected.

Chronic Obstructive Lung Disease / 428
Definition
Combined emphysema and chronic bronchitis.

Derangements of Structure and Function
Chronic inflammation of bronchioles leads to trapped air in lungs.

Nonuniform ventilation of alveoli reduces efficiency of ventilation.

Enlargement of air spaces and reduction of capillary bed reduces efficiency of gas exchange.

Loss of lung elasticity requires active expiratory effort.

Prevention and Treatment of Emphysema
Refrain from smoking and inhalation of injurious agents.

Treatment cannot restore damaged lung but can prevent further progression and may improve pulmonary function.

Emphysema as a Result of Alpha$_1$ Antitrypsin Deficiency
Antitrypsin prevents lung damage from lysosomal enzymes released from leukocytes in lung.

Deficiency permits enzymes to damage lung tissue.

Bronchial Asthma / 434
Pathogenesis
Spasmodic contraction of bronchial smooth muscle narrows air passages.

Treatment
Drugs that relax bronchospasm or prevent release of mediators from mast cells.

Many cases caused by allergy.

Neonatal Respiratory Distress Syndrome / 435
Pathogenesis
Inadequate surfactant impedes normal lung expansion and promotes collapse.

Premature infants, infants born by cesarean section, and infants by diabetic mothers predisposed to syndrome.

Treatment
Administration of corticosteroids to mother may stimulate lung maturation in fetus and reduce likelihood of syndrome. No specific treatment available.

Adult Respiratory Distress Syndrome / 435
Pathogenesis
Systemic disease with shock and impaired lung perfusion.

Direct lung damage: trauma, gastric aspiration, inhalation of irritants or toxic gases.

Derangement
Damaged alveolar capillaries leak fluid and protein.

Impaired surfactant production from damaged alveolar lining cells.

Formation of hyaline membranes.

Treatment
Correct predisposing conditions.

Administer oxygen under positive pressure.

Pulmonary Fibrosis / 436
Pathogenesis
Collagen diseases.

Pneumoconioses:

Silicosis.

Asbestosis (also predisposes to lung carcinoma and pleural mesothelioma).

Various other injurious substances inhaled in course of occupations.

Treatment

No specific treatment. Prevent occupational exposure.

Lung Carcinoma / 436
Pathogenesis

A smoking-related neoplasm.

Incidence in women now exceeds breast carcinoma.

Arises from mucosa of bronchi and bronchioles.

Classification and Prognosis

Several histologic types, which differ in their prognosis.

Poor prognosis as a result of early spread to distant sites.

Treatment

Depends on histologic type. Generally by resection.

Small cell carcinoma treated by chemotherapy and radiation.

16

The Breast

Learning Objectives

1. Describe the normal structure and physiology of the breast. List and define the common developmental abnormalities.
2. Explain the applications and limitations of mammography in the diagnosis and treatment of breast disease.
3. List the three common breast diseases that present as a lump in the breast, and explain how they are differentiated by the physician.
4. Describe the clinical manifestations of breast carcinoma. Explain the methods of diagnosis and treatment.

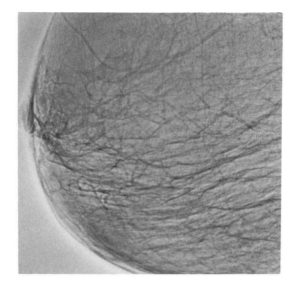

Chapter 16 ■ Contents

The female breasts are each composed of about twenty lobes of glandular tissue embedded in fibrous and adipose tissue. Each lobe consists of clusters of glands, called *lobules,* connected by a series of branching ducts that converge to form large ducts that extend to the nipple. The breasts are modified sweat glands that have become specialized to secrete milk. Before puberty, breast tissue in both sexes consists only of branching ducts and fibrous tissue without glandular tissue or fat. In the female, they enlarge at puberty in response to estrogen and progesterone produced by the ovaries, whereas the unstimulated male breasts retain their prepubertal form. Postpubertal changes in the female include proliferation of glandular and fibrous tissue and accumulation of adipose tissue within the breasts. Variations in the size of the postpubertal breasts of nonpregnant women are due primarily to variations in the amount of fat and fibrous tissue in the breasts rather than to differences in the amount of glandular tissue.

The breasts are fixed to the chest wall by bands of fibrous tissue called *suspensory ligaments,* which extend from the skin of the breast to the connective tissue covering the muscles of the chest wall.

The breasts have an abundant blood supply and a rich lymphatic drainage. Lymphatic channels drain from each breast into groups of lymph nodes located in the armpit, or axilla *(axillary lymph nodes),* above the clavicle *(supraclavicular lymph nodes),* and beneath the sternum *(mediastinal lymph nodes).*

The breasts are extremely responsive to hormonal stimulation. Mild cyclic hyperplasia followed by involution of breast tissue occurs normally during the menstrual cycle. The glandular and ductal tissues of the breast become markedly hypertrophic under the hormonal stimulus of pregnancy and lactation, and the breast undergoes regression in the postpartum period. After the menopause, sex-hormone levels decline and the breasts gradually decrease in size. Figure 16–1 illustrates the histologic appearance of breast tissue under varying hormonal conditions.

Structure and Physiology of the Breast

Monthly breast self-examination is recommended for all women. Examination of the breasts by the woman herself or by her physician is performed in a standard manner. First, the breasts are inspected with the arms at the sides, then as the arms are elevated and lowered, and finally with the hands on the hips. One looks for irregularities in the contours of the breasts or nipples or abnormalities in the skin of the breasts. Next, the breasts are systematically palpated by compressing the breast tissue gently against the chest wall with the fingertips. The examination is begun at the periphery of the breast, and all parts of the breast are palpated in a clockwise direction until finally the tissues under the nipple are examined. Then the breast and nipple are compressed to assure that no discharge or blood can be expressed from the nipple. Last, one palpates in both armpits for the presence of enlarged lymph nodes or other abnormalities.

Examination of the Breasts

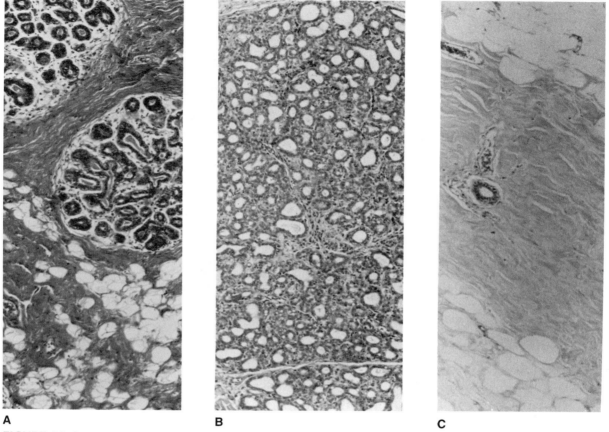

A　　　　　　　　　　　　　　　　　　**B**　　　　　　　　　　　　　　　　　　**C**

FIGURE 16–1

Photomicrographs illustrating the appearance of breasts under varying hormonal conditions (original magnification × 40). **A,** Normal nonpregnant breast. Two lobules of glandular tissue appear in the upper half of the photograph. **B,** Glandular hyperplasia in pregnancy. **C,** Postmenopausal atrophy.

Mammograms

A *mammogram* is a special type of x-ray examination that allows the physician to visualize the internal structure of the breast and recognize abnormalities that may not be detected by clinical examination. In a mammogram, the fibrous and glandular tissue of the breast appear as interlacing white strands. The less-dense fatty tissue, which transmits x-rays readily, appears dark (figure 16–2). Cysts and tumors within the breast appear as dense white masses surrounded by the less-dense dark tissue of the adjacent normal breast. Cysts and benign tumors appear well circumscribed, whereas malignant tumors often have irregular margins that indicate infiltration of the tumor into the surrounding breast tissue. These same criteria are used to distinguish between benign and malignant tumors on gross examination when a biopsy specimen is examined. Malignant tumors also frequently contain

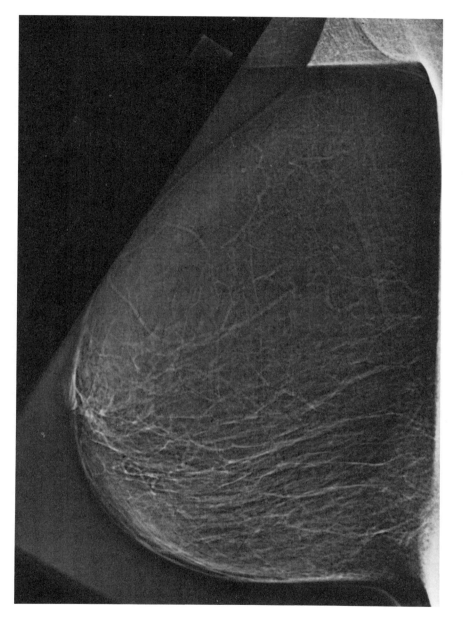

FIGURE 16–2

Normal mammogram.

fine flecks of calcium that indicate calcification within the carcinoma. This is another feature suggestive of malignancy when seen on the mammogram.

The mammogram is most useful for examining the breasts of post-menopausal women because they contain more fat and less glandular tissue than the breasts of younger women. A dense tumor within a postmenopausal breast usually contrasts sharply with the less-dense fatty tissue and is more easily identified. In contrast, a mammogram is less useful for examining the breasts of younger women, which appear much denser because they contain much more glandular and fibrous tissue. Consequently, it is more difficult to recognize a tumor in such a breast because there is less contrast between the tumor and the surrounding dense breast tissue.

Periodic mammograms are recommended for all women as a screening procedure. Mammograms can detect early breast cancers much sooner than they could be felt by physical examination of the breasts, and early detection followed by prompt treatment while a tumor is still small greatly increases the woman's chance of survival. The current recommendations are for an initial baseline mammogram between ages thirty-five and forty, followed by repeat mammograms every one or two years until age fifty, and yearly examinations thereafter.

Abnormalities of Breast Development

Accessory Breasts and Nipples

Embryologically the breasts develop from columns of cells called *mammary ridges,* which extend along the anterior body wall from the armpits to the upper thighs (figure 16–3). Most of the ridges disappear in the course of prenatal development except for the parts in the midthoracic region, which give rise to the breasts and nipples. Sometimes, persons have extra breasts or nipples. These are most commonly found in the armpits or on the lower chest below and medial to the normal breasts, but they may appear anywhere along the course of the embryonic mammary ridges (figure 16–4). Extra nipples and breast tissue may be a source of embarrassment to the subject, but usually they do not cause other problems. Occasionally, however, accessory breast tissue may cause symptoms, as illustrated by the following case:

CASE 16–1

A twenty-two-year-old woman visited a medical clinic for an examination and Pap smear. In the course of the examination, bilateral soft masses of tissue were palpated in both armpits. Each mass measured about 5 cm in diameter, and they became quite prominent when the subject raised her arms above her head. On further questioning, she stated the lumps had been present for some time. They often became tender just before the onset of her menstrual period, and the overlying skin sometimes became irritated by rubbing against her clothing. She was advised that the lumps were masses of extra breast tissue and could be removed surgically if they continued to cause problems.

Unequal Development of the Breasts

The fully developed breasts are usually similar in size and shape, but not identical. Occasionally, one breast may fail to develop as much as its counterpart and may be significantly smaller than the opposite breast. Moreover, any condition that causes the breasts to enlarge may accentuate the dispro-

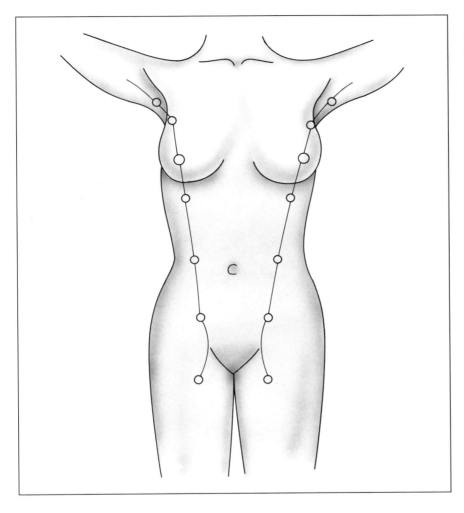

FIGURE 16–3

FIGURE 16–3

Common sites of accessory breasts and nipples, which may form anywhere along the course of the embryonic mammary ridges.

portion. This possibility must be considered when prescribing medications, as illustrated by the following case:

CASE 16–2

A twenty-year-old woman visited a medical clinic seeking contraceptive pills. Examination revealed that the left breast was much smaller than the right, which the subject masked by padding the left brassiere cup. The rest of the examination was normal. She was advised that contraceptive pills could be prescribed. However, owing to the effect of the hormones contained in these pills on the glandular tissues of the breast, slight breast enlargement could result. Such enlargement might accentuate the difference in the size of the two breasts. The client decided not to use contraceptive pills and chose to be fitted with a diaphragm instead.

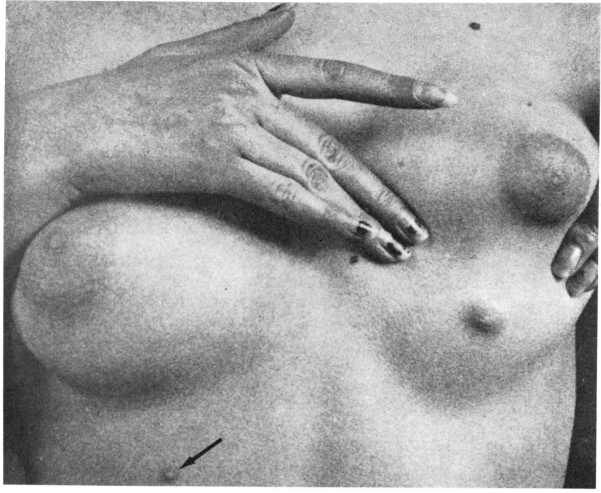

FIGURE 16–4

A fifteen-year-old girl with an extra nipple below right breast *(arrow)* and an extra breast with nipple just below normal left breast. (*From:* Haagensen, C. D. 1971. *Disease of the breast,* 2d ed. Philadelphia, W. B. Saunders. Used by permission.)

Breast Hypertrophy

Sometimes at puberty, one or both female breasts overrespond to hormonal stimulation and may enlarge excessively. True breast hypertrophy is due primarily to overgrowth of fibrous tissue, not glandular tissue or fat. The subject may experience considerable back and shoulder discomfort owing to the excessive weight of the breasts. If symptoms are severe, the excessive breast tissue may be surgically resected, after which the breasts may be reconstructed so they have a more normal size and shape.

Gynecomastia

Occasionally at puberty the ductal and fibrous tissue of the adolescent male breast may begin to proliferate, forming a distinct nodule of breast tissue under the nipple. This condition, which is called **gynecomastia** (*gyne* = woman + *mastos* = breast), may affect one or both breasts. It appears to result from a temporary imbalance of male and female hormones that sometimes occurs in the male at puberty. Normally, the male secretes both male and female hormones, but male hormones predominate and "cancel out" the effects of the female hormones. Gynecomastia results when there is a temporary increase in estrogen relative to male hormones. The condition is not serious but may cause considerable emotional distress to the affected youth. Treatment usually consists of surgical removal of the excess breast tissue.

Benign Cystic Change in the Breast

Benign cystic change in breast tissue, often called benign cystic disease or benign fibrocystic disease, it a very common condition. It is characterized by focal areas of proliferation of glandular and fibrous tissue in the breast associated with localized dilatation of ducts, resulting in the formation of various-sized cysts within the breast. Cystic change appears to be caused by irregularities in the response of the breast tissue to the normal cyclic variations of each menstrual cycle. Clinically, a breast cyst may feel very firm and may appear to be a solid tumor. Ultrasound examination of the breast is often very helpful in distinguishing a cystic from a solid mass in the breast (figure 16–5). Often, if the physician believes the mass to be a cyst rather than a solid tumor, an attempt is made to aspirate the cyst. A needle is introduced into the breast under local anesthesia. If a cyst is present, the fluid is aspirated and the mass disappears. If no fluid can be obtained, surgical excision is performed.

Fibroadenoma

Fibroadenoma is a benign, well-circumscribed tumor of fibrous and glandular breast tissues that is seen most commonly in young women. It is readily cured by simple surgical excision (figure 16–6).

Carcinoma of the Breast

Breast carcinoma is a very common tumor. There are more than 100,000 new cases each year, and it is estimated that one out of every ten women will eventually develop a breast carcinoma. There is some tendency for breast carcinoma to run in families, and a woman is at higher-than-normal risk if her mother or sister has had a breast carcinoma. Hormonal factors also influence the risk of breast carcinoma. Women who have never borne children or had their first child after age thirty are at increased risk, as are women who have had early onset of menses (menarche) or late menopause. A small proportion of breast carcinomas are hereditary and can be traced to inheritance of

FIGURE 16–5

Benign cyst of breast.
A, Cyst viewed in cross-section. Cyst is filled with fluid that escapes when cyst is incised. **B,** Ultrasound examination of breast, revealing breast cyst (dark area near center of photograph).

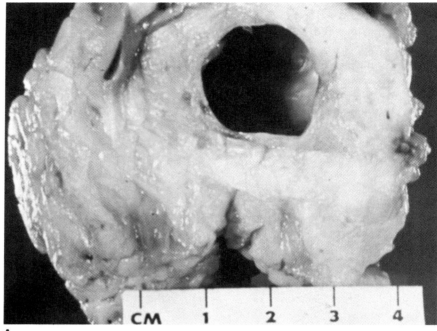

A

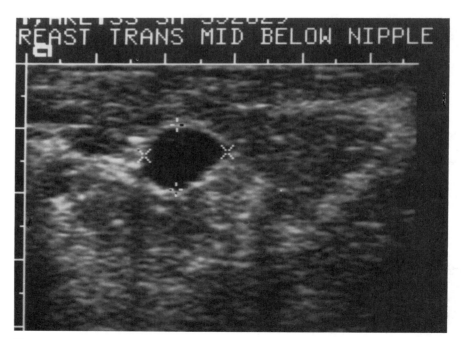

B

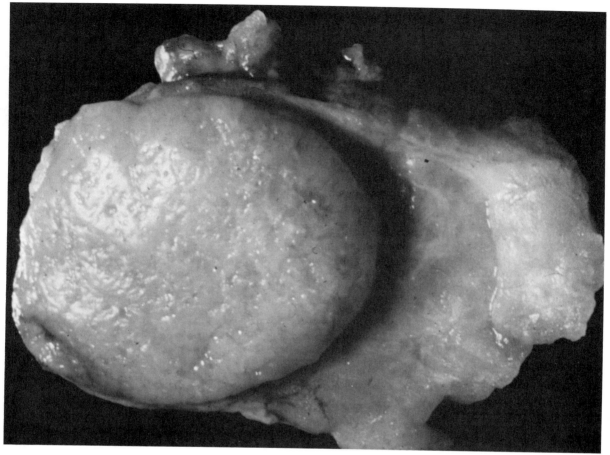

FIGURE 16–6

Benign fibroadenoma of breast. Tumor is well circumscribed and readily separates from adjacent normal breast tissue.

a mutant cancer susceptibility gene. Two genes have been identified and designated as the *BRCA1* (breast carcinoma 1) gene, and the *BRCA2* (breast carcinoma 2) gene. Inheritance of either a mutant *BRCA1* gene or a mutant *BRCA2* gene greatly increases breast cancer risk in a woman carrying one of these mutant genes. (The role of tumor suppressor genes on cell functions and the effect of an inherited mutation were considered in chapter 10.)

Breast cancers are classified according to the site of origin, the presence or absence of invasion, and the degree of differentiation of the tumor cells. More than 90 percent of carcinomas arise from the epithelium of the ducts and are called *ductal carcinomas*. The rest arise from the lobules and are designated *lobular carcinomas*. Initially, a carcinoma remains confined for a time within the duct or lobule in which it arose and is called a *noninfiltrating* or *in situ* ductal or lobular carcinoma. Eventually, however, the tumor breaks through the ducts or lobules and extends into the adjacent breast tissue, becoming an *invasive ductal* or *lobular carcinoma.* Histologically, the degree of differentiation of the tumor also is specified. A *well-differentiated carcinoma* is composed of cells that resemble the epithelium of the ducts or lobules in which the tumor arose, whereas a *poorly differentiated tumor* is composed of bizarre cells in haphazard arrangement that appear immature and quite different from normal breast epithelial cells.

In its early stages, a breast carcinoma is too small to be detected by breast examination but can often be demonstrated by mammography, sometimes as early as two years before it becomes large enough to form a palpable lump within the breast. As the tumor continues to grow, it infiltrates the breast tissue more extensively, and left untreated, eventually metastasizes to regional lymph nodes and distant sites. Five-year survival rates and the problem of late metastases are discussed in chapter 10. Early diagnosis allows prompt treatment and improves the cure rate. For this reason, all women are encouraged to examine their breasts regularly and to consult their physicians if an abnormality is detected. Routine screening mammograms also are highly recommended, as noted earlier.

Many breast carcinomas induce fibrosis in the surrounding normal breast tissue that is being invaded by the tumor cells, as though the body were trying to defend itself by laying down fibrous tissue to contain the tumor. Consequently, many breast cancers are very firm and have a puckered, scarred appearance with irregular margins that blend into the surrounding breast tissue. This appearance is due more to the proliferation of fibrous tissue in response to the tumor than to the tumor cells themselves. Nevertheless, this appearance is quite characteristic of many breast cancers and aids in identifying a carcinoma by mammography (figure 16–7). Not all breast carcinomas have such a characteristic appearance. In many instances, the mammogram identifies only an abnormal or suspicious area within the breast that could be an early carcinoma but is not conclusive, and a biopsy is necessary to establish the exact diagnosis.

Clinical Manifestations

The most common initial manifestation of breast carcinoma is a lump in the breast. It is often first detected by the patient herself in a monthly examination of her breasts. Sometimes the carcinoma may also cause secondary changes in the overlying skin or the nipple. The neoplasm may infiltrate the suspensory ligaments, exerting traction on the ligaments and causing them to shorten. Because the ligaments attach to the skin of the breast, shortening of the ligaments causes the overlying skin to retract as well (figure 16–8). Consequently, skin or nipple retraction generally indicates the presence of an infiltrating carcinoma deeper within the breast (figure 16–9).

If the tumor infiltrates and plugs the lymphatic vessels that drain lymph from the skin, the overlying skin will become edematous. (Lymphatic obstruction as a cause of edema is considered in chapter 12.) Skin edema produces a rather characteristic appearance in which the normal cutaneous

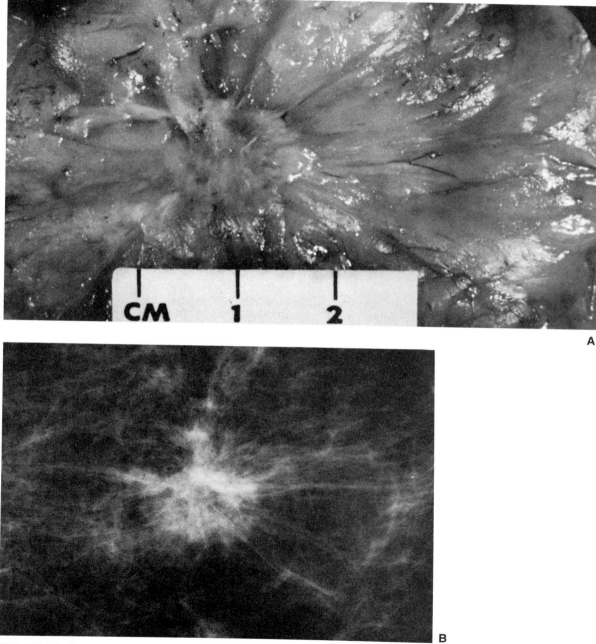

A

B

FIGURE 16–7

Breast carcinoma. **A,** Cross-section of breast biopsy. Tumor appears as firm, poorly circumscribed mass that infiltrates the surrounding fatty breast tissue. **B,** Appearance of breast carcinoma in a mammogram. Tumor appears as a white area with infiltrating margins. Note that the same criteria used to identify breast carcinoma on gross examination are used to recognize malignancy in the mammogram.

FIGURE 16–8

Mechanism of skin or nipple retraction in breast carcinoma. **A,** Normal breast. *Horizontal lines* represent suspensory ligaments extending from chest wall to skin. **B,** Tumor growing in breast causes shortening of suspensory ligaments, which leads to skin retraction.

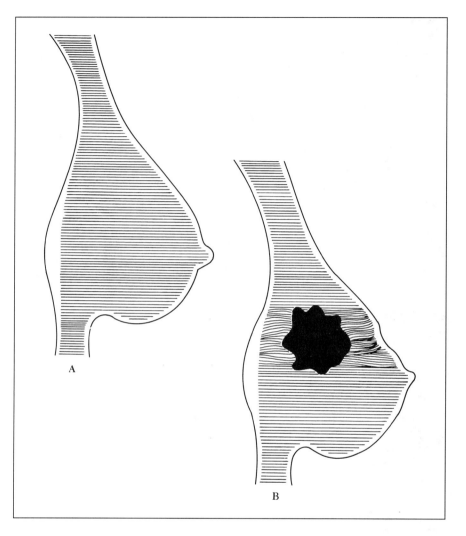

hair follicles stand out sharply as multiple small depressions within the edematous skin. The appearance has been compared to the skin of an orange and is usually called the *"orange-peel" sign* (figure 16–9A). Unfortunately, this finding indicates an advanced carcinoma that has already invaded lymphatic vessels and has probably also metastasized to regional lymph nodes. The likelihood of curing the cancer is much reduced at this stage.

If the patient delays in consulting her physician and a breast cancer is not treated, the tumor will eventually infiltrate the entire breast and will become fixed to the chest wall. The tumor will also metastasize widely. Although a far-advanced cancer often can be controlled for a time by various methods of treatment, there is no longer a possibility of cure (figure 16–10).

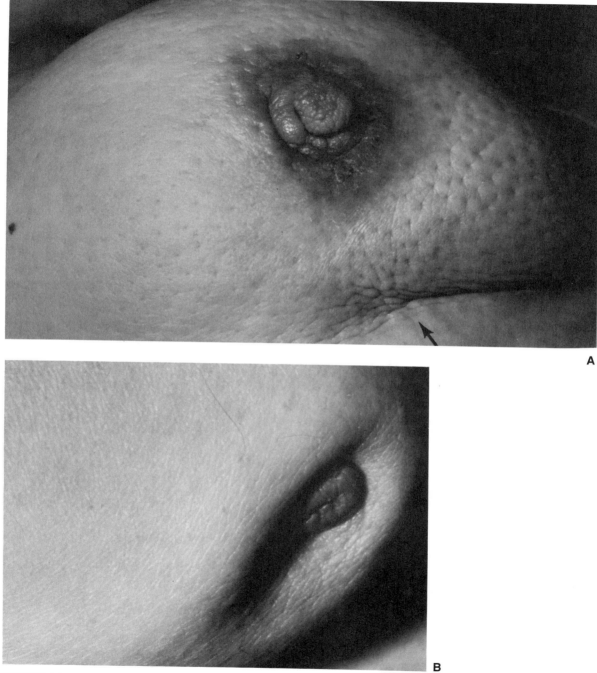

FIGURE 16–9

Changes in breast caused by carcinoma. **A,** Skin retraction *(arrow)* and orange-peel appearance of skin *(upper right).*
B, Nipple retraction.

FIGURE 16–10

Advanced breast carcinoma. Tumor involves entire breast and is fixed to the chest wall. Patient also has widespread metastases.

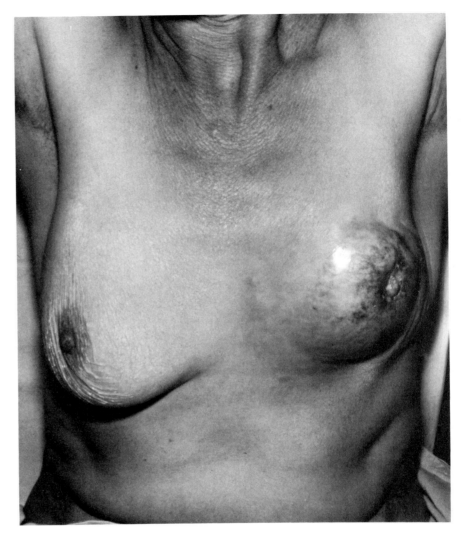

Treatment

There is continuing controversy concerning the best method for treating breast carcinoma. One widely accepted method of treatment is a surgical procedure called *modified radical mastectomy* or *total mastectomy with axillary lymph node dissection.* As the names indicate, the procedure consists of resecting the entire breast along with the axillary tissues that contain the lymph nodes draining the breast, but leaving the pectoral muscles overlying the chest wall.

A second method of treatment consists of removing only part of the breast along with the tumor (*partial mastectomy*) or removing only the tumor along with a small amount of adjacent breast tissue (*lumpectomy*). In these procedures, axillary lymph nodes also are removed, as in a total mastectomy. A course of radiotherapy is then administered to the breast in order to eradicate any carcinoma remaining within the breast that was not removed by surgical procedure. This treatment offers the advantage of preserving the breast but has the disadvantage of possible complications related to the radiotherapy.

Whichever method of treatment is selected, part of the tumor obtained at the time of breast biopsy or mastectomy is tested for the presence of estrogen and progesterone receptors, as described in the next section. In many cases, other specialized studies also are performed on the tumor cells, including the determination of their nuclear DNA content and their growth rate, as determined by measuring the rate at which the tumor cells are synthesizing DNA.

Determination of the hormone receptor status of the tumor has two purposes:

1. To provide information on prognosis. Tumors containing hormone receptors are better differentiated than those lacking receptors, and patients with tumors containing hormone receptors have a more favorable clinical course.
2. As a guide to further treatment.

The axillary lymph nodes are removed primarily so that they can be examined histologically in order to determine whether the tumor has spread beyond the breast. If the axillary lymph nodes contain metastatic carcinoma, it is likely that the tumor has already spread beyond the breast and axillary lymph nodes and a course of adjuvant chemotherapy is administered (described in chapter 10). The adjuvant therapy may consist either of an antiestrogen drug, such as Tamoxifen, that impedes tumor growth by blocking the effect of estrogen, on tumor cells, or of an anticancer chemotherapy drug that destroys tumor cells by blocking some aspect of their growth, metabolism, or cell division. If the axillary lymph nodes are free of tumor, the patient has a very favorable prognosis. Often no further treatment is required if the tumor is small and well differentiated. Adjuvant therapy in patients with unaffected axillary lymph nodes is usually reserved for those with large, poorly differentiated tumors.

Estrogen and Progesterone Receptors in Breast Carcinoma

A breast carcinoma is derived from cells whose growth and functions are influenced by various hormones: estrogen, progesterone, growth hormone, prolactin, and adrenal corticosteroids. Many breast tumors require these hormones for their continued growth and may undergo temporary regression if the body's hormonal balance is changed. Deliberate alteration of the body's hormones is often called *hormonal manipulation* and may be accomplished by withdrawing a required hormone or by blocking its action.

Not all breast tumors undergo regression in response to hormonal manipulation, but laboratory tests can be used to determine whether or not the tumor cells require estrogen and progesterone. The tests analyze the tumor cells obtained at the time of breast biopsy or mastectomy for the presence of specific cytoplasmic proteins that combine with estrogen or progesterone. The

FIGURE 16–11

Action of estrogen receptor. **A,** Estrogen enters cytoplasm and binds to estrogen receptor protein. **B,** Estrogen receptor complex enters nucleus. **C,** Complex attaches to nuclear chromatin, activating mRNA synthesis. Messenger RNA directs protein synthesis on ribosomes in cytoplasm.

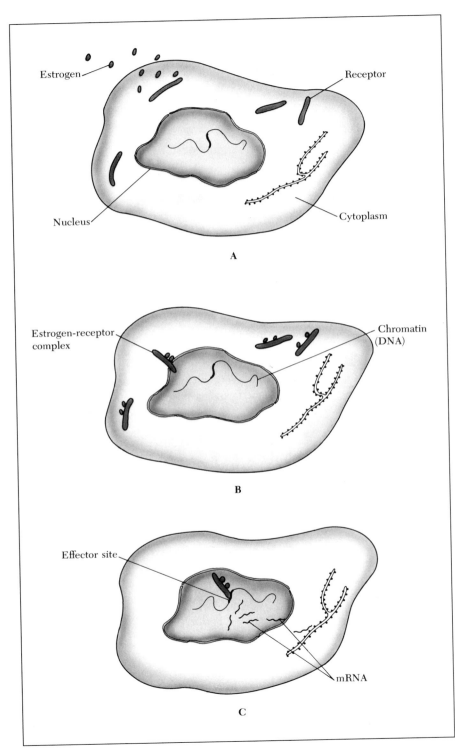

protein that combines with estrogen is called *estrogen receptor protein* or simply *estrogen receptor* (ER). The higher the content of estrogen-binding protein, the greater the likelihood that the tumor will respond to hormone treatment. A similar assay is used to determine the concentration of *progesterone receptor protein,* or simply *progesterone receptor* (PR). The presence of progesterone receptors in addition to estrogen receptors in the tumor increases the likelihood of response to hormonal manipulation. Approximately 60 percent of all breast tumors are estrogen receptor positive, and most estrogen receptor positive tumors are also positive for progesterone receptors. Response to hormonal manipulation is unlikely if the tumor cells lack hormone receptors.

Figure 16–11 illustrates how estrogen interacts with its receptor protein, and a similar mechanism applies to progesterone as well. In order for a cell to respond to estrogen, the hormone must enter the cell and combine with the estrogen receptors in the cytoplasm. The hormone-protein complex then moves into the nucleus and attaches to the nuclear DNA, where it stimulates the growth and other metabolic activities of the cell.

Unfortunately, a significant number of patients treated by total mastectomy or partial mastectomy and radiation will eventually develop widespread carcinoma and will require further treatment. The methods of treatment selected for an individual patient depend upon many factors, including the hormone receptor status of the tumor, the location of the metastases, the age of the patient, and the length of time that has elapsed between the initial treatment and the development of metastases. In general, initial treatment is by means of a drug (Tamoxifen) that blocks the effect of estrogen; so the tumor cells are no longer stimulated by the hormone. Both premenopausal and postmenopausal patients whose tumors are hormone receptor positive are likely to respond. Some patients respond initially to this treatment, but the drug later loses its effectiveness and other treatment methods must be used. If this occurs, other types of hormonal manipulation may be tried or anticancer drugs may be administered. Anticancer chemotherapy is much more toxic than antiestrogen drugs or other types of hormonal manipulation and usually is reserved for patients who fail to respond to hormonal manipulation. Usually, these are patients whose tumors lack estrogen receptors.

Sarcoma of the Breast

Sarcoma of the breast is rare in comparison with breast carcinoma. It may raise from the fibrous tissue or blood vessels within the breast. Sarcomas often form large, bulky tumors that may metastasize widely (figure 16–12). Treatment is by surgical resection of the involved breast.

A Lump in the Breast as a Diagnostic Problem

Many times, a physician faces the difficult problem presented by a patient who has a lump in her breast. It may have been detected either by the patient herself or by the physician in the course of a routine physical examination. The lump could be a benign cyst, a benign fibroadenoma, a carci-

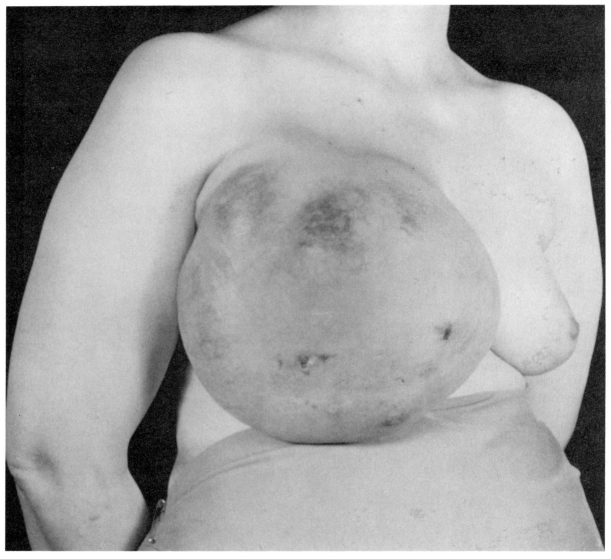

FIGURE 16–12

Large sarcoma of right breast. Note edema of right arm caused by the extension of tumor to lymphatics and veins in axilla.

noma, or one of many other, less-common diseases of the breast. Certain clinical features may suggest to the physician the probability that the breast lesion is benign or malignant, and mammograms of the breast may provide helpful information. However, the only way to be certain is to perform an aspiration biopsy or needle biopsy of the mass, or to completely excise the mass. This can be examined by a pathologist, who can make an exact diagnosis. If the lesion is benign, limited conservative treatment is all that is required. If the lesion proves to be malignant, the surgeon can perform a more extensive surgical operation.

Questions for Review

1. What are the three common diseases of the breast that may be manifested as a lump in the breast? How are they distinguished from one another by a physician?

2. What is a mammogram? How is it used by a physician?

3. What are estrogen receptors in tumor cells? How is an estrogen receptor analysis used in management of patients with breast carcinoma?

4. What is gynecomastia?

5. What methods are used to treat breast carcinoma?

Supplementary Readings

Berg, J. W., and Robbins, G. F. 1966. Factors influencing short and long term survival of breast cancer patients. *Surgery, Gynecology, and Obstetrics* 122:1311–16. A classic article on factors influencing prognosis. Information on late recurrences.

Cooper, G. M. 1992. *Elements of human cancer.* Boston: Jones and Bartlett Publishers. A readable book on various aspects of human cancer. Good sections on breast cancer.

Cotran, R., Kumar, V., and Robbins, S. 1994. *Robbins pathologic basis of disease.* 5th ed. Philadelphia: Saunders. A standard pathology textbook. Good section on breast disease.

Dupont, W. D., and Page, D. L. 1985. Risk factors for breast cancer in women with proliferative breast disease. *New England Journal of Medicine* 312:146–51. Women with benign breast disease in whom atypical epithelial hyperplasia was demonstrated are at increased risk of breast cancer.

Hetelekidis, S., Schnitt, S. J., Morrow, M., and Harris, J. R. 1995. Management of ductal carcinoma in situ. *CA: A Cancer Journal for Clinicians* 45:244–53. Reviews the current methods of treating this condition, current concepts regarding diagnosis, and the natural history of this disease.

Homer, M. J. 1984. Nonpalpable breast abnormalities. A realistic view of the accuracy of mammography in detecting malignancies. *Radiology* 153:831–32. Mammography will detect early breast cancer before it is palpable in the breast, but about 80 percent of radiologically suspicious lesions prove to be benign.

Hortobagyi, G., and Buzdar, A. U. 1995. Current status of adjuvant systemic chemotherapy for primary breast cancer: Progress and controversy. *CA: A Cancer Journal for Clinicians* 45:199–226. A review article on the current status of adjuvant chemotherapy and controversies surrounding chemotherapy.

Lipsztein, R., et al. 1985. Sequelae of breast radiation. *Journal of the American Medical Association* 253: 3582–84. Discusses the advantages and disadvantages of breast radiation.

Page, D. L., and Anderson, T. J. 1988. *Diagnostic histopathology of the breast.* New York: Churchill-Livingstone. A detailed treatment of histopathology of benign and malignant breast disease.

Wold, L. E., Ingle, J. N., Pisansky, T. M. 1995. Prognostic factors for patients with carcinoma of the breast. *Mayo Clinic Proceedings* 70:678–79. Reviews standard accepted prognostic factors and new prognostic factors. A major goal is to use prognostic factors to accurately predict which women with lymph node negative breast carcinoma will benefit from adjuvant chemotherapy.

Woods, J. 1986. Breast reconstruction: Current state of the art. *Mayo Clinic Proceedings* 61:579–85. Describes the patients suitable for breast reconstruction, the types of procedures available, and the results of reconstruction.

Chapter 16 ■ Outline Summary

Structure and Physiology / 447
Structure
Glands and branching ducts in fibrofatty tissue.

Fixed to chest wall by suspensory ligaments.

Abundant blood supply and lymphatic drainage.

Physiology
Responsive to hormonal stimulation.

Undergo cyclic changes.

Hypertrophy of glands in pregnancy.

Involution after menopause.

Examination of the Breasts / 447
Clinical Examination
Inspection.

Palpation.

Examination of axillary tissues.

Mammogram
Application: may identify lesions not detected on clinical examination.

Limitation: less useful for examining dense breast tissue of younger women.

Abnormalities of Breast Development / 450
Accessory Breasts and Nipples
Breasts develop from mammary ridges extending from axillae to groins.

Extra breasts and nipples occur occasionally.

Unequal Development of Breasts
Breasts may not develop equally.

Disproportion accentuated if breasts enlarge.

Breast Hypertrophy
Overgrowth of fibrous tissue.

Treated by surgical resection of excessive tissue.

Gynecomastia
Enlargement of male breast.

Temporary hormonal imbalance at puberty.

Treated by surgical resection.

Benign Cystic Disease / 453
Pathogenesis
Irregular cyclic response of breast to hormones.

May appear as solitary lump.

Treatment
Aspiration of surgical excision.

Fibroadenoma / 453
Appearance
Well-circumscribed tumor of glands and fibrous tissue.

Common in young women.

Treatment
Surgical excision.

Carcinoma of Breast / 453
Nature of Problem
Common malignant tumor in women.

Prone to late recurrence (see chapter 10).

Early diagnosis and treatment improves cure rate.

Appearance of Carcinoma
Often has characteristic gross appearance.

Mammogram assists in diagnosis.

Clinical Manifestations
Lump in breast.

Nipple or skin may be retracted owing to pull on suspensory ligaments.

Skin edema: caused by plugging of lymphatics.

Fixation of tumor to chest wall: late manifestation.

Treatment
Modified radical mastectomy or partial mastectomy/lumpectomy followed by breast radiation.

Examine axillary nodes for tumor; administer adjuvant chemotherapy if nodes are affected.

Estrogen Receptors in Breast Cancer
Estrogen receptors (ER) in cytoplasm fix hormone, move to nucleus, and stimulate cell functions.

Estrogen receptor positive tumor that has metastasized often responds to hormone treatment. Estrogen receptor negative tumors usually do not.

Sarcoma of the Breast / 463
Frequency
A rare tumor.

Often large and bulky.

Treated by surgical resection.

Lump in the Breast as a Diagnostic Problem / 463
Diagnostic Possibilities
Cystic disease.

Fibroadenoma.

Carcinoma.

Other less common conditions.

Diagnostic Approach
Clinical evaluation.

Mammogram.

Biopsy.

17

The Female Reproductive System

Learning Objectives

1. Describe the common infections of the genital tract and relate them to sexually transmitted diseases.
2. Describe the clinical manifestations and complications of endometriosis.
3. List the common causes of irregular uterine bleeding.
4. Describe the common diseases of the cervix, endometrium, myometrium, and vulva.
5. List the common cysts and tumors of the ovary.
6. Explain the pathogenesis, clinical manifestations, and treatment of toxic shock syndrome.
7. Categorize the common methods of artificial contraception, explain how they prevent conception, and describe their possible side effects.
8. Describe the abnormalities of the genital tract that most commonly develop in women whose mothers took diethylstilbestrol during pregnancy.

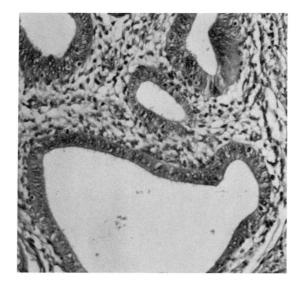

Chapter 17 ▪ Contents

Infections of the genital tract are common. Frequently involved sites are the vagina, the cervix, and the fallopian tubes. In addition, certain virus infections of the genital tract cause highly characteristic lesions called **condylomas**.

Vaginitis

Vaginal infections are common. They frequently cause vaginal discharge, together with vulvovaginal itching and irritation. There are three major causes:

1. The fungus *Candida albicans*
2. The protozoan parasite *Trichomonas vaginalis*
3. A small gram-negative bacterium called *Gardnerella* (*Hemophilus*) *vaginalis,* in conjunction with various anaerobic vaginal bacteria

Candida vaginitis is considered along with other fungal infections in chapter 6. The protozoan parasite. *Trichomonas vaginalis* is considered with the parasitic infections in chapter 7. The third common type of vaginitis, often called *nonspecific vaginitis,* is usually associated with a profuse, foul-smelling vaginal discharge. Highly specific methods of treatment are available for each type of vaginitis.

Cervicitis

Mild chronic inflammation of endocervical glands is very common in women who have had children. Cervicitis causes few symptoms and is of little clinical significance. More severe cervical inflammation may result from a gonococcal infection (described in chapter 8) or a chlamydial infection (described in chapter 6). Both infections are sexually transmitted and may be followed by spread of the infection into the fallopian tubes and adjacent tissues.

Salpingitis and Pelvic Inflammatory Disease

Salpingitis means an inflammation of the fallopian tube (*salpinx* = tube). The more general term **pelvic inflammatory disease,** or simply *PID,* refers to any infection that affects the fallopian tubes and adjacent tissues. Sometimes the ovaries are infected along with the fallopian tubes. Most cases are secondary to the spread of a cervical gonorrheal or chlamydial infection through the uterus into the fallopian tubes and surrounding tissues. Less commonly, other pathogenic organisms are involved. An acute pelvic infection causes severe lower abdominal pain and tenderness, together with elevated temperature and leukocytosis.

Both gonorrheal and nongonorrheal salpingitis respond to appropriate antibiotic therapy; healing of the inflammation, however, may be associated with scarring and obstruction of the tubal lumen. Sterility may result if the tubal obstruction is bilateral (figure 17–1). Sometimes, even if the tubes are not completely occluded, the scarring may delay the transport of a fertilized ovum through the tube and lead to implantation of the ovum in the fallop-

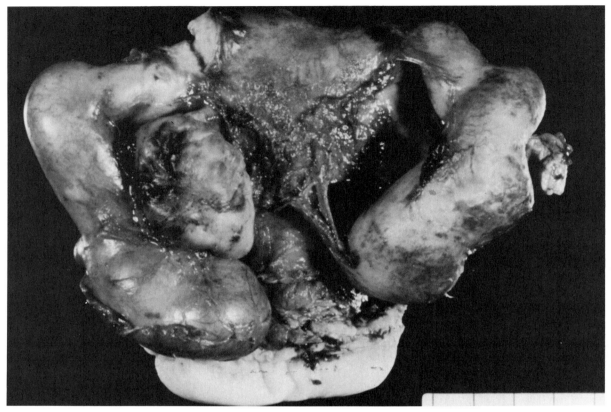

FIGURE 17–1

Chronic pelvic inflammatory disease. Resected uterus, tubes, and left ovary viewed from behind. Tubes are swollen and fimbriated ends are occluded. There are numerous adhesions between tubes and uterus.

ian tube rather than in the endometrial cavity. This condition is called an **ectopic pregnancy** and is considered in chapter 18.

Condylomas of the Genital Tract

Condylomas, sometimes called *venereal warts,* are benign, warty, tumor-like overgrowths of squamous epithelium caused by a virus that is spread by sexual contact. They vary in size from a few millimeters to more than 1 centimeter in diameter and are frequently multiple. Condylomas develop most often on the vulvar labia, around the vaginal orifice, and around the anus (see chapter 6, figure 6–10), but they may also occur in the vagina and on the cervix. Treatment consists of destruction of the lesions, which may be accomplished by application of a strong chemical (podophyllin), by electrocoagulation, by freezing (*cryocautery*), or by surgical excision.

The term **endometriosis** refers to the presence of endometrium in any location outside the endometrial cavity (figure 17–2). Ectopic deposits (*ecto* = outside) of endometrium may occasionally be encountered in the wall of the uterus (figure 17–3), in the ovary (figure 17–4), or elsewhere in the pelvis. Sometimes, endometrial tissue is found in the appendix or in the rectum. The reason that endometrial deposits occur in unusual locations is unknown, although many theories have been proposed. Some cases seem to be caused by reflux of bits of shed endometrium along with menstrual blood through the fallopian tubes into the peritoneal cavity during menstruation (retrograde menstruation), which then implant and grow in the pelvis. This does not provide a complete explanation, however, because retrograde menstruation is common but implantation of menstrual endometrium carried through the tubes into the peritoneal cavity is infrequent.

Endometrial deposits respond to normal hormonal stimuli and therefore undergo cyclic menstrual desquamation and regeneration. Because the misplaced endometrial tissue does not communicate with the endometrial cavity, the "menstruating" tissue is not discharged through the vagina. Old blood and desquamated material are retained in the ectopic sites, leading to considerable scarring and causing crampy pain during menstrual periods. Obstruction of the fallopian tubes by scarring may cause sterility.

Endometriosis

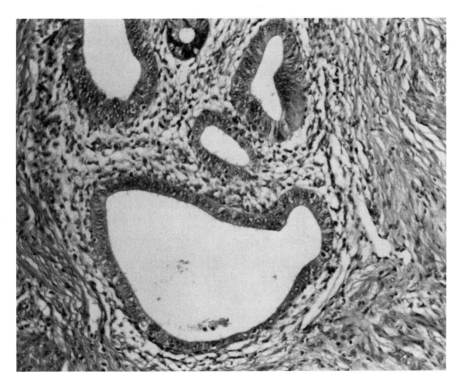

FIGURE 17–2

Photomicrograph of endometriosis in uterine wall. Normal endometrial glands and stroma are surrounded by uterine muscle. (Original magnification × 100.)

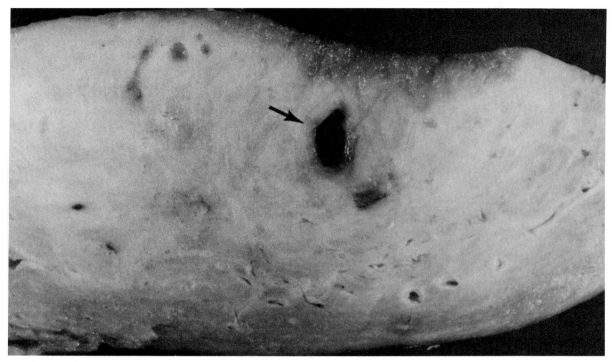

FIGURE 17–3

Cross-section of resected uterus illustrating a cystic deposit of endometriosis filled with old blood located in the uterine wall (*arrow*).

Diagnosis of endometriosis is usually established by visualizing the ectopic deposits within the pelvis with a lighted tubular instrument called a *laparoscope* (described in chapter 1). The laparoscope is inserted into the abdominal cavity through a small incision in the umbilicus. Treatment consists of removing or destroying the deposits surgically or impeding the progression of endometriosis by administering drugs or hormones. Three methods of hormone treatment are commonly used:

1. Synthetic hormones having progesterone activity, which completely suppress the menstrual cycles.
2. Birth-control pills, which suppress ovulation, so the endometrium becomes thin and atrophic and menstrual periods are very light. The endometriosis is similarly suppressed, retarding its progression and associated scarring.
3. Administration of drugs, such as danazol, that suppress the output of gonadotropins from the pituitary gland. This in turn leads to a decline in ovarian function, similar to that occurring in the menopause. The deposits of endometriosis, deprived of cyclic estrogen-progesterone stimulation, undergo regression.

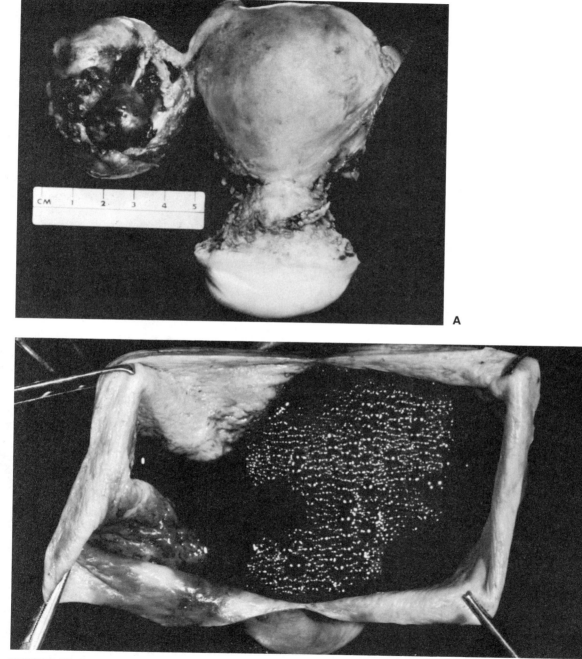

FIGURE 17–4

A, Endometriosis of ovary, appearing as areas of hemorrhage within enlarged ovary. **B,** Large cyst of ovary caused by endometriosis; cyst has been opened to reveal cyst contents consisting of old blood and debris derived from endometrium lining the cyst.

Cervical Polyps

Occasionally, benign polyps arise from the cervix. Usually, they are small and do not cause symptoms, but some may be quite large (figure 17–5). Sometimes the tip of the polyp becomes eroded and causes bleeding. Treatment consists of surgical removal of the polyp.

Cervical Dysplasia and Cervical Carcinoma

Abnormal growth and maturation of cervical squamous epithelium is called *cervical dysplasia* (described in chapter 2). Dysplastic changes range from mild disturbances of epithelial maturation to severe cellular abnormalities. Mild dysplasia may result from cervical inflammation or other causes and

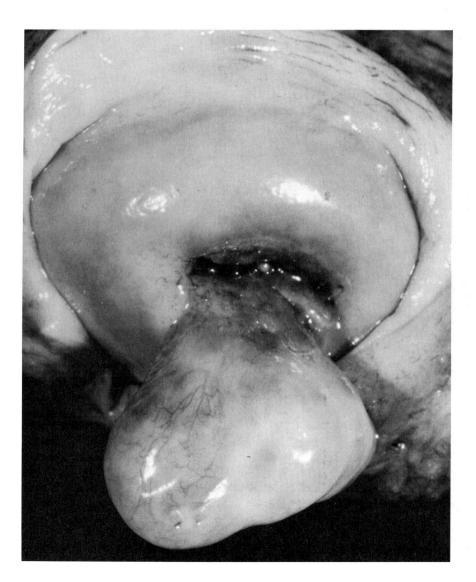

FIGURE 17–5

Large cervical polyp.

may regress spontaneously. Severe dysplasia usually does not regress and may progress to in situ carcinoma and eventually to invasive carcinoma after a variable period of time. Most physicians regard cervical dysplasia and in situ carcinoma as very closely related, constituting different stages in a progressive spectrum of epithelial abnormalities. Indeed, many physicians classify both dysplasia and in situ carcinoma under the general term *cervical intraepithelial neoplasia,* which is usually abbreviated CIN and is graded I, II, and III. In this terminology, mild dysplasia is called CIN I, moderate dysplasia is termed CIN II, severe dysplasia and in situ carcinoma are classified together and designated CIN III.

Persons infected with some strains of papilloma virus, the same virus that causes genital condylomas, are at increased risk of developing cervical dysplasia and cervical carcinoma. The dysplasia–cancer-causing strains can infect the cervical epithelial cells, and the viral DNA becomes incorporated into the cell's DNA, which induces cell dysfunction leading to cervical dysplasia and cervical carcinoma.

Diagnosis and Treatment

The cellular abnormalities indicative of dysplasia or carcinoma develop first in the cells at the junction between the squamous epithelium covering the exterior of the cervix and the columnar epithelium lining the cervical canal. This region is called the *squamocolumnar junction* or *transition zone* and is usually located at the external opening (*external os*) of the cervix. Abnormal cells indicative of dysplasia or carcinoma can be identified by means of a Pap smear prepared from material obtained from around the external os and endocervical canal, as described in chapter 10.

An abnormal Pap smear requires further evaluation, which is usually accomplished by means of a binocular magnifying instrument called a **colposcope.** This instrument provides the physician with a greatly magnified view of the cervix and endocervical canal. In cervical dysplasia and carcinoma, one can often identify characteristic abnormalities in the cervical epithelium and underlying blood vessels and can define the location and extent of the abnormal epithelium. Then multiple biopsy specimens are taken from the abnormal-appearing areas, and material is also obtained from the endocervical canal. Treatment depends on the results of the biopsies. Dysplasia and in situ carcinoma are usually treated by destruction of the abnormal epithelium by freezing (*cryocautery*), by laser light, by surgical excision of the abnormal area, or sometimes by removal of the uterus (*hysterectomy*). Invasive carcinoma is treated either by radiation or by resection of the uterus, fallopian tubes, ovaries, and adjacent tissues (*radical hysterectomy*).

Dysplasia and in situ carcinoma can be cured by proper treatment and carry an excellent prognosis. In situ carcinoma may remain localized within the epithelium of the cervix for as long as ten years before eventually becoming invasive. Once invasion has occurred, however, the neoplasm is much harder to treat and the results are less satisfactory. The tumor may extend through the cervix into the adjacent tissues and may infiltrate the rectum and bladder. The ureters, which lie on each side of the cervix, also may be invaded and obstructed by the neoplasm. Metastatic spread to regional lymph nodes and distant sites also is common.

Endometrial Hyperplasia, Polyps, and Carcinoma

Occasionally, the endometrium of the uterus may undergo *benign hyperplasia*, which is often associated with irregular uterine bleeding (figure 17–6). *Benign polyps* in the endometrium also are common (figure 17–7). Sometimes an endometrial polyp may cause uterine bleeding if the tip becomes inflamed or ulcerated. *Endometrial adenocarcinoma* has been increasing in frequency. This condition also is manifested by irregular uterine bleeding or postmenopausal bleeding. Endometrial carcinoma is often related to prolonged or excessive stimulation of the endometrium by estrogen. The rising incidence of the neoplasm seems to have been related to frequent and long-term use of estrogens to control menopausal symptoms. Because physicians have become aware of this association, use of estrogens

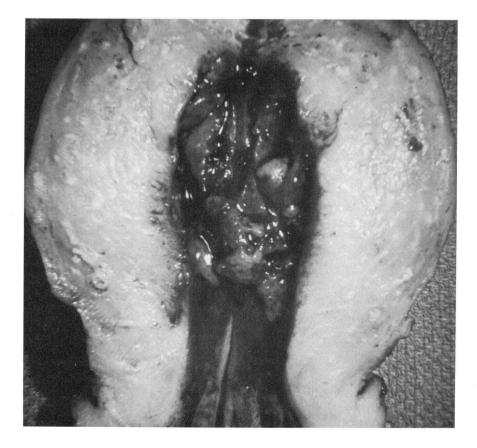

FIGURE 17–6

Benign endometrial hyperplasia. Uterus opened to reveal polypoid masses of hyperplastic endometrium filling endometrial cavity.

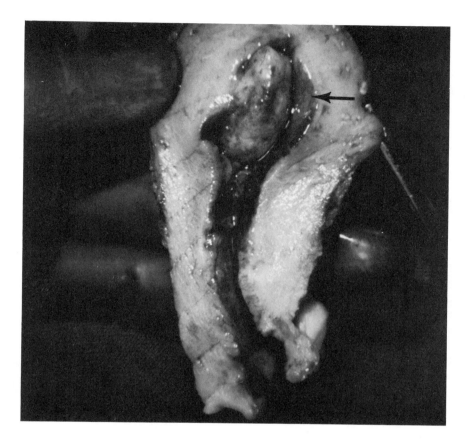

FIGURE 17–7

Cross-section of resected uterus revealing a large endometrial polyp filling endometrial cavity (*arrow*).

in the menopause has been reduced and the incidence of endometrial carcinoma seems to be declining.

Uterine Myomas

Benign smooth-muscle tumors called **myomas** arise in the wall of the uterus (figures 17–8A, B). They are frequently encountered and are said to occur in approximately 30 percent of women over thirty years of age. Occasionally, myomas may be responsible for excessive or irregular uterine bleeding or may produce symptoms related to pressure on the adjacent bladder or rectum (figure 17–9). Hysterectomy is performed if the myomas are producing symptoms.

Irregular Uterine Bleeding

Excessive or irregular uterine bleeding is a common gynecologic problem. Most cases in younger women result from a disturbance in the normal cyclic interaction of estrogen and progesterone upon the endometrium. This is

FIGURE 17–8A

Uterus opened to reveal a large spherical myoma protruding into endometrial cavity.

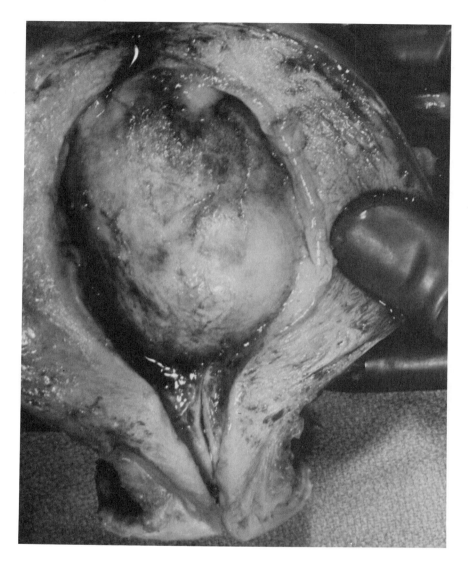

usually called *dysfunctional uterine bleeding.* In older women, bleeding can be the result of many causes.

Dysfunctional Uterine Bleeding

Normally, the first half of the menstrual cycle is characterized by proliferation of endometrial glands and stroma under the influence of estrogen produced by the ovarian follicle. At about midcycle, ovulation occurs and the follicle discharges its egg. Then the follicle becomes a *corpus luteum,* which produces both progesterone and estrogen. Under the influence of progesterone, the endometrium becomes a secretory phase in preparation for

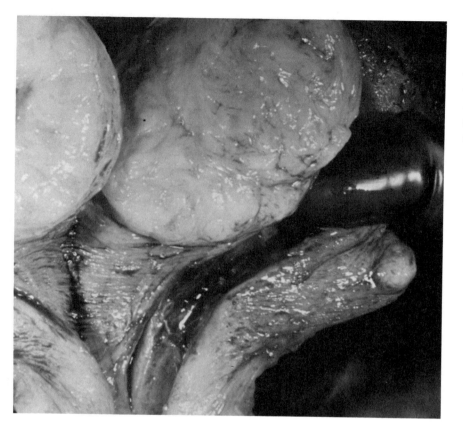

FIGURE 17–8B

Cross-section of myoma illustrating a well-circumscribed tumor without evidence of necrosis—features suggesting a benign neoplasm.

receiving a fertilized ovum. If no pregnancy occurs, the corpus luteum begins to decline and estrogen-progesterone levels begin to drop. The secretory endometrium is deprived of its hormonal support and is shed along with a small amount of blood, constituting the menstrual flow, after which a new cycle begins.

Most cases of dysfunctional uterine bleeding occur because the follicle fails to mature to the point of ovulation and, consequently, no corpus luteum forms. As a result, the endometrium is subjected to continuous estrogen stimulation and responds by shedding in an irregular manner associated with irregular uterine bleeding, instead of shedding all at once as in a normal period. This condition is also called *anovulatory bleeding* (*ana* = without + ovulation). It tends to arise at both extremes of reproductive life: when normal menstrual cycles are being established at puberty and near menopause when ovarian function is declining. Less commonly, irregular bleeding is the result of continuous secretion of progesterone from a corpus luteum that fails to involute. This prolongs the secretory phase of the endometrium, which sometimes sheds irregularly.

Dysfunctional uterine bleeding is treated by administering hormones to restore the proliferative-secretory sequence in the endometrium that is char-

FIGURE 17–9

Enlarged, irregularly shaped uterus containing multiple myomas, which bulge from the uterus. Cervix is at *bottom* of photograph.

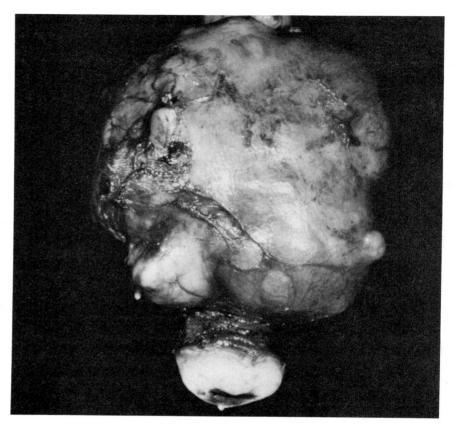

acteristic of a normal menstrual cycle. In one common treatment, the patient is given a synthetic steroid hormone having progesterone activity. The hormone induces secretory changes in the endometrium and stops the bleeding. The hormone treatment is the stopped, and the endometrium sheds as in a normal period. Frequently, the next cycle is normal and no further treatment is required.

Other Causes of Uterine Bleeding

Other conditions that may cause endometrial bleeding include benign endometrial hyperplasia, endometrial and cervical polyps, uterine myomas, and uterine carcinoma.

Diagnosis and Treatment

Irregular bleeding is always a cause for concern when it occurs in an older woman nearing the end of her reproductive years or after the menopause, because it may be the result of an endometrial carcinoma. Bleeding in older women is usually treated by dilating the cervix with various metal dilators and then scraping out the lining of the uterus with a long-handled scoop-like instrument called a *curette*. This procedure is called *dilatation and curettage* or simply **D and C.** The tissue removed is examined microscopically by the pathologist. If the endometrial tissue is not malignant, no further treatment is needed. If endometrial carcinoma is detected on histologic examination, further treatment is required. Usually this consists of hysterectomy, sometimes preceded by a course of radiation therapy.

Dysmenorrhea

Dysmenorrhea means painful menstruation. There are two types: *primary dysmenorrhea,* in which the pelvic organs are normal, and *secondary dysmenorrhea,* which results from various diseases of the pelvic organs, such as endometriosis.

Primary dysmenorrhea is the more common type. The pain is crampy, begins just prior to menstruation, and lasts for one or two days after onset of the menstrual flow. Usually, menstrual periods are painless for the first year or two after onset of menses during adolescence, because early menstrual cycles are usually anovulatory and primary dysmenorrhea does not occur unless ovulation occurs. Dysmenorrhea does not usually become a problem until regular ovulatory menstrual cycles are established.

Crampy menstrual pain is caused by a class of compounds called **prostaglandins,** complex unsaturated fatty-acid derivatives that are synthesized in many locations throughout the body and have many functions. The name derives from the prostate gland, where these substances were first identified. Prostaglandins are synthesized within the endometrium under the influence of progesterone produced by the ovary during the secretory phase of the cycle. They are released when the endometrium breaks down during menstruation. They then diffuse into the myometrium, where they stimulate intense, spasmodic myometrial contractions, causing the characteristic crampy menstrual pain. Dysmenorrhea does not occur if cycles are anovulatory, because no corpus luteum forms and no progesterone is produced to stimulate prostaglandin synthesis.

Treatment consists of aspirin or another anti-inflammatory drug, which is administered prior to onset of menses. These drugs suppress the synthesis of prostaglandins within the endometrium. Primary dysmenorrhea can also be treated very effectively with oral contraceptive pills, which prevent dysmenorrhea by suppressing ovulation.

Cysts and Tumors of the Ovary

The ovary gives rise to a wide variety of cysts and tumors, and only the more common ones are considered here. Benign ovarian cysts are common. They arise either from ovarian follicles or from corpora lutea that have failed to regress normally and instead become converted into fluid filled cysts. Follicle cysts and corpus luteum cysts are often called *functional cysts* because they represent a derangement of the normal maturation and involution of a follicle or corpus luteum. Functional cysts do not usually become very large, and most regress spontaneously.

Endometrial deposits in the ovary may form cysts lined by endometrium and filled with old blood and debris. These are called **endometrial cysts.**

True ovarian neoplasms may arise in one or both ovaries. They may be either benign or malignant, cystic or solid. Benign cystic teratomas, often called **dermoid cysts,** commonly develop in the ovary. These tumors arise from unfertilized ova that have undergone neoplastic change. They often contain skin, hair, teeth, bone, parts of gastrointestinal tract, thyroid, and other tissues growing in a jumbled fashion (figure 17–10). Sometimes teeth and bone contained in dermoid cysts can be detected in x-ray films of the pelvis (figure 17–11; see also chapter 10, figure 10–16). A dermoid cyst apparently represents an attempt of an unfertilized ovum to realize its potential by producing diverse tissues like those in a fetus. In contrast with the frequency of benign ovarian teratomas, malignant teratomas of the ovary are quite rare.

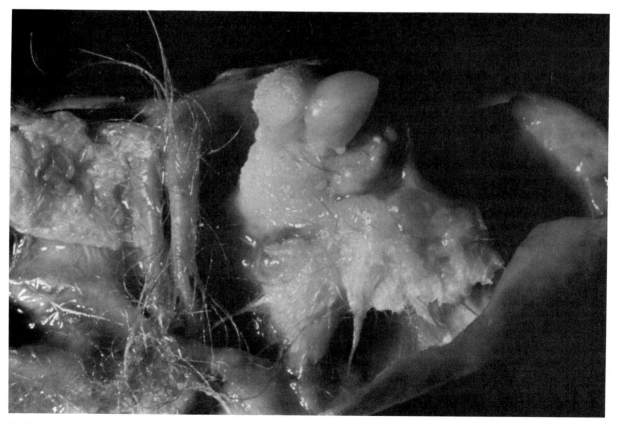

FIGURE 17–10

Opened dermoid cyst of ovary with contents evacuated. Cyst contains a well-formed jawbone with two teeth (*center* of photograph). Note hair arising from skin that lines the cyst.

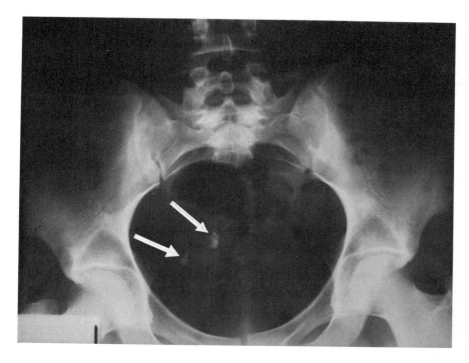

FIGURE 17–11

X-ray of pelvis illustrating teeth (*arrows*) contained within dermoid cyst.

Another groups of ovarian tumors are those arising from the epithelial cells on the surface of the ovary, and the epithelium of the tumor cells may resemble the epithelium found in other parts of the genital tract. If the tumor epithelium resembles the cells lining the fallopian tube, the tumor is classified as a serous tumor. If the tumor epithelium resembles the mucus-secreting epithelium of the endocervix, it is called a mucinous tumor; and, if the tumor epithelium resembles endometrium, it is termed an endometroid tumor. Many of the serous and mucinous tumors are cystic, and the term *serous cystadenoma* or *serous cystadenocarcinoma* is used. A mucinous tumor is designated as either a *mucinous cystadenoma* or a *mucinous cystadenocarcinoma.* Most of the ovarian tumors with endometrium-like epithelium are malignant and are called *endometroid carcinomas.* Another common ovarian tumor arises from the fibrous connective tissue cells of the ovary and is called a *fibroma.*

A few ovarian tumors produce sex hormones. One type arises from the estrogen-producing cells lining the follicles (granulosa cells) and the closely associated cells adjacent to the follicle cells (called theca cells). These cells produce estrogen and so does a tumor arising from these cells, which is called a **granulosa cell tumor** or **granulosa-theca cell tumor.** The tumor may induce endometrial hyperplasia owing to excessive endometrial stimulation from the estrogen produced by the tumor. A granulosa cell tumor in a postmenopausal woman may induce irregular uterine bleeding. A few rare types of ovarian tumor produce male sex hormones instead of estrogen and may induce masculinization.

Some ovarian tumors may become quite large, as illustrated by the following case.

CASE 17–1

A young women who was seven months pregnant had noted marked enlargement of the abdomen that she attributed to the pregnancy. Examination by her physician revealed a large cystic mass lying above and posterior to the pregnant uterus. At operation, a large benign cystic tumor of the ovary was encountered. It contained 15 L of fluid and weighed 35 pounds (figure 17–12). The day after the operation, the patient went into labor and delivered a premature infant who was transferred to the pediatric intensive care unit. Both mother and infant did well after the operation.

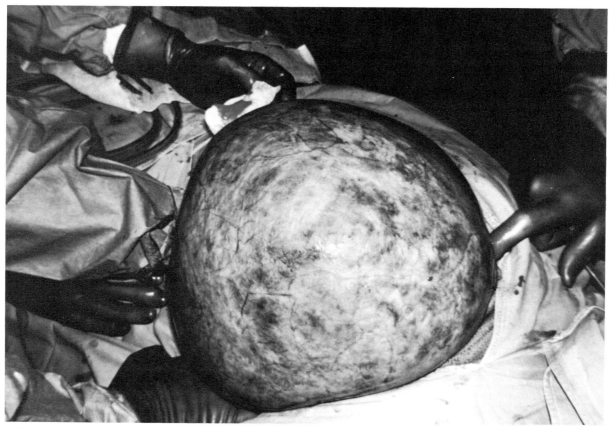

FIGURE 17–12

Large benign ovarian cyst weighing 35 pounds identified at operation in a pregnant woman (case 17–1).

Vulvar Dystrophy

The epithelium of the vulva may exhibit irregular areas of thickening and inflammation that appear as white patches. Histologically, the affected epithelium is heavily keratinized and the epithelial cells show variable abnormalities of maturation. Clinically, the condition is associated with intense itching and tenderness of the affected areas. The descriptive term *leukoplakia* (*leuko* = white + *plakia* = patch) has often been applied to this lesion but has been discarded in favor of a newer term, *vulvar dystrophy* (*dys* = abnormal + *trophe* = growth). In some cases, vulvar dystrophy progresses gradually over a period of years into in situ carcinoma and eventually into invasive carcinoma. Consequently, many physicians consider vulvar dystrophy a precancerous lesion. Various types of local treatment are frequently effective, but if significant precancerous changes are present in the epithelium, the affected areas are generally removed surgically.

Carcinoma of the Vulva

Vulvar carcinoma is occasionally found in both premenopausal and postmenopausal women, frequently arising in areas of vulvar dystrophy (figure 17–13). Treatment consists of resection of the vulva (*vulvectomy*) along with the inguinal lymph nodes, which receive lymphatic drainage from the vulva.

Toxic shock syndrome (TSS) is a disease that was first recognized in menstruating women who used high-absorbency tampons. However, no tampon can be considered entirely free from risk.

Clinically, the disease is characterized by elevated temperature, vomiting and diarrhea, muscular aches and pains, a fall in blood pressure (often to shock levels), and various other systemic manifestations. A characteristic feature of the disease is an erythematous (sunburnlike) skin rash that is followed by flaking and peeling of the affected skin (somewhat like the peeling that occurs after a severe sunburn).

The clinical manifestations of toxic shock syndrome are caused by a toxin produced by a penicillin-resistant *Staphylococcus aureus* that grows in the vagina of the affected patients. The menstrual blood and secretions provide an excellent culture medium that fosters the growth of the staphylococci and the production of toxin. Tampons apparently promote the development of TSS in two ways. First, they prevent drainage of menstrual products from the vagina and thereby favor growth of the staphylococci. Second, tampons are foreign bodies and may injure the vaginal lining, causing small superficial ulcerations of the vaginal mucosa. Absorption of toxins could occur rapidly through such injured areas.

Treatment of toxic shock syndrome consists of general supportive measures to sustain the patient until the effects of the toxin have worn off. There is no way to counteract or neutralize the toxin. Tampon use should be

FIGURE 17–13

Large, partially ulcerated carcinoma of vulva. The white appearance of the skin adjacent to the carcinoma is caused by preexisting vulvar dystrophy.

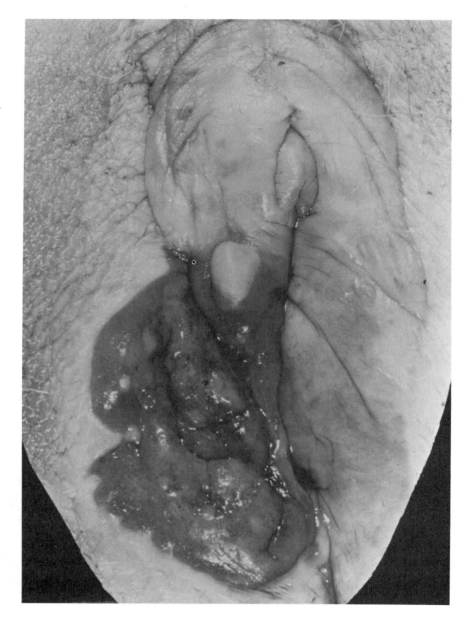

promptly discontinued. Antibiotics are often prescribed to eradicate the staphylococci, but the antibiotics do not shorten the course of the disease.

Women can completely eliminate the risk of toxic shock syndrome by not using tampons and can reduce their risk by using tampons only intermittently during the menstrual period. If a woman has had toxic shock syndrome, she should probably never again use tampons, because the recurrence rate among tampon users is about 30 percent.

Natural sea sponges ("menstrual sponges") have been promoted as an alternative to tampons. However, there are no studies to indicate that menstrual sponges are less risky than tampons, and cases of toxic shock syndrome have been associated with use of sponges as well as tampons. Moreover, the sponges may cause other problems because they have been found to contain sand, bacteria, and other potentially harmful substances.

Rarely, toxic shock syndrome occurs in nonmenstruating women and in men. These cases are a result of staphylococcal infections in other parts of the body, such as the skin, kidneys, or bone, with liberation of toxins from the infected site into the circulation.

Contraception

Methods of contraception fall into two major groups: "natural" methods and artificial methods. *Natural family planning* methods attempt to prevent pregnancy by avoiding intercourse around the time of ovulation when pregnancy is more likely to occur. These methods have no side effects or medical complications but require a high degree of motivation and are generally less effective than artificial methods. In contrast, *artificial methods* act by preventing the union of sperm and egg, preventing ovulation, or preventing implantation of the fertilized ovum. Many of these methods are highly effective, but some have potentially serious side effects.

Diaphragms and *condoms* are mechanical devices that are usually used in conjunction with a spermacidal foam or jelly. They function by preventing the union of sperm and egg; they are highly effective when used correctly and have no serious side effects.

Recently, a "condom for women" has been marketed. The device consists of a soft plastic tube closed at one end. Two flexible plastic rings are located at opposite ends of the tube. When the device is inserted into the vagina, its closed upper end is held in place against the cervix by the upper plastic ring, much like a diaphragm that covers the cervix, and the plastic tube lines the vagina. The open, lower end of the tube, encircled by the lower plastic ring, is positioned outside the vagina.

A vaginal *contraceptive sponge* functions much like a diaphragm. It is a soft, flat polyurethane disk with a central depression. The sponge contains a spermacide called nonoxynol-9. Inserted high in the vagina against the cervix before intercourse, the sponge blocks sperm from entering the cervix and the spermacide destroys any sperm that come in contact with the sponge. *Contraceptive suppositories* are another popular contraceptive methods. The suppository is inserted in the vagina before intercourse, where it dissolves and releases a spermacide. Suppositories reduce the chance of conception but are less effective than the preceding methods because they are not used along with mechanical devices that cover the cervix.

Most *contraceptive pills* consist of a synthetic estrogen combined with a compound having progesterone activity (progestin). "The pill" prevents ovulation by suppressing release of gonadotrophic hormones from the pituitary and is almost 100-percent effective but does have side effects. The estrogen in the pill promotes increased synthesis of blood coagulation factors, predisposing to formation of blood clots within the circulatory system. Women who smoke cigarettes and women over thirty-five years of age are at especially high risk. Some women on the pill develop high blood pressure. The elevated pressure probably results from an increased synthesis of a blood protein (called *renin substrate*) induced by the estrogen in the pill, which interacts with renin produced by the kidney to yield *angiotensin,* a potent blood-pressure-raising compound described in chapter 19. Women on the pill are closely observed for this complication, and the pill is discontinued if the blood pressure starts to rise.

A second less frequently used type of contraceptive pill contains only a progestin and may have fewer side effects than the combined estrogen-progesterone pill. The progestin acts by changing the character of the cervical mucus, which impedes sperm penetration, changes the character of the endometrium so that a fertilized egg is unable to become implanted, and may suppress ovulation in some patients. A recently marketed implantable form of a progestin contraceptive consists of silicone rubber rods containing a progestin which is inserted under the skin. The progestin is slowly released from the implant into the circulation over a period of several years, eliminating the need for daily pill taking.

An **intrauterine device** (IUD) is a small, flexible plastic structure that is inserted into the uterine cavity by a physician (figure 17–14). A string

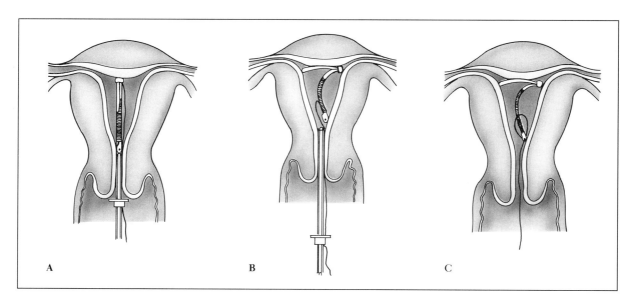

FIGURE 17–14

Technique of inserting one type of IUD (copper 7 device). Other devices are inserted in a similar manner. **A,** Device is retracted into insertion tube, and tube is introduced through cervix to fundus of uterus. **B,** Tube is retracted, allowing plastic device to resume its original configuration. **C,** Tube is withdrawn. String attached to IUD protrudes through cervix into vagina.

attached to the device extends through the cervix into the vagina. The string serves two purposes. The woman can assure herself that the device is still within the uterine cavity by feeling the string. It also facilitates removal of the IUD by the physician when it is no longer needed.

Intrauterine devices do not prevent conception but act by preventing implantation of the fertilized ovum. Most of the devices are no longer marketed because of declining sales and because of concerns about lawsuits initiated by women who may have experienced complications from use of the devices.

A formerly popular device, the *copper 7 IUD,* which was named from its shape and the copper wire wound around its stem, has been withdrawn from the market. There are only two intrauterine contraceptive devices available currently. One, called the *Paragard®*, is a T-shaped plastic device with copper wire wound around both the stem and the side arms that replaces the copper 7 IUD. The effectiveness of copper-wound devices is related primarily to the contraceptive effect of the copper, which is released slowly within the endometrium as the copper wire gradually dissolves. The device must be replaced every four years because the effectiveness of the device declines as the copper wire dissolves. The other IUD, also a T-shaped plastic device, is called the *Progestasert®*, so named because a reservoir in the stem of the device contains progesterone that diffuses slowly from the IUD over a period of a year. The device must then be replaced with a new one. Much of its effectiveness depends on the slow release of progesterone, which alters the endometrium, inhibiting implantation of the fertilized ovum (figure 17–15).

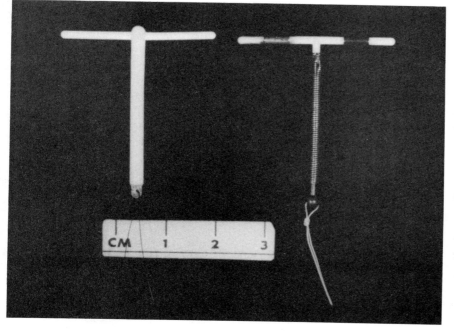

FIGURE 17–15

Intrauterine devices. *Left,* Progestasert®. *Right,* Paragard®. Approximate length 3 cm.

Two major problems are associated with use of an IUD. The first is an increased incidence of uterine and tubal infections, which may be followed by tubal scarring and impaired fertility. Some women have developed serious chronic pelvic infections caused by anaerobic bacteria that sometimes infect a uterus containing an IUD. A second problem relates to tubal pregnancies. Because an IUD prevents implantation only within the uterus and does not prevent either ovulation or fertilization, implantation may occur within the tube.

If a woman becomes pregnant while wearing an IUD, the pregnancy may be in the tube rather than in the uterus. The incidence of ectopic pregnancies in *Progestasert®* users is much higher than in users of other IUDs, possibly because the progesterone diffusing from the device not only changes the endometrium, but also slows tubal motility, predisposing to tubal implantations. (Chapter 18 discusses tubal pregnancy and the significance of previous tubal infection as a predisposing factor.)

Effects of Prenatal Exposure to Diethylstilbestrol (DES)

Diethylstilbestrol (DES) and similar nonsteroidal estrogens were in widespread use from about 1946 to 1970 for treating mothers who were prone to spontaneous abortion and for treating various other obstetric problems. Subsequently, it was found these drugs often caused developmental abnormalities in the genital tracts of women whose mothers took these drugs in pregnancy and induced malignant tumors in a small percentage of cases.

The developmental abnormalities most commonly found consist of constricting fibrous bands involving the cervix or upper vagina. They are often associated with projecting ridges composed of epithelium and stroma. Sometimes the ridges form irregular polypoid masses projecting from the cervix or they may appear as collarlike structures that completely encircle the cervix. In another common abnormality called *adenosis,* small foci of columnar epithelium are interspersed within the normal cervical and vaginal squamous epithelium. The areas of adenosis appear bright red in contrast with the pale pink appearance of the surrounding normal stratified squamous epithelium.

The foregoing developmental abnormalities are not considered precancerous. They may eventually become less conspicuous or even disappear completely. The more serious DES-induced abnormality is an unusual type of carcinoma arising from the cervix or vagina. It is called *clear cell adenocarcinoma* because the neoplastic cells have a very pale (clear) cytoplasm. Apparently, DES induces some abnormality of the genital tract that predisposes to the later development of cancer. Fortunately, the incidence of this serious complication is quite low. It is estimated to occur in not more than about one per thousand exposed women, and the actual incidence may be considerably lower. Nevertheless, because of this risk, periodic pelvic examination and biopsy of any suspicious lesion is recommended for all DES-exposed women.

Questions for Review

1. What parts of the female genital tract may be affected by gonorrheal infection? How does gonorrhea lead to sterility?

2. What is the difference between in situ and invasive cervical carcinoma? How is the Pap smear used in the diagnosis of carcinoma?

3. A patient consults her physician because of irregular uterine bleeding. What are some of the diseases of the genital tract that cause this bleeding?

4. What is endometriosis? What symptoms does it produce? What are some complications that may be associated with endometriosis?

5. What is a dermoid cyst?

6. What is toxic shock? How does tampon use predispose to this syndrome? What role do staphylococci play?

7. How do contraceptive pills and IUDs exert their contraceptive effects? What medical problems may be associated with their use?

8. What is vulvar dystrophy? What symptoms does it cause? What are its complications?

Supplementary Readings

Boston Women's Health Book Collective Staff. 1992. *The new our bodies, ourselves.* New York: Simon and Schuster. Covers a wide range of subjects dealing with sexual anatomy, physiology, and pathology in a clear and concise manner. A useful reference.

Crum, C. P., et al. 1984. Human papillomavirus, type 16, and early cervical neoplasia. *New England Journal of Medicine* 310:880–83. Human papillomavirus, type 16, is associated with flat warts of the cervix, which is precursor to invasive cervical cancer.

Davis, J. P., et al. 1980. Toxic-shock syndrome. *New England Journal of Medicine* 303:1429–35. A good review article.

Hatcher, R. A. 1994. *Contraceptive technology 1994–1996.* New York: Irvington. A standard reference. Updated annually.

Herbst, A. L., et al. 1975. Effects of maternal DES ingestion on the female genital tract. *Hospital Practice* 10:51–57. Describes the adverse effects of DES. Written by the physician who first reported the association of DES with genital tract cancer.

Kurman, R. J., ed. 1994. *Blaustein's pathology of the female genital tract.* 4th ed. New York: Springer. A standard reference. Documents relation of certain strains of papillomavirus to condylomas and cervical neoplasms. Good sections on ovarian cysts and tumors.

Kurman, R. J., Henson, D. E., Herbst, A. L., et al. 1994. Interim guidelines for management of abnormal cervical cytology. *Journal of the American Medical Association* 271:1866–69. Reviews current management approaches and described applications and limitations of the Bethesda cytology classification system.

Lu, P., and Ory, S. J. 1995. Endometriosis: Current management. *Mayo Clinic Proceedings* 70:453–63. A review of the clinical features, theories of pathogenesis, and current methods of treatment.

Reeves, W. C., Rawls, W. E., and Brinton, L. A. 1988. Epidemiology of genital papillomaviruses and cervical cancer. *Reviews of Infectious Diseases* 11:426–39. Genital papillomavirus causes dysplastic lesions, and most invasive cervical cancer contains papillomavirus DNA. Virus appears to integrate into cell DNA.

Robboy, S. J., et al. 1981. Prenatal diethylstilbestrol (DES) exposure: Recommendations for the diethylstilbestroladenosis (DESAD) project for the identification and management of exposed individuals. NIH Publication No. 81-2049. Washington, DC: U.S. Department of Health and Human Services. Describes the DES-induced genital tract abnormalities and methods of screening exposed women for clear cell carcinoma.

Scully, R. E. 1977. Ovarian tumors. *American Journal of Pathology* 87:686–720. A comprehensive review article.

Shands, K. et al. 1980. Toxic-shock syndrome in menstruating women. *New England Journal of Medicine* 303:1436–42. A review of the subject.

Smith, D. C., et al. 1975. Association of exogenous estrogen and endometrial cancer. *New England Journal of Medicine* 293:1164–67. One of the early definitive studies relating endometrial cancer to use of estrogens to control menopausal symptoms.

Chapter 17 ■ Outline Summary

Infections of the Genital Tract / 469
Vaginitis
Manifestations: vaginal discharge, itching, and irritation.

Causes:

Candida albicans: chapter 6.

Trichomonas vaginalis: chapter 7.

Gardnerella (*Hemophilus*) *vaginalis* in conjunction with anaerobic bacteria (nonspecific vaginitis).

Cervicitis
Mild chronic inflammation: common and of little clinical significance.

More severe inflammation often caused by gonococci or *Chlamydia*. May spread to infect tubes and adjacent tissues (pelvic inflammatory disease).

Salpingitis and Pelvic Inflammatory Disease
Definitions:

Salpingitis: tubal infection.

Pelvic inflammatory disease (PID): more general term referring to infection of tubes and adjacent tissues as well.

Manifestations and complications:

Usually caused by gonococcal or chlamydial infection spreading from cervix.

Causes lower abdominal pain and tenderness, elevated temperature, and leukocytosis.

Tubal scarring following healing may cause sterility or predispose to ectopic pregnancy.

Condylomas of Genital Tract
Virus warts of genital tract.

Can be destroyed by chemicals, electrocoagulation, freezing (cryocautery), or excision.

Endometriosis / 471
Clinical Manifestations
Deposits of endometrium outside normal location in endometrial cavity.

Ectopic endometrium responds to hormonal stimuli; undergoes menstrual desquamation and regeneration.

Secondary scarring may obstruct fallopian tubes and cause infertility.

Cervical Polyps / 474
Polyps
Usually small.

Erosion of tip may cause bleeding.

Cervical Dysplasia and Cervical Carcinoma / 474
Concept of Cervical Intraepithelial Neoplasia
Varies from mild to severe.

Mild dysplasia may regress; severe dysplasia may progress to carcinoma.

Dysplasia and in situ carcinoma closely related.

Genital viral infections may predispose to neoplasia.

Diagnosis and Treatment
Pap smear shows abnormal cells.

Colposcopy localizes abnormalities.

Biopsies establish diagnosis.

Treatment depends on extent of disease.

Dysplasia and in situ carcinoma treated by cryocautery, excision, or hysterectomy. Results excellent.

Invasive carcinoma treated by radiation or radical surgery. Results less satisfactory.

Endometrial Hyperplasia, Polyps, and Carcinoma / 476
Benign Hyperplasia
May cause irregular uterine bleeding.

Benign Polyps
Common lesion.

May bleed if tip eroded.

Endometrial Carcinoma
Estrogen use in menopause increases incidence.

Causes irregular uterine bleeding or postmenopausal bleeding.

Uterine Myomas / 477
Incidence and Manifestations
Very common: in approximately 30 percent of women over thirty.

May cause uterine bleeding or pressure symptoms on bladder or rectum.

Treated by hysterectomy.

Irregular Uterine Bleeding / 477
Pathogenesis
Dysfunctional uterine bleeding: caused by failure of ovulation.

Other causes: must rule out carcinoma in older women by dilatation and curettage.

Dysmenorrhea / 481
Primary Dysmenorrhea
Onset about one or two years after menarche, when regular menstrual cycles established.

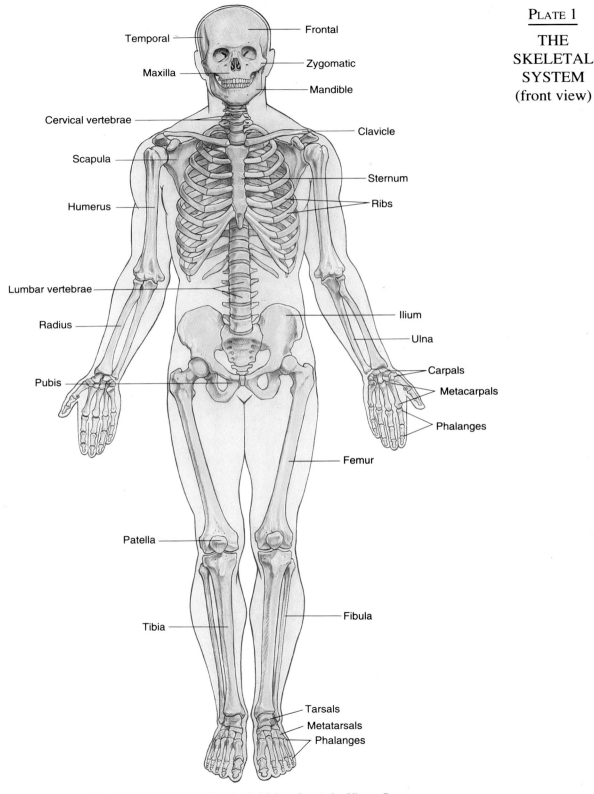

Temporal

Maxilla

Cervical vertebrae

Scapula

Humerus

Lumbar vertebrae

Radius

Pubis

Patella

Tibia

Frontal

Zygomatic

Mandible

Clavicle

Sternum

Ribs

Ilium

Ulna

Carpals

Metacarpals

Phalanges

Femur

Fibula

Tarsals

Metatarsals

Phalanges

Plate 1

THE
SKELETAL
SYSTEM
(front view)

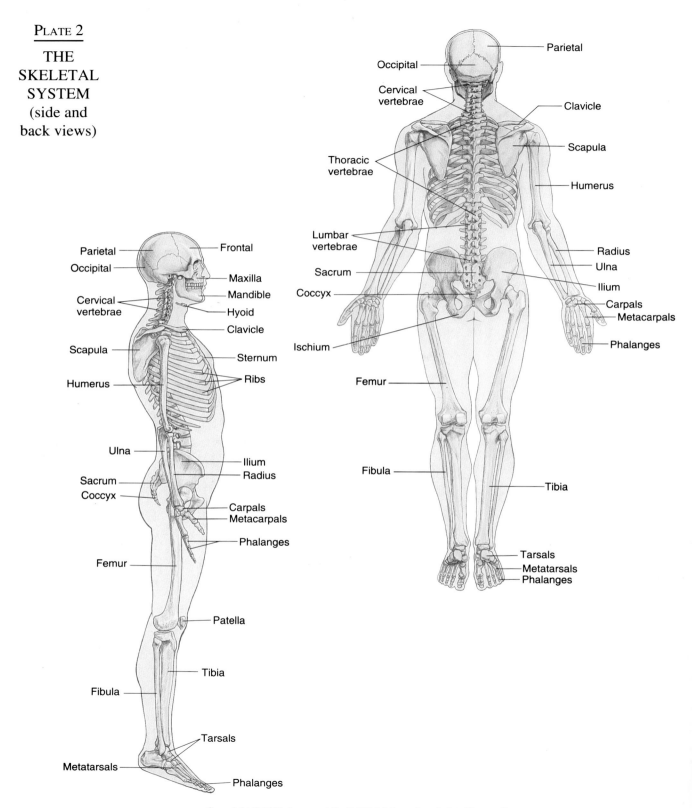

PLATE 2

THE
SKELETAL
SYSTEM
(side and
back views)

Parietal

Occipital

Cervical
vertebrae

Thoracic
vertebrae

Lumbar
vertebrae

Sacrum

Coccyx

Ischium

Femur

Fibula

Clavicle

Scapula

Humerus

Radius

Ulna

Ilium

Carpals

Metacarpals

Phalanges

Tibia

Tarsals

Metatarsals

Phalanges

Parietal

Occipital

Cervical
vertebrae

Scapula

Humerus

Ulna

Sacrum

Coccyx

Femur

Fibula

Metatarsals

Frontal

Maxilla

Mandible

Hyoid

Clavicle

Sternum

Ribs

Ilium

Radius

Carpals

Metacarpals

Phalanges

Patella

Tibia

Tarsals

Phalanges

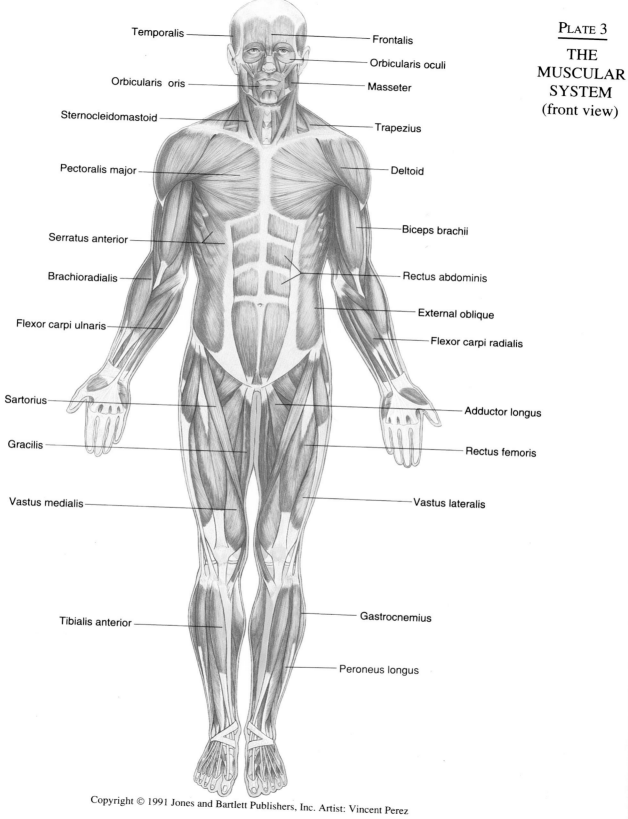

PLATE 3

THE
MUSCULAR
SYSTEM
(front view)

Temporalis

Frontalis

Orbicularis oculi

Orbicularis oris

Masseter

Sternocleidomastoid

Trapezius

Pectoralis major

Deltoid

Serratus anterior

Biceps brachii

Brachioradialis

Rectus abdominis

Flexor carpi ulnaris

External oblique

Flexor carpi radialis

Sartorius

Adductor longus

Gracilis

Rectus femoris

Vastus medialis

Vastus lateralis

Tibialis anterior

Gastrocnemius

Peroneus longus

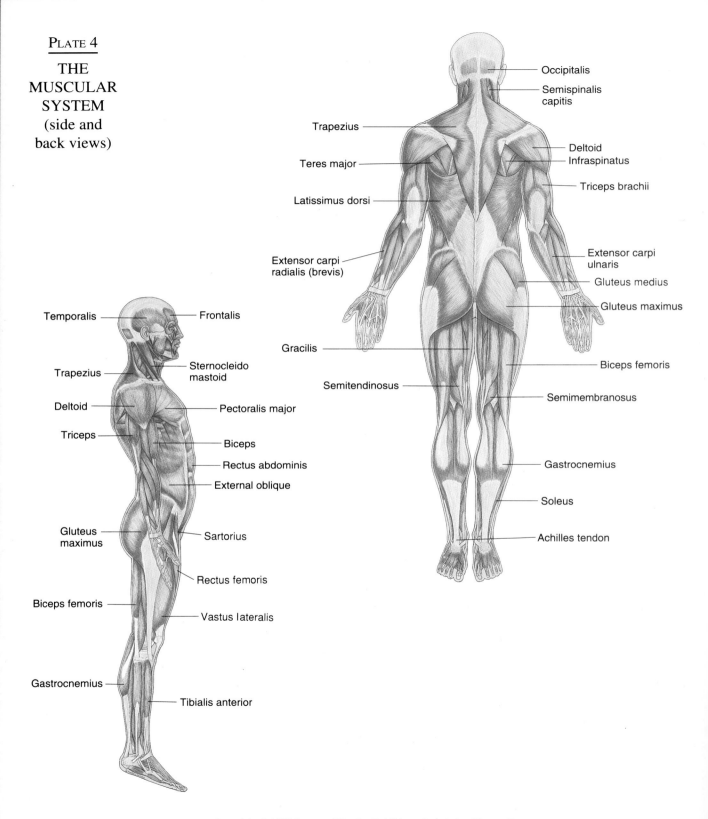

PLATE 4

THE MUSCULAR SYSTEM
(side and back views)

Occipitalis

Semispinalis capitis

Trapezius

Deltoid

Infraspinatus

Teres major

Triceps brachii

Latissimus dorsi

Extensor carpi ulnaris

Extensor carpi radialis (brevis)

Gluteus medius

Gluteus maximus

Temporalis

Frontalis

Gracilis

Trapezius

Sternocleido mastoid

Biceps femoris

Deltoid

Pectoralis major

Semitendinosus

Semimembranosus

Triceps

Biceps

Rectus abdominis

External oblique

Gluteus maximus

Sartorius

Gastrocnemius

Rectus femoris

Soleus

Biceps femoris

Vastus lateralis

Achilles tendon

Gastrocnemius

Tibialis anterior

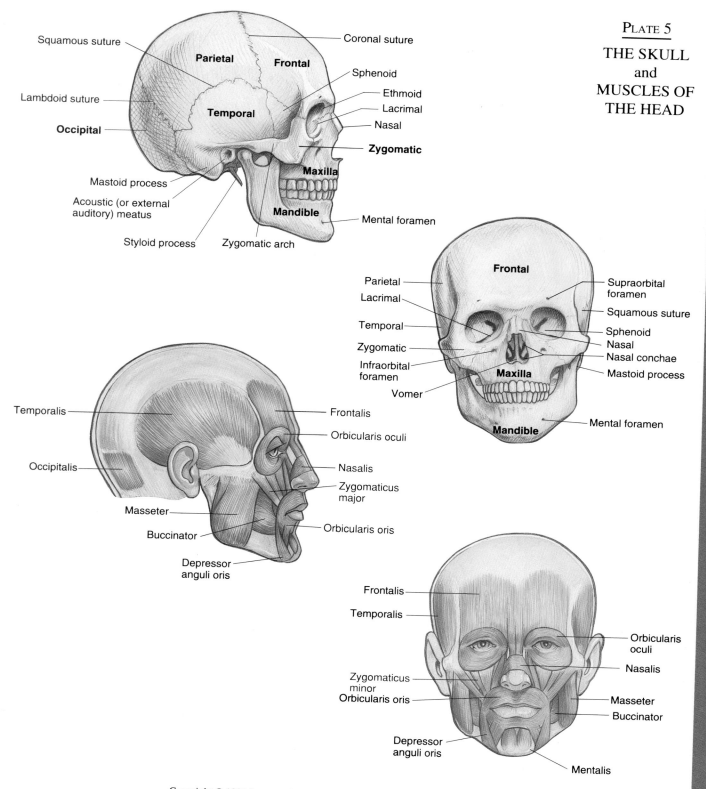

PLATE 5

THE SKULL
and
MUSCLES OF
THE HEAD

Squamous suture

Parietal

Frontal

Coronal suture

Sphenoid

Ethmoid

Lacrimal

Nasal

Zygomatic

Lambdoid suture

Temporal

Occipital

Maxilla

Mastoid process

Acoustic (or external
auditory) meatus

Mandible

Mental foramen

Styloid process

Zygomatic arch

Parietal

Frontal

Supraorbital
foramen

Lacrimal

Squamous suture

Temporal

Sphenoid

Zygomatic

Nasal

Infraorbital
foramen

Nasal conchae

Mastoid process

Maxilla

Vomer

Mandible

Mental foramen

Temporalis

Frontalis

Orbicularis oculi

Occipitalis

Nasalis

Zygomaticus
major

Masseter

Orbicularis oris

Buccinator

Depressor
anguli oris

Frontalis

Temporalis

Orbicularis
oculi

Nasalis

Zygomaticus
minor

Orbicularis oris

Masseter

Buccinator

Depressor
anguli oris

Mentalis

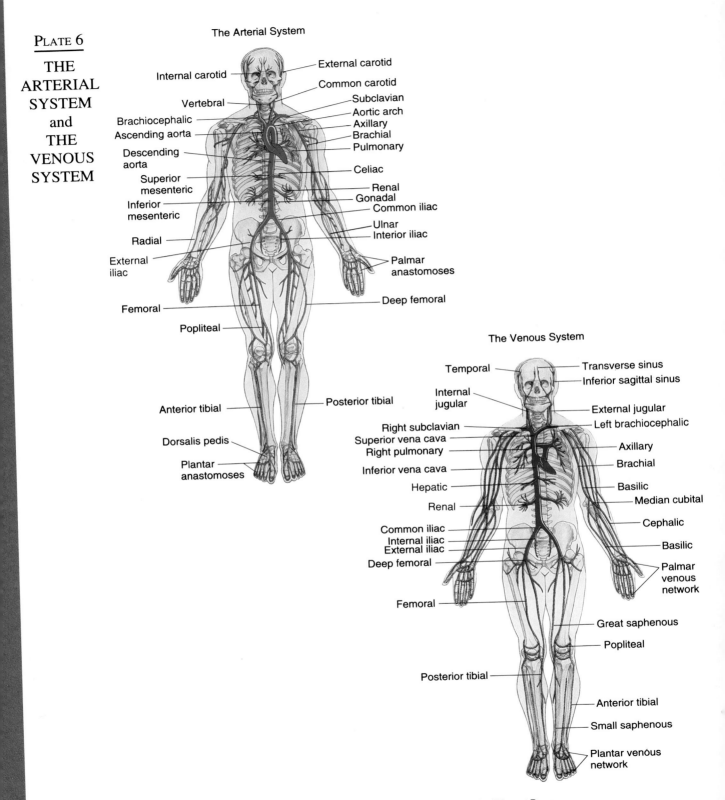

PLATE 6

THE
ARTERIAL
SYSTEM
and
THE
VENOUS
SYSTEM

The Arterial System

Internal carotid
External carotid
Common carotid
Vertebral
Subclavian
Brachiocephalic
Aortic arch
Ascending aorta
Axillary
Brachial
Descending aorta
Pulmonary
Superior mesenteric
Celiac
Inferior mesenteric
Renal
Gonadal
Common iliac
Ulnar
Interior iliac
Radial
External iliac
Palmar anastomoses
Femoral
Deep femoral
Popliteal
Anterior tibial
Posterior tibial
Dorsalis pedis
Plantar anastomoses

The Venous System

Temporal
Transverse sinus
Inferior sagittal sinus
Internal jugular
External jugular
Right subclavian
Left brachiocephalic
Superior vena cava
Axillary
Right pulmonary
Brachial
Inferior vena cava
Basilic
Hepatic
Median cubital
Renal
Cephalic
Common iliac
Internal iliac
External iliac
Basilic
Deep femoral
Palmar venous network
Femoral
Great saphenous
Popliteal
Posterior tibial
Anterior tibial
Small saphenous
Plantar venous network

PLATE 7

THE
ARTERIAL-
VENOUS
SYSTEM

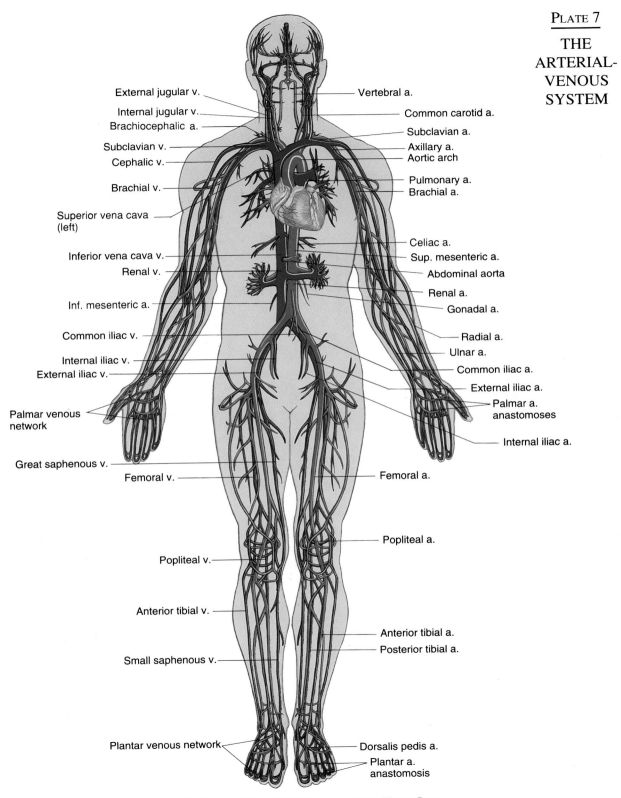

External jugular v. ———— Vertebral a.

Internal jugular v. ———— Common carotid a.

Brachiocephalic a. ———

Subclavian v. ———— Subclavian a.

Cephalic v. ———— Axillary a.
———— Aortic arch

Brachial v. ———— Pulmonary a.
———— Brachial a.

Superior vena cava ————
(left)

Inferior vena cava v. ———— Celiac a.
———— Sup. mesenteric a.

Renal v. ———— Abdominal aorta

———— Renal a.

Inf. mesenteric a. ———— Gonadal a.

Common iliac v. ———— Radial a.

Internal iliac v. ———— Ulnar a.

External iliac v. ———— Common iliac a.

———— External iliac a.

Palmar venous ———— Palmar a.
network   anastomoses

———— Internal iliac a.

Great saphenous v. ————

Femoral v. ———— Femoral a.

———— Popliteal a.

Popliteal v. ————

Anterior tibial v. ————

———— Anterior tibial a.
———— Posterior tibial a.

Small saphenous v. ————

Plantar venous network ———— Dorsalis pedis a.

———— Plantar a.
anastomosis

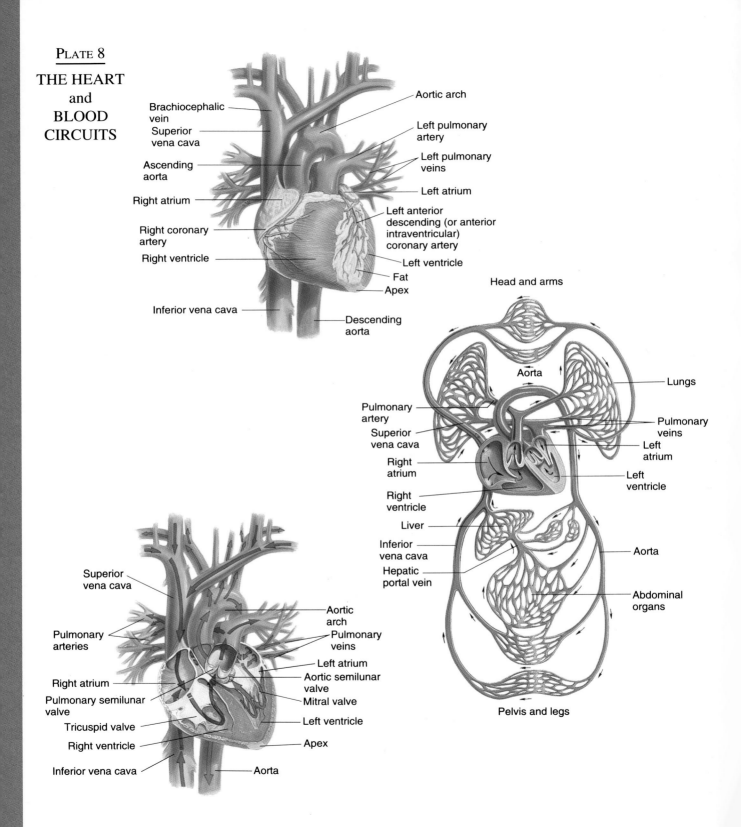

PLATE 8

THE HEART
and
BLOOD
CIRCUITS

Brachiocephalic vein
Superior vena cava
Ascending aorta
Right atrium
Right coronary artery
Right ventricle
Inferior vena cava

Aortic arch
Left pulmonary artery
Left pulmonary veins
Left atrium
Left anterior descending (or anterior intraventricular) coronary artery
Left ventricle
Fat
Apex
Descending aorta

Head and arms

Aorta
Lungs
Pulmonary artery
Pulmonary veins
Superior vena cava
Left atrium
Right atrium
Left ventricle
Right ventricle
Liver
Inferior vena cava
Aorta
Hepatic portal vein
Abdominal organs

Pelvis and legs

Superior vena cava
Pulmonary arteries
Right atrium
Pulmonary semilunar valve
Tricuspid valve
Right ventricle
Inferior vena cava

Aortic arch
Pulmonary veins
Left atrium
Aortic semilunar valve
Mitral valve
Left ventricle
Apex
Aorta

PLATE 9

THE
ENDOCRINE
SYSTEM

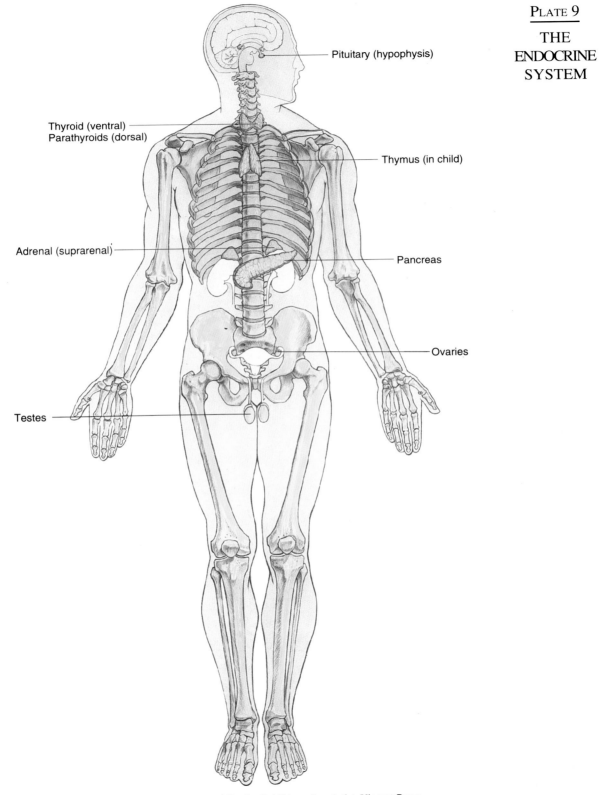

Pituitary (hypophysis)

Thyroid (ventral)
Parathyroids (dorsal)

Thymus (in child)

Adrenal (suprarenal)

Pancreas

Ovaries

Testes

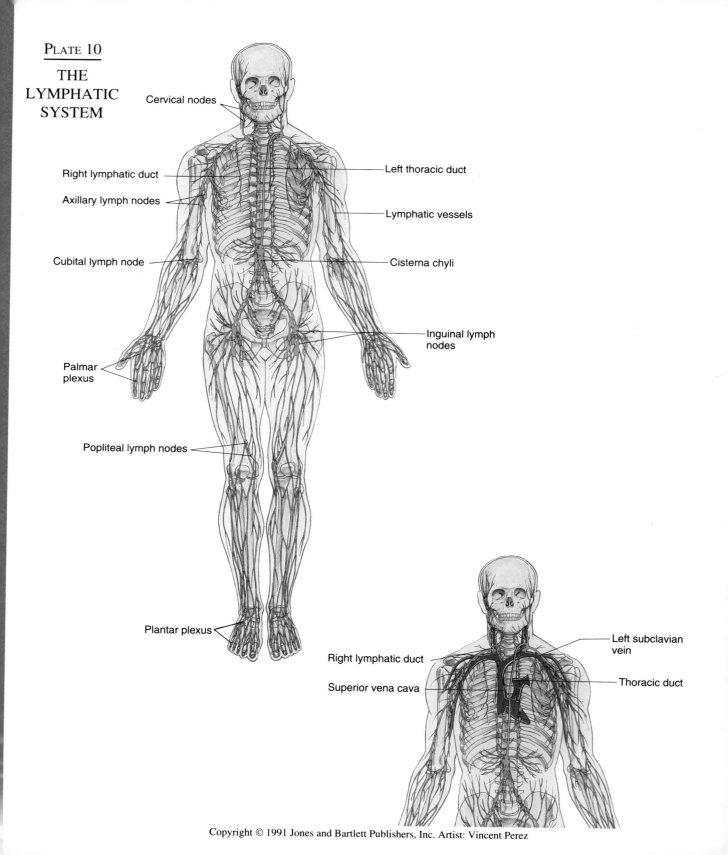

PLATE 10

THE
LYMPHATIC
SYSTEM

Cervical nodes

Right lymphatic duct

Axillary lymph nodes

Cubital lymph node

Palmar
plexus

Popliteal lymph nodes

Plantar plexus

Left thoracic duct

Lymphatic vessels

Cisterna chyli

Inguinal lymph
nodes

Right lymphatic duct

Superior vena cava

Left subclavian
vein

Thoracic duct

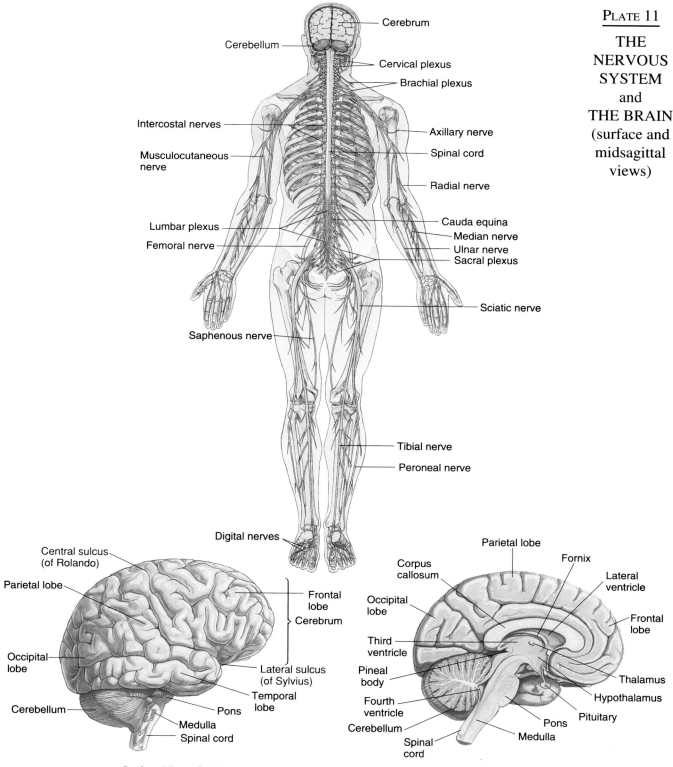

PLATE 11

THE
NERVOUS
SYSTEM
and
THE BRAIN
(surface and
midsagittal
views)

Cerebrum

Cerebellum

Cervical plexus

Brachial plexus

Intercostal nerves

Musculocutaneous
nerve

Axillary nerve

Spinal cord

Radial nerve

Lumbar plexus

Femoral nerve

Cauda equina

Median nerve

Ulnar nerve

Sacral plexus

Sciatic nerve

Saphenous nerve

Tibial nerve

Peroneal nerve

Digital nerves

Central sulcus
(of Rolando)

Parietal lobe

Occipital
lobe

Cerebellum

Frontal
lobe

Cerebrum

Lateral sulcus
(of Sylvius)

Temporal
lobe

Pons

Medulla

Spinal cord

Surface View of the Brain

Parietal lobe

Corpus
callosum

Fornix

Lateral
ventricle

Occipital
lobe

Frontal
lobe

Third
ventricle

Pineal
body

Thalamus

Hypothalamus

Fourth
ventricle

Pituitary

Cerebellum

Pons

Spinal
cord

Medulla

Midsagittal View of the Brain

PLATE 12

THE
VISCERA

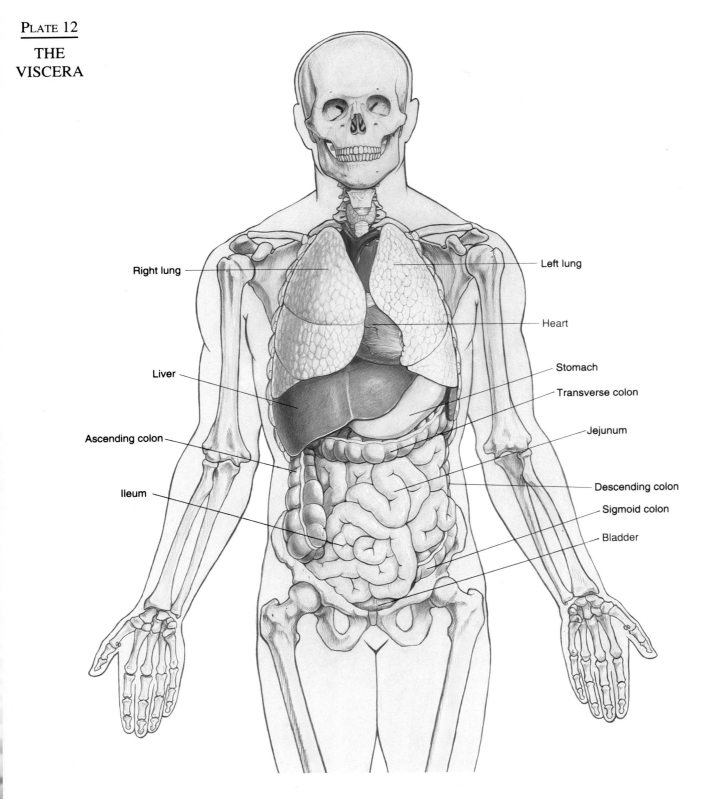

Right lung

Left lung

Heart

Liver

Stomach

Transverse colon

Jejunum

Ascending colon

Descending colon

Sigmoid colon

Ileum

Bladder

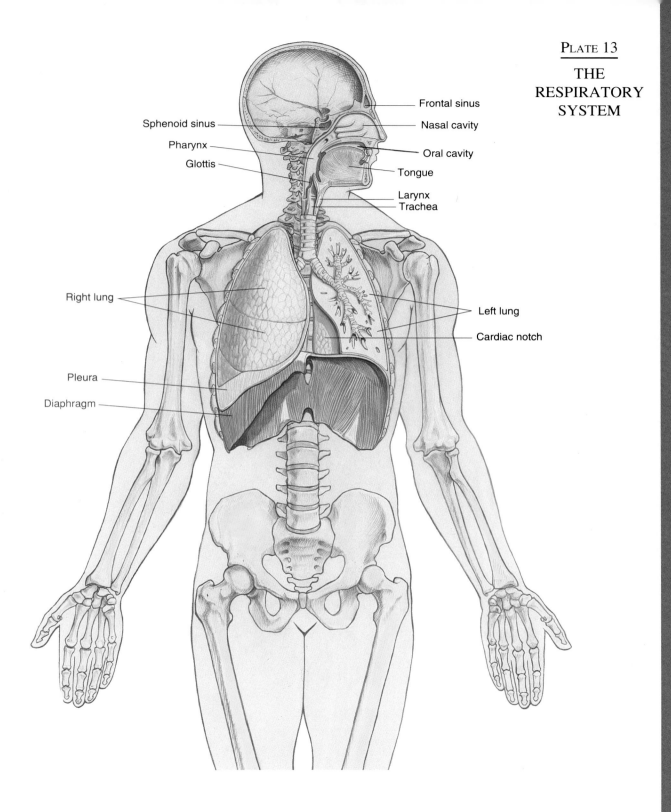

PLATE 13

THE
RESPIRATORY
SYSTEM

Frontal sinus

Sphenoid sinus

Nasal cavity

Pharynx

Oral cavity

Glottis

Tongue

Larynx
Trachea

Right lung

Left lung

Cardiac notch

Pleura

Diaphragm

PLATE 14

THE
DIGESTIVE
SYSTEM

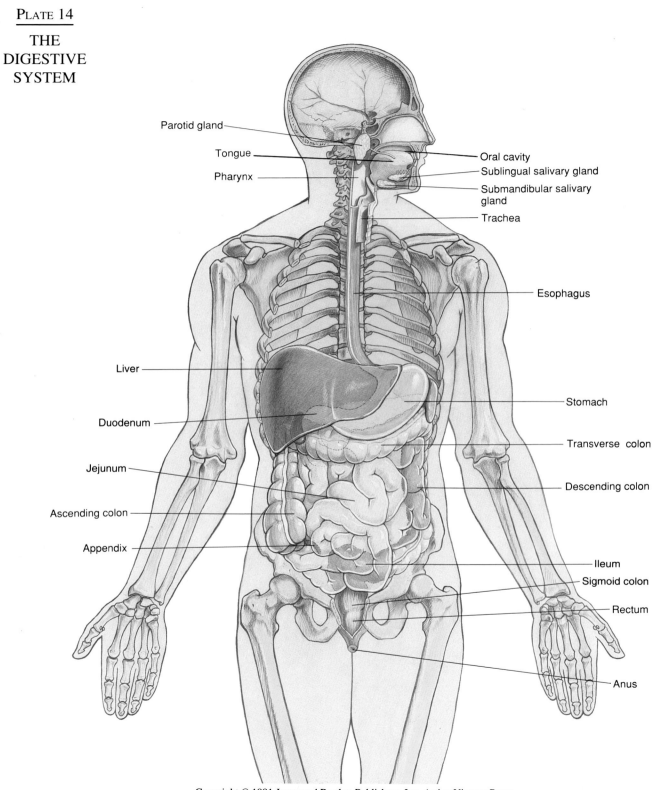

Parotid gland

Tongue

Pharynx

Oral cavity

Sublingual salivary gland

Submandibular salivary
gland

Trachea

Esophagus

Liver

Duodenum

Jejunum

Ascending colon

Appendix

Stomach

Transverse colon

Descending colon

Ileum

Sigmoid colon

Rectum

Anus

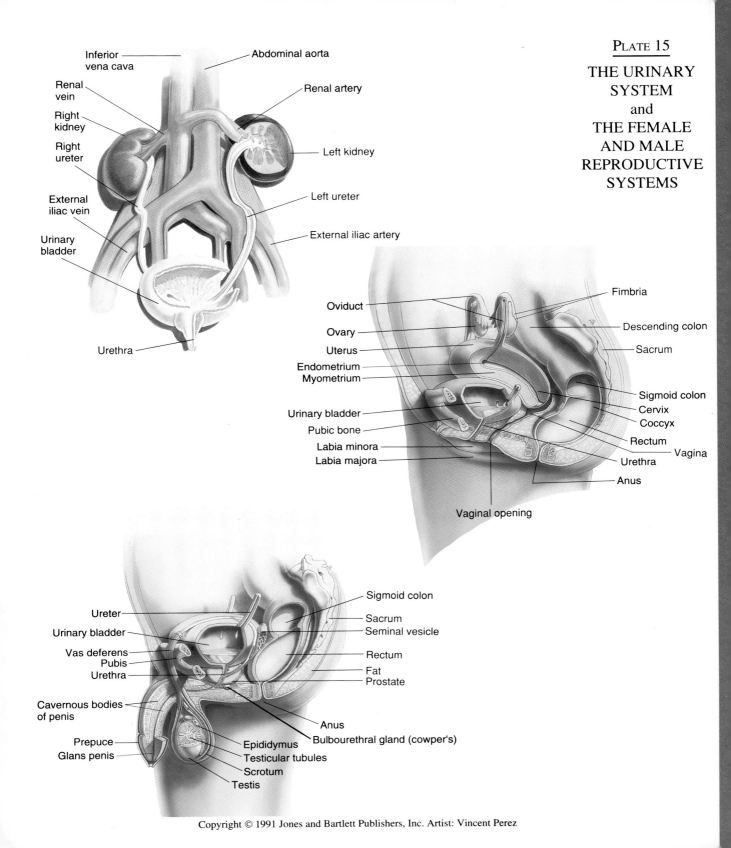

Inferior vena cava

Abdominal aorta

Renal vein

Renal artery

Right kidney

Left kidney

Right ureter

Left ureter

External iliac vein

External iliac artery

Urinary bladder

Urethra

PLATE 15

THE URINARY
SYSTEM
and
THE FEMALE
AND MALE
REPRODUCTIVE
SYSTEMS

Oviduct

Fimbria

Ovary

Descending colon

Uterus

Sacrum

Endometrium
Myometrium

Urinary bladder

Sigmoid colon

Pubic bone

Cervix

Labia minora

Coccyx

Labia majora

Rectum

Vagina

Urethra

Anus

Vaginal opening

Ureter

Sigmoid colon

Urinary bladder

Sacrum

Seminal vesicle

Vas deferens

Pubis

Rectum

Urethra

Fat

Prostate

Cavernous bodies
of penis

Anus

Prepuce

Bulbourethral gland (cowper's)

Glans penis

Epididymus

Testicular tubules

Scrotum

Testis

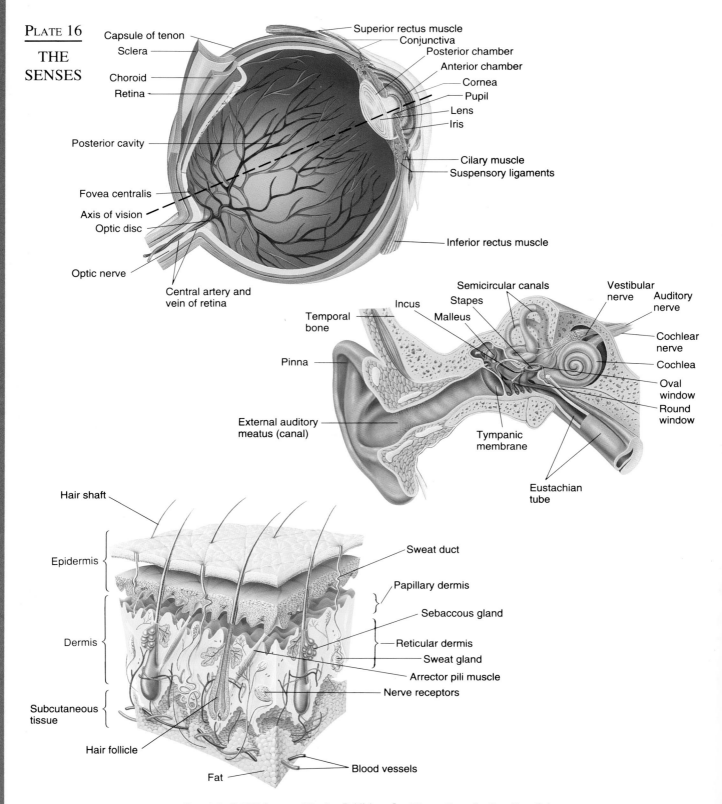

PLATE 16

THE SENSES

Capsule of tenon
Sclera
Choroid
Retina
Posterior cavity
Fovea centralis
Axis of vision
Optic disc
Optic nerve
Central artery and vein of retina

Superior rectus muscle
Conjunctiva
Posterior chamber
Anterior chamber
Cornea
Pupil
Lens
Iris
Cilary muscle
Suspensory ligaments
Inferior rectus muscle

Temporal bone
Pinna
External auditory meatus (canal)

Semicircular canals
Stapes
Incus
Malleus
Vestibular nerve
Auditory nerve
Cochlear nerve
Cochlea
Oval window
Round window
Tympanic membrane
Eustachian tube

Hair shaft
Epidermis
Dermis
Subcutaneous tissue
Hair follicle
Fat

Sweat duct
Papillary dermis
Sebaccous gland
Reticular dermis
Sweat gland
Arrector pili muscle
Nerve receptors
Blood vessels

Prostaglandins synthesized under influence of progesterone during secretory phase of cycle are released from endometrium during menses and stimulate myometrial contractions, causing pain.

Treated by prostaglandin inhibitors (aspirin or other anti-inflammatory drugs) or by birth-control pills, which suppress ovulation.

Secondary Dysmenorrhea
As a result of disease of pelvic organs, such as endometriosis.

Treatment consists of correcting basic cause whenever possible.

Cysts and Tumors of the Ovary / 481
Cysts Derived from Follicle or Corpus Luteum
Develop frequently.

Usually regress spontaneously.

Endometrial Cysts
Dermoid Cysts
Contain various tissues.

Bone in dermoid may be identified.

Cystadenoma and Cystadenocarcinoma
Granulosa Cell Tumor
Estrogen produced by tumor causes endometrial hyperplasia.

May cause postmenopausal bleeding.

Male Hormone-Producing Tumors
Diseases of the Vulva / 485
Vulvar Dystrophy
Irregular white patches on vulvar skin (leukoplakia).

Intense itching.

May progress to carcinoma.

Local treatment usually effective.

Carcinoma of the Vulva
Occasionally found in postmenopausal women.

Often preexisting vulvar dystrophy.

Treated by vulvectomy.

Toxic Shock Syndrome (TSS) / 485
Incidence
Occurs most commonly in women using high-absorbency tampons.

Estimated ten to fifteen cases per 100,000 women of menstrual age per year.

Clinical Manifestations
Elevated temperature, vomiting, diarrhea.

Erythematous rash.

Pathogenesis
Toxin-producing *Staphylococcus* grows in vagina.

Menstrual blood is good culture medium.

Tampons hinder drainage and may injure vaginal mucosa.

Treatment
Supportive.

Discontinue tampon use.

Antibiotics to eradicate staphylococci.

Advise no further tampon use.

Contraception / 487
Natural Family Planning
Avoid intercourse around time of ovulation.

Less effective than artificial methods.

Artificial Contraception
Diaphragms and condoms: effective and no side effects.

Contraceptive pills: suppress ovulation but have side effects.

Increased tendency to thromboembolic complications, especially in cigarette smokers.

Hypertension develops in some patients.

Intrauterine contraceptive devices (IUDs): prevent implantation.

Increased incidence of tubal infections.

Increased incidence of tubal pregnancies.

Effects of Prenatal Exposure to Diethylstilbestrol (DES) / 490
Benign Lesions
Fibrous ridges and polypoid projections from cervix and vaginal vault.

Adenosis: patches of glandular epithelium interspersed in cervicovaginal squamous epithelium.

Malignant Lesions
Clear cell carcinoma develops in small percentage of exposed women.

Periodic gynecologic examination of exposed women recommended.

18

Prenatal Development and Diseases Associated with Pregnancy

Learning Objectives

1. Explain the processes of fertilization, implantation, and early development of the ovum, including the origin of the decidua, fetal membranes, and the placenta.
2. Describe how amnionic fluid is formed and eliminated. Identify the conditions leading to abnormal amounts of amnionic fluid.
3. Explain the causes and effects of spontaneous abortion and ectopic pregnancy.
4. Identify and explain the problems that may result if pregnancy occurs after failure of contraceptive pills or an intrauterine device.
5. Describe the mechanism and clinical manifestations of the problems associated with abnormal attachment of the placenta within the uterus and abnormal attachment of the umbilical cord.
6. Differentiate identical and fraternal twins. Describe how zygosity can be determined from examination of the placenta.
7. List the disadvantages of a twin pregnancy.
8. Classify the types of gestational trophoblast disease. Explain their prognoses and describe the methods of treatment.
9. Explain the pathogenesis, clinical manifestations, diagnostic criteria, and methods used to treat hemolytic disease of the newborn.

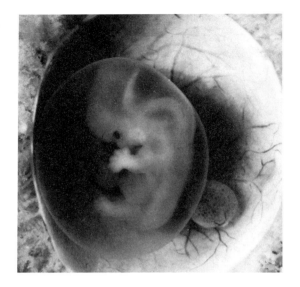

Chapter 18 ■ Contents

Fertilization

The tadpolelike *sperm* consists of three parts: a head, a middle piece, and a tail (figure 18–1). The sperm head contains genetic material. It is partially covered by a thin, membranelike structure called the *head cap,* which contains enzymes that enable the sperm head to penetrate the ovum at the time of fertilization. The middle piece contains the enzymes that provide the energy required to propel the sperm, and the tail is the propulsive portion. Sperm can travel several millimeters per minute by their own propulsive efforts, but they are also passively transported by rhythmic contractions of the uterine muscles that aspirate them upward into the uterus and fallopian tubes.

The *ovum* is expelled from the follicle at ovulation. It is surrounded by a thin layer of acellular material called the **zona pellucida** to which are attached clusters of cells from the follicle that are called **granulosa cells** (figure 18–2). The ovum is swept into the fallopian tube by the beating of the cilia covering the tubal epithelium and is propelled down the tube by the peristaltic contractions of the smooth muscle in the tubal wall. Fertilization is possible when intercourse occurs reasonably close to the time of ovulation. The enzymes in the head cap of the sperm disperse the cluster of granulosa cells and permit the sperm head to penetrate the zona pellucida. Once the sperm has penetrated, the ovum completes its second meiotic division (oogenesis is described in chapter 3). Sperm penetration causes the zona pellucida to become impermeable to penetration by other sperm, assuring that only one sperm can enter

Fertilization and Prenatal Development

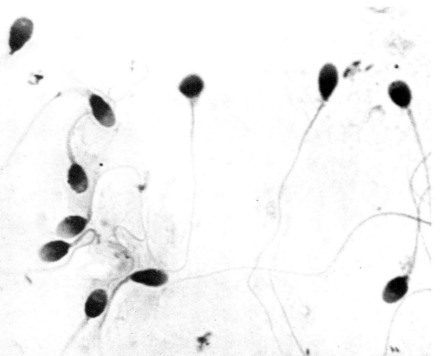

FIGURE 18–1

Normal sperm in vaginal secretions. The darkly staining head containing the genetic material is covered by a lightly staining head cap. The long, narrow tail provides propulsion. (Original magnification × 1000.)

FIGURE 18–2

Mature ovum with adherent granulosa cells. The nucleus is seen near the center of the cell. The homogeneous band surrounding the ovum is the *zona pellucida.* (Original magnification × 400.)

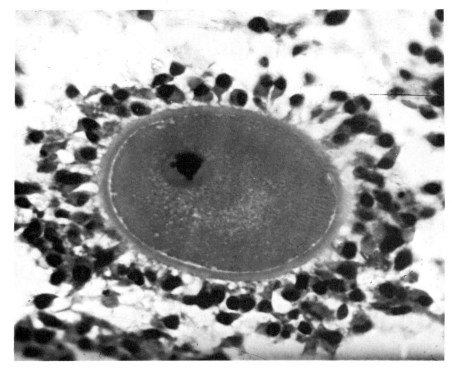

the egg. Fusion of the sperm head and egg nucleus (each containing twenty-three chromosomes) restores the genetic component of the cell to forty-six chromosomes, and the fertilized ovum is now termed a **zygote.**

Early Development of the Fertilized Ovum

As the fertilized ovum passes along the fallopian tube, it undergoes a series of mitotic divisions. The first cell division is completed about thirty hours after fertilization. Subsequent divisions occur in rapid succession and convert the zygote into a small, mulberry-shaped ball of cells called a **morula,** which is enclosed within the zona pellucida. The morula reaches the endometrial cavity by about the third day. Soon fluid begins to accumulate in the center of the morula, and a central cavity forms. At this stage of development, the structure is called a **blastocyst.** The cells of the blastocyst begin to differentiate into two different groups of cells: the **inner cell mass,** which will form the embryo, and a peripheral rim of cells called the **trophoblast,** which will give rise to the fetal membranes and will contribute to the formation of the placenta.

The blastocyst lies free within the endometrial cavity for several days. Then the zona pellucida degenerates, exposing the trophoblast. The blastocyst begins to burrow into the endometrium by the end of the first week after fertilization and soon becomes completely embedded (figure 18–3).

Soon after implantation, the inner cell mass becomes a flat structure called the **germ disk,** which differentiates into the three germ layers: ectoderm, mesoderm, and entoderm. Each of the layers will give rise to specific tissues and organs as described in chapter 2. A fluid-filled sac called the **amnionic sac** forms between the ectoderm of the germ disk and the surrounding trophoblast, and a second sac called the **yolk sac** forms on the opposite side of the germ disk. The interior of the blastocyst cavity then becomes lined by a layer of primitive connective-tissue cells (**mesoderm**) that also covers the external surfaces of the amnionic sac and yolk sac. As soon as the blastocyst cavity acquires a connective-tissue lining, it is called the *chorionic cavity* and its wall is called the *chorion.* The entire sac with its enclosed amnion, yolk sac, and developing embryo is called the **chorionic vesicle.** Fingerlike columns of cells called **chorionic villi** extend from the chorion and anchor the chorionic vesicle in the endometrium.

The chorionic cavity continues to enlarge, and the chorionic vesicle increases in size and complexity. By the end of the second week after fertilization, the small germ disk with its surrounding amnion and yolk sac projects into the chorionic cavity, suspended from the wall of the chorion by a mass of connective tissue called the **body stalk** (figure 18–4).

By the fourth week after fertilization, the organ systems begin to form, and the embryo, which had been flat, becomes cylindrical. The central part of the germ disk grows more rapidly than the periphery, owing to the beginning formation of the nervous system. As a result, the germ disk flexes and bulges

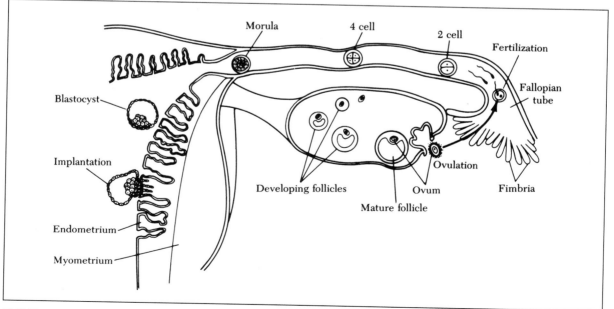

FIGURE 18–3

Summary of the maturation of the ovum, fertilization, and early development of the fertilized ovum.

FIGURE 18–4

Appearance of the chorionic vesicle at the end of the second week after ovulation, illustrating the relation of the germ disk to the amnion, chorion, body stalk, and chorionic cavity.

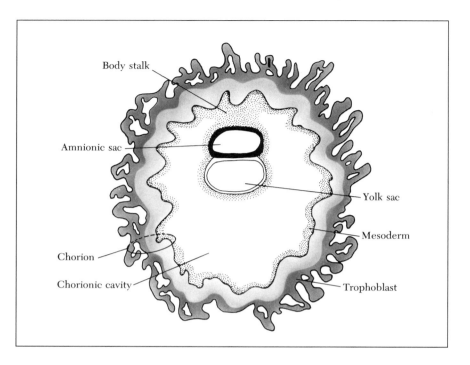

Body stalk

Amnionic sac

Yolk sac

Mesoderm

Chorion

Chorionic cavity

Trophoblast

into the amnionic cavity. The amnionic sac, which is attached to the lateral margins of the germ disk, follows the changing contour of the embryo and is reflected around the embryo. Part of the yolk sac also becomes enfolded within the embryo when flexion occurs (figure 18–5). The enclosed part will give rise to the intestinal tract and other important structures. The lateral margins of the germ disk also fuse in the midline to form the ventral (anterior) body wall. The fusion is incomplete in the middle of the body wall where the umbilical cord is attached, and part of the yolk sac that was not included within the embryo protrudes through the defect. It persists for a time but soon degenerates.

In Vitro Fertilization and Embryo Transfer

Some women ovulate normally but are infertile because their fallopian tubes are obstructed by scarring that cannot be corrected surgically or because both fallopian tubes have been removed as a consequence of previous ectopic pregnancies. In such cases, it is sometimes possible to achieve a pregnancy by fertilizing the patient's ovum, allowing it to develop outside her body, and then implanting the embryo in her uterus.

The egg is aspirated from the patient's ovary just prior to the expected ovulation with the aid of a long, tubular telescope-like device called a **laparoscope.** The instrument is passed into the abdominal cavity through a small incision made at the umbilicus so that the physician can visualize the ovaries and pelvic organs and aspirate the ovarian follicle. The ovum, sus-

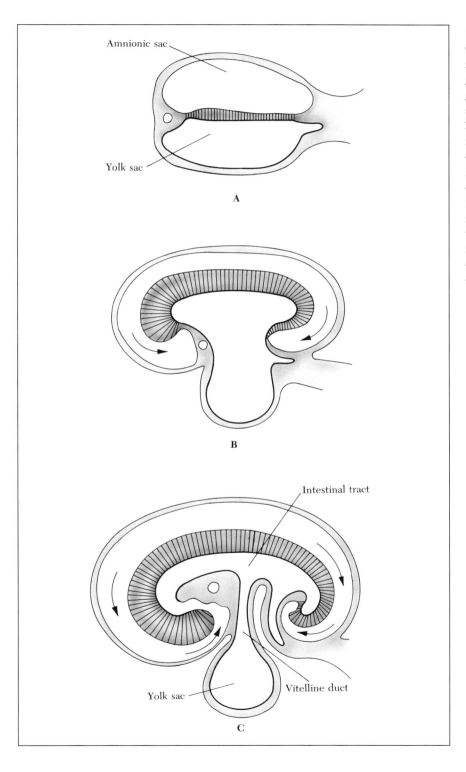

FIGURE 18–5

Changes in shape of embryo resulting from more rapid growth of germ disk. **A,** Flat germ disk with amnionic sac above and yolk sac below. **B,** Embryo begins to bulge into amnionic sac. **C,** Flexion completed. Part of yolk sac is included in the body of the embryo and will form the intestinal tract. The embryo now has a cylindrical configuration. Part of the yolk sac remains connected to the embryo by a narrow vitelline duct.

Amnionic sac

Yolk sac

A

B

Intestinal tract

Yolk sac

Vitelline duct

C

pended in a suitable culture medium, is fertilized by the husband's sperm, and the fertilized egg is allowed to develop to the eight-cell or sixteen-cell stage of division. Then it is inserted into the uterus through a thin catheter passed through the cervix into the endometrial cavity, where the fertilized ovum becomes implanted and continues its development.

In some cases, these procedures have led to the birth of full-term healthy infants, but most attempts have been unsuccessful. Failures have occurred for several reasons: because an ovum could not be collected from the ovary, or could not be fertilized, or failed to divide normally after fertilization, or failed to implant after being introduced into the uterine cavity. Moreover, some implanted embryos have had an abnormal number of chromosomes and have been aborted spontaneously. There is some concern that in vitro fertilization and embryo transfer will increase the incidence of birth defects, because the multiple steps and "handling" of the ovum required to achieve fertilization and early embryonic development may damage it or disrupt its growth. These techniques probably do increase the frequency of chromosome abnormalities, but the abnormal embryos are usually unable to survive and are aborted.

Stages of Prenatal Development

It is customary to subdivide prenatal development into three main periods:

1. The preembryonic period
2. The embryonic period
3. The fetal period

The first three weeks after fertilization are the *preembryonic period.* During this time the blastocyst becomes implanted and the inner cell mass differentiates into the three germ layers that will eventually form specific tissues within the embryo.

The *embryonic period* extends from the third through the seventh week. This is the time when the developing organism begins to assume a human shape and is called an **embryo.** This is also the time when all the organ systems are formed. Consequently, it is a very critical period of development. At this stage, drugs ingested by the mother, radiation, some viral infections, and various other factors may disturb embryonic development and lead to congenital abnormalities, as described in chapter 9.

The *fetal period* extends from the eighth week until the time of delivery. The developing organism is no longer called an embryo; the term **fetus** is now applied. As the fetus grows, it becomes larger and heavier, but there are no major changes in its basic structure comparable to those in the embryonic period. Initially, the fetal head is disproportionately large and the body appears quite scrawny because subcutaneous fat has not yet been deposited (figure 18–6). Shortly before delivery, subcutaneous fat begins to accumulate and the body begins to fill out. Figure 18–7 illustrates the progressive changes in the size of the fetus in relation to the duration of the gestation.

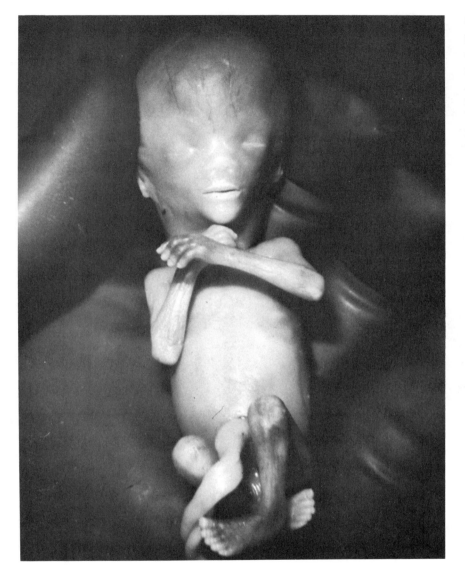

FIGURE 18–6

Small, well-formed fetus at end of first trimester. At this stage, the fetus weighs only 30 g but is completely formed. Its small size can be appreciated by comparing fetus with the fingers of the gloved hand that holds it.

Duration of Pregnancy

The total duration of pregnancy from fertilization to delivery is called the *period of gestation*. This is approximately thirty-eight weeks when dated from the time of ovulation. Usually, however, the actual date of ovulation is not known and the length of gestation is calculated from the beginning of the last normal menstrual period. Expressed in this way, the duration of pregnancy is forty weeks, because the first day of the calculation is actually about two weeks before the date of conception. The gestation calculated in this way

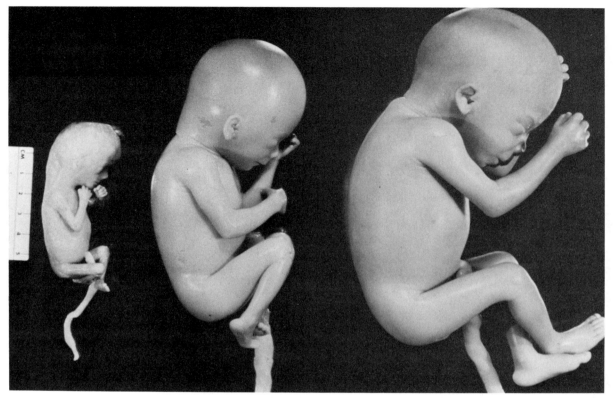

FIGURE 18–7

Progressive change in size of the fetus at various stages of gestation. *Left,* Three and one-half months (32 g). *Center,* Four and one-half months (230 g). *Right,* Five and one-half months (420 g).

may also be expressed as 280 days, as ten lunar (28-day) months, or nine calendar (31-day) months. Sometimes the nine calendar months are subdivided into three periods called *trimesters,* each of three months' duration.

Decidua, Fetal Membranes, and Placenta

Figure 18–8 demonstrates the relation of the embryo to the surrounding amnionic sac and chorion about seven weeks after fertilization. Figure 18–9 diagrammatically illustrates these relations in both early and late pregnancy.

The Decidua

The endometrium of pregnancy is called the **decidua.** Special names are applied to the parts of the decidua in which the chorionic vesicle is embedded, as indicated in figure 18–9. The part beneath the chorionic vesicle is called the *decidua basalis,* the part that is stretched over the vesicle is called the *decidua capsularis,* and the part that lines the rest of the endometrial

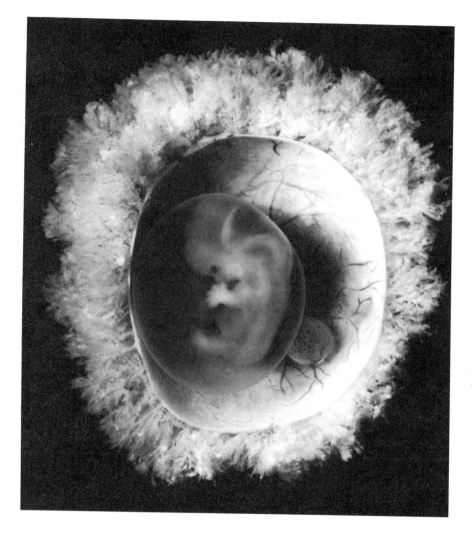

FIGURE 18-8

Relation of the embryo to the amnionic sac, yolk sac, and chorionic cavity at about seven weeks after conception. The chorionic sac has been bisected. At this stage, villi still arise from the entire periphery of the chorion and the amnionic sac (surrounding the embryo) does not completely fill the chorionic cavity. The embryo is attached to the chorion by the umbilical cord (not shown in the photograph). The yolk sac is located at the right of the amnionic sac, between the amnion and the chorion. (Photograph courtesy of the Carnegie Institution of Washington.)

cavity is called the *decidua parietalis* (*parietes* = wall). As the embryo and its surrounding amnionic sac continue to increase in size, the thin capsular decidua becomes stretched and thinned. Eventually, it fuses with the decidua parietalis on the opposite wall of the uterus.

The Chorion and Chorionic Villi

At first, the chorionic villi arise from the entire periphery of the chorion, but soon the villi arising from the superficial part of the chorion become compressed by the decidua capsularis and atrophy. This part of the chorion, which is devoid of villi, is called the *chorion laeve* (*laeve* = smooth). In contrast, the villi arising from the deeper portion of the chorion adjacent to the decidua basalis proliferate actively. This part of the chorion is called the

FIGURE 18–9

A, Relation of the fetus to the decidua, fetal membranes, and chorion in early pregnancy. The part of the yolk sac not incorporated within the fetus lies between the amnion and the chorion. **B,** Relationships in late pregnancy. The amnionic sac envelops the fetus. The amnion has fused with the chorion, and the chorionic cavity has been obliterated. The decidua capsularis has fused with the chorion laeve and has become adherent to the decidua parietalis on the opposite wall of the uterus.

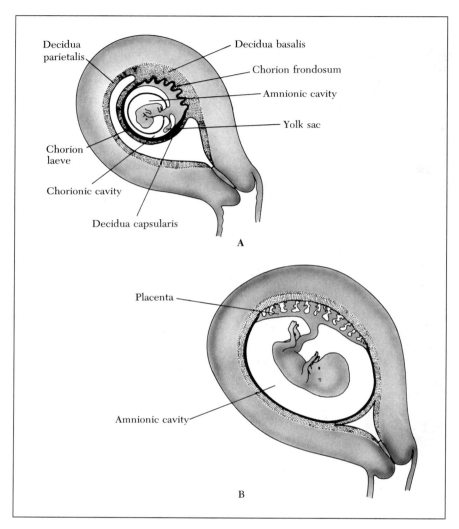

chorion frondosum because of the frondlike appearance of the villi. These villi project into the large blood vessels within the decidua basalis through which the maternal blood flows. Blood vessels that form within the villi as they grow become connected with blood vessels that are forming in the chorion and the body stalk, as well as within the body of the embryo. As soon as the embryo's heart begins to beat, blood begins to flow through this developing network of vessels.

The Amnionic Sac

The **amnionic sac** is enclosed within the chorion. At first the sac is much smaller than the chorionic cavity (see figure 18–8), but the enlarging sac expands into the chorionic cavity and soon surrounds the developing embryo. Eventually the amnionic sac completely fills the chorionic cavity and fuses with the chorion. The sac functions as a buoyant, temperature-controlled environment that protects the fetus throughout pregnancy and assists in opening the cervix during childbirth.

The Yolk Sac

In the human being, the yolk sac never contains yolk, but it performs other important functions. Part of the yolk sac becomes incorporated into the body of the embryo to form the intestinal tract. The part that is not included within the embryo persists for a time but eventually atrophies.

The Placenta

The **placenta** is a flattened, disk-shaped structure weighing about 500 g. It has a dual origin, both fetal and maternal (figure 18–10). The chorion and the villi are formed from the trophoblast, which is of fetal origin, and the decidua basalis in which the villi are anchored is derived from the endometrium. The fused amnion and chorion extend from the margins of the placenta to form the fluid-filled sac that encloses the fetus and that ruptures at the time of delivery. The fetus is connected to the placenta by the *umbilical cord,* which contains two arteries and a single vein. The vessels follow a spiral course in the cord and then divide on the surface of the placenta to send branches into the chorionic villi. Blood returning from the villi is collected into large veins on the surface of the placenta that join to form the single *umbilical vein* that enters the cord. The maternal surface of the placenta, which is attached to the uterus, is divided by incomplete partitions into compartments called **cotyledons** (figure 18–10B).

Circulation of Blood in the Placenta

The placenta has a dual circulation of blood (figure 18–11). The *fetoplacental circulation* delivers arterial blood low in oxygen from the fetus to the chorionic villi through the two umbilical arteries. It returns oxygenated blood to the fetus in the single umbilical vein. The *uteroplacental circulation* delivers oxygenated arterial blood from the mother into the large placental blood spaces that are located between the villi and are called the *intervillous spaces.* The blood spurts into the intervillous spaces from the many uterine arteries that penetrate the basal portion of the placenta. It flows back into the maternal circulation through veins that penetrate the basal part of the placenta. The arrangement of the two circulations in the placenta brings the maternal and fetal blood into close approximation. In this way, oxygen and nutrients can be exchanged between the maternal and fetal circulations, but there is no actual intermixing of fetal and maternal blood.

Endocrine Function of the Placenta

The placenta synthesizes two steroid hormones, *estrogen* and *progesterone,* and two protein hormones called **human placental lactogen (HPL)** and

FIGURE 18–10

The normal placenta. **A,** The fetal surface. The umbilical cord vessels subdivide on the surface to supply the chorionic villi. **B,** The maternal surface. Incomplete partitions of decidua subdivide the placenta into structures called *cotyledons,* imparting a cobblestone appearance to this surface.

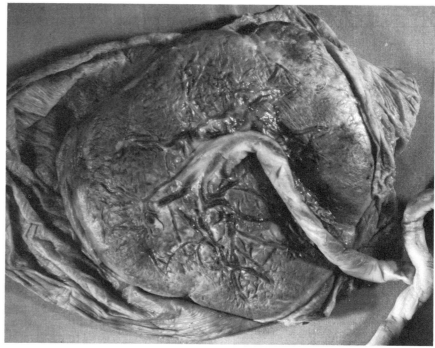

A

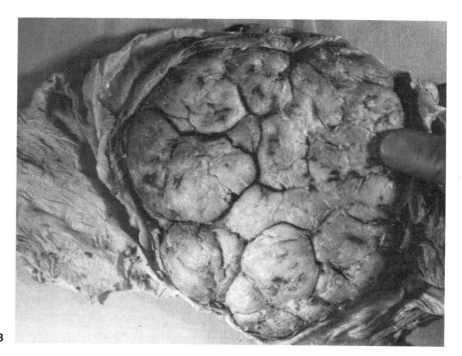

B

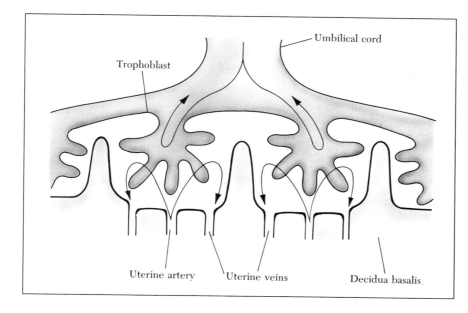

FIGURE 18–11

Dual circulation of blood in the placenta. Fetal blood circulates through villi and maternal blood circulates around villi, but circulations do not intermix.

human chorionic gonadotrophin (HCG). HPL stimulates maternal metabolic processes, and HCG is quite similar to the gonadotrophic hormones produced by the pituitary gland. Tests that detect HCG are called *pregnancy tests*. The newer, very sensitive tests, which are performed on blood or urine, become positive as early as ten to twelve days after fertilization, even before the woman misses her first period.

Amnionic Fluid

Amnionic fluid is produced both by filtration and by excretion, and its quantity varies with the stage of pregnancy. During the early part of pregnancy, the amnionic fluid is formed chiefly by filtration of fluid into the amnionic sac from maternal blood as it passes through the uterus and from fetal blood passing through the placenta. Additional fluid diffuses directly through the fetal skin and from the fetal respiratory tract. Later, when the fetal kidneys begin to function in the last part of pregnancy, the fetus urinates into the amnionic fluid and fetal urine becomes the major source of this fluid.

Both filtration and fetal urine continually add to the volume of fluid, but the additions are counterbalanced by losses of amnionic fluid into the fetal gastrointestinal tract. Normally, the fetus swallows as much as several hundred milliliters of fluid per day. This fluid is absorbed from the fetal intestinal tract into the fetal circulation, transferred across the placenta into the mother's circulation, and eventually excreted by the mother in her urine.

Polyhydramnios and Oligohydramnios

Polyhydramnios is a condition in which the volume of amnionic fluid is markedly increased. There are two common causes:

1. A congenital maldevelopment of the fetal brain called **anencephaly** (described in chapter 26), which disturbs the normal swallowing mechanism, so the fetus is unable to swallow amnionic fluid
2. A congenital obstruction of the fetal upper intestinal tract that blocks the entry of swallowed fluid into the small intestine where it can be absorbed

Oligohydramnios is a marked reduction in the volume of amnionic fluid. It occurs either because the fetal kidneys have failed to develop and no urine is formed, or because a congenital obstruction blocks the urethra so urine cannot be excreted.

Spontaneous Abortion ("Miscarriage")

Most spontaneous abortions occur early in pregnancy. The actual incidence is difficult to establish but is estimated to be from 10 to 20 percent of all pregnancies. Many spontaneous abortions are a result of chromosomal abnormalities or maldevelopment of the embryo that rendered it incapable of survival. Others result from defective implantation of the fertilized ovum within the endometrial cavity. In many cases, the cause of spontaneous abortion in early pregnancy cannot be determined.

Occasionally, intrauterine fetal death occurs late in pregnancy. This is generally caused by partial detachment of the placenta from the wall of the uterus, which is called *placental abruption,* or by obstruction of the blood supplied through the umbilical cord. Compression of the blood vessels in the umbilical cord, shutting off the blood supply to the fetus, may occur if the cord becomes knotted or wrapped tightly around the infant's neck or limbs (figure 18–12). If the placenta becomes separated or the cord becomes obstructed, the fetus no longer receives oxygen and nutrients from the mother and it dies. A dead fetus is usually expelled promptly, but occasionally it is retained within the uterine cavity for several weeks or months.

Cocaine abuse in pregnancy also has been shown to cause intrauterine fetal death. Cocaine increases maternal heart rate, constricts arterioles, and raises blood pressure. The constriction of uterine arterioles reduces uterine blood flow and impairs oxygen supply to the fetus. In some patients, the high pressure within the uterine arterioles may cause one of the vessels to rupture. As a result, a large hemorrhage forms between the uterine wall and the placenta and partially separates the placenta from the uterus (placental abruption), which severely compromises oxygenation of fetal blood.

If a dead fetus is retained for some time within the uterine cavity, products of degenerated fetal tissue diffuse into the maternal circulation. This material has thromboplastic activity and may induce a hemorrhagic disease in the mother owing to depletion of maternal blood-coagulation factors that occurs when the coagulation mechanism is activated by the thromboplastic

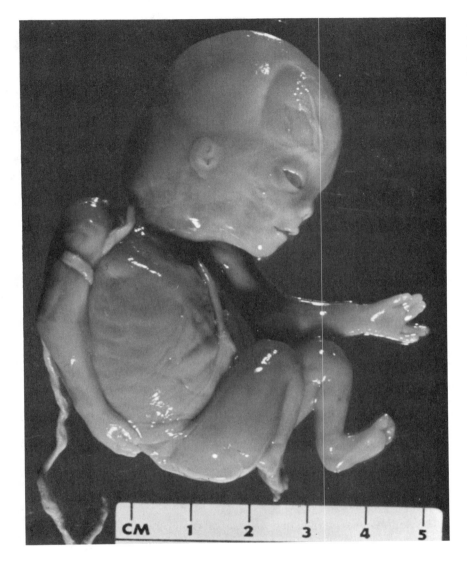

FIGURE 18–12

Fetus spontaneously aborted late in pregnancy, owing to interruption of blood supply through the umbilical cord. The cord extended around back of neck and had become tightly wrapped around upper arm, shutting off circulation and leading to intrauterine death.

material. A retained dead fetus is one cause of **disseminated intravascular coagulation,** which is discussed in the section on blood coagulation in chapter 11.

Ectopic Pregnancy

An ectopic pregnancy (*ecto* = outside) is the development of an embryo outside its normal location within the uterine cavity. Most ectopic pregnancies occur in the fallopian tubes, but on rare occasions a fertilized ovum develops in the ovary or abdominal cavity. Normally, fertilization occurs in the fallopian tube and the fertilized ovum then proceeds into the endometrial cavity, where implantation takes place at the end of the first week after fertilization. Implantation may take place in the fallopian tube, however, if transport of the ovum is delayed. Two factors predispose to this complication:

1. A previous infection in the fallopian tubes. Often this is followed by scarring and fusion of tubal folds, which retards the passage of the fertilized egg through the tube.
2. Failure of the muscular contractions of the tubal wall to propel the ovum through the tube.

Frequently, the conditions that predispose to a tubal pregnancy affect both fallopian tubes. Consequently, a woman who has had one tubal pregnancy is more likely to develop an ectopic pregnancy in the opposite tube.

Consequences of Tubal Pregnancy

An ectopic pregnancy in the fallopian tube gradually distends the tube. The embryo may develop normally for a time but rarely survives for more than a few months. The invading trophoblast erodes tubal blood vessels, causing bleeding into the lumen and wall of the tube and sometimes into the tissues surrounding it.

A woman with an ectopic pregnancy experiences signs and symptoms of early pregnancy and misses her expected menstrual period, as with a normal intrauterine pregnancy. She may also complain of some abdominal pain and tenderness caused by distention of the tube and irritation of the pelvic peritoneum caused by bleeding in the tube wall and adjacent tissues. She may also experience slight vaginal bleeding if blood leaks from the tubal implantation site, escapes into the uterus, and is discharged into the vagina.

Rupture of the tube can occur at any time (figure 18–13). This catastrophe is accompanied by severe abdominal pain and profuse intraabdominal bleeding caused by disruption of large tubal blood vessels at the site of rupture. If the patient is not treated promptly, tubal rupture may prove fatal because of the severe hemorrhage that occurs.

The following case illustrates some of the common clinical features encountered in a patient with a ruptured ectopic pregnancy.

CASE 18–1

A thirty-four-year-old woman consulted her physician because of recent onset of severe abdominal pain. Her last normal menstrual period had been two and one-half months earlier. For the previous two weeks, she had experienced mild abdominal pain and slight intermittent vaginal bleeding. On examination, she exhibited evidence of severe blood loss and her abdomen was diffusely tender. A diagnosis of ruptured ectopic pregnancy was made and an operation was performed immediately. A large amount of blood was found within the abdominal cavity as a result of a ruptured ectopic pregnancy in the midportion of the left fallopian tube. The ruptured tube was removed and the severe blood loss was treated by four blood transfusions. The patient made a satisfactory recovery.

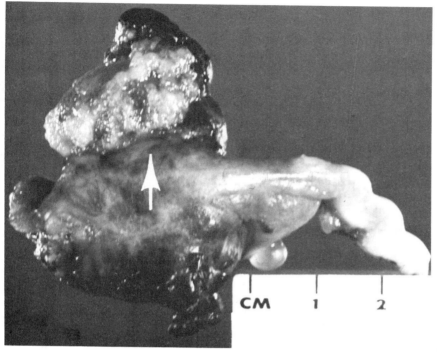

A

FIGURE 18–13

Ectopic pregnancy in right fallopian tube. **A,** A mass of placental tissue protrudes through tear in the wall of the greatly distended tube (*arrow*). **B,** Embryo contained within intact amniotic sac.

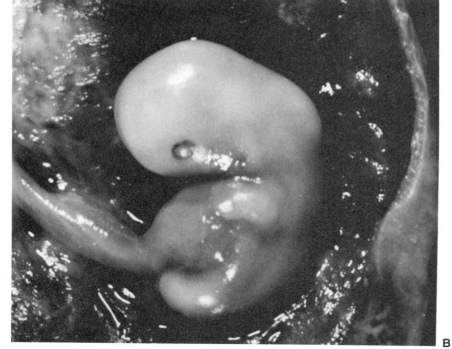

B

Because of the potential life-threatening risk of a ruptured tubal pregnancy, a physician always considers the possibility of a tubal pregnancy in any woman of reproductive age who exhibits any symptoms suggesting a tubal pregnancy. A pelvic examination reveals an area of tenderness adjacent to the uterus and may also reveal a fullness or mass caused by the swollen tube. A positive pregnancy test confirms the pregnancy, and an ultrasound examination demonstrates that the chorionic vesicle indicative of pregnancy is not within the uterus. If these findings indicate that a tubal pregnancy is likely, a laparoscopic examination is performed, which allows the physician to visualize the fallopian tubes and ovaries, and to identify the unruptured pregnancy within the fallopian tube.

Although a ruptured tubal pregnancy is usually treated by resection of the torn fallopian tube along with the ectopic pregnancy, it is often possible to remove the ectopic pregnancy without resecting the tube if the tube has not yet ruptured. Sometimes, the ectopic pregnancy can be dislodged from its tubal attachment by manipulating the tube, and then expressing the ectopic pregnancy from the tube through the fimbriated end. Usually, it is necessary to incise the distended tube, evacuate the ectopic pregnancy, and then close the tubal incision.

Recently, a nonsurgical treatment has been used successfully in some patients. This treatment destroys the tubal pregnancy by giving the patient a single oral dose of an antimetabolite drug called methotrexate. (Antimetabolite drugs destroy rapidly dividing cells by interrupting their metabolic processes and are used to treat patients with cancer, as described in chapter 10.)

Pregnancy Subsequent to Failure of Artificial Contraception

Failure of Contraceptive Pills

Estrogen-progestin contraceptive pills are highly effective when used properly, but occasional pregnancies do occur, usually owing to failure to take the pills regularly or at the proper time. If a woman becomes pregnant while taking oral contraceptives, the developing embryo is exposed to the synthetic estrogen and progestin compounds during the critical early states of embryonic development. This exposure may lead to congenital malformations. The risk is low, but women must be advised of the possibility.

Failure of an Intrauterine Device

Intrauterine devices (IUD) are no longer a popular method of contraception, and most of these devices are no longer marketed. Some women, however, are still using IUDs. In about 2 percent of women, an intrauterine device fails to prevent implantation and pregnancy occurs. This event may lead to serious and sometimes life-threatening complications. The IUD predisposes to infection of the pregnant uterus that in some cases is followed without warning by a serious and sometimes fatal bloodstream infection (*septicemia*). Because of this hazard, the IUD should be removed as soon as the pregnancy is diagnosed. This can usually be accomplished without great difficulty if the string is visible. Often the pregnancy continues normally after the IUD has been removed, but sometimes removal disturbs the implantation site and leads to spontaneous abortion. If the IUD cannot be removed or if the string has retracted inside the uterus, most physicians recommend that the pregnancy be terminated. If the woman decides to continue the pregnancy, she must be closely observed throughout her pregnancy because of the increased risk of serious infection.

Velamentous Insertion of the Umbilical Cord

Abnormal Attachment of the Umbilical Cord and Placenta

Sometimes the umbilical cord vessels are not gathered together normally, and the cord attaches to the membranes attached to the placenta (fetal membranes) rather than to the placenta itself. When this occurs, the umbilical vessels must travel for a distance within the fetal membranes before reaching the placenta (figure 18–14). This is called a **velamentous insertion** of the cord (*velum* = veil). The abnormality may be very hazardous to the fetus if the vessels are located in the membranes that extend over the cervix, because these vessels may be compressed or ruptured in the course of labor or delivery. If one of the vessels ruptures, the circulation between the fetus and placenta is disrupted and the fetus bleeds to death through the ruptured vessel. Because the maternal and fetal circulations are not interconnected, however, the flow of maternal blood through the intervillous space is not disturbed and the mother does not suffer any adverse effects. Even if the vessels crossing the cervix do not rupture, they may be compressed by the fetal head during delivery, causing fetal death by shutting off the circulation through the umbilical vessels.

Placenta Previa

Normally, the placenta attaches high on the anterior or posterior uterine wall. If the placenta becomes attached in the lower part of the uterus, it may cover the cervix. This is called a **placenta previa** (figure 18–15). The term literally means a placenta blocking the exit from the uterus (*pre* = before + *via* = pathway). A placenta that completely covers the cervix is called a *central placenta previa*. If only the edge of the placenta encroaches on the cervix, the abnormality is designated a *partial placenta previa*. The patient with a placenta previa experiences episodes of bleeding during the last part of pregnancy, as a consequence of partial separation of the placenta from the uterine wall. Normally, the lower part of the uterus undergoes gradual dilatation during the last part of pregnancy in preparation for childbirth. The abnormally located placenta is unable to stretch to conform to the contour of the expanding lower part of the uterus, and parts of the placenta therefore tear loose. The tearing disrupts the large uterine vessels that penetrate

FIGURE 18–14

Velamentous insertion of umbilical cord. Note the vessels traversing the membranes to reach the placenta.

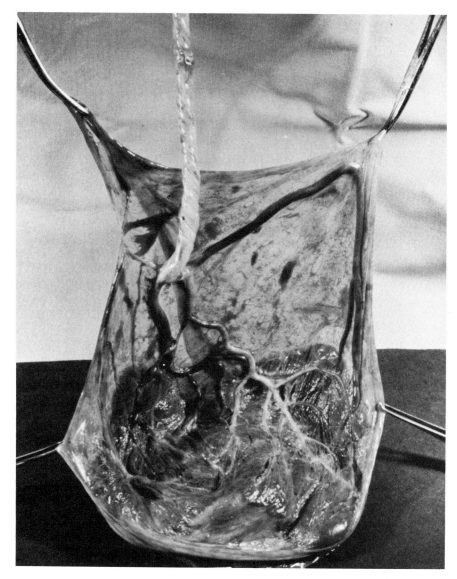

the basal part of the placenta to supply the intervillous spaces (see figure 18–11). In contrast with a velamentous insertion of the cord, which places only the infant in jeopardy, placenta previa is hazardous to the mother as well. The mother may bleed to death if a large part of the placenta is torn from the uterine wall. Large areas of placental disruption may also prevent proper oxygenation of fetal blood passing through the placenta, leading to the death of the fetus.

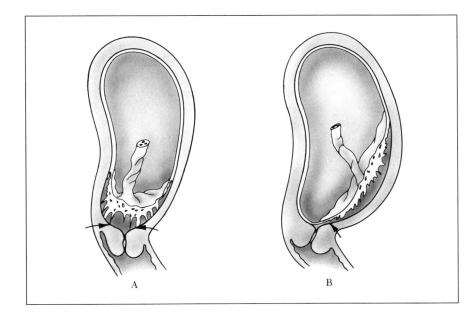

FIGURE 18–15

Types of placenta previa. **A,** Central placenta previa. **B,** Partial placenta previa. *Arrows* indicate the usual locations where the placenta tears from its attachment to the lower part of the uterus late in pregnancy.

Because the placenta blocks the cervix, vaginal delivery is not possible without the risk of severe hemorrhage and injury to the cervix. Delivery is generally accomplished by cesarean section.

Twins and Multiple Pregnancies

Normally, about 1 percent of all pregnancies are twins (approximately one in one hundred). Twins may be either identical (*monozygotic*) or fraternal (*dizygotic*). Approximately 0.01 percent of pregnancies (approximately one in ten thousand) are triplets. Quadruplets, quintuplets, and sextuplets are very rare. The incidence of all types of multiple pregnancies is much higher than normal when ovulation is induced by administration of gonadotrophic hormones or other drugs.

Fraternal Twins

Seventy percent of twins are fraternal and result from fertilization of two separate ova by two different sperm. Fraternal twins are no more alike than brothers and sisters, but they share a family resemblance because they are born of the same parents. Each fertilized ovum implants separately, and each twin forms its own placenta and fetal membranes. Frequently, the margins of the two placentas grow together and fuse, but each fetus remains enclosed within its own amnion and chorion. A fused placenta of this type is called a *diamnionic dichorionic placenta.*

Identical Twins

Thirty percent of twins are identical and result from the splitting of a single fertilized ovum. Splitting may occur at various times after fertilization, as illustrated in figure 18–16. In about 30 percent of monozygotic twin pregnancies, the fertilized ovum splits before the inner cell mass forms. Each half of the zygote implants separately, forms a complete embryo, and develops its own placenta. The two placentas may remain separate or may become fused to form a *diamnionic dichorionic placenta* in the same manner as that for fraternal twins.

More commonly (in almost 70 percent of monozygotic twin pregnancies), the inner cell mass divides after the blastocyst has formed but before implantation takes place. In this instance, each half of the inner cell mass

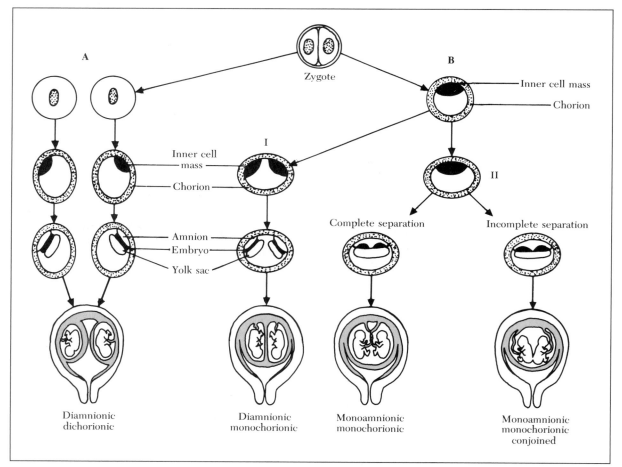

FIGURE 18–16

Stages at which twinning can occur, and types of placenta associated with each stage of twinning.

forms a complete embryo and develops its own amnion and yolk sac, but both develop within a single chorionic cavity. This gives rise to a placenta called a *diamnionic monochorionic placenta.*

Rarely, the inner cell mass divides after the amnionic sac has already formed. When this occurs, the two embryos develop within a single amnionic cavity and form a *monoamnionic monochorionic placenta.* If the division of the inner cell mass is incomplete, conjoined (Siamese) twins are formed.

Determination of Zygosity of Twins from Examination of Placenta

It is often desirable to know at the time of birth whether the twins are identical or fraternal. If they are of different sexes, they must be fraternal; but, if they are the same sex, they could be either fraternal or identical. Sometimes the zygosity of the twins can be determined by examining the placenta. If there are two separate placentas, the twins must have implanted separately. A single placenta with two amnionic sacs, however, could be either a *monochorionic placenta* or a *dichorionic placenta.* It is possible to distinguish between these two types of placentas by gross and microscopic examination of the partition between the two amnionic sacs, because the structure of the partition indicates how it was formed. Figure 18–17 compares the arrangement of fetal membranes of twins implanted separately (dichorionic placenta) with that of twins developing within a single chorionic cavity (monochorionic placenta). As the amnionic sacs gradually enlarge, the membranes eventually establish contact and form a midline partition between the two sacs (figure 18–18). If the placenta is monochorionic, the dividing septum consists only of two amnions without intervening chorions; in a dichorionic placenta, four separate membranes can be identified in the partition: two outer amnions and two inner chorions (figure 18–19). A diamnionic monochorionic placenta always indicates identical twins, as does the rare monoamnionic monochorionic placenta. If the placenta is diamnionic dichorionic or if there are two separate placentas, the twins could be either identical or fraternal. All fraternal twins have a diamnionic dichorionic placenta or separate placentas, but so do 30 percent of identical twins.

Twin Transfusion Syndrome

The placental circulations of identical twins are frequently joined by multiple *vascular anastomoses* (interconnecting blood vessels), and consequently there is normally some intermixing of blood from the two fetuses in the placentas (figure 18–20). Sometimes the placental anastomoses are such that an excess of blood from the fetoplacental circulation from one infant (called the *donor twin*) flows into the circulation of the second twin (called the *recipient*). If this occurs, the donor twin may become anemic and the recipient twin may become overloaded with blood (*polycythemic*). Some degree of twin-to-twin transfusion is relatively common and is reported in about 15 percent of all twin births. Minor differences in the blood volumes of the two

FIGURE 18–17

Comparison of the formation of the placentas and fetal membranes in twins. **A,** Separate implantations leading to the formation of a dichorionic placenta. **B,** Twins developing in a single chorionic cavity and forming a monochorionic placenta. A dichorionic placenta can be encountered with either identical or fraternal twins. A monochorionic placenta is characteristic of identical twins.

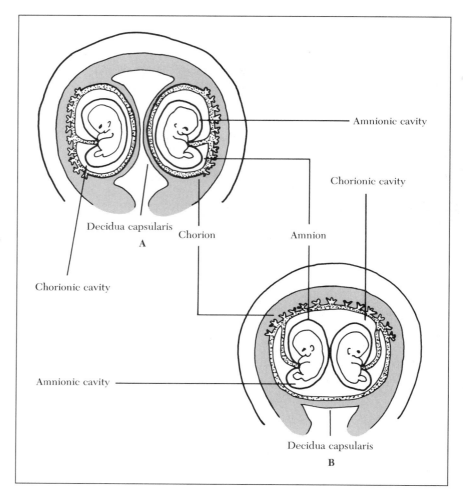

twins can be tolerated, but large disproportions are harmful to both twins (figure 18–21). The severe anemia may be fatal to the donor twin, and the circulation of the recipient twin may become so overloaded by the great excess of blood that the polycythemic twin dies of heart failure.

Blighted Twins

Sometimes one fetus in a multiple pregnancy fails to develop normally or dies early in pregnancy but is retained within the uterus until the surviving fetus is delivered at term. One fetus of a multiple pregnancy that fails to develop is called a *blighted twin,* as illustrated by the following case.

CASE 18–2

A thirty-year-old woman delivered normal, well-formed female twins prematurely at thirty-six weeks' gestation. Examination of the placenta after delivery revealed a third amnionic sac containing a compressed

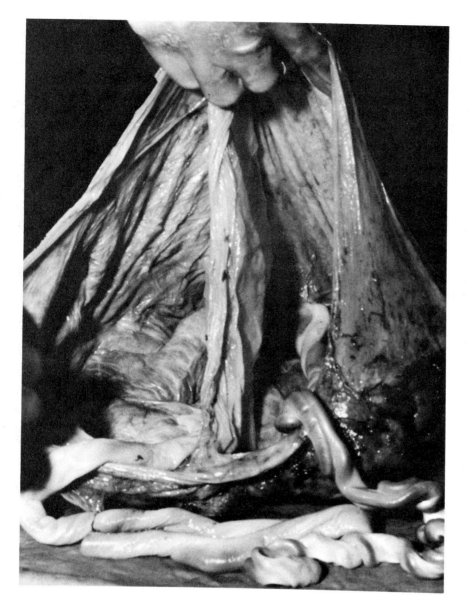

FIGURE 18–18

Partition between amnionic sacs in twin pregnancy. Examination of the partition may indicate zygosity of twins.

degenerated fetus measuring 13 cm in length (figure 18–22). The partition between the amnionic sacs consisted of double amnions and double chorions. In this triplet pregnancy, one fetus died at about seventeen weeks' gestation and was retained within the uterus until the delivery of the two remaining infants at thirty-six weeks. Each fetus was enclosed within its own amnion and chorion. Consequently the zygosity of the surviving twins could not be determined from examination of the placenta, because a diamnionic dichorionic placenta can be associated with either identical or fraternal twins.

FIGURE 18–19

Relation of membranes composing the partition between amnionic sacs in a diamnionic dichorionic placenta. **A,** Undissected partition between amnionic sacs. **B,** Dissection of partition reveals two amnions (A) and two chorions (C). **C,** Photomicrograph of partition reveals four layers, confirming the gross examination. (Original magnification × 40.)

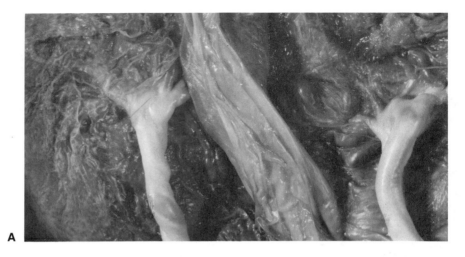

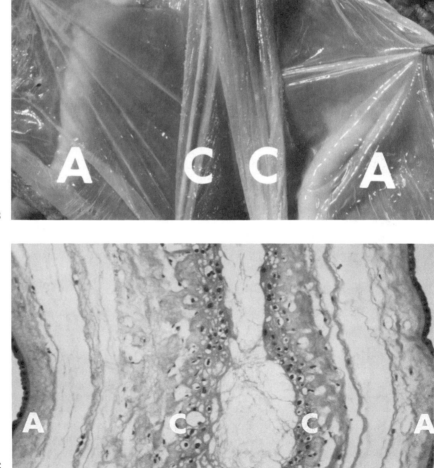

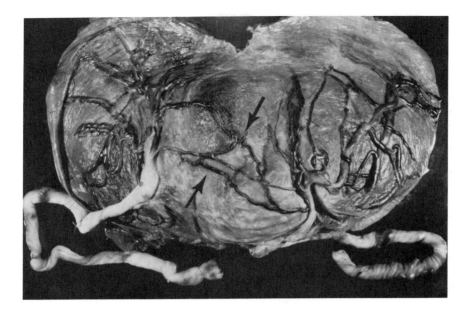

FIGURE 18–20

Placenta of identical twins with amnions removed, revealing interconnecting blood vessels (*arrows*).

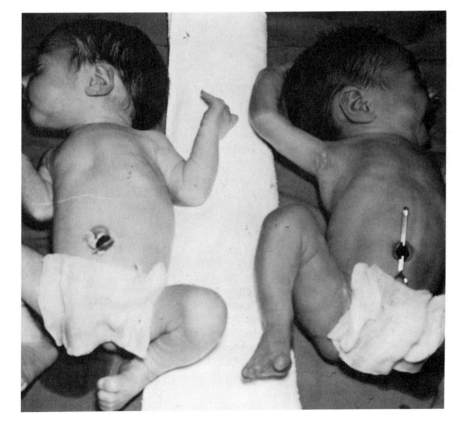

FIGURE 18–21

Identical twins exhibiting twin transfusion syndrome. One twin is pale and anemic. The other appears ruddy and contains an excess of blood. Both twins survived.

FIGURE 18–22

Triplet placenta. Two infants were born prematurely at thirty-six weeks. The third fetus (*arrow*) died early in pregnancy and was retained in the uterus until delivery of the surviving twins (case 18–2).

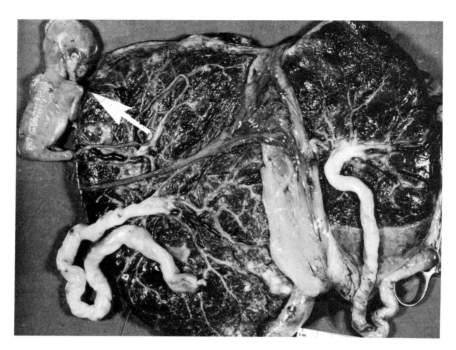

Conjoined Twins

Incomplete separation of the inner cell mass leads to a variable degree of union between two **conjoined twins.** The twins may be joined at the head, thorax, abdomen, or pelvis, the union being face to face, side to side, or back to back. The extent of union is variable but often quite considerable, and often the twins share common internal organs to such a degree that it is not possible to separate them surgically. The conjoined twins are generally equal in size and are often well formed except for their failure to separate.

The following case illustrates some of the clinical features associated with conjoined twins:

CASE 18–3

Conjoined twin girls were born to a twenty-five-year-old woman at term. The infants lived only a few hours. Their combined weight was eight pounds, ten ounces, and they were joined at the lower thorax and upper abdomen. A single umbilical cord supplied both fetuses, and there was a large defect in the lower abdominal wall covered with a thin membrane that ruptured during delivery (figure 18–23). The infants shared a common heart but had separate great vessels entering and leaving the heart. They also shared a single liver but had separate gallbladders and biliary ducts. Each twin had a separate esophagus and stomach, but they shared a common pancreas and duodenum. The remainder of the small bowel and colon were separate. Other organs were separate and normally formed.

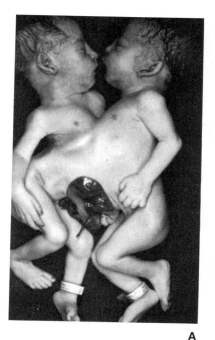

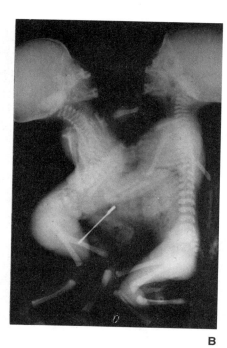

A   **B**

FIGURE 18–23

A, Conjoined twins sharing common organs and exhibiting a large congenital defect in the abdominal wall (case 18–3). **B,** X-ray demonstrating extreme curvature of spine. This resulted from twisting of the spine so that the twins, linked in face-to-face position, could fit within the confines of the crowded uterus.

Disadvantages of Twin Pregnancies

Twins are at a disadvantage compared with singletons. Because they are overcrowded within the uterus, a twin is always smaller than a single infant at a comparable stage of gestation. Overdistention of the uterus frequently promotes premature onset of labor, leading to delivery of premature infants having a reduced chance of survival. Congenital malformations occur twice as often in twins as in singletons, and vascular anastomosis within the placental circulation may lead to a twin transfusion syndrome.

Sometimes, when a pregnancy does not develop normally, the embryo dies and is absorbed, but the trophoblastic cells covering the villi continue to grow at an excessive rate. Masses of abnormal proliferating trophoblastic tissues may invade the uterus, spread into the vagina, and even metastasize to distant sites. In such cases, the trophoblast is behaving like a neoplasm. The general term *gestational trophoblast disease,* which is often applied to this condition, includes two separate entities. The more benign form of this condition is called a **hydatidiform mole.** The villi, which are covered by proliferating trophoblast, become converted into large cystic structures resembling masses of grapes (figure 18–24). The unusual name given to this condition is derived from its gross appearance. A *hydatid* is a fluid-filled vesicle, and a *mole* is a

Hydatidiform Mole and Choriocarcinoma

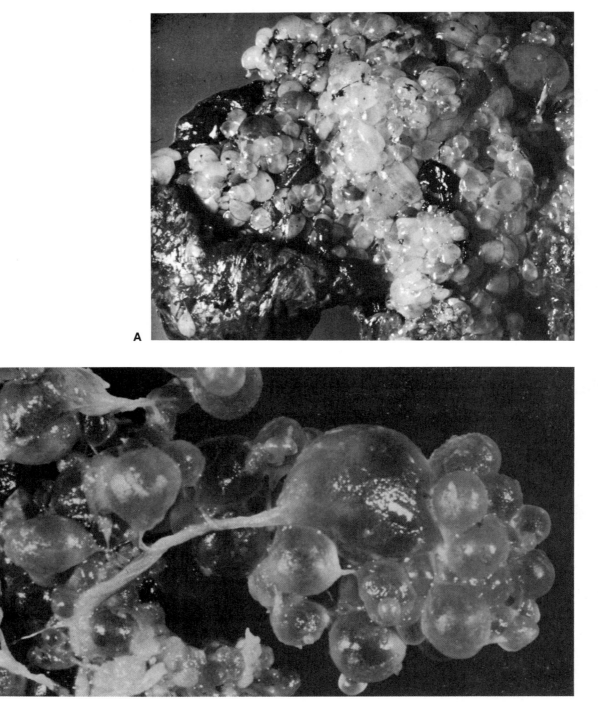

A

B

FIGURE 18–24

Hydatidiform mole. **A,** Placenta converted into a large mass of cysts. **B,** Closer view of hydropic villi.

shapeless mass of tissue. The mole may invade and overdistend the uterus but usually does not metastasize.

Because of the increased volume of the placenta caused by the multiple cystic villi, the patient with a hydatidiform mole experiences an enlargement of the uterus that is much greater than would be expected in relation to the duration of the pregnancy. The mole also exhibits invasive properties, eroding maternal blood vessels and causing irregular uterine bleeding. The overdistention of the uterus caused by the mole may precipitate uterine contractions leading to the expulsion of pieces of the mole.

The more malignant form of gestational trophoblast disease is called a **choriocarcinoma.** It consists entirely of proliferating neoplastic trophoblast without cystic villi and it may metastasize widely.

Treatment of hydatidiform mole consists of evacuation of the uterus by curettage, followed by anticancer chemotherapy if the mole recurs. Choriocarcinoma is usually treated vigorously by several courses of anticancer chemotherapy. Both conditions can usually be cured by adequate treatment.

Hemolytic Disease of the Newborn (Erythroblastosis Fetalis)

Erythroblastosis fetalis is a hemolytic anemia in the newborn infant, which results from sensitization of the mother to a "foreign" blood group antigen present in the red cells of the fetus. The mother reacts by forming antibody that crosses the placenta and damages the infant's red cells, resulting in accelerated destruction of the red cells. The infant attempts to "keep up" with the increased blood destruction by increasing the rate of red cell production (*compensatory hematopoiesis*). The severity of the hemolytic disease depends on the intensity of the blood destruction in the infant. Often, if the hemolytic process is extremely severe, the infant dies in the uterus in the last trimester of pregnancy.

The severely affected infant is extremely anemic and very edematous. This severe form of erythroblastosis is often called *hydrops fetalis,* the term *hydrops* referring to the severe edema in the affected infant (figure 18–25). The edema is the result of heart failure and impaired hepatic plasma-protein synthesis, which are caused by the severe anemia. If the hemolytic process is less intense, the infant may be born alive but will be moderately or severely anemic. Infants with mild disease may appear normal at birth but become anemic and jaundiced soon afterward.

Changes in Hemoglobin and Bilirubin After Delivery

Figure 18–26 illustrates the typical changes in hemoglobin and bilirubin levels after delivery in an infant with hemolytic disease. Anemia invariably develops or increases in severity after delivery; jaundice also develops rapidly. The anemia is aggravated by a decline in the rate of compensatory hematopoiesis after delivery. In the uterus, hematopoiesis is stimulated by both the increased blood destruction and the low oxygen tension in the fetal blood. After delivery, respiration is established and the arterial oxygen ten-

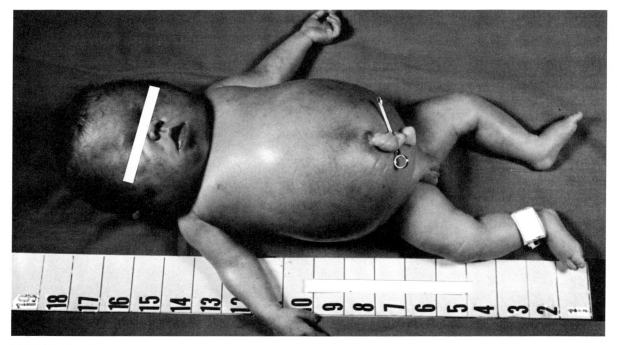

FIGURE 18–25

Stillborn infant with fetal hydrops. Because the fetus was head down in the uterus, the edema is more marked in the face than in the legs and feet. The abdomen is swollen because the liver and spleen are enlarged, and fluid has accumulated in the peritoneal cavity.

sion in the infant's blood rises. Low intrauterine oxygen tension no longer stimulates hematopoiesis and the rate of compensatory hematopoiesis declines. However, blood destruction continues at the same rate. The increasing severity of the anemia reflects the greater postnatal disproportion between blood production and blood destruction.

The accelerated blood destruction in hemolytic disease also causes jaundice. The high rate of red cell breakdown leads to production of large amounts of bile pigment. Before delivery, the bile pigment crosses the placenta into the maternal circulation and is excreted by the mother. After delivery, the infant is called upon to excrete the large amount of pigment formerly handled by the mother, but its liver is still relatively inefficient in conjugating and excreting bilirubin. As a result, the level of unconjugated bilirubin in the infant's blood rises rapidly. This condition is called *hyperbilirubinemia* (*hyper* = elevated + bilirubin + *heme* = blood) and is hazardous to the infant. The high levels of unconjugated bilirubin are toxic to the nervous system, causing necrosis and degeneration of brain tissues (called *kernicterus*).

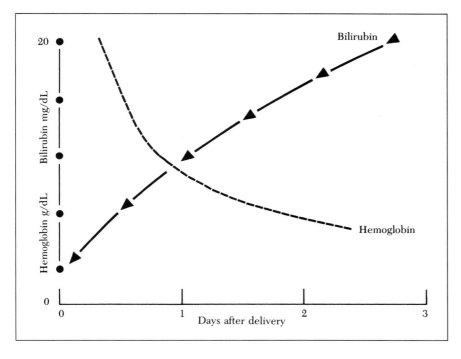

FIGURE 18–26

Changes in hemoglobin and bilirubin concentration that take place in infant with hemolytic disease after delivery.

Rh Hemolytic Disease

Most cases of hemolytic disease are the result of maternal-fetal Rh incompatibility. The Rh system is a relatively complex system consisting of a series of allelic genes that determine multiple Rh antigens on the red cells. The Rh antigen most important clinically is an antigen named the *D antigen* in one terminology and the *Rh$_o$ antigen* in another terminology. (The subscript *o* refers to original, meaning that it was the first Rh antigen recognized.) The presence of the D (Rh$_o$) antigen is considered to be determined by the allelic genes *D* and *d,* giving three possible genotypes: *DD, Dd,* and *dd.* For clinical purposes, persons whose red cells possess the D (Rh$_o$) antigen are considered Rh positive, regardless of the presence or absence of other Rh antigens, and persons lacking the D antigen (genotype *dd*) are considered Rh negative. An Rh-positive person may be either homozygous (*DD*) or heterozygous (*Dd*). Consequently, two heterozygous Rh-positive parents may have an Rh-negative child if each parent passes a *d* gene to the offspring. It is also possible for a heterozygous Rh-positive father and Rh-negative mother to have an Rh-negative child.

In the vast majority of cases of hemolytic disease, the mother is D (Rh$_o$) negative, the infant is D (Rh$_o$) positive, and the antibody is anti-D (anti-Rh$_o$). The first Rh-positive infant born to an Rh-negative mother is usually normal because a woman rarely forms Rh antibody during her first pregnancy. However, once the mother has been sensitized to Rh-positive fetal cells and has formed Rh antibody, Rh hemolytic disease will develop in any subsequent pregnancy in which the fetus is Rh positive.

Hemolytic Disease as a Result of Other Blood Group Antigens

Hemolytic disease may occasionally result from sensitization of the mother to another antigen in the Rh system or from sensitization to an antigen in one of the other blood group systems. The essential feature required for the pathogenesis of hemolytic disease is maternal-fetal blood group incompatibility, and this may be caused by any of a number of blood group antigens.

Diagnosis of Hemolytic Disease in the Newborn Infant

From a knowledge of the pathogenesis of the disease, it follows that the diagnosis of hemolytic disease can be made when the following features are demonstrated.

1. Blood group differences between mother and child. The child has a blood group antigen lacking in the mother's blood. In the most common type of hemolytic disease, the mother lacks the D (Rh_o) antigen, which is present in the cells of the infant.
2. Sensitization of the mother to the "foreign" antigen in the infant's cells. Diagnosis requires demonstrating the presence of an antibody in the mother's blood directed against the "foreign" antigen. Usually this is anti-D (Rh_o).
3. Passage of antibody across the placenta into the infant's blood, with fixation of the antibody to the surface of the infant's cells. This is demonstrated by means of the direct Coombs test performed on the infant's blood. This test detects antibody-protein coating on the surface of the infant's red cells.
4. Evidence of increased destruction of the infant's cells. Determination of the hemoglobin and bilirubin levels in the infant's blood indicates the intensity of the hemolytic process.

Diagnosis of hemolytic disease is summarized in table 18–1. When the foregoing criteria have been met, the diagnosis of hemolytic disease is established with certainty. In routine clinical practice, this information can be obtained promptly without great difficulty. Generally, blood typing of the mother and studies to determine the presence of antibodies are performed routinely during pregnancy by the physician, who generally knows before delivery whether the mother has been sensitized and is likely to deliver an affected infant. When the infant is born, a sample of blood from the umbilical cord (which is the infant's blood) is sent to the laboratory for a direct Coombs test and determination of blood type as well as hemoglobin and bilirubin levels. The Coombs test and blood typing indicate whether the infant is affected, and the hemoglobin and bilirubin levels indicate the severity of the hemolytic disease.

Characteristic feature	Means of recognition	
Production of antigenic fetal cells	Maternal-fetal blood group differences; mother lacks antigen present in fetal cells	**TABLE 18–1**
Maternal sensitization	Mother's blood contains antibody against antigenic cells	*Diagnosis of hemolytic disease*
Transplacental passage of maternal antibody	Positive direct Coombs test on cord blood	
Increased blood destruction in newborn infant	Decreased hemoglobin in cord blood; elevated bilirubin	

Treatment of Hemolytic Disease

A common and widely used treatment of erythroblastosis is **exchange transfusion.** The infant with hemolytic disease is in jeopardy because its body is saturated with passively transferred maternal antibody. The antibody is the cause of the hemolytic anemia and jaundice, and several months are required before the antibody can be completely eliminated from the infant's circulation. The rationale of exchange transfusion is to provide the infant with a population of cells that will not be destroyed by the antibody. In the usual case of hemolytic disease caused by Rh incompatibility, a transfusion of Rh-negative blood is given. At the same time, exchange transfusion provides the infant with bilirubin-free plasma to replace the jaundiced plasma, thereby helping to prevent severe elevation of potentially toxic, unconjugated bilirubin. It should be emphasized that the exchange transfusion has no effect on the infant's own blood type. The transfused Rh-negative cells will be gradually eliminated and replaced by the infant's own Rh-positive cells. The purpose of the exchange transfusion is to tide the infant over an acute, life-threatening situation. This is accomplished by decreasing the rate of red cell destruction through transfusion of cells not subject to hemolysis and by lowering the concentration of potentially toxic unconjugated bilirubin in the infant's plasma.

Exchange transfusion may be compared to replacing the contents of a barrel of salt water with fresh water without emptying and refilling the barrel. This can be accomplished by withdrawing a pail of salt water from the barrel and replacing it with an equal quantity of fresh water. If this is repeated many times, the salt concentration of the water in the barrel is gradually reduced, until eventually the barrel is filled with virtually fresh water. An exchange transfusion is an application of the same principle. The usual method of exchange transfusion is to introduce a catheter into the umbilical vein. A small quantity of the infant's own blood is withdrawn and replaced with an equal quantity of blood lacking the sensitizing antigen (usually Rh-negative blood). The process of withdrawing a small quantity of blood and replacing it with an equal quantity of exchange blood is continued until about 500 mL of blood has been administered. At the conclusion of the exchange transfusion, about 85 percent of the infant's own cells will have been replaced by the transfused cells.

Fluorescent Light Therapy for Hyperbilirubinemia

The elevated level of unconjugated bilirubin that causes kernicterus can be reduced by exposing the unclothed jaundiced infant to fluorescent lights continuously for several days. The infant is turned frequently so that the skin receives maximum exposure to the fluorescent light. The eyes are covered to protect them from the bright light. The light exposure acts by converting the toxic unconjugated bilirubin into less-toxic compounds that are not as hazardous to the infant. This procedure, which is called **phototherapy,** has reduced the need for exchange transfusions.

Intrauterine Fetal Transfusion

Exchange transfusion can be used to treat only those infants who survive long enough to be born alive. It cannot be used to salvage severely affected infants, who often die in utero late in pregnancy. It is possible to identify fetuses who are severely affected with erythroblastosis by means of **amniocentesis.** A needle is inserted through the maternal abdominal wall, through the uterus, and into the amnionic cavity, and a small quantity of amnionic fluid is withdrawn. The amnionic fluid of infants affected with hemolytic disease often contains increased amounts of bile pigments; a rough correlation exists between the severity of the hemolytic disease and the amount of pigments in the amnionic fluid. If study of the fluid indicates that the infant is severely affected and may not survive, a blood transfusion may be administered to the fetus while it is still within the uterus. It is not necessary to inject the blood into a fetal vein. Blood can be introduced into the infant's peritoneal cavity from which it will be adequately absorbed. Newer, sophisticated ultrasound-guided techniques also have been developed that allow direct intrauterine transfusion of blood into the umbilical vein by means of a needle introduced into the amnionic sac. All these methods of intrauterine transfusion require highly specialized techniques and carry a risk to the infant. They are used only in extremely desperate situations in which the infant is likely to die if transfusion is not performed.

Prevention of Rh Hemolytic Disease with Rh Immune Globulin

Postpartum Administration

As previously stated, the first Rh-positive infant born to an Rh-negative mother is usually normal because Rh antibodies are rarely formed during the first pregnancy. The antigenic Rh-positive cells that induce sensitization do not usually enter the maternal circulation until after the delivery. When the placenta begins to separate from the uterus and is eventually expelled, the barrier separating the maternal and fetal circulations is disrupted, and some of the Rh-positive fetal cells within the villi may be expressed into the uterine blood vessels and may enter the mother's circulation. In general, the larger the volume of fetal blood entering the mother's circulation, the greater the likelihood of sensitization to Rh antigen; and, once sensitization has occurred, Rh hemolytic disease will develop in any subsequent pregnancy in which the fetus is Rh positive.

Rh immune globulin is a gamma globulin containing a high concentration of Rh antibody. When administered to an unsensitized Rh-negative mother within seventy-two hours after delivery of an Rh-positive fetus, it is extremely effective in preventing the formation of Rh antibody. The Rh antibody in the gamma globulin suppresses the mother's own ability to form Rh antibody in response to the fetal Rh-positive cells. The antibody apparently coats the Rh-antigen sites on the surface of the fetal red cells in the mother's bloodstream. Consequently, the mother's immune system can no longer "recognize" the cells as containing a "foreign" antigen and does not respond by forming antibody. In addition, the antibody-coated cells are rapidly eliminated from the maternal circulation, so they do not persist long enough to induce sensitization. Rh immune globulin is recommended for all Rh-negative mothers who have not already formed Rh antibodies and who have given birth to an Rh-positive infant. It is of no value if the mother has already formed antibodies. Unsensitized Rh-negative patients should also receive Rh immune globulin after an abortion or ectopic pregnancy because these conditions also may induce sensitization. The risk is low, however, if the gestation is less than twelve weeks.

The standard dose of Rh immune globulin is sufficient to "neutralize" and eliminate about one ounce of fetal blood. In the very uncommon situation in which a larger volume of fetal blood enters the maternal circulation, more Rh immune globulin is required. Special laboratory tests can detect and quantitate the volume of fetal blood in the mother's circulation, enabling the physician to determine how much additional Rh immune globulin to administer.

The incidence of Rh hemolytic disease has been greatly reduced by the routine use of Rh immune globulin, but the disease has not been completely eliminated. There are two reasons why the disease persists:

1. A very small number of Rh-negative women form Rh antibody in their first pregnancy, apparently because of prior contact with Rh antigen from an unrecognized abortion, transfusion of Rh-positive blood, or other cause.
2. Rh immune globulin is not 100-percent effective. About 1.5 percent of Rh-negative women will form antibodies in a subsequent Rh-positive pregnancy despite postpartum administration of Rh immune globulin. (About 15 percent of Rh-negative women would be expected to form antibodies if no treatment were administered.)

Combined Antepartum and Postpartum Administration

One of the reasons why postpartum administration of Rh immune globulin does not always prevent Rh sensitization is that small numbers of fetal Rh-positive red cells occasionally enter the mother's circulation late in pregnancy through small breaks in the placental villi. When this occurs, the antigenic fetal cells may induce sensitization prior to delivery, rendering postpartum administration of Rh immune globulin ineffective.

In an effort to further reduce the failure rate of Rh immune globulin, many physicians recommend that an injection of Rh immune globulin be given at about twenty-eight weeks' gestation, in addition to the postpartum injection. Combined antepartum and postpartum administration reduces the incidence of sensitization to about 0.5 percent, compared with a 1.5-percent incidence when only postpartum administration is employed. There are some drawbacks to this approach. When Rh immune globulin is used prior to delivery, it is given to all Rh-negative mothers, many of whom are carrying an Rh-negative fetus and do not need it. Only mothers with Rh-positive fetuses would receive the postpartum injection.

When Rh immune globulin is given during pregnancy, the antibody does cross the placenta and attach to the fetal red cells, causing a direct Coombs test on the infant's cells to be weakly positive. However, the quantity of antibody sufficient to eliminate the antigenic red cells from the mother's circulation is not sufficient to damage the red cells in the fetal circulation.

ABO Hemolytic Disease

In most cases, hemolytic disease of infants is the result of sensitization to a "foreign" antigen, which provokes the formation of a new antibody. However, a very mild type of hemolytic disease may occasionally be caused by ABO blood group differences between mother and infant. In **ABO hemolytic disease,** the mother is group O (and has anti-A and anti-B antibodies in her serum), and the infant is either group A or group B. The A or B antigen of the fetus stimulates the maternal ABO antibodies, increasing the titer and changing the character of the antibodies so that they are capable of crossing the placenta and becoming fixed to the cells of the infant. ABO hemolytic disease may be encountered in a first pregnancy because it is caused by a pre-existing antibody capable of being stimulated by an ABO-incompatible pregnancy. This is in contrast with most other types of hemolytic disease, in which a first pregnancy is required to provoke sensitization before antibody can be formed in a subsequent pregnancy.

Questions for Review

1. Why do spontaneous abortions occur? What are the consequences of prolonged retention of a dead fetus within the uterine cavity?

2. What is an ectopic pregnancy? What factors predispose to development of an ectopic pregnancy in the fallopian tube? What are the consequences of a tubal pregnancy?

3. What is the difference between a hydatidiform mole and a choriocarcinoma?

4. What is hemolytic disease of the newborn? How does it affect the infant? How does it affect the mother? Why do severely affected infants become edematous?

5. In infants with hemolytic disease, why does jaundice increase after delivery? Why does anemia become more severe after delivery?

6. How does the physician make a diagnosis of hemolytic disease? How is the disease treated?

7. How does ABO hemolytic disease differ from Rh hemolytic disease?

8. What are some of the adverse effects of an intrauterine contraceptive device? How does an IUD prevent pregnancy?

9. What structures contribute to the formation of the placenta? What are the main functions of the placenta?

10. Describe some of the important abnormalities of the placenta and umbilical cord that may have an unfavorable effect on pregnancy.

11. What is the source of amnionic fluid? What factors regulate the total volume of amnionic fluid?

12. Why does a pregnancy test become positive? When does it become positive?

13. What are the possible causes and the significance of polyhydramnios? of oligohydramnios?

Supplementary Readings

Acker, D., et al. 1983. Abruptio placentae associated with cocaine use. *American Journal of Obstetrics and Gynecology* 146:220–21. One of the early reports of this serious cocaine-induced complication.

Centers for Disease Control. 1995. Ectopic pregnancy: United States, 1990–1992. *Morbidity and Mortality Weekly Reports* 44:46–48. Approximately 2 percent of all pregnancies are ectopic, and ectopic pregnancies account for 9 percent of pregnancy-related deaths. Current tendency is to treat many ectopic pregnancies in an outpatient setting by laparoscopic salpingectomy or salpingostomy or by methotrexate chemotherapy.

Collins, J. A. 1994. Reproductive technology: The price of progress (Editorial). *New England Journal of Medicine* 331:270–71. Discusses the very high cost of the various methods used to achieve conception in infertile couples.

Davey, M. G., and Zipursky, A. 1979. McMaster conference on prevention of Rh immunization. *Vox Sanguinis* 36:50–64. A summary of practices and recommendations.

Freda, V. J., et al. 1978. Rh disease: How near the end? *Hospital Practice* 13:61–69. Discusses the prevention of Rh hemolytic disease by means of Rh immune globulin and the reasons why sensitization sometimes occurs in spite of administration of Rh immune globulin.

Grannum, P. A., et al. 1986. In utero exchange transfusion by direct intravascular injection in severe erythroblastosis fetalis. *New England Journal of Medicine* 314:1431–34. Current status of intrauterine fetal transfusions.

Neumann, P. J., et al. 1994. The cost of a successful delivery after in vitro fertilization. *New England Journal of Medicine* 331:239–43. The cost of a successful delivery after in vitro fertilization ranges from $67,000 to $114,000 and, in some unusual cases, can be as high as $800,000.

NIH Consensus Conference. 1995. Effect of corticosteroids for fetal maturation on perinatal outcomes. *Journal of the American Medical Association* 273:413–18. Administration of corticosteroids to mothers at risk of premature birth (24–34 weeks gestation) improves infant survival by reducing neonatal respiratory distress syndrome.

O'Rahilly, R., and Müller, F. 1987. *Developmental stages in human embryos.* Washington, DC: Carnegie Institution of Washington. A comprehensive reference on prenatal development based on the material in the Carnegie collection.

Ory, S. J. 1992. New options for diagnosis and treatment of ectopic pregnancy. *Journal of the American Medical Association* 267:534–37. A review of current methods of diagnosis and treatment.

Rodeck, C. H., et al. 1981. Direct intravascular fetal blood transfusion by fetoscopy in severe rhesus isoimmunization. *Lancet* 1:625–27. Blood administered directly into an umbilical vessel either at the umbilicus or at the placental cord insertion.

Stovall, T. G., et al. 1991. Single does methotrexate for treatment of ectopic pregnancy. *Obstetrics and Gynecology* 77:754–57. In selected cases, the ectopic pregnancy can be destroyed by administration of the antimetabolite methotrexate, rather than by laparoscopic salpingostomy or salpingectomy. This method is still somewhat experimental. Its applications and limitations are still being defined.

Stroup, M. 1977. Rh system: Genetics and function. *Mayo Clinic Proceedings* 52:141–44. Basic concepts of the genetics of the Rh system and the complexity of the Rh antigen.

Wilcox, A. J., Weinberg, C. R., and Baird, D. D. 1995. Timing of sexual intercourse in relation to ovulation. *New England Journal of Medicine* 333:1517–21. In a carefully studied group of women who were planning to become pregnant, the likelihood of conception from a single intercourse increased from 8 percent six days before ovulation to 36 percent on the day of ovulation. There were no pregnancies from intercourse on the day after ovulation and more than six days before ovulation. The fertile period lasts about six days and ends on the day of ovulation. Sperm in the reproductive tract can fertilize for as many as five days, but ova have an extremely short survival after ovulation.

Woods, J. R., et al. 1987. Effects of cocaine on uterine blood flow and fetal oxygenation. *Journal of the Ameri-*

can Medical Association 257:957–61. Cocaine alters fetal oxygenation by reducing uterine blood flow and impairing oxygen transfer to the fetus.

Chapter 18 ▪ Outline Summary

Fertilization and Prenatal Development / 497
Fertilization

Sperm contains genetic material and enzymes to penetrate egg.

Sperm has motility and is also transported by aspiration.

Ovum expelled, surrounded by zona pellucida and granulosa cells.

Union occurs in fallopian tube.

Only one sperm can enter egg.

Early Development

Zygote develops into small ball of cells.

Fluid accumulates and blastocyst forms.

Inner cell mass forms embryo.

Trophoblast forms placenta and membranes.

Implantation occurs at end of first week.

Amnionic sac, yolk sac, and germ disk form.

Germ disk rounds up to form tubular embryo by fourth week.

In Vitro Fertilization and Embryo Transfer

Applicable to infertility as a result of tubal scarring or absence of tubes from previous surgery.

Follicle aspirated by laparoscopy just prior to ovulation.

Ovum fertilized and allowed to develop in culture medium outside body to eight-cell or sixteen-cell stage; then introduced into uterus by catheter passed through cervix.

Low success rate and possibility of chromosomally abnormal embryos, which are aborted spontaneously.

Stages of Prenatal Development

Preembryonic period: implantation and differentiation of blastocyst.

Embryonic period: third through seventh week.

Human shape develops and organ systems form, a critical period of development.

Fetal period: eighth week until term. Increase in size but no major changes.

Duration of Pregnancy

Dated from conception: thirty-eight weeks.

Dated from last menstrual period: forty weeks.

Frequently expressed in trimesters.

Decidua, Fetal Membranes, and Placenta / 504
Decidua

Decidua basalis: under chorionic vesicle.

Decidua capsularis: over chorionic vesicle.

Decidua parietalis: lines rest of uterus.

Chorion

Chorion laeve: superficial smooth chorion.

Chorion frondosum: bushy chorion that will form placental villi.

Amnionic Sac

Enclosed within chorion.

Forms protective environment for fetus.

Yolk Sac

Never contains yolk in human.

Forms intestinal tract and other structures.

Placenta

Provides oxygen and nutrition for fetus.

Fetus connected to placenta by umbilical cord.

Double circulation of blood in placenta.

Fetoplacental circulation: from fetus to villi.

Uteroplacental circulation: maternal blood circulates around villi.

No normal intercommunication between circulations.

Endocrine function of placenta:

Makes estrogen and progesterone.

Makes HCG and HPL.

Pregnancy tests detect HCG.

Amnionic Fluid / 509
Formation and Excretion

Chiefly a filtration from maternal blood early in pregnancy.

Mostly fetal urine later in pregnancy.

Fetus swallows fluid, which is absorbed, transferred to maternal circulation, and excreted by mother.

Normally, balance maintained between secretion and excretion of fluid.

Polyhydramnios

Fetus unable to swallow; so fluid accumulates in sac.

Congenital obstruction of fetal upper intestinal tract; so fluid cannot be absorbed from intestinal tract.

Oligohydramnios

Fetal kidneys fail to develop: no urine formed.

Congenital obstruction of urethra: no urine escapes into amnionic fluid.

Spontaneous Abortion / 510
Incidence

Occurs in 10 to 20 percent of all pregnancies.

Early abortion often as a result of chromosomal abnormalities incompatible with survival, or defective implantation.

Late abortions usually caused by detachment of placenta or obstruction of blood supply through cord.

Cocaine abuse disturbs blood flow to placenta and may cause placental abruption and intrauterine fetal death.

Complications

Disseminated intravascular coagulation syndrome: see chapter 12.

Ectopic Pregnancy / 511
Predisposing Factors of Tubal Pregnancy

Previous tubal infection.

Disturbed tubal motility.

Frequently both fallopian tubes predisposed.

Consequences

Tube ruptures within a few months.

May cause profuse bleeding from torn blood vessels.

Pregnancy Subsequent to Failure of Artificial Contraception / 514
Failure of Contraceptive Pills

Pills effective if used properly.

Synthetic estrogens, progestins in pills may induce congenital abnormalities in developing embryo.

Failure of Intrauterine Device (IUD)

Predisposes to infection.

Remove IUD as soon as pregnancy diagnosed.

Advise patient of risks if IUD cannot be removed.

Abnormal Attachment of Umbilical Cord and Placenta / 515
Velamentous Insertion of Cord

Cord attaches to membranes, and vessels must travel in membranes to reach placenta.

Vessels may tear or be compressed during labor; may be fatal to infant, but no effect on mother.

Placenta Previa

Central placenta previa: placenta covers entire cervix.

Partial placenta previa: margin of placenta covers cervix.

Causes episodes of bleeding late in pregnancy.

Hazardous to both mother and infant.

Cesarean section delivery required.

Twins and Multiple Pregnancies / 517
Twin Transfusion Syndrome

Vascular anastomoses connect placental circulations of identical twins.

One twin may receive excess blood while the other becomes anemic.

Minor disproportions in blood may be tolerated, but severe disproportions may be fatal to both twins.

Blighted Twins

One twin dies; other survives to term.

Dead twin may be compressed and degenerates.

Conjoined (Siamese) Twins

Variable union between identical twins.

Separation often not possible after birth.

Disadvantages of Twin Pregnancy

Twins smaller for gestational age.

Premature onset of labor.

Higher incidence of congenital malformations.

Twin transfusion syndrome.

Hydatidiform Mole and Choriocarcinoma / 525
Hydatidiform Mole

"Benign" form.

Villi form cystic structures.

May invade and overdistend uterus.

Treated by emptying uterus.

Chemotherapy if mole recurs.

Choriocarcinoma

More malignant form.

Consists of neoplastic trophoblast without villi.

Treated by anticancer chemotherapy.

Hemolytic Disease of the Newborn / 527
Pathogenesis and Clinical Manifestations

Infant sensitizes mother to blood group antigen.

Maternal antibody damages fetal cells.

Infant increases blood production to compensate.

Variable severity.

Hydrops fetalis: severe anemia and edema.

Anemia and jaundice.

Mild disease with few symptoms.

Changes in Hemoglobin and Bilirubin After Delivery

Anemia increases because blood destruction continues and compensatory hematopoiesis declines.

Jaundice develops because of inefficient excretion of bilirubin by newborn infant's liver.

Severe jaundice causes brain damage (kernicterus).

Rh Hemolytic Disease / 529
The Rh System

Determined by series of allelic genes.

Individual whose red cells contain D antigen is Rh positive. May be homozygous or heterozygous.

Most cases of Rh hemolytic disease as a result of Rh-negative mother with Rh-positive infant.

Rarely occurs in first pregnancy.

Diagnosis of Hemolytic Disease

Blood group differences between mother and infant (e.g., mother Rh negative and fetus Rh positive).

Mother has formed antibodies (e.g., anti-D).

Antibody coats infant's cells (positive direct Coombs test).

Evidence of increased blood destruction.

Treatment of Hemolytic Disease

Exchange transfusion.

Provides population of cells not attacked by maternal antibody.

Provides plasma low in bilirubin.

Does not change infant's blood type.

Fluorescent light therapy.

Converts unconjugated bilirubin into less-toxic compound.

Reduces need for exchange transfusion.

Intrauterine fetal transfusion.

Used to salvage infants who would die prior to delivery.

Blood instilled into fetal peritoneal cavity or umbilical cord using special techniques.

Prevention of Rh Hemolytic Disease

Rh immune globulin administered to mother eliminates antigenic fetal cells.

Incidence of Rh hemolytic disease greatly reduced.

Not 100-percent effective.

Some physicians recommend injections late in pregnancy as well as after delivery to further reduce incidence of sensitization.

ABO Hemolytic Disease

Fetal A or B antigens stimulate maternal ABO antibodies.

Causes mild hemolytic disease.

May be encountered in first pregnancy.;

19

The Urinary System

Learning Objectives

1. Describe the normal structures of the kidneys and their functions.
2. Explain the pathogenesis of glomerulonephritis, nephrosis, nephrosclerosis, and glomerulosclerosis. Describe the clinical manifestations of each of these disorders.
3. Describe the clinical manifestations and complications of urinary tract infections.
4. List the causes of renal tubular injury. Describe the manifestations of tubular injury and the treatments for each disorder.
5. Explain the mechanism for formation of urinary tract calculi. Describe the complications of stone formation. Explain the manifestations of urinary tract obstruction.
6. Differentiate the major forms of cystic disease of the kidney and their prognoses. Name the more common kinds of tumors affecting the urinary tract.
7. Describe the causes, clinical manifestations, and treatment of renal failure.
8. Describe the principles and techniques of hemodialysis.

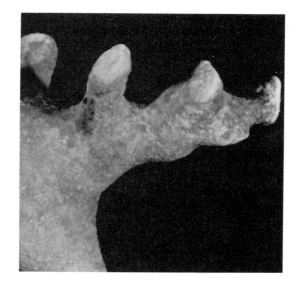

Chapter 19 ■ Contents

The urinary system (figure 19–1A) consists of

1. The *kidneys,* which produce the urine
2. An *excretory duct system* (renal calyces, renal pelves, and ureters) that transports the urine
3. The *bladder,* where the urine is stored
4. The *urethra,* which conveys the urine from the bladder for excretion

The Kidneys

The *kidneys* are paired, bean-shaped organs located along the back body wall below the diaphragm and adjacent to the vertebral column. Their structure is illustrated in figure 19–1B. The region where the blood vessels enter and leave and where the ureter exits to descend to the bladder is called the *hilus of the kidney.* The expanded upper end of the ureter is the *renal pelvis* (plural, *pelves*). The pelvis divides into several large branches called the *major calyces* (singular, *calyx*), and these in turn subdivide to form the *minor calyces.* The renal substance is divided into an outer *cortex* and an inner *medulla.* The cone-shaped masses of renal tissue in the medulla that

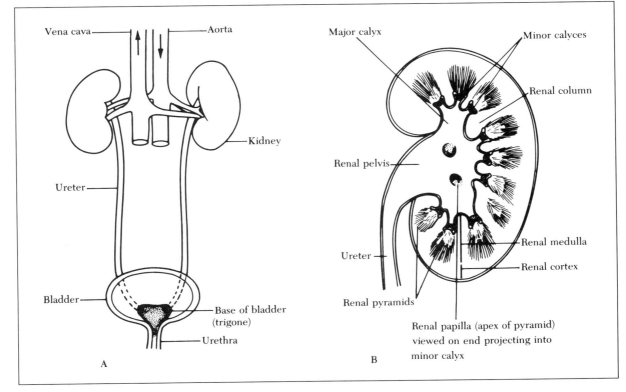

FIGURE 19–1

A, Components of the urinary system. **B,** Structure of the kidney in cross-section.

project into the minor calyces are called the *renal pyramids,* and the tip of each pyramid is called the *renal papilla.* Columns of cortical tissue that extend into the medulla between the pyramids are called the *renal columns.*

The calyces and pelves convey the urine into the ureters, which extend downward to enter the posterior wall of the bladder near its base, as illustrated in figure 19–1A. Each ureter enters the bladder at an angle so that, when the bladder contracts, its muscular wall compresses the ureters as they run obliquely through it, somewhat like a one-way valve. This prevents backflow of urine into the ureters during voiding (urination). The ureteral openings in the bladder are also partially covered by folds of mucosa that help prevent retrograde flow of urine.

The Ureters

The *ureters* are muscular tubes that propel the urine into the bladder by wavelike contractions of their muscular walls **(peristalsis).** Urine is discharged into the bladder in spurts. It does not drain by gravity.

The Bladder and Urethra

The *urinary bladder* is the distensible reservoir for urine. It is lined by transitional epithelium continuous with that which lines the remainder of the urinary tract. The opening of the *urethra* is located at the base of the bladder, and the ureteral openings are located on either side and behind the urethral opening. The triangular area at the base of the bladder bounded by the two ureteral orifices posteriorly and the urethral orifice anteriorly is called the *trigone* of the bladder (*tri* = three).

Function of the Kidneys

The kidneys are important excretory organs, functioning along with the lungs in excreting the waste products of food metabolism. Carbon dioxide and water are end-products of carbohydrate and fat metabolism. Protein metabolism produces urea, as well as various acids, which only the kidneys can excrete. The kidneys also play an important role in regulating mineral and water balance by excreting minerals and water that have been ingested in excess of the body's requirements, and conserving minerals and water as required. It has been said that the internal environment of the body is determined not by what a person ingests but rather by what the kidneys retain.

The kidneys serve an endocrine function as well. Specialized cells in the kidneys elaborate a hormone called *erythropoietin,* which regulates red blood cell production in the bone marrow, and another humoral substance called **renin,** which takes part in the regulation of the blood pressure.

The Nephron

The basic structural and functional unit of the kidneys are the **nephrons,** which consist of a glomerulus and a renal tubule. There are about one million nephrons in each kidney. The *glomerulus* is a tuft of capillaries supplied by an *afferent glomerular artery*. The capillaries of the glomerulus then recombine into an *efferent glomerular artery,* which in turn breaks up into a network of capillaries that supply the *renal tubule.*

The histologic structure of the glomerulus and related structures is illustrated schematically in figure 19–2. The expanded proximal end of the tubule is called **Bowman's capsule.** The tuft of capillaries that make up the glomerulus is pushed into Bowman's capsule much as one would push a fist into a balloon. The layer of Bowman's capsule cells, which is pushed in (*invaginated*), becomes closely applied to the capillaries of the glomerulus and is called the *visceral layer of Bowman's capsule* or simply the *glomerular epithelium.* The cells of this layer have long, footlike cytoplasmic processes and are usually called *podocytes* (*podos* = foot) (figure 19–2A). The outer layer of Bowman's capsule is called the *parietal layer of Bowman's capsule,* or simply the *capsular epithelium.* The space between the two layers, into which the urine filters, is called *Bowman's space.*

The capillary tuft is held together and supported by groups of modified connective-tissue cells that are located between the capillaries and are concentrated in the region where the afferent and efferent glomerular arterioles enter and leave the glomerulus. This region is called the *vascular pole of the glomerulus.* Because of their location, the cells are called **mesangial cells** (*meso* = middle + *angio* = vessel). Also located at the vascular pole is a specialized cluster of cells called the **juxtaglomerular apparatus** (*juxta* = near to), which regulates blood flow through the glomerulus. It also plays a role in regulating blood pressure by producing renin, as described in a later section. The juxtaglomerular apparatus consists of three parts:

1. The *macula densa,* a condensation of cells in the distal part of the renal tubule where it is in contact with the vascular pole of the glomerulus
2. The *juxtaglomerular cells,* which are specialized cells containing renin and are located in the wall of the afferent glomerular artery
3. A group of cells interposed between the vascular pole of the glomerulus and the macula densa (figure 19–2B)

Water and soluble material filter from the blood through the glomerular capillaries into Bowman's space. When visualized by electron microscopy, the membrane through which the filtrate passes can be seen to consist of three layers, as depicted in figure 19–3. The *inner layer* is formed by the endothelium of the glomerular capillaries. The cytoplasm is very thin and is perforated by many small holes called *fenestrations* (*fenestra* = window). Most of the fenestrations are open but some, called *pseudofenestrations* (*pseudo* = false), are covered by a thin membrane containing a central knob. This layer is freely permeable to water and to many large molecules. The *middle layer* is the porous basement membrane that supports the capillary endothelium. The *outer layer* is composed of the podocytes. Their highly branched cytoplasmic processes are called **foot processes,** and their terminal branches are called **pedicels** ("little feet"). The pedicels are attached to the basement membrane, and the pedicels of one cell interdigitate with others from the

FIGURE 19–2

Structure of glomerulus and Bowman's capsule. **A,** Anterior half of Bowman's capsule removed to reveal capillary tuft covered by podocytes (schematic). **B,** Cross-section through glomerulus to reveal structure of glomerular filter and juxtaglomerular apparatus.

Proximal tubule
Nucleus of podocyte
Bowman's space
Glomerular capillaries covered by podocytes
Capsular epithelium
Afferent glomerular artery
Vascular pole of glomerulus
Efferent glomerular artery

A

FIGURE 19–3 (OPPOSITE)

Schematic representation of fine structure of glomerular filter as visualized by electron microscope. **A,** Segment of glomerular capillaries. **B,** Cross-section through the center of the glomerulus including part of Bowman's capsule.

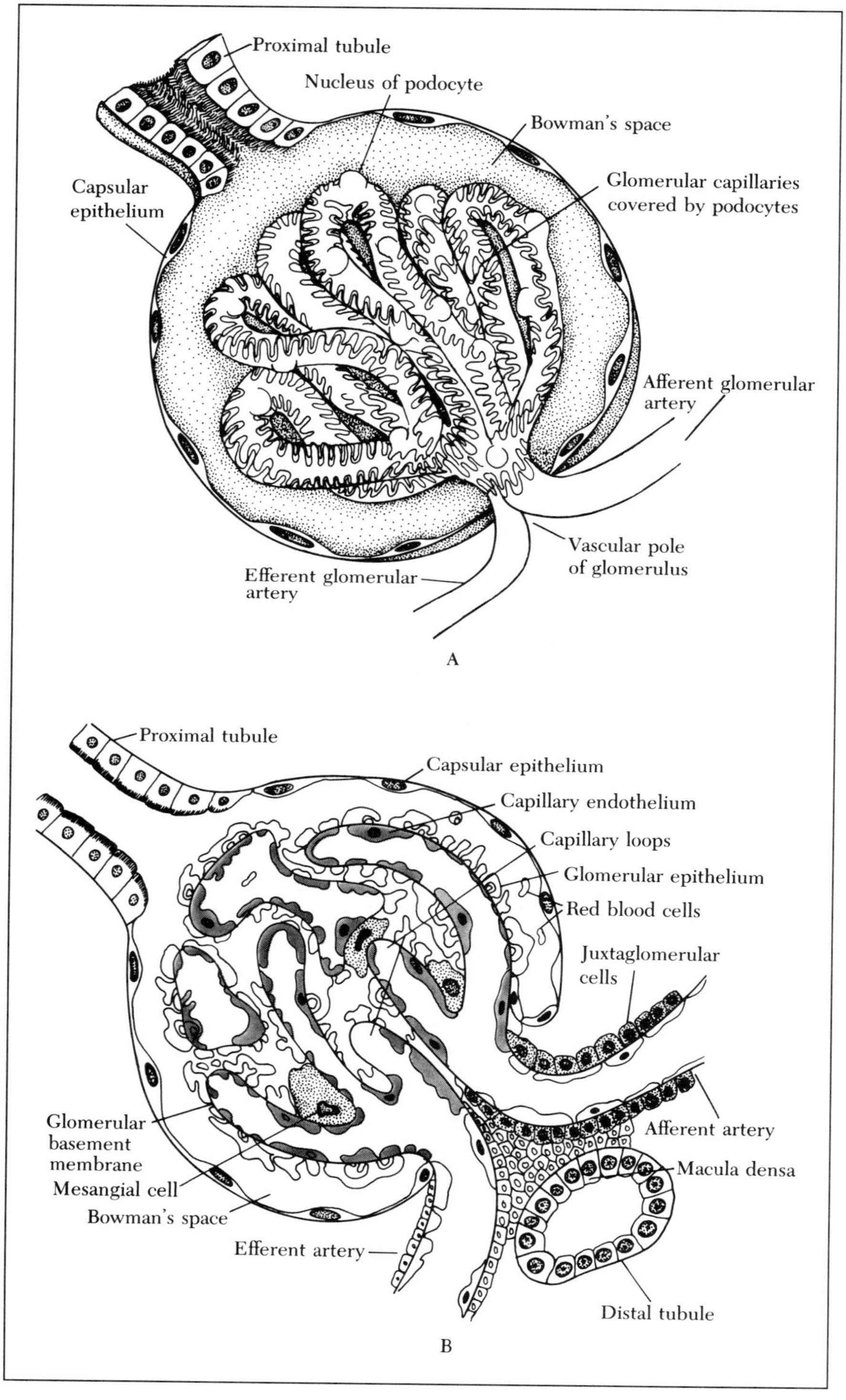

Proximal tubule
Capsular epithelium
Capillary endothelium
Capillary loops
Glomerular epithelium
Red blood cells
Juxtaglomerular cells
Glomerular basement membrane
Mesangial cell
Bowman's space
Efferent artery
Afferent artery
Macula densa
Distal tubule

B

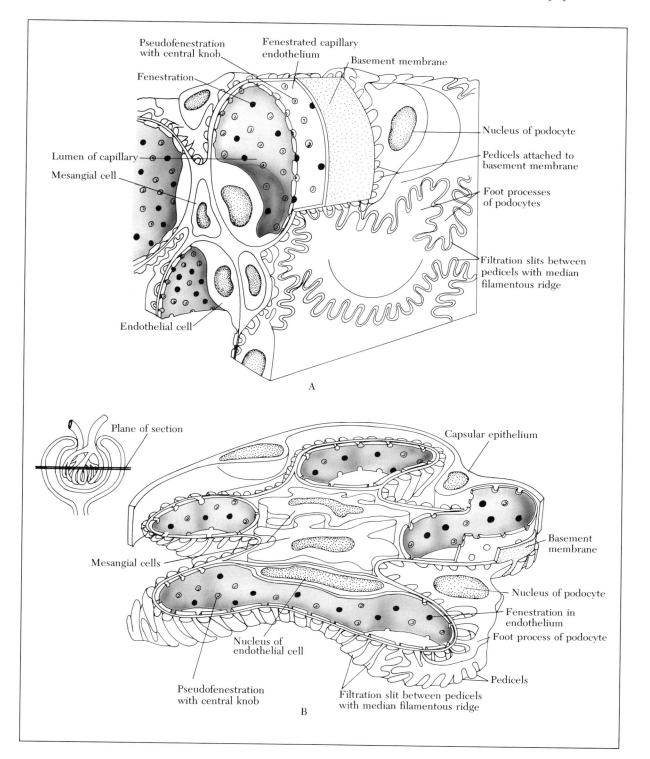

Pseudofenestration with central knob

Fenestrated capillary endothelium

Basement membrane

Fenestration

Nucleus of podocyte

Lumen of capillary

Pedicels attached to basement membrane

Mesangial cell

Foot processes of podocytes

Filtration slits between pedicels with median filamentous ridge

Endothelial cell

A

Plane of section

Capsular epithelium

Mesangial cells

Basement membrane

Nucleus of podocyte

Fenestration in endothelium

Foot process of podocyte

Nucleus of endothelial cell

Pseudofenestration with central knob

Pedicels

Filtration slit between pedicels with median filamentous ridge

B

same cell or adjacent cells. The narrow spaces between adjacent interdigitating pedicels are called **filtration slits.** Each slit is covered by a thin membrane called a **filtration membrane** and is reinforced by a filamentous ridge. The filtration membranes are less porous than the other layers of the glomerular filter and perform much of the filtration.

The renal tubules are long tubes that measure as much as 4 cm in length. The proximal end of the tubule is invaginated by the glomerulus, and its distal end empties into a collecting tubule. The tubule is divided into three parts (figure 19–4):

1. The proximal convoluted tubule
2. The loop of Henle
3. The distal convoluted tubule

FIGURE 19–4

Structure of the renal tubule, illustrating its relation to the glomerulus and the collecting tubules. The epithelium characteristic of each part of the renal tubule and the collecting tubule also is illustrated.

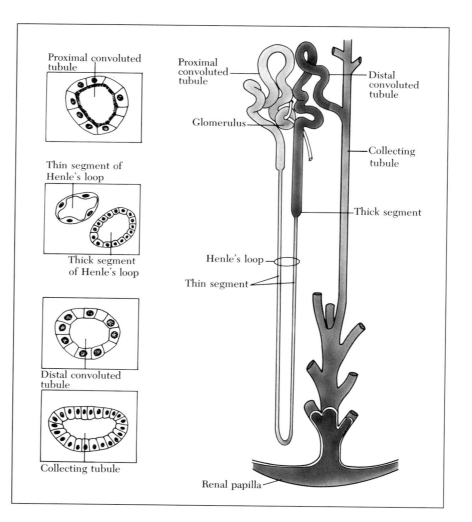

The *proximal convoluted tubule* is the greatly coiled first part of the tubule, its convolutions being located very close to the glomerulus. The *loop of Henle* is a U-shaped segment composed of descending and ascending limbs joined by a short segment. The descending limb and proximal half of the ascending limb are lined by flat epithelial cells, forming the *thin segment of Henle's loop*. The distal part of the ascending limb, called the *thick segment of Henle's loop*, is lined by tall columnar epithelium similar to that lining the distal tubule. The loop descends from the cortex into the medulla and then bends back sharply, returning to the cortex close to the vascular pole of its own glomerulus, where it becomes continuous with the distal convoluted tubule. The *distal convoluted tubule* is much shorter than the proximal tubule. It empties into a *collecting tubule,* which passes through the medulla to drain into one of the minor calyces at the apex of a renal pyramid (*renal papilla*).

The renal tubules selectively reabsorb water, minerals, and other substances that are to be conserved, and excrete unwanted materials that are eliminated. Urine is the glomerular filtrate that remains after most of the water and important constituents have been reabsorbed by the renal tubules, and other substances excreted by the renal tubules have been added.

Renal Regulation of Blood Pressure and Blood Volume

The kidneys play a major part in regulating both the blood pressure and the blood volume by secreting a substance called **renin.** Renin is released in response to a drop in blood pressure, a reduction in blood volume, or a low concentration of sodium in the blood plasma. It produces effects that tend to restore these alterations toward normal (figure 19–5). Renin interacts with a blood protein called *renin substrate* in two stages to yield a product called **angiotensin.** *Angiotensin I* is converted into **angiotensin II,** a powerful vasoconstrictor that raises the blood pressure by causing the peripheral arterioles to constrict. Angiotensin II also stimulates the adrenal cortex to secrete a steroid hormone called **aldosterone,** which increases reabsorption of sodium chloride and water by the kidneys. As a result, the blood volume is increased by the greater volume of salt and water entering the circulation and the blood pressure rises because there is more fluid within the vascular system. Thus, renin regulates blood pressure both by controlling the degree of arteriolar vasoconstriction and by regulating the volume of fluid within the circulation. The system is self-regulating because renin secretion declines as blood pressure, volume, and sodium concentration are restored to normal.

Requirements for Normal Renal Function

The functions of the two kidneys reflect the sum of the functions of their individual nephrons. For a nephron to function normally, the following conditions must be satisfied:

1. There must be free flow of blood through the glomerular capillaries.

FIGURE 19–5

Role of the kidneys in regulation of blood pressure and blood volume, as described in text.

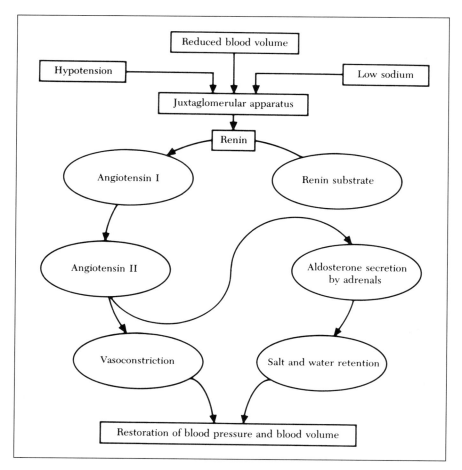

2. The glomerular filter must function normally. An adequate volume of filtrate must be produced, but the filter must restrict passage of blood cells and proteins.
3. The tubules must be able to selectively reabsorb important substances from the filtrate and to excrete other constituents into the filtrate.
4. The urine formed by the nephron must be able to flow freely from the kidney into the bladder and out the urethra.

Derangement of any of these functions results in kidney disease.

Developmental Disturbances

The urinary system develops from several different components. The kidneys form from masses of primitive connective tissue (*mesoderm*) located along the back body wall of the embryo. The bladder develops as an offshoot of the lower end of the intestinal tract. The ureters, renal pelves, renal calyces

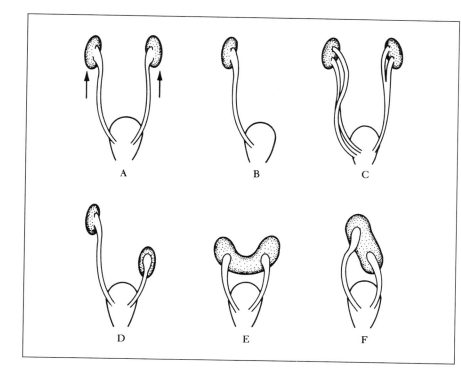

FIGURE 19–6

Common congenital abnormalities of kidneys and urinary tract. **A,** Normal ascent of kidneys. **B,** Unilateral renal agenesis resulting from failure of one ureteric bud to form. **C,** Various types of duplications of ureters and renal pelves resulting from formation of an extra ureteric bud (*left*) or premature splitting of a single ureteric bud (*right*). **D,** Failure of one kidney to ascend to normal position. **E,** Horseshoe kidney resulting from fusion of lower poles of kidneys. **F,** Fusion of lower pole of one kidney to upper pole of opposite kidney which has failed to ascend normally.

(the urinary drainage system), and the renal collecting tubules derive from paired tubular structures called *ureteric buds*. Each bud grows upward from the developing bladder and connects with the kidney that is forming on the corresponding side. The kidneys begin their development within the pelvis. Later, as the embryo grows, the kidneys and their excretory ducts come to occupy a higher location, until eventually they ascend to reach their final positions in the upper lumbar region (figure 19–6A).

Sometimes this developmental process is disturbed and congenital malformations result. Three of the more common developmental abnormalities are:

1. Failure of one or both kidneys to develop, which is called *renal agenesis*
2. Formation of extra ureters and renal pelves, which are called *duplications of the urinary tract*
3. *Malpositions* of one or both kidneys, which is often associated with fusion of the two kidneys

Renal agenesis (*a* = without + *genesis* = formation) may affect one or both kidneys. *Bilateral renal agenesis* is uncommon. It often accompanies other congenital malformations and is incompatible with postnatal life. In contrast, *unilateral renal agenesis* (figure 19–6B) is a relatively common condition that has an incidence of about one in a thousand persons, about the same frequency as cleft palate. When one kidney is absent, the other kidney enlarges and is able to carry out the functions of the missing kidney; so the affected person is usually not inconvenienced by the abnormality. The recognition of this condition, however, is of great importance to the clinician who is treating an individual with kidney disease, because one can never assume that the patient has two kidneys. Before a surgeon performs a kidney operation, diagnostic studies must always be performed first in order to ascertain that the patient has two kidneys. Such precautions are essential to prevent inadvertent removal of a solitary kidney.

Duplications of the urinary tract may be unilateral or bilateral. Sometimes a kidney has an extra renal pelvis and ureter that drains separately into the bladder (*complete duplication*). Sometimes double ureters draining the kidney unite to form a single ureter just before entering the bladder (*partial duplication*). Duplications result from abnormal prenatal development of the ureteric buds. A complete duplication results when an extra ureteric bud develops and gives rise to a separate excretory system draining the kidney on the affected side. If the ureteric bud branches after it has formed, only the upper part of the excretory system is duplicated; the lower part of the ureter is not duplicated and enters the bladder normally (figure 19–6C).

Abnormalities of position and *fusion* of the kidneys may occur if both kidneys remain in the pelvis where they began their development or if they ascend only part way (figure 19–6D). Kidneys that fail to ascend normally are in very close approximation as they develop and may become fused. One of the more common fusion abnormalities is a union of the lower poles of the two kidneys to form a U-shaped mass of renal tissue called a *horseshoe kidney* (figure 19–6E). In other cases, when the kidneys ascend abnormally, the upper pole of one kidney may become fused to the lower pole of the other (figure 19–6F).

Renal duplications, malpositions, and fusions often are of little clinical significance. At times, however, drainage of urine may be impeded by the abnormalities, causing the urine to stagnate and predisposing the patient to urinary infections. Another important developmental abnormality called *congenital polycystic kidney disease* is considered in the section on renal cysts.

Glomerulonephritis

Glomerulonephritis is an inflammation of the glomeruli caused by an antigen-antibody reaction within the glomerular capillaries. The interaction of antigen and antibody activates complement and liberates mediators that attract polymorphonuclear leukocytes. The actual glomerular injury is caused by destructive lysosomal enzymes that are released from the leukocytes that have accumulated within the glomeruli.

The antigen-antibody reaction within the glomeruli may take place in two ways. In most cases, the antigen and antibody interact within the circulation, forming small clumps called *immune complexes*. These are deposited in the walls of the glomerular capillaries as the blood filters through the glomeruli. Glomerulonephritis that occurs in this way is called *immune-complex glomerulonephritis.* Less commonly, the glomerular inflammation is caused by an autoantibody directed against the basement membranes of the glomerular capillaries. This type of glomerulonephritis is called *antiglomerular basement membrane (anti-GBM) glomerulonephritis.*

Immune-Complex Glomerulonephritis

Immune-complex glomerulonephritis usually develops as a complication about two weeks after infection by certain beta streptococci, the same type of organism that causes the familiar streptococcal sore throat. However, glomerular inflammation occurs only in a small percentage of patients with streptococcal infections. In affected subjects, the body responds to the streptococcal infection by forming antistreptococcal antibodies that interact in the bloodstream with soluble antigens from the streptococci to form immune complexes. Some of the antigen-antibody complexes are small enough to pass completely through the walls of the glomerular capillaries and be excreted in the urine. Larger complexes, however, pass through the endothelium and basement membranes of the glomerular capillaries but become trapped between the filtration slits of the glomerular epithelial cells, where they induce an inflammatory reaction.

Acute glomerulonephritis may at times follow other bacterial infections or viral infections. The mechanism of glomerular injury is similar to that of poststreptococcal glomerulonephritis. Immune complexes composed of a bacterial or viral antigen and its corresponding antibody interact in the circulation and are trapped in the glomeruli, where they produce inflammation and injury by activating complement and attracting leukocytes.

The signs and symptoms of glomerulonephritis are related to the changes within the glomeruli. Many glomeruli are completely blocked by inflammation, so less blood is filtered and less urine is excreted. As urinary output is reduced, waste products are retained and accumulate in the blood. Other glomeruli, damaged by lysosomal enzymes, are no longer able to function as efficient filters. Protein and red cells leak through the damaged glomerular capillary walls and are excreted in the urine. Frequently, masses of red cells and protein accumulate within the tubules and become molded to the shape of the renal tubules before finally being excreted. These structures, which are called *urinary casts,* are an important indication of glomerular injury.

In most cases, glomerulonephritis subsides spontaneously and the patient recovers completely without residual kidney damage. Occasionally, the disease is so severe that the patient dies of renal insufficiency. In some patients, the glomerulonephritis never heals completely. The disease becomes chronic, progresses slowly, and eventually causes renal failure. Patients with chronic poststreptococcal glomerulonephritis who develop a streptococcal sore throat or other streptococcal infection may experience recurrent episodes of acute glomerulonephritis. This is analogous to the situation in rheumatic fever, in which recurrent beta-streptococcal infections are sometimes followed by recurrent episodes of rheumatic fever.

Anti-GBM Nephritis

Glomerulonephritis caused by autoantibodies directed against glomerular basement membranes (anti-GBM nephritis) is a type of autoimmune disease. It is a relatively uncommon cause of acute glomerulonephritis. In some patients, the anti-GBM antibodies may also injure the basement membranes of the pulmonary capillaries and may cause intrapulmonary hemorrhage as well as acute glomerulonephritis.

It is possible to distinguish immune-complex glomerulonephritis from anti-GBM glomerulonephritis by special studies performed on kidney tissue obtained by renal biopsy. Immune-complex glomerulonephritis is characterized by large, irregular, lumpy deposits composed of antigen, antibody, and complement. These deposits form along the outer surface of the glomerular basement membranes, where the complexes have been trapped between the filtration slits of the glomerular epithelial cells. In contrast, anti-GBM nephritis is characterized by a relatively uniform layer of antibody and complement deposited along the inner surface of the glomerular basement membranes.

The following case illustrates the clinical features of glomerulonephritis that lead to renal failure and demonstrates the use of renal biopsy.

CASE 19–1

A fifty-one-year-old man was admitted to the hospital because of cough, chest pain, and weight loss. Physical examination was essentially normal. Urine contained 1 + albumin and many red cells. Blood urea nitrogen was 87 mg/dL (normal range 10–20 mg/dL). Blood pH was reduced to 7.2 (normal range 7.35–7.45). Plasma bicarbonate was reduced to 15 mEq/L (normal range 24–28 mEq/L). A renal biopsy revealed an active glomerulonephritis (figure 19–7). By means of special studies, immunoglobulins and complement were identified uniformly attached to the glomerular basement membranes. The lesion was interpreted as glomerulonephritis secondary to antiglomerular basement membrane antibodies. The patient was referred to another center for dialysis and further treatment.

Nephrotic Syndrome

The term **nephrotic syndrome** refers to a group of abnormalities characterized by a severe loss of protein in the urine. Urinary excretion of protein is so great that the body is unable to manufacture protein fast enough to keep up with the losses and the concentration of protein in the blood plasma falls. This, in turn, causes significant edema owing to the low plasma osmotic pressure (chapter 12). Nephrotic syndrome may be produced by a number of different types of renal diseases. The basic cause is injury to the glomerulus that allows proteins to leak through the damaged basement membrane. Because the albumin molecule is much smaller than the globulin molecule, a disproportionately large amount of albumin is lost in the urine. The osmotic pressure of the plasma falls to such an extent that excessive amounts of fluid leak from the capillaries into the interstitial tissues and body cavities. Patients with the nephrotic syndrome have marked leg edema, and often fluid collects in the abdominal cavity (called **ascites**); sometimes fluid also accumulates in the pleural cavities (called **hydrothorax**).

The nephrotic syndrome occurs most frequently in children, usually owing to relatively minimal abnormality of unknown cause in the foot processes and filtration slits of the glomerular epithelial cells. Nephrotic syndrome caused by this type of glomerular abnormality responds to corticosteroid therapy, and most children recover completely, as illustrated by the following case:

> A six-year-old boy complained of abdominal discomfort. His mother noted that his face, abdomen, scrotum, and legs were very edematous. His urine contained large amounts of protein and a few casts. His serum protein and serum albumin were both much lower than normal. Additional studies of serum proteins by electrophoresis were also consistent with nephrotic syndrome. The child was hospitalized, placed on a low-sodium diet, and treated with adrenal corticosteroid hormones. The edema gradually subsided, and the corticosteroids were gradually discontinued. He was discharged after a two-week hospitalization.

CASE 19–2

In contrast to the favorable outcome in children, the nephrotic syndrome in adults is usually a manifestation of progressive, more serious renal disease in which there are marked structural changes in the glomeruli. Some cases result from chronic progressive glomerulonephritis; others result from glomerular damage resulting from long-standing diabetes, as described later, or from a connective-tissue disease affecting the kidney, such as lupus erythematosus. Some other relatively uncommon types of kidney disease involving the glomeruli may also produce nephrotic syndrome.

Arteriolar nephrosclerosis (sometimes called simply **nephrosclerosis**) is a complication of severe hypertension. Because of the extreme elevation of the systemic blood pressure, the small arterioles and arteries throughout the body are called upon to carry blood at a much higher pressure than normal. As a result, the blood vessels undergo severe degenerative changes characterized by thickening and narrowing of the lumens; this reduces blood flow through the narrowed arterioles. The name of the disease, which means literally "sclerosis of the arterioles of the nephrons," refers to these characteristic renal vascular changes. Glomerular filtration is reduced because the arterioles are greatly narrowed. The renal tubules, which are also supplied by the glomerular arterioles, also undergo degenerative changes. Eventually the kidneys become shrunken and scarred as a result of reduction of their blood supply (figure 19–8). Patients with severe nephrosclerosis may die from renal insufficiency, as well as from the effects of the severe hypertension.

Arteriolar Nephrosclerosis

FIGURE 19–7

A, Photomicrograph illustrating effects of severe glomerulonephritis, which has caused severe glomerular injury and scarring (case 19–1). **B** (*Opposite*) Normal glomerulus for comparison. (Original magnification × 400.)

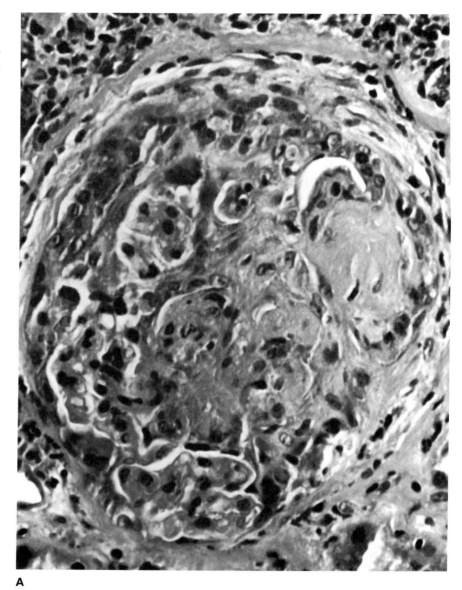

A

Diabetic Nephropathy

Persons with long-standing diabetes mellitus often develop progressive renal damage. The glomerular basement membranes exhibit characteristic nodular and diffuse thickening called diabetic **glomerulosclerosis** (figure 19–9), which disturbs glomerular function. Usually there is also severe sclerosis of the glomerular arterioles, impairing the flow of blood to the glomeruli and tubules. Sometimes the general term *diabetic nephropathy* (*nephros* = kidney + *path* = disease) is used when referring to both the glomerular and the arteriolar lesions.

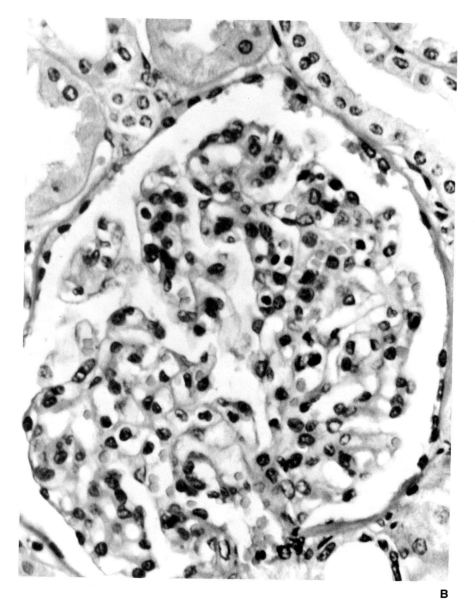

B

Clinically, the condition is characterized by progressive impairment of renal function that may eventually lead to renal failure. Protein leaks through the diseased glomeruli and is lost in the urine. In some patients, so much protein is lost that the nephrotic syndrome develops. There is no specific treatment that can arrest the progression of the disease. A renal transplant may be required if the patient develops renal failure. (Diabetes mellitus and its complications are considered in chapter 22.)

FIGURE 19–8

Irregular scarring of kidney as a result of nephrosclerosis.

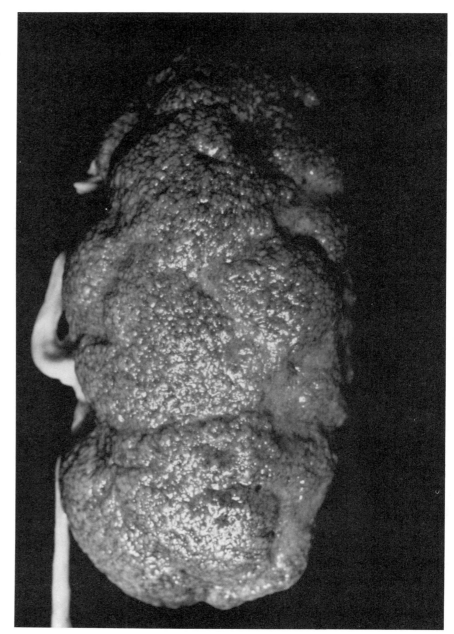

Infections of the Urinary Tract

Urinary tract infections are common and may be either acute or chronic. An infection that affects only the bladder is called **cystitis** (*cystis* = bladder). If the upper urinary tract is infected, the term is **pyelonephritis** (*pyelo* = pelvis + *nephros* = kidney + *itis* = inflammation). Most infections are caused by gram-negative intestinal bacteria. These organisms often con-

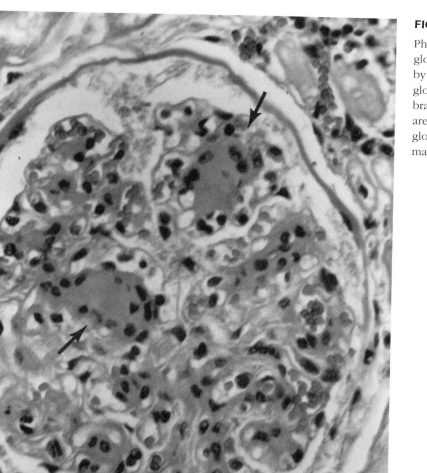

FIGURE 19–9

Photomicrograph showing glomerular damage caused by diabetes. Nodular areas of glomerular basement membrane thickening (*arrows*) are characteristic of diabetic glomerulosclerosis. (Original magnification × 400.)

taminate the perianal and genital areas and gain access to the urinary tract by ascending the urethra.

Free urine flow, large urine volume, and complete emptying of the bladder protect against urinary tract infections because any bacteria that enter the bladder are soon flushed out during urination instead of being retained to multiply in the bladder urine. An acid urine is an additional defense against infection, because most bacteria grow poorly in an acid environment. On the other hand, several conditions predispose to urinary tract infections:

1. Any condition that impairs free drainage of urine increases the likelihood of infection, because stagnation of urine favors multiplication of any bacteria that enter the urinary tract.
2. Injury to the mucosa of the urinary tract, as by a kidney stone (*calculus*) or foreign body, disrupts the protective epithelium, permitting bacteria to invade the deeper tissues and set up an infection.
3. Introduction of a catheter or instrument into the bladder may carry bacteria into the urinary tract when the catheter or instrument is introduced and may also injure the bladder mucosa.

Cystitis

Cystitis is more common in women than in men, probably because the short female urethra allows infectious organisms to enter the bladder more easily. Young, sexually active women are especially predisposed because sexual intercourse promotes transfer of bacteria from the distal urethra into the bladder and may cause minor injury to the mucosa at the base of the bladder (trigone). Cystitis is also common in older men who cannot empty their bladders completely because of an enlarged prostate gland (described in chapter 20). The urine remaining in the bladder after voiding favors multiplication of bacteria and may lead to infection.

The manifestations of cystitis result from congestion and inflammation of the bladder (vesical) mucosa. The patient complains of burning pain on urination and a desire to urinate frequently. The urine contains many bacteria and leukocytes. Cystitis is not usually a serious problem and generally responds promptly to antibiotics. Sometimes, however, the infection may spread into the upper urinary tract to affect the renal pelvis and kidney.

Pyelonephritis

Most cases of pyelonephritis are secondary to spread of infection from the bladder (*ascending pyelonephritis*), but occasionally the organisms are carried to the kidneys through the bloodstream (*hematogenous pyelonephritis*). The symptoms of pyelonephritis are those of an acute infection, together with localized pain and tenderness over the affected kidney. Histologically, the infected portion of the kidney is infiltrated by masses of leukocytes and bacteria, and many of the renal tubules in the inflamed area are filled with leukocytes (figure 19–10). Because cystitis and pyelonephritis are frequently associated, the patient also experiences urinary frequency and pain on urination; the urine contains many bacteria and leukocytes. Treatment is with appropriate antibiotics, together with measures directed at correcting any abnormalities in the lower urinary tract that may impede drainage of urine and predispose to infection.

Most episodes of pyelonephritis respond promptly to treatment. If part of the kidney is severely damaged by the infection, the injured area heals by

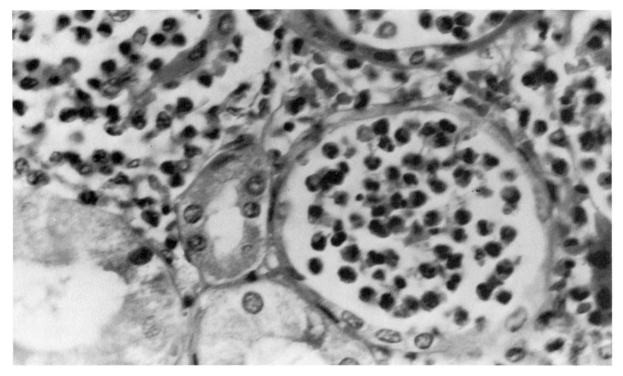

FIGURE 19–10

Photomicrograph illustrating histologic effects of acute pyelonephritis. Many tubules are dilated and filled with neutrophils. (Original magnification × 400.)

scarring. The main danger of pyelonephritis lies in the tendency of the disease to become chronic and recurrent. With each subsequent attack, more kidney tissue may be destroyed and healed by scarring. After many episodes of infection, the kidneys may become markedly scarred and shrunken, until the patient eventually exhibits manifestations of renal insufficiency.

Vesicoureteral Reflux and Infection

Normally, effective mechanisms prevent urine from flowing upward from the bladder into the ureters during urination. Sometimes, however, these mechanisms are defective, permitting urine to flow retrograde (*reflux*) into one or both ureters when the bladder contracts during urination. This condition is called **vesicoureteral reflux.** It predisposes to urinary tract infection by preventing complete emptying of the bladder. The urine forced into the ureters during voiding flows back into the bladder at the completion of urination; so residual urine remains in the bladder (figure 19–11). Bacteria also may be carried into the upper urinary tract by the reflux of urine; this predisposes to pyelonephritis.

FIGURE 19–11

Vesicoureteral reflux.
A, Urine is forced up one ureter during voiding (*right side of illustration*) because of defective function of vesicoureteral valve. **B,** Urine flows back into bladder after voiding, which prevents complete emptying of bladder and predisposes to infection.

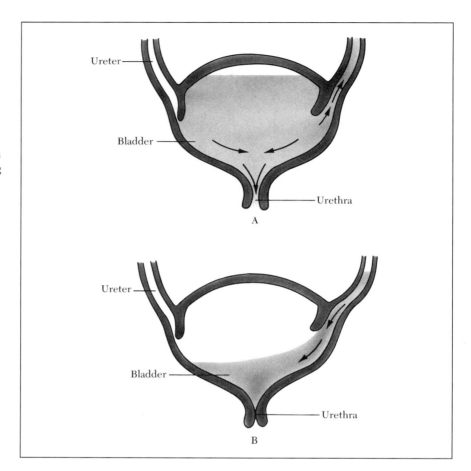

Ureter

Bladder

Urethra

A

Ureter

Bladder

Urethra

B

Calculi

Stones may form anywhere in the urinary tract. They are usually called **calculi** (singular, *calculus*), which is a Latin word meaning "little stone" or "pebble." Most are composed either or uric acid or of a mixture of calcium salts. Three factors predispose to stone formation: increased concentration of salts in the urine, infection of the urinary tract, and urinary tract obstruction.

A greatly increased excretion of salts in the urine causes the urine to become supersaturated, and the salts may precipitate to form calculi, especially if the urine is concentrated. For example, in the disease called **gout** (described in chapter 27), excretion of uric acid is often greatly increased, which may cause uric acid to precipitate from the urine and form uric acid calculi. In conditions characterized by hyperfunction of the parathyroid glands, which regulate calcium metabolism (described in chapter 25), excessive calcium is excreted in the urine, often with the subsequent formation of urinary tract calculi composed of calcium salts.

Infection predisposes to calculi primarily by reducing the solubility of the salts in the urine. Clusters of bacteria also serve as sites where urinary salts may crystallize to form the stone.

Obstruction of the outflow of urine predisposes to stone formation by causing stagnation of urine, and urinary salts tend to precipitate out. Stagnation also predisposes to infection, which further increases the likelihood of stone formation.

Most calculi are small, but occasionally they may gradually increase in size to form large branching structures that adopt the contour of the renal pelvis and calyces where they have formed. This kind of structure is called a **staghorn calculus** because it vaguely resembles the antlers of a male deer (figure 19–12). Smaller stones sometimes pass into the ureter. The smooth muscle of the ureter contracts spasmodically to propel the stone along the ureter, causing **renal colic**—paroxysms of intense flank pain radiating into the groin. Frequently, the rough edges of the stone injure the lining of the ureter, causing red blood cells to appear in the urine. Many stones can be passed through the ureter and excreted in the urine, but some become impacted in the ureter and must be removed. This usually can be accomplished by inserting a cystoscope into the bladder and then passing a specially designed catheter-like instrument through the cystoscope into the ureter. The instrument is constructed to snare the stone, which is then pulled through the ureter into the bladder and extracted through the cystoscope.

In the past, stones forming in the pelvis or calyces that were too big to pass through the ureter had to be removed surgically. Now methods are available that can break up the stones into small pieces that can be excreted in the urine, avoiding an operation. This type of stone-breaking procedure is called *lithotripsy* (*litho* = stone + *tripsy* = crushing). One technique entails the insertion of a small tube under x-ray guidance to create a small track extending from the skin of the flank directly into the pelvis or calyx of the affected kidney. The track is then stretched so that it is wide enough to pass a cystoscope-like device called a nephroscope into the kidney pelvis. Next, a probe capable of delivering pulses of ultrasonic waves is inserted through the nephroscope and brought into direct contact with the calculus. Finally, a series of ultrasonic waves are delivered through the probe, shattering the stone into small bits that are eventually excreted in the urine. The procedure is called *percutaneous ultrasonic lithotripsy* because the ultrasonic-wave-generating instrument that shatters the calculus is introduced through the skin (*per* = through + *cutaneous* = skin).

An even more spectacular method of fragmenting calculi requires positioning the anesthetized patient in a large, water-filled stainless steel tub, somewhat like a large bathtub, which is equipped to generate electrically produced shock waves and contains x-ray equipment capable of visualizing the location of the stone within the kidney. The shock-wave-generating equipment is focused very precisely on the kidney stone, and multiple shock waves are produced that travel unobstructed through the water and patient's body until they strike the stone, which is fragmented into fine par-

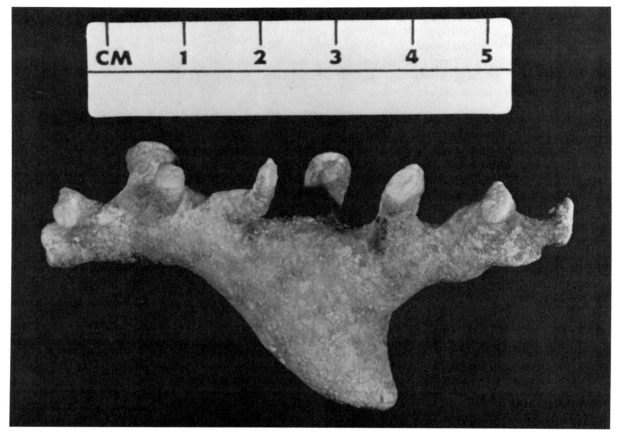

FIGURE 19–12

Large staghorn calculus of kidney.

ticles that can be excreted. This procedure is called *extracorporeal shock wave lithotripsy* because the shock waves that fragment the calculus are generated outside the patient's body (*extra* = outside + *corpus* = body).

Sometimes stones form in the bladder. Usually this stone formation is secondary to the combined effect of infection and stasis of urine, which decrease the solubility of dissolved salts in the urine. Sometimes bladder calculi can be removed through the bladder by means of a cystoscope. The stones are first broken up by an instrument passed through the cystoscope into the bladder and are then flushed out.

Foreign Bodies

It is not uncommon for people to insert various foreign bodies into the urethra and bladder either accidentally or as a means of sexual stimulation. Such objects must be removed because they may induce infection and may perforate the bladder wall. Frequently, the objects can be removed by means of a cystoscope passed into the bladder through the urethra. Sometimes, however, it is necessary to perform an operation in which the bladder is opened and the object is removed. The following two cases illustrate some of the clinical problems presented by intravesical (*intra* = within + *vesica* = bladder) foreign bodies (figure 19–13).

> An elderly woman was admitted to the hospital emergency room complaining of lower abdominal pain and burning on urination. An x-ray of the abdomen revealed a rectal thermometer lying horizontally within her bladder. A cystoscope was inserted into the bladder, and the thermometer was manipulated into a vertical position and then extracted through the urethra.

CASE 19–3

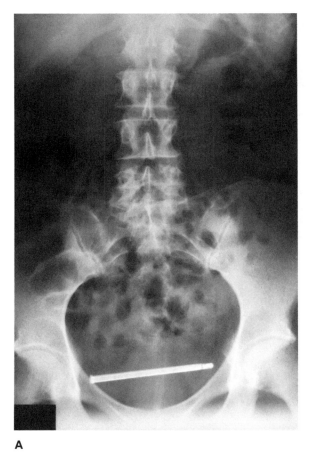

A

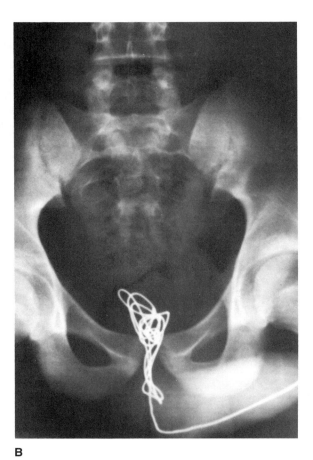

B

FIGURE 19–13

X-ray films illustrating foreign bodies in bladder. **A,** Thermometer (case 19–3). **B,** Electrical wire (case 19–4).

CASE 19–4

A fifteen-year-old boy inserted a long piece of stiff electrical wire into his bladder through his penis. The wire coiled within the bladder and could not be extracted. It was necessary to open the bladder and remove the wire through the bladder. Fortunately, neither the urethra nor the bladder were damaged by the wire, and the patient made an uneventful recovery.

Obstruction

In order for urine to be excreted normally, the urinary drainage system that transports the urine must permit free flow of urine. Obstruction or marked narrowing of the system at any point (*stricture*) leads the system proximal to the blockage to dilate progressively owing to the pressure of the retained urine. Dilatation of the ureter is called **hydroureter.** Dilatation of the renal pelvis and calyces is called **hydronephrosis** (*hydro* = water + *nephros* = kidney + *osis* = condition) (figure 19–14). The distention of the calyces and pelvis in turn causes progressive atrophy of the kidney on the affected side, owing to the high pressure of the urine within the obstructed drainage system. Eventually, if the obstruction is not relieved, the affected kidney is reduced to a thin shell of atrophic parenchyma covering the overdistended pelvis and calyces.

Which part of the drainage system is affected by the obstruction depends on the location of the block. Obstruction to the outflow of urine from the bladder, as by an enlarged prostate gland or stricture in the urethra, leads to bilateral hydronephrosis and hydroureter, as well as causing overdistention of the bladder (figure 19–15A). Hydronephrosis and hydroureter are unilateral if the obstruction is located low in the ureter, as might be caused by an obstructing calculus impacted in the ureter or an obstructing tumor of the ureter (figure 19–15B). If the obstruction is located at the junction of the renal pelvis and ureter, as might be caused by scarring of the ureter in this area, a unilateral hydronephrosis develops, but the ureter on the affected side is of normal caliber (figure 19–15C).

Stagnation of urine secondary to obstruction of the drainage system may lead to further complications. Stagnation predisposes to infection and to stone formation caused by precipitation of urinary salts. A cycle may become established in which hydronephrosis leads to infection and urinary calculi; these in turn may increase the degree of urinary tract obstruction and cause further progression of the hydronephrosis.

Diagnosis of urinary tract obstruction is usually made by means of a pyelogram or by CT scan (procedures described in chapter 1). These procedures demonstrate the dilatation of the urinary tract. Treatment is directed toward relieving the obstruction by appropriate means before the kidneys are irreparably damaged.

Renal Tubular Injury

The blood supply to the renal tubules is derived from the efferent glomerular artery, and minor degrees of tubular injury are seen in many diseases affecting the renal glomeruli. Renal tubular injury in the absence of glomeru-

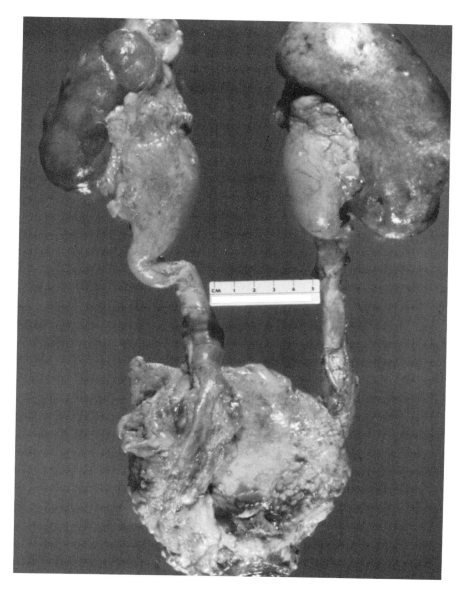

FIGURE 19–14

Bilateral hydronephrosis and hydroureter caused by obstruction of bladder (vesical) neck.

lar disease may be encountered in two situations: tubular necrosis as a result of impaired renal blood flow and tubular necrosis caused by toxic drugs and chemicals. Any condition associated with shock and marked drop in the blood pressure leads to impaired blood flow to the kidneys, which often causes degeneration and necrosis of renal tubules. Drugs and chemicals that are ingested or absorbed by the body are excreted by the kidneys. Thus, they may cause direct toxic injury to the tubular epithelium.

Acute tubular necrosis causes severe impairment of renal function characterized by a marked decrease in urine output (*oliguria*) or complete sup-

FIGURE 19–15

Possible locations and results of urinary tract obstruction. *Arrows* indicate sites of obstruction. **A,** Bilateral hydronephrosis and hydroureter with dilatation of the bladder caused by urethral obstruction. **B,** Unilateral hydroureter and hydronephrosis caused by obstruction in the distal ureter. **C,** Unilateral hydronephrosis caused by obstruction at the ureteropelvic junction.

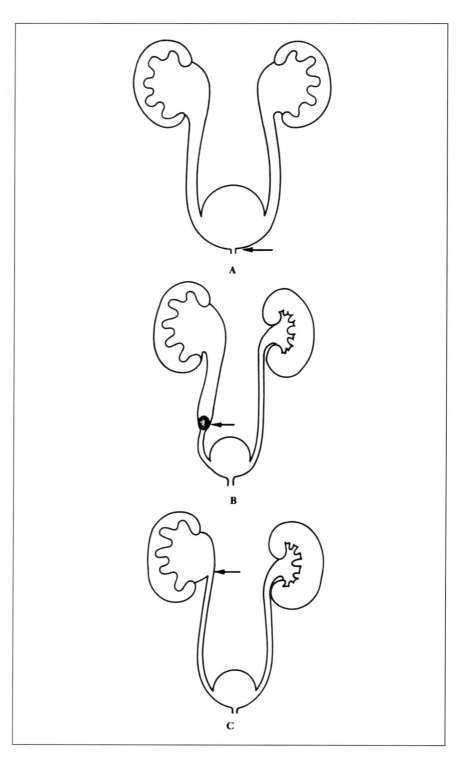

pression of urine formation (*anuria*). This condition is called *acute renal failure*. The reason why urine output is reduced is not well understood. Apparently, marked constriction of renal arterioles reduces blood flow to the kidneys and decreases glomerular filtration. Other factors also may contribute to the reduction of urine output. Many of the tubules are blocked by casts and necrotic debris. The damaged tubular epithelium also has lost its capacity for selective tubular reabsorption, and the glomerular filtrate diffuses back through the damaged tubular epithelium into the adjacent peritubular blood vessels. After a period of several weeks, tubular function is slowly restored by regeneration of the damaged epithelium, but several months may be required before renal function returns completely to normal. During the period of acute renal failure, waste products must be removed from the blood by means of dialysis (described in a later section) until tubular function has been restored.

Solitary Cysts

Renal Cysts

Solitary cysts of the kidney are relatively common. They vary in diameter from a few millimeters to about 15 centimeters. They are not associated with impairment of renal function and are of no significance to the patient (figure 19–16).

Multiple Cysts

Several different conditions are associated with the formation of multiple cysts throughout both kidneys. The most common and clinically most important of these conditions is *congenital polycystic kidney disease* (*poly* = many). The condition develops in about one in a thousand persons, is transmitted as a Mendelian dominant trait, and apparently results from faulty development of the renal tubules and collecting tubules. The cysts gradually increase in size, causing progressive enlargement of both kidneys. As the cysts expand, they compress and destroy adjacent renal tissue until eventually almost no normal kidney tissue remains, and renal failure supervenes (figure 19–17). Sometimes small numbers of cysts also form in the liver, but usually they do not disturb liver function.

Because renal tissue is destroyed slowly, renal insufficiency does not usually occur until the patient reaches middle age, and some patients do not experience problems until they are in their sixties. Many persons with congenital polycystic kidney disease are free of symptoms until onset of renal failure but some experience periodic urinary tract infections or episodes of bloody urine (*hematuria*) caused by bleeding into one of the enlarging cysts. Some patients also develop hypertension, which often accompanies renal failure.

Polycystic kidney disease can often be suspected by physical examination, which reveals the greatly enlarged kidneys. The diagnosis can be confirmed in several ways. Ultrasound examination or CT scan of the abdomen reveals the large cystic kidneys. An intravenous pyelogram (IVP) reveals the distortion of the pelves and calyces caused by the cysts.

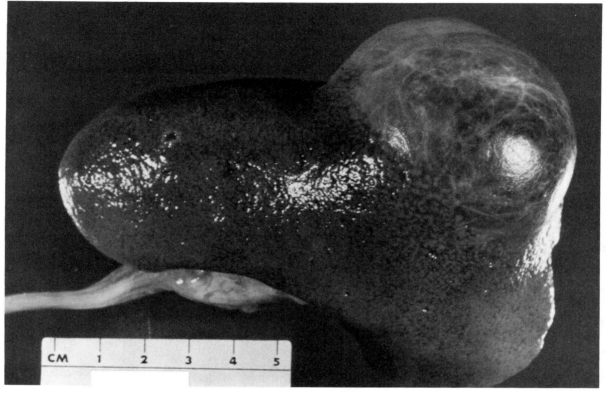

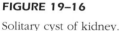

FIGURE 19–16

Solitary cyst of kidney.

There is no specific treatment. When the kidneys fail, dialysis treatments or a kidney transplant may be required.

The following case illustrates some of the characteristic features of congenital polycystic kidney disease.

CASE 19-5

A sixty-seven-year-old man was admitted to the hospital after having sustained a severe heart attack. Marked enlargement of both kidneys was detected on physical examination, and there was also clinical and laboratory evidence of severe renal insufficiency. The patient had seven brothers and sisters, four of whom had died between the ages of forty and sixty of renal failure as a result of congenital polycystic kidneys. The patient eventually died in the hospital of heart failure in conjunction with chronic renal failure. The autopsy revealed greatly enlarged polycystic kidneys. There were also a few cysts within the liver.

Tumors of the Urinary Tract

Tumors may arise from the epithelium of the renal tubules in the cortex of the kidney, from the transitional epithelium lining the urinary tract, or rarely from remnants of embryonic tissue within the kidney.

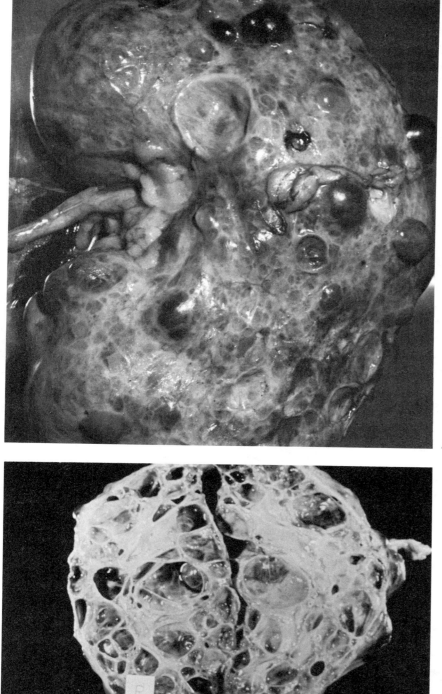

A

B

FIGURE 19–17

Congenital polycystic kidney disease, which eventually leads to renal failure in middle age (case 19–5). **A,** External surface of kidney. **B,** Cross-section of kidney illustrating cut surfaces, which exhibit multiple cysts. No normal renal tissue remains.

Renal Cortical Tumors

Benign tumors called *renal cortical adenomas* sometimes arise within the kidney. Usually, they are small and of no clinical significance. Malignant tumors, called *renal cortical carcinomas,* are more common (figure 19–18). Often, the first manifestation of a cortical carcinoma is blood in the urine (*hematuria*) as a result of ulceration of the epithelium of the pelvis or calyces caused by the growing tumor. Often, the tumor eventually invades the renal vein and gives rise to distant metastases. The tumor can be diagnosed by means of a pyelogram (described in chapter 1), which reveals the distortion of the pelvis and calyces caused by the tumor, or by means of the CT scan, which demonstrates a mass within the kidney. Treatment is by resection of the kidney (*nephrectomy*).

Transitional Cell Tumors

Almost all tumors arising from the transitional epithelium of the urinary tract are malignant and are called *transitional cell carcinomas.* Most arise from bladder epithelium, are of low-grade malignancy, and carry a good prognosis. The tumors are often quite vascular and they tend to bleed; so hematuria may be the first manifestation of the neoplasm. Bladder tumors can be visualized by means of a cystoscope inserted into the bladder through the urethra and often can be resected by means of a similar type of instrument inserted through the urethra. Sometimes it is necessary to resect part of the bladder in order to remove the tumor completely.

Embryonic Tumor

An unusual, highly malignant tumor sometimes arises from persisting remnants of embryonic tissue in the kidneys of infants and young children. Histologically, the tumor resembles the structure of an embryonic kidney, and it is called a **Wilms's tumor.** The neoplasm often metastasizes widely. Treatment is by nephrectomy followed by radiotherapy and anticancer chemotherapy.

Diagnostic Evaluation of Kidney and Urinary Tract Disease

A variety of methods are used to detect disease of the kidneys and urinary tract, to evaluate the degree to which renal function is disturbed, and to define the type of disease present.

Urinalysis

The most widely used diagnostic test is an examination of the urine, which is called a **urinalysis.** The examination is useful for detecting whether or not urinary tract disease is present and for detecting other systemic diseases that alter renal function. The examination includes determinations of urine pH (acidity) and specific gravity (a measure of urine concentration) and simple

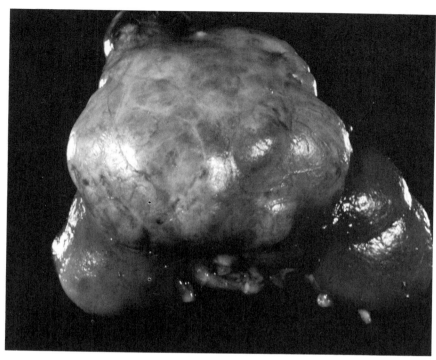

A

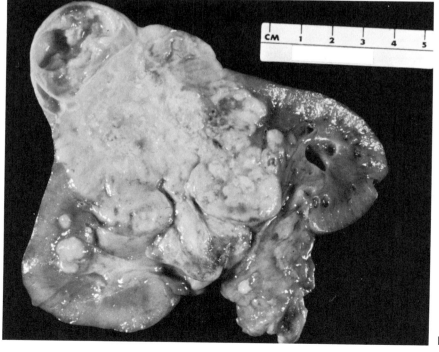

B

FIGURE 19–18

Large renal cortical carcinoma. **A,** External surface, illustrating tumor bulging from middle of kidney. **B,** Cross-section of kidney and tumor.

tests for glucose and protein. The urinalysis may also include tests for bile pigment, acetone, and other constituents that may appear in the urine in association with various diseases. A sample of the urine is also centrifuged, and the sediment is examined microscopically. If the urinalysis is normal, renal disease is unlikely. Alternatively, the presence of red cells and protein in the urine may indicate that damage to the glomerular filter has permitted these substances to leak into the glomerular filtrate or that bleeding is occurring somewhere in the urinary tract. *Renal casts,* which are collections of protein and cells molded into the shape of the kidney tubules, are an indication of glomerular disease. Leukocytes and bacteria in the urinary sediment indicate urinary tract infection.

Additional tests may be performed on the urine, as indicated by the patient's clinical condition. If a urinary tract infection is suspected, for example, the urine is cultured for pathogenic bacteria and sensitivity tests are performed if bacteria are present.

Clearance Tests

Impairment of renal function can be recognized by measuring the concentration in the blood of various substances, such as urea and creatinine, which are waste products excreted by the kidneys. Elevated levels indicate impaired renal function, and the degree of elevation is a measure of the degree of impairment. Even before elevated levels of waste products are present in the blood, impaired renal function can be detected by means of renal function tests called **clearance tests.** Clearance tests provide a rough estimate of the degree of kidney damage, and periodic clearance tests can be used to follow the progress of renal disease. A gradual fall in the renal clearance of a substance means that renal function is declining.

Clearance tests measure the ability of the kidneys to remove various substances from the blood and excrete them in the urine. To determine the clearance of a substance, one calculates how much blood plasma must flow through the kidney each minute and be completely cleared of the substance in order to provide the quantity of the substance that appears in the urine within the same period of time. For example, if the concentration of a substance in the plasma is 1 mg per milliliter (mg/mL) and 50 mg of the substance is excreted in the urine in 1 minute, then 50 mL of blood must flow through the kidneys each minute and be cleared of the substance to obtain a urinary excretion of 50 mg per minute (mg/min).

Clearance is expressed in milliliters of plasma cleared of the constituent per minute and is expressed by the following formula:

$$\text{Clearance} = \frac{UV}{P}$$

where U is the concentration of the substance excreted in milligrams per milliliter of urine; V is the volume of urine excreted, expressed in milliliters per minute; and P is the concentration of the substance in the plasma expressed in milligrams per milliliter.

The most frequently used clearance test measures the clearance of the waste product **creatinine,** which is derived from the breakdown of a compound present in muscle, called *phosphocreatine*. To determine creatinine clearance, the urine output is measured for a specific period of time and the average output per minute is calculated. The concentrations of creatinine in the urine and in the blood also are determined, and clearance is calculated by means of the standard formula. For example, if the urine output is 2 mL/min, the concentration of creatinine in the urine is 0.15 mg/mL, and the concentration of creatinine in the blood is 0.003 mg/mL, the creatinine clearance is

$$\frac{UV}{P} = \frac{0.15 \times 2}{0.003} = \frac{0.3}{0.003} = 100 mL/min$$

Additional Techniques

Many other specialized procedures can be used to study the kidneys and urinary tract, including various x-ray examinations, ultrasound examinations, and cystoscopy. These examinations are described in chapter 1. Their specific diagnostic applications have also been considered in conjunction with the various renal and urinary tract diseases in which they provide useful information. X-ray examination of the abdomen, for example, can identify the size and location of the kidneys and can detect radiopaque calculi in the kidneys or urinary tract. CT scans and pyelograms can detect anatomic abnormalities within the kidneys, such as cysts and tumors, and many abnormalities of the urinary drainage system, such as hydronephrosis. Other specialized procedures using radioisotopes can measure renal blood flow and renal excretory function. Renal arteriograms, with the use of techniques similar to those used to study the coronary arteries, can determine the caliber of the renal arteries, can detect segmental areas of narrowing in the renal arteries, and can identify areas of increased vascularity within the kidney, which often occur when a tumor is present.

Sometimes the clinician cannot make an exact diagnosis concerning the type of renal disease without resorting to biopsy of the kidney. This can be accomplished without undue difficulty or serious risk to the patient by introducing a small biopsy needle through the skin of the flank directly into the substance of the kidney. A small bit of kidney tissue is removed for histologic study. Examination of the biopsy material by the pathologist often permits an exact diagnosis as to the nature and extent of the renal disease, which serves as a guide to proper treatment.

Renal Failure (Uremia)

Renal failure may be either acute or chronic and may result from any of several causes. *Acute renal failure* is caused by necrosis of renal tubules, which can be caused by impairment of blood flow to the kidneys or by the effects of toxic drugs. Renal function usually returns after a variable period of time.

In contrast, *chronic renal failure* is a gradual deterioration of renal function resulting from progressive renal disease. More than 50 percent of all cases of chronic renal failure result from chronic glomerulonephritis. Chronic pyelonephritis, congenital polycystic kidney disease, nephrosclerosis, and diabetic nephropathy make up most of the remainder.

Normally, each kidney has about one million nephrons. In chronic renal failure, renal function declines as the population of nephrons decreases. Eventually the kidneys are no longer able to perform their normal regulatory and excretory functions. The patient experiences severe derangements of electrolytes and acid-base balance owing to the loss of renal regulatory function. In addition, various acids and minerals that would normally be excreted by the kidneys are retained. Renal failure is sometimes called **uremia.** This term refers to the characteristic retention of urea in the blood when the kidneys fail. **Urea** is a normal by-product of protein metabolism and is excreted in the urine. It is not a toxic compound and is only one of many substances that accumulate in the blood when the kidneys fail. The amount of urea in the blood, however, correlates with the degree of retention of other waste products and with the clinical manifestations of deteriorating renal function. Therefore, measurement of the concentration of urea in the blood (blood urea nitrogen test, or BUN) provides a rough estimate of the severity of the kidney failure. Another commonly used measure of renal functional impairment is the level of creatinine in the blood.

Symptoms of renal failure are nonspecific. They begin to appear when about 80 percent of renal function has been lost and are quite pronounced by the time renal function has fallen to 5 percent of normal. Symptoms include weakness, loss of appetite, nausea, and vomiting. Production of red cells by the bone marrow decreases, and the patient becomes moderately anemic. Waste products are not eliminated and increase to toxic levels. Excess salt and water are retained by the failing kidneys, resulting in weight gain as a result of retained fluid ("water weight"). The blood volume increases, owing to fluid retention, and the blood pressure also tends to rise as the intravascular volume increases. If untreated, the patient in chronic renal failure eventually lapses into coma, may have convulsions, and eventually dies.

The outlook for patients with renal failure has improved dramatically in recent years because of two effective methods of treatment:

1. **Hemodialysis,** which removes waste products from the patient's blood (*heme* = blood)
2. **Renal transplantation,** using kidneys from living related donors or recently deceased persons (cadaver donors)

Hemodialysis

Hemodialysis substitutes for the functions of the kidneys. Waste products from the patient's blood diffuse across a semipermeable membrane into a solution (the *dialysate*) on the other side of the membrane. The rate of diffusion is determined by several factors: the concentration of the substances on the two sides of the membrane, the rate of blood flow and flow of the dialysate through the dialyzer, and the characteristics of the dialyzer membrane. Waste products, which are present in high concentrations in the patient's blood, diffuse from the blood into the dialysate because of differences in the concentration on the two sides of the membrane. Usually, the patient's blood is dialyzed by an "artificial kidney" machine. This type of hemodialysis is called *extracorporeal hemodialysis* (*extra* = outside + *corpus* = body) because the blood is transported outside the patient's body for dialysis in the artificial kidney and then returned by means of a system of tubes connected to the patient's circulatory system. Less commonly, the patient's own *peritoneum* (the membrane lining the abdominal cavity) is used as the dialyzing membrane. This procedure is called **peritoneal dialysis.**

Extracorporeal Hemodialysis

Extracorporeal hemodialysis is the most commonly used type. Most people who use the term *hemodialysis* are referring to extracorporeal hemodialysis, and this shorter term is used in the following discussion.

Every year many new patients with advanced renal disease begin hemodialysis. Some will continue on dialysis indefinitely. Others will rely on hemodialysis until a kidney becomes available for transplantation.

In hemodialysis, the patient's blood flows along one side of a synthetic semipermeable membrane that restricts the passage of blood cells and protein but permits the passage of water and small molecules. The dialysate flows on the other side of the membrane in a direction opposite to the flow of blood. This type of flow pattern, which is called *countercurrent dialysis* (*counter* = against + *current* = blood flow), promotes more efficient removal of waste products than when dialysate and blood flow in the same direction.

During dialysis, plastic tubes connect the patient's circulation to the dialyzer in the artificial kidney machine. One tube transmits blood to the dialyzer unit where the blood is cleansed and excess fluid is removed, and the other tube conveys the blood from the dialyzer back to the patient's circulation. Before dialysis begins, the clotting time of the patient's blood is prolonged by administration of heparin to prevent the blood from clotting as it flows through the dialyzer. Usually, dialysis treatments last four or five hours and treatments are administered three times per week. Dialysis can be performed in the hospital, in special centers for ambulatory patients, or at home with the assistance of a family member who has been given special training along with the patient.

In order to perform hemodialysis on a regular basis, one of the patient's arteries and a large vein must be easily accessible so that the tubes that transport blood to and from the dialyzer unit can easily be connected to the patient's blood vessels. Several methods have been devised to gain access to the patient's circulation (figure 19–19). A commonly used method consists of surgically interconnecting the radial artery in the wrist and an adjacent vein, forming an artificial communication called an *arteriovenous fistula* (figure 19–19A). Once the fistula has been created, arterial blood is short-circuited directly into the vein instead of flowing through the periph-

FIGURE 19–19

Procedures used to facilitate access to a patient's circulatory system for hemodialysis. **A,** Arteriovenous fistula created between radial artery and adjacent (cephalic) vein. **B,** Permanently implanted tubes in radial artery and cephalic vein project through the skin and are interconnected between dialysis treatments. **C,** Graft of synthetic material or bovine artery connects patient's brachial artery and cephalic vein.

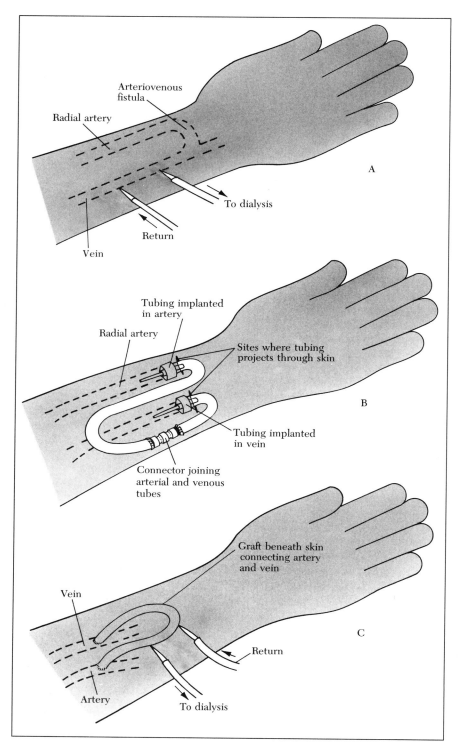

eral capillaries. The vein, which now receives blood directly under high pressure, becomes much larger and develops a thick wall.

Once it has been determined that long-term dialysis will be needed, the arteriovenous fistula is created several months prior to the first dialysis treatment so that the vein has time to enlarge and thicken. When the vein has become suitable for use, dialysis treatments are begun. Two needles are inserted through the skin directly into the vein. One needle is attached to the tube that delivers blood to the dialyzer, and the second needle is attached to the tube that returns the blood to the patient.

Less commonly, other procedures are used to gain access to the patient's circulation for dialysis. Various types of arteriovenous shunts can be created. In one procedure, two plastic tubes are permanently implanted, one in the radial artery and another in an adjacent vein. Both tubes protrude through the skin and are joined by a short connecting piece (figure 19–19B). During dialysis, the connector is removed and the implanted arterial and venous tubes are attached to the tubes that convey blood to and from the dialyzer. At the completion of dialysis, the arteriovenous communication is reestablished until the next treatment. In another method, an arteriovenous fistula is created by connecting a large artery and vein in the forearm by a graft made either from synthetic material or from a specially treated segment of a cow's artery (called a *bovine graft*). The graft is placed beneath the skin, and needles are inserted through the skin directly into the graft to connect the patient's circulation to the dialyzer (figure 19–19C).

There are many types of artificial kidney machines. Many are quite compact, and portable units are available. Improvements in the design and operation of the machines are being made continually. The essential component of the artificial kidney machine is the *dialyzer*. Attached to it are the tubes that carry blood to and from the patient and the tubes that carry dialysate to and from the unit. There are three basic types of dialyzers: coil dialyzers, parallel plate dialyzers, and hollow fiber dialyzers (figure 19–20). In a *coil dialyzer*, the blood flows through a tube made of synthetic semipermeable membrane material. The tube is wrapped around a mesh screen to form a coil, and the dialysate flows around the coil. In a *plate dialyzer*, blood flows within a synthetic semipermeable membrane between the plates, and the dialysate flows in the opposite direction outside the membrane. A *hollow fiber dialyzer*, which is quite compact and efficient and is the most commonly used type, consists of a bundle of hollow synthetic fibers through which the blood passes. The dialysate circulates around the outside of the fibers in the opposite direction.

Peritoneal Dialysis

Peritoneal dialysis uses the patient's own peritoneum as the dialyzing membrane (figure 19–21). In order to perform peritoneal dialysis, a large plastic tube must first be inserted into the patient's abdominal (peritoneal) cavity and fixed in position by suturing it to the skin. The dialysis procedure consists of instilling several liters of dialysis fluid through the tube into the peritoneal cavity and allowing the fluid to remain within the peritoneal

FIGURE 19–20

Types of dialyzers, as described in text. **A,** Coil dialyzer. **B,** Plate dialyzer. **C,** Hollow fiber dialyzer.

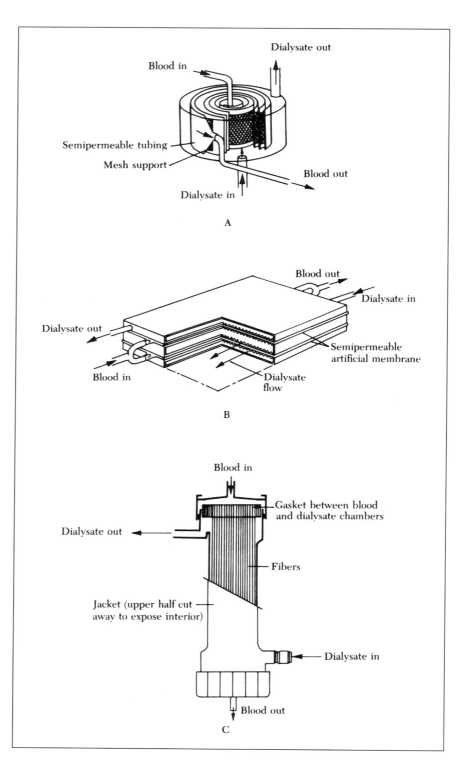

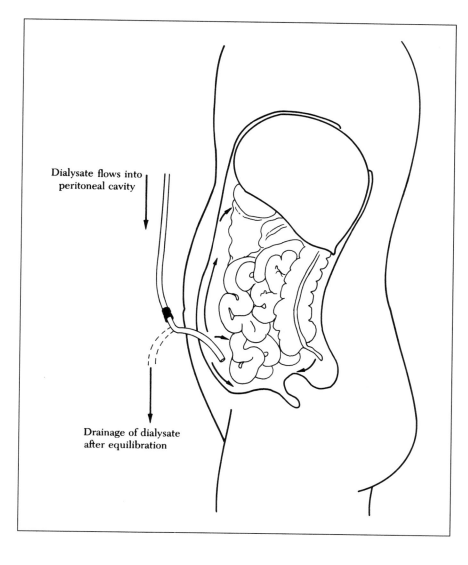

Dialysate flows into
peritoneal cavity

Drainage of dialysate
after equilibration

FIGURE 19–21

Principle of peritoneal dialysis. Dialysate fills peritoneal
cavity. Waste products diffuse
(*arrows*) from blood vessels
beneath peritoneum into
dialysate. Fluid is drained
after equilibration.

cavity for a variable period of time. During this time, waste products diffuse
across the peritoneum from the underlying blood vessels into the dialysis
fluid that fills the peritoneal cavity. Dialysis fluid is then withdrawn and
fresh fluid is instilled. The procedure is repeated periodically by a machine
that drains and refills the peritoneal cavity many times over a twenty-four-
hour period.

Another, similar method is called *continuous ambulatory peritoneal dialysis*. In this procedure, two liters of fluid remain within the peritoneal cavity all the time. The patient replaces the fluid with fresh dialysis fluid four

or five times a day. Patients carry out their usual activities when they are not draining and refilling their peritoneal cavities.

Peritoneal dialysis is used less frequently than extracorporeal hemodialysis because the procedure has two major drawbacks. Peritoneal dialysis is much less efficient at removing waste products. The procedure also carries the risk of peritonitis, which can result if bacteria gain access to the peritoneal cavity around the tube that extends from the skin surface directly into the peritoneal cavity.

Renal Transplantation

When the kidneys fail, a normal kidney sometimes can be transplanted from either a close relative or a recently deceased person (cadaver donor).

Unless the transplanted kidney comes from an identical twin whose tissues contain identical HLA antigens, the transplant will invariably contain foreign HLA antigens that the patient lacks. (The HLA system is considered in chapter 3.) Consequently, the patient's immunologic defenses will respond to the foreign antigens and attempt to destroy (*reject*) the foreign kidney unless the patient's immune system is suppressed by drugs or other agents (described in chapter 5).

The likelihood that a transplanted kidney will survive depends on how closely the HLA antigens match those of the patient. The more closely they resemble one another, the better the chances of survival. More than 90 percent of transplanted kidneys survive for five years when the transplanted kidney is obtained from a close relative whose HLA antigens very closely resemble those of the patient. The survival rate of cadaver transplants has improved greatly in recent years and now is almost as good as transplants from living related donors.

In the transplant operation, the transplanted kidney is usually placed in the iliac area outside the peritoneal cavity. The renal artery of the transplanted kidney is connected to the internal iliac (hypogastric) artery, the renal vein is connected to the iliac vein, and the ureter is connected to the bladder (figure 19–22). In the great majority of patients, the transplant is successful and "takes over" for the patient's own nonfunctional kidneys. Some patients, however, reject the transplant despite intensive immunosuppressive therapy. Most rejections occur within the first few months after transplantation. Should this occur, the patient resumes dialysis treatments until another kidney suitable for transplantation becomes available.

Although a well-functioning transplanted kidney permits the patient to lead a relatively normal life, the patient with a renal transplant may have other problems. Immunosuppressive drugs must be continued indefinitely to prevent rejection of the foreign kidney, and adverse side effects sometimes result from these drugs. The immunosuppressed patient is also more susceptible to infection, because the body's immune defenses have been weakened so that the transplant can survive. Occasionally, the disease that destroyed the patient's own kidneys, such as glomerulonephritis, also destroys the function of the transplanted kidney.

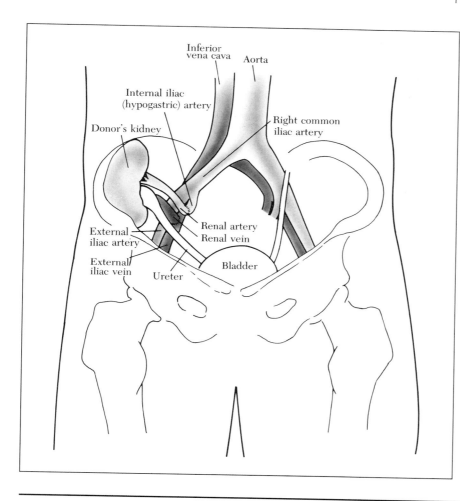

FIGURE 19–22

Method of kidney transplantation in an adult. Transplanted kidney is placed in iliac region. Artery and vein of transplant are connected to patient's iliac artery and vein, and ureter of transplant is connected to the bladder.

Questions for Review

1. What is the difference between glomerulonephritis and pyelonephritis? What is the relation between glomerulonephritis and beta-streptococcal infection? What factors predispose to urinary tract infection?

2. What is the difference between nephrotic syndrome and nephrosclerosis? Why does edema develop in a patient with nephrosis?

3. What are the common causes of urinary tract obstruction? What are its effects on the kidneys and lower urinary tract?

4. What conditions lead to renal tubular necrosis? What are its clinical manifestations?

5. What is uremia? What are its manifestations? How is it treated? What is the role of urea in producing the clinical manifestations of uremia?

6. What methods does the clinician use to establish a diagnosis of renal disease?

7. What is congenital polycystic kidney disease? What are its clinical manifestations? What is its pattern of inheritance? How is it treated?

8. What is the difference between acute and chronic renal failure?

9. What is the difference between hemodialysis and peritoneal dialysis? How is the patient's circulation connected to the artificial kidney for hemodialysis?

10. Why does a kidney transplant from a donor who is a close relative usually have a greater likelihood of survival than does a cadaver transplant?

11. How does diabetes affect the kidneys? What are the clinical manifestations?

Supplementary Readings

Berkow, E., ed. 1992. *The Merck manual of diagnosis and therapy*. 16th ed. (Genitourinary disorders, pp. 1645–1752.) Rahway, N.J.: Merck and Co. A well-written, concise treatment of the subject.

Charig, C. R., et al. 1986. Comparison of treatment of renal calculi by open surgery, percutaneous nephrolithotomy, and extracorporeal shockwave lithotripsy. *British Medical Journal* 292:879–82. Advantages and limitations of various methods are compared. Shock wave lithotripsy had lowest morbidity and was the most cost-effective method.

Coe, F. L., et al. 1988. Pathophysiology of kidney stones and strategies for treatment. *Hospital Practice* 23:185–200. A review article.

Friedman, E. A. 1982. Diabetic nephropathy is a hyperglycemia nephropathy. *Archives of Internal Medicine* 142:1269–70. Renal failure as a result of diabetic nephropathy is a common problem in insulin-dependent diabetes and can largely be prevented by rigid control of the hyperglycemia.

Ganong, W. F. 1993. *Review of medical physiology*. 16th ed. pp. 635–71. Norwalk, Conn.: Appleton & Lange. Aspects of renal function relating to renal disease.

Kirkpatrick, C. H., and Rowlands, D. T. 1992. Transplantation immunology. *Journal of the American Medical Association* 268:2952–58. A discussion of transplantation antigens, transplant rejection, transfusions as immunosuppressive agents, and immunosuppressive therapy.

Levinsky, N. G. 1977. Pathophysiology of acute renal failure. *New England Journal of Medicine* 196:1453–57. Describes pathogenesis of the syndrome, which involves both tubular and vascular mechanisms.

Mulley, A. G. 1986. Shock-wave lithotripsy: Assessing a slam-bang technology. *New England Journal of Medicine* 314:845–47. Lithotripsy is a well-engineered, highly selective application of brute force. Applications in fracturing gallstones also described.

See also sections in standard textbooks of medicine, pathology, and urology listed in General References.

Chapter 19 ▪ Outline Summary

Structure and Function of Urinary Tract / 541
Kidneys
Bean-shaped organs below diaphragm adjacent to vertebral column.

Divided into outer cortex and inner medulla.

Latter contains pyramids and renal columns.

Excretory Duct System
Ureter conveys urine to bladder by peristalsis.

Pelvis: expanded upper end of ureter.

Major calyces: subdivisions of pelvis.

Minor calyces: subdivisions of major calyces into which renal papillae (apices of pyramids) discharge.

Bladder
Stores urine.

Discharges urine into urethra during voiding.

Anatomic configuration of bladder and ureters normally prevents reflux of urine into ureters during voiding.

Function of the Kidneys
Excretory organ.

Regulates mineral and water balance.

Produces erythropoietin and renin.

The Nephron
Composed of glomerulus and renal tubule.

Material filtered by three-layered glomerular filter.

Inner: fenestrated capillary endothelium.

Middle: basement membrane.

Outer: capillary epithelial cells (with foot processes and filtration slits).

Mesangial cells: hold capillary tuft together.

Renal Regulation of Blood Pressure and Blood Volume
Renin released in response to reduced blood volume, low blood pressure, or low sodium concentration.

Angiotensin II formed.

Functions as vasopressor.

Stimulates aldosterone secretion.

Requirements for Normal Renal Function
Free flow of blood through glomeruli.

Normal glomerular filter.

Normal tubular function.

Normal outflow of urine.

Developmental Disturbances / 548
Normal Development
Kidneys develop from mesoderm along back body wall of embryo.

Bladder derived from lower end of intestinal tract.

Excretory ducts (ureters, calyces, pelves) develop from ureteric buds that extend from bladder into developing kidneys.

Kidneys develop in pelvis and ascend to final position.

Developmental Abnormalities

Renal agenesis.

Bilateral: rare and associated with other congenital abnormalities. Usually incompatible with postnatal life.

Unilateral: relatively common and usually asymptomatic.

Duplications of the urinary tract.

As a result of abnormal development of ureteric buds.

Complete duplication: extra ureter and renal pelvis.

Incomplete duplication: only upper part of excretory system duplicated.

Malpositions.

Caused by failure of kidneys to ascend to normal position.

Kidneys may be fused.

Horseshoe kidney: fusion of lower poles.

Fusion of upper pole of one kidney to lower pole of other kidney.

Glomerulonephritis / 550

Immune-Complex Glomerulonephritis

Usually follows beta-streptococcal infection.

Circulating antigen-antibody complexes are filtered by glomeruli and incite inflammation.

Most patients recover completely.

Anti-GBM Glomerulonephritis

An autoimmune disease.

Autoantibodies directed against glomerular basement membranes.

Nephrotic Syndrome / 552

Clinical Features

Loss of protein in urine exceeds body's capacity to replenish plasma proteins.

Low plasma protein leads to edema and ascites.

Prognosis

In children: minimal glomerular change, with complete recovery.

In adults: manifestation of more severe progressive renal disease.

Arteriolar Nephrosclerosis / 553

Pathogenesis

Develops in hypertensive patients.

Renal arterioles undergo thickening.

Glomeruli and tubules undergo secondary degenerative changes.

Diabetic Nephropathy / 554

Pathogenesis and Structural Changes

A complication of long-standing diabetes.

Nodular and diffuse thickening of glomerular basement membranes (glomerulosclerosis).

Usually coexisting nephrosclerosis.

Manifestations

Impaired renal function.

Nephrotic syndrome may result from protein loss in urine.

May lead to renal failure.

Urinary Tract Infections / 556

Pathogenesis

Usually caused by gram-negative bacteria ascending the urethra.

Free urine flow, large urine volume, complete emptying of bladder, and acid urine protect against infection.

Impaired drainage of urine, injury to mucosa of urinary tract, and introduction of catheters of instruments into bladder predispose to infection.

Manifestations

Cystitis: bladder infection.

Causes pain and burning on urination; bacteria and leukocytes in urine.

Common in young, sexually active women and older men who are unable to empty their bladders completely owing to enlarged prostate.

Usually responds promptly to antibiotics.

Pyelonephritis: infection of upper urinary tract.

Usually ascending infection. May be hematogenous.

Stagnation of urine or obstruction or both predispose.

Usually responds to antibiotics.

Some cases become chronic and may lead to kidney failure.

Role of Vesicoureteral Reflux in Urinary Tract Infections / 559

Urine normally prevented from flowing retrograde into ureters during voiding.

Failure of mechanism allows bladder urine to reflux into ureter during voiding.

Urine forced into ureter flows back into the bladder after voiding, preventing complete emptying of bladder.

Reflux predisposes to urinary tract infection because of residual urine.

Urinary Tract Calculi / 560
Predisposing Factors
Increased concentration of salts in urine.

Uric acid in gout.

Calcium salts in hyperparathyroidism.

Infections: alter solubility of salts.

Urinary tract obstruction: promotes stasis and infection.

Clinical Manifestations
Renal colic associated with passage of stone.

Obstruction of urinary tract causes hydronephrosis-hydroureter proximal to obstruction.

Predisposes to infection.

Foreign Bodies in the Urinary Tract / 562
Incidence and Manifestations
Usually inserted by patient.

May injure bladder.

Predispose to infection.

Treatment
Usually removed by cystoscopy.

Occasionally necessary to open bladder by surgical operation.

Obstruction of Urinary Tract / 564
Pathogenesis
Blockage of urine outflow leads to progressive dilatation of urinary tract proximal to obstruction.

Eventually causes compression atrophy of kidneys.

Manifestations
Hydroureter: dilatation of ureter.

Hydronephrosis: dilatation of pelvis and calyces.

Common Causes
Bilateral: obstruction of bladder neck by enlarged prostate or urethral stricture.

Unilateral: ureteral stricture, calculus, or tumor.

Complications
Stone formation.

Infection.

Diagnosis and Treatment
Pyelograms or CT scans or both demonstrate dilatation of drainage system.

Treat cause of obstruction.

Renal Tubular Injury / 564
Pathogenesis
Caused by toxic chemicals.

As a result of reduced renal blood flow.

Clinical Manifestations
Oliguria or anuria.

Tubular function gradually recovers.

Treated by dialysis until function returns.

Renal Cysts / 567
Solitary Cysts
Relatively common.

Usually asymptomatic.

Multiple Cysts: Congenital Polycystic Kidney Disease
Incidence one per thousand.

Mendelian dominant transmission.

Cysts enlarge and destroy renal function.

Onset of renal insufficiency in middle age or later.

May be complicated by infections or bleeding into cysts.

Relatively common cause of renal failure.

Tumors of the Urinary Tract / 568
Renal Cortical Tumors
Arise from epithelium of renal tubules.

Adenomas small and asymptomatic.

Carcinomas more common.

May cause hematuria as first manifestation.

Tumor may invade renal vein and metastasize through bloodstream.

Treated by nephrectomy.

Transitional Cell Tumors
Arise from transitional epithelium lining urinary tract.

Most are of low-grade malignancy and have good prognosis.

Hematuria may be first manifestation.

Diagnosis by cystoscopy.

Treated by resecting tumor.

Wilms's Tumor
Uncommon, highly malignant renal tumor of infants and children.

Arises from embryonic cells in kidney.

Treated by nephrectomy, radiotherapy, and chemotherapy.

Diagnostic Evaluation of Kidney and Urinary Tract Disease / 570
Urinalysis
Detects abnormalities in urine.

Widely used screening test.

Urine Culture and Sensitivity Tests
Where appropriate.

Blood Chemistry Tests

Measure retention of waste products normally excreted by kidneys.

Urea and creatinine commonly measured.

Degree of elevation correlates with degree of renal insufficiency and clinical condition.

Clearance Tests

Measure ability of kidneys to remove constituent from blood and excrete it in the urine.

Calculated by formula: Clearance = UV/P.

U = concentration of substance excreted in urine in milligrams per milliliter.

V = volume of urine excreted in milliliters per minute.

P = concentration of substance in plasma in milligrams per milliliter.

Creatinine clearance commonly used to monitor renal function.

X-ray Studies

X-ray of abdomen: determines size and location of kidneys, radiopaque calculi.

Pyelograms: evaluate drainage system and distortion of calyces caused by renal cysts or tumors.

CT scan: detects renal cysts, tumors, hydronephrosis.

Arteriogram: detects abnormalities of renal blood flow, narrowing of renal arteries, increased renal vascularity associated with tumors.

Ultrasound Examination

Identifies cysts and tumors.

Cystoscopy

Visualizes interior of bladder.

Renal Biopsy

Small biopsy of kidney obtained by needle inserted into kidney through flank.

Invasive procedure performed when nature of renal disease uncertain.

Histologic diagnosis serves as guide for proper treatment.

Renal Failure (Uremia) / 573

Classification

Acute:

Caused by tubular necrosis from impaired renal blood flow or toxic drugs.

Renal function returns when tubules regenerate.

Chronic:

As a result of progressive chronic kidney disease.

No recovery of renal function.

Manifestations

Nonspecific symptoms.

Anemia: as a result of reduced red cell production.

Toxic manifestations: caused by retained waste products.

Retention of salt and water.

Hypertension.

Treatment

Extracorporeal hemodialysis.

Patient's circulation connected to artificial kidney machine (dialyzer).

Access to patient's circulation facilitated by creation of arteriovenous fistula between radial artery and adjacent vein or by means of shunt between artery and vein.

Blood cleansed and excess fluid removed.

Several types of dialyzers used.

Treatments last from four to five hours three times per week.

Peritoneal dialysis.

Patient's own peritoneum used as dialyzing membrane.

Indwelling tube placed in peritoneal cavity and fixed to skin.

Dialysis fluid fills peritoneal cavity, is allowed to equilibrate, and is then drained. Cycles repeated.

Less efficient than hemodialysis and carries risk of peritonitis.

Kidney transplantation.

Kidney obtained from close relative or recently deceased person (cadaver donor).

Survival of transplant depends on similarity of HLA antigens between donor and recipient.

The Male Reproductive System

Learning Objectives

1. Differentiate between benign prostatic hyperplasia and prostatic carcinoma, describing clinical manifestations and methods of treatment.
2. List the three most common types of testicular cancer, describe their manifestations, and explain the methods of treatment.
3. Name the anatomic structures of the male reproductive system. Describe their functions as they relate to the diseases affecting them.

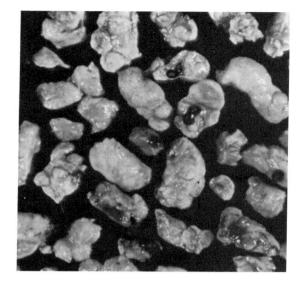

Chapter 20 ▪ Contents

The components of the male reproductive system are the *penis,* the *prostate* and certain accessory glands, the *testes,* and a duct system for transporting sperm from the testes to the urethra. The transport duct system begins as the *epididymides* (singular, *epididymis*), which are closely applied to the testes, and continues as the two *vasa deferentia* (singular, *vas deferens*). The two vasa extend upward in the *spermatic cords* and enter the prostatic urethra as the *ejaculatory ducts.* The urethra is divided into a long *penile urethra* and a short segment transversing the prostate gland, called the *prostatic urethra.* It is conventional to speak of the distal penile urethra as the *anterior urethra* and the prostatic urethra and adjacent proximal part of the penile urethra as the *posterior urethra.* Figure 20–1 illustrates the anatomy of the male reproductive system. A working knowledge of how these structures are interrelated is necessary in order to understand the spread of inflammatory disease in the male reproductive tract and the various complications that may result.

The prostate is a spherical gland about 5 cm in diameter that surrounds the urethra just below the base of the bladder. It is composed of numerous branched glands arranged in two major groups intermixed with masses of smooth muscle and fibrous tissue. The *inner group of glands* surrounds the

Structure and Function of the Male Reproductive Organs

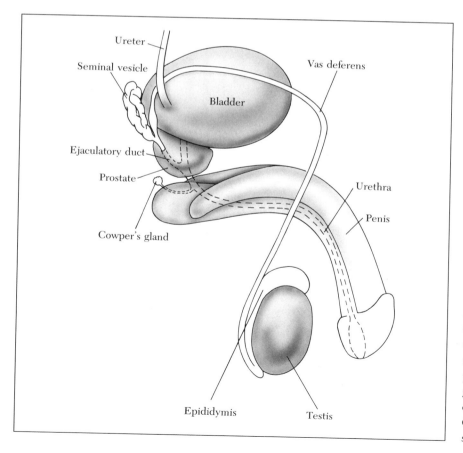

FIGURE 20–1

Side view of male reproductive system. Seminal fluid consists of sperm mixed with secretions of seminal vesicles, prostate gland, and Cowper's glands. The testes, excretory ducts, seminal vesicles, and Cowper's glands are paired structures.

urethra as it passes through the prostate, and the *outer,* or *main, group* of glands makes up the bulk of prostatic glandular tissue (figure 20–2). The prostate secretes a thin alkaline fluid containing a high concentration of an enzyme secreted by the prostatic epithelial cells. The prostatic secretions are discharged into the urethra during ejaculation through very fine ducts that open near the orifices of the ejaculatory ducts. Secretions mix with sperm and the secretions of the seminal vesicles to form the *seminal fluid.*

Gonorrhea and Nongonococcal Urethritis

Gonorrhea is a relatively common disease. The gonococcus, spread by sexual contact, initially causes an acute inflammation of the anterior urethra. However, the inflammation may spread into the posterior urethra, prostate, seminal vesicles, and epididymides. The gonococcus may also cause an acute inflammation of the rectal mucosa. Occasionally, healing of the gonorrheal inflammation in the posterior urethra may be associated with considerable scarring, leading to narrowing of the urethra and thus to urinary tract obstruction. Inflammatory obstruction of the vasa deferentia may block sperm transport and lead to sterility. *Nongonococcal urethritis,* caused by chlamydia, causes an acute urethritis and clinically is very similar to gonorrhea. (The sexually transmitted diseases are considered in chapter 8.)

Prostatitis

Acute prostatitis develops when an acute inflammation of the bladder or urethra spreads into the prostate. It may follow a gonococcal infection of the posterior urethra. *Chronic prostatitis* is a mild chronic inflammation of the prostate that is quite common and causes few symptoms.

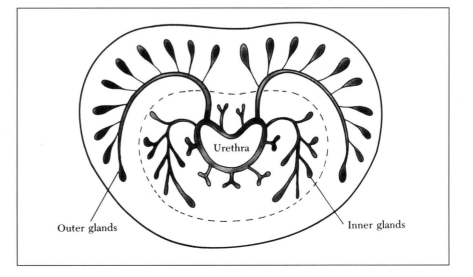

FIGURE 20–2

Diagrammatic cross-section of prostate indicating the arrangement of inner and outer groups of glands.

Moderate enlargement of the prostate gland is relatively common in elderly men and usually involves the inner group of glands surrounding the urethra (figure 20–3). The hyperplasia results from stimulation of the gland by a potent male sex hormone called *dihydrotestosterone* which is formed in the prostate from testosterone by a prostatic enzyme called 5-alpha reductase. Prostatic enlargement is significant only if it obstructs the bladder neck, leading to incomplete emptying of the bladder, or causes complete urinary tract obstruction. An enlarged obstructing prostate causes difficulty in urinating and may lead to various other complications caused by urinary retention and stagnation of urine in the bladder, such as cystitis, pyelonephritis, hydronephrosis, and stone formation.

An obstructing prostate that prevents complete emptying of the bladder is treated surgically. It is possible to relieve the urinary obstruction by "reaming out" the enlarged part of the gland that is encroaching on the urethra and blocking outflow of urine. This is usually accomplished by a procedure called a **transurethral resection of the prostate** (usually called simply TUR). A hollow tubular instrument is inserted through the penis into the urethra, and the site of the obstruction is visualized. Then, by means of a snarelike cutting instrument, pieces of the enlarged prostate are shaved off and removed (figure 20–4). This procedure enlarges the urethral opening so

Benign Prostatic Hyperplasia

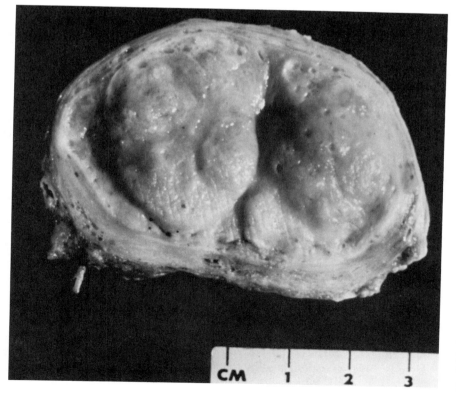

FIGURE 20–3

Cross-section of prostate, showing nodules of hyperplastic tissue compressing the urethra as it passes through the prostate.

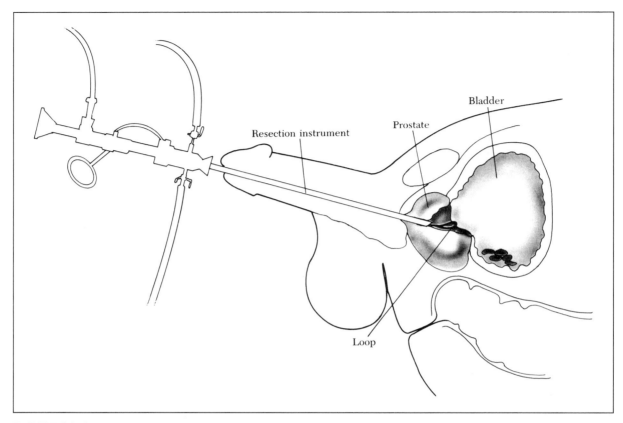

FIGURE 20–4

Principle of transurethral resection of prostate.

that the patient can void normally. The resected tissue is examined histologically by the pathologist to establish the diagnosis of benign prostatic hyperplasia and exclude prostatic carcinoma as a cause of the obstruction (figure 20–5). The lining of the urethra covering the enlarged prostate is removed along with the obstructing part of the gland, but the epithelial lining soon regenerates and the continuity of the urethral lining is restored. Figure 20–6 illustrates the appearance of the base of the bladder and prostate in a patient on whom a transurethral resection had been performed several years earlier.

Nonsurgical treatment of benign hyperplasia that can shrink the gland and relieve obstructive symptoms in many patients also is available. A drug called *finasteride,* which can be taken orally, inhibits the prostatic reductase enzyme that converts testosterone into dihydrotestosterone. As a result, the prostate is no longer stimulated by dihydrotestosterone, and it decreases in

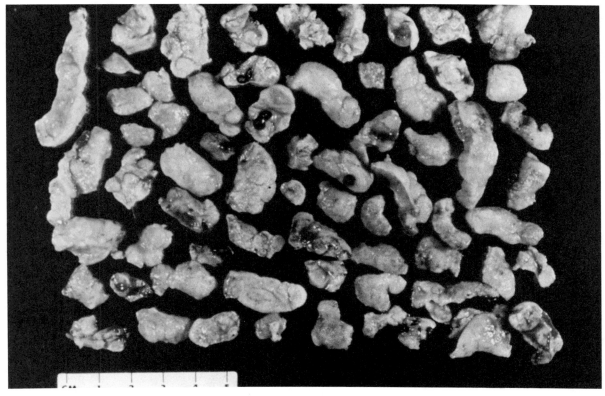

FIGURE 20–5

Appearance of tissue removed by transurethral resection.

size. Continuous administration of the drug is required, however, in order to maintain the suppression of dihydrotestosterone synthesis within the gland.

Various other medical and surgical methods for treating this common condition also are being investigated.

Carcinoma of the Prostate

Carcinoma of the prostate is a common tumor in elderly men. It usually originates in the outer group of prostatic glands, in contrast with benign prostatic hyperplasia, which involves the inner group of glands surrounding the urethra. The initial symptoms are often caused by urinary tract obstruction resulting from encroachment of the tumor-infiltrated prostate on the neck of the bladder and on the urethra. Frequently, the tumor also infiltrates the tissues surrounding the prostate and metastasizes to the bones of the spine and pelvis.

The tumor cells often secrete *acid phosphatase,* as do normal prostatic epithelial cells, and the enzyme leaks into the bloodstream. Many patients

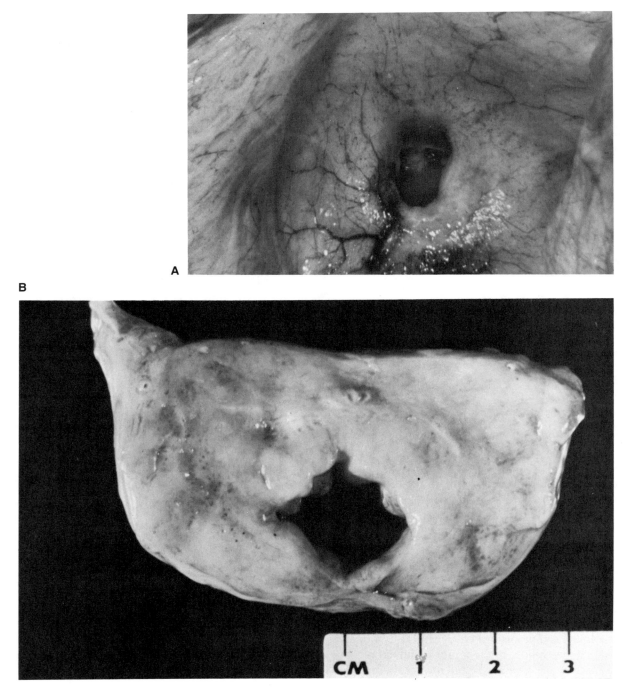

FIGURE 20–6

A, Appearance of base of bladder several years after transurethral resection of prostate, illustrating large urethral opening created by the resection. **B,** Cross-section of prostate, showing enlarged opening. Compare with figure 20–3.

with prostatic carcinoma have high levels of this enzyme in their blood, which is a valuable diagnostic test for prostatic carcinoma.

Another substance called **prostate-specific antigen** (PSA) also is secreted by prostatic epithelial cells, and elevated levels appear in the blood of many patients with prostatic cancer. The test is not specific for prostate cancer, however, because patients with prostatic hyperplasia and other types of benign prostatic disease also may have higher-than-normal levels.

Patients in the early stages of prostate carcinoma may be completely free of symptoms, and the tumors are identified only by routine rectal examination as an area of irregularity or nodularity on the posterior surface of the prostate when palpated through the rectum by the examiner's finger. In other patients, the first manifestations may appear when the growing tumor partially obstructs the bladder neck, causing the same type of symptoms as in patients with benign prostatic hyperplasia. Diagnosis of prostatic carcinoma is established by needle biopsy of the prostate, in which the needle is inserted into the abnormal area in the prostate through the rectum or perineum. Sometimes ultrasound examination is used to locate dense areas in the prostate, which assists in selecting the site for biopsy.

Treatment depends on the degree of differentiation of the tumor and how far the cancer has advanced when first detected. A small, localized prostatic carcinoma can be treated by removal of the entire prostate and surrounding tissues. This procedure is called a radical prostatectomy (figure 20–7). Although this operation may eradicate the tumor, it usually also disrupts the nerve supply to the penis, which leads to permanent inability to achieve an erection of the penis (*impotence*). In other cases, the tumor is treated by irradiation rather than surgery. Radical prostatectomy alone or combined with radiation therapy appears to improve survival in many patients. There is considerable con-

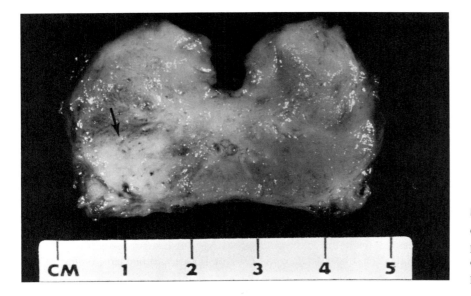

FIGURE 20–7

Cross-section of resected prostate illustrating a small carcinoma arising from outer prostate glands (*arrow*).

troversy, however, about the effectiveness of radical surgery or radiation therapy in elderly men with localized well-differentiated carcinoma of the prostate. Many of these tumors grow very slowly, and it may be ten or more years before the tumor produces symptoms of urinary tract obstruction or metastases to the skeletal system. Many physicians believe that treatment does not improve survival in this group of patients, that the treatment causes more disability and complications than the tumor, and that a slowly growing prostatic carcinoma in an elderly man is best left alone.

When a prostatic carcinoma has advanced to the stage when it has spread beyond the prostate and has metastasized, it is often possible to induce regression of the tumor by altering the level of male sex hormones in the body. Most prostatic carcinomas are dependent on the male sex hormone for their continued growth. Therefore, many advanced prostatic tumors can be treated effectively either by surgical removal of the testes, eliminating the source of the male sex hormone, or by administration of female sex hormone, which indirectly suppresses output of testosterone. Alternatively, one can administer drugs that suppress output of pituitary gonadotropic hormone, thereby inhibiting testicular testosterone secretion. Either castration or hormone treatment usually causes regression of the tumor.

Carcinoma of the Testis

Testicular tumors are uncommon and usually develop in young men. Most arise from the germinal epithelium of the testicular tubules and are malignant. There are several different types. The type with the most favorable prognosis is called a **seminoma.** (This term is another exception to standard terminology. It means literally a tumor of semen-producing epithelium. In this case, the term refers to a malignant neoplasm, not a benign tumor.) Another type of testicular tumor is a *malignant teratoma,* which is composed of many different types of malignant tissues, as described in chapter 10. Some other testicular tumors resemble placental trophoblastic tissue. One tumor of this type is called an *embryonal carcinoma.* Another is called a *choriocarcinoma,* which is the same kind of tumor that arises from trophoblastic tissue in the uterus, as described in chapter 18. Testicular cancers are treated by extensive surgical resection of the testicle, the spermatic cord, and sometimes the regional lymph nodes as well. In some cases, radiation and anticancer chemotherapy also are used.

The neoplastic cells of many testicular tumors produce **human chorionic gonadotrophin** (HCG), which is the same hormone made by the placenta in pregnancy. Consequently, a pregnancy test given to a man with testicular cancer may be positive. Some testicular tumors also produce another substance called **alpha fetoprotein** (AFP), which is a protein produced by the fetus early in prenatal development but not normally found in the adult. If a testicular carcinoma produces these substances, the concentrations fall after successful treatment of the tumor and rise again if the tumor recurs. Consequently, the physician can monitor the response of the testicular tumor to treatment by serial determinations of HCG and AFP, in the same way that carcinoembryonic antigen analyses are used to evaluate the response to treatment of other malignant tumors, as described in chapter 10. (Determination of the concentration of AFP in amnionic fluid is also used to detect certain congenital abnormalities of the nervous system. This application is considered in chapter 26.)

Carcinoma of the penis is uncommon; it is almost never encountered in a circumcised male (figure 20–8). It is generally considered that the secretions that accumulate under the foreskin of the penis are carcinogenic and this accumulation is prevented by circumcision. However, other factors also may account for the low incidence of carcinoma in circumcised males. Some strains of the papilloma virus, the same virus that appears related to cervical dysplasia and carcinoma in women, may also play a role in causing penile cancer. Possibly the papilloma virus grows well beneath an intact foreskin but does not thrive if the foreskin has been removed.

Treatment usually consists of partial or complete resection of the penis.

Carcinoma of the Penis

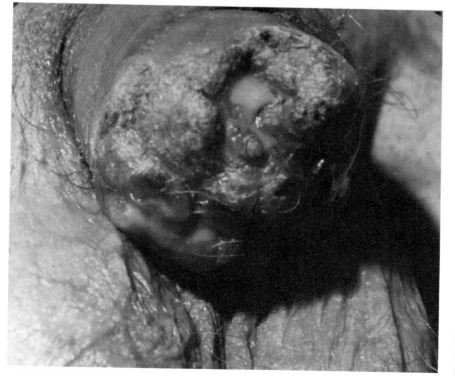

FIGURE 20–8

Large carcinoma of penis involving foreskin.

Questions for Review

1. What are the components of the male reproductive system?

2. What is benign prostatic hyperplasia? What are its clinical manifestations? How is it treated?

3. How does administration of female sex hormones affect prostatic carcinoma? What is the effect of castration on prostatic carcinoma?

4. A young man has a positive pregnancy test. Under what circumstances could this occur?

5. What factors predispose to the development of carcinoma of the penis? How may the disease be prevented?

Supplementary Readings

Brawer, M. K., and Lange, P. H. 1989. Prostate-specific antigen and premalignant change: Implications for early detection. *CA: A Cancer Journal for Clinicians* 39:361–75.

Cooner, W. H., et al. 1988. Clinical application of transrectal ultrasonography and prostate-specific antigen in the search for prostate cancer. *Journal of Urology* 139:758–61.

Fleming, C., Wasson, J. H., Albertsen, P. C., et al. 1993. A decision analysis of alternative treatment strategies for clinically localized prostate cancer. *Journal of the American Medical Association* 269:2650–58. Radical prostatectomy and radiation therapy may benefit some men but appear harmful for patients older than seventy years.

Javadpour, N. 1980. Germ cell tumors of the testis. *CA: A Cancer Journal for Clinicians* 30:242–54. A comprehensive review.

Krahn, M. D., Mahoney, J. E., Eckman, M. H., et al. 1994. Screening for prostate cancer. *Journal of the American Medical Association* 272:773–80. Screening unselected men from ages fifty to seventy with prostatic specific antigen test and transrectal ultrasound did not improve health outcomes and increased costs dramatically.

Littrup, P. J., Lee, F., and Mettlin, C. 1992. Prostatic cancer screening: Current trends and future implications. *CA: A Cancer Journal for Clinicians* 42:198–211. There is no clear evidence that any screening test can decrease mortality.

Lu-Yao, G. L., McLerran, D., and Wennberg, J. E. 1993. An assessment of radical prostatectomy. *Journal of the American Medical Association* 269:2633–36. Radical prostatectomy carries a significant morbidity and mortality, especially in older men.

Monda, J. M., and Oesterling, J. E. 1993. Medical treatment of benign prostatic hyperplasia: 5 α-Reductase inhibitors and α-adrenergic antagonists. *Mayo Clinic Proceedings* 68:670–79. Both medical treatments are effective for treating prostatic hyperplasia.

Persky, L. 1986. Carcinoma of the penis. *CA: A Cancer Journal for Clinicians* 36:258–73. Treatment consists of either partial or complete removal of the penis and may also require resection of groin and pelvic lymph nodes.

Stamey, T. A., 1987. Prostate-specific antigen as a serum marker for adenocarcinoma of the prostate. *New England Journal of Medicine* 317:909–12. Discusses the diagnostic utility of this tumor marker.

Whitmore, W. 1994. Management of clinically localized prostatic cancer: An unresolved problem. *Journal of the American Medical Association* 269:2676–77. Aggressive treatment may benefit selected patients, but the benefits are sufficiently marginal to make watchful waiting a reasonable alternative for many patients.

Zincke, H., et al. 1987. Treatment options for patients with stage D_1 adenocarcinoma of prostate. *Urology* 30: 307–15. Describes results on 306 patients with advanced prostate cancer treated by prostatectomy followed by hormonal or radiation therapy or both. More than 87 percent ten-year survivals.

See also sections in standard textbooks in urology, listed in the General References.

Chapter 20 ■ Outline Summary

Components of the Male Reproductive System / 589
Penis
Transport Ducts
Prostate
  Inner glands: may give rise to benign hyperplasia.

  Outer glands: may give rise to carcinoma.

Gonorrhea and Nongonococcal Urethritis / 590
Gonorrhea
  A common disease spread by sexual contact.

  May spread to posterior urethra and transport ducts.

  Obstruction of vasa may cause sterility.

Nongonococcal Urethritis
Symptoms similar to gonorrhea.

Caused by *Chlamydia*.

Prostatitis / 590
Acute Prostatitis
Spread of infection from bladder or urethra.

May be secondary to gonococcal infection.

Chronic Prostatitis
Mild chronic inflammation.

Causes few symptoms.

Benign Prostatic Hyperplasia / 591
Manifestations
Enlarged prostate obstructs outflow of urine.

Predisposes to infection, calculi, and hydronephrosis.

Treatment
Transurethral resection most commonly used procedure.

Carcinoma of the Prostate / 593
Manifestations
Early case may be asymptomatic.

May obstruct bladder neck and cause symptoms of obstruction like benign prostatic hyperplasia.

Often metastasizes to pelvic and vertebral bone.

Diagnosis
Rectal examination indicates abnormality.

Prostate-specific antigen or acid phosphatase or both often elevated.

Prostate biopsy, sometimes assisted by ultrasound examination of prostate.

Treatment
Surgery:
Conservative transurethral resection.
Radical prostatectomy.
Hormones: suppress tumor growth.

Carcinoma of the Testis / 596
Classification
Seminoma.

Malignant teratoma.

Choriocarcinoma.

Treatment
Resection of testicle and associated structures.

Chemotherapy.

Methods Used to Monitor Response to Therapy
Chorionic gonadotropins (HCG).

Alpha fetoprotein (AFP).

Carcinoma of the Penis / 597
Manifestations and Pathogenesis
Rare in circumcised male.

Secretions accumulating under foreskin may be carcinogenic.

Papilloma virus may play a role.

Treatment
Partial or complete amputation of penis.

Removal of inguinal lymph nodes also usually performed.

The Liver and the Biliary System

Learning Objectives

1. Describe the normal structure of the liver and explain the functions of the liver as they relate to the major diseases of the liver.
2. List the major causes of liver injury and describe their effects on hepatic function.
3. Compare the three major types of viral hepatitis in terms of their pathogenesis, incubation period, incidence of complications, and frequency of carriers. Explain the diagnostic tests used to identify each type of viral infection and describe methods of prevention.
4. Explain the adverse effects of excess alcohol intake on liver structure and function.
5. Explain how gallstones are formed and describe their causes and effects.
6. Compare the three major causes of jaundice.

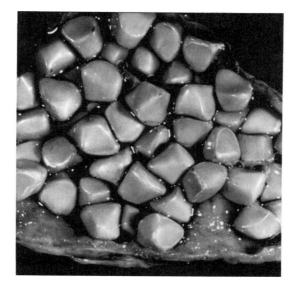

Chapter 21 ▪ Contents

The liver weighs about 1500 g and is the largest organ in the body. It has a roughly triangular shape and is located beneath the diaphragm in the upper abdomen. It is a complex organ with many functions. These are concerned primarily with the following:

1. Metabolism of ingested carbohydrates, protein, and fat delivered through the portal circulation
2. Synthesis of various substances, including plasma proteins and proteins taking part in blood clotting
3. Storage of vitamin B_{12} and other materials
4. Detoxification and excretion of various substances

The liver has a double blood supply. About three-quarters of the blood flow is provided by the *portal vein,* which drains the spleen and gastrointestinal tract. Portal blood is rich in nutrients absorbed from the intestines but low in oxygen content. The rest of the blood, which comes from the *hepatic artery,* has a high oxygen content but is low in nutrients. Blood flowing from the hepatic artery and the portal vein mixes as it flows through the liver and is eventually collected into the *right* and *left hepatic veins,* which drain into the inferior vena cava.

The liver cells are arranged in the form of long, wide plates interconnected at various angles to form a lattice. The *hepatic sinusoids* occupy the spaces between the plates (figure 21–1A).

Branches of the hepatic artery, portal vein, bile ducts, and lymphatic vessels travel together within the liver and are called the **portal tracts** (figure 21–1B). The terminal branches of both the hepatic artery and the portal vein discharge their blood into the hepatic sinusoids. In histologic sections, the liver plates appear as cords surrounded on each side by sinusoids that converge toward the central veins. The portal tracts appear at the periphery. This anatomic configuration, which is called a **liver lobule,** is illustrated diagrammatically in figure 21–2A.

Blood flow in the liver is from portal tracts through the sinusoids into central veins (figure 21–2B). Consequently, the liver cells nearest the portal tracts receive the most oxygen and nutrients, and those nearest the central veins are much less well supplied. Because of their relatively poor nutritional state, the liver cells nearest the central veins are more vulnerable to injury from toxic agents or circulatory disturbances, as occurs in shock and heart failure, than are the cells nearer the portal tracts.

The small terminal bile channels are called **bile canaliculi.** They are located between adjacent liver cords and drain into the bile ducts traveling in the portal tracts. The direction of the bile flow is opposite that of the blood flow in the sinusoids (figure 21–2B). The bile ducts gradually converge to form larger ducts, which finally unite as the large *right* and *left hepatic ducts.* The two hepatic ducts join to form the *common hepatic duct.* The gallbladder joins the common hepatic duct by means of the *cystic duct* to form the *common bile duct* that enters the duodenum.

FIGURE 21–1

Photomicrographs showing cellular structure of normal liver. **A,** Low-magnification photomicrograph illustrating plates of liver cells, which appear as cords in histlogic sections, and sinusoids between plates (cords), which drain into central veins. *Arrow* indicates central vein. (Original magnification × 25.) **B,** Higher magnification illustrating portal tract. *Arrow* indicates bile duct. Branch of hepatic artery is located at left of bile duct and branch of portal vein is below. (Original magnification × 400.)

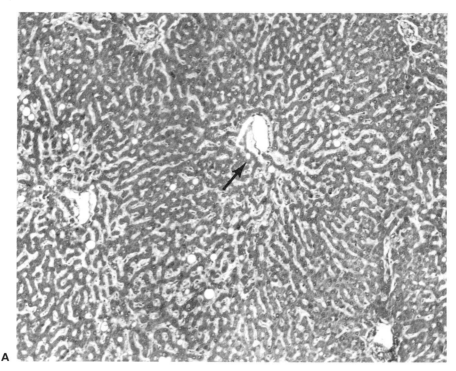

A

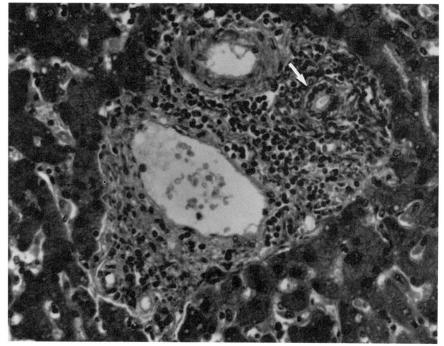

B

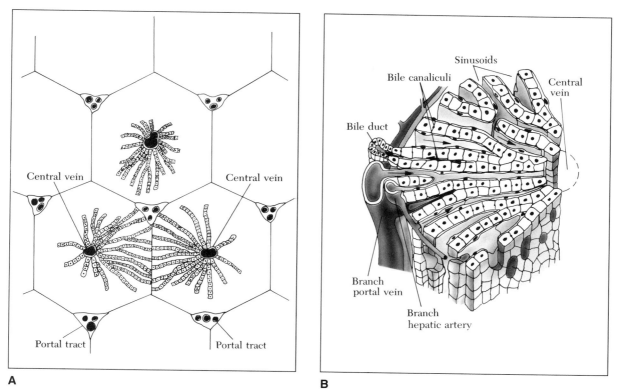

FIGURE 21–2

A, Concept of liver lobule, consisting of cords of cells radiating toward central vein with portal tracts at periphery. Lobules are outlined in diagram. **B,** Blood flow in sinusoids toward central vein; flow of bile toward portal tract.

Formation and Excretion

Bile pigment is a product of the breakdown of red blood cells. Red cells normally survive for about four months. The worn-out erythrocytes are broken down by the reticuloendothelial cells throughout the body. The iron derived from the hemoglobin is conserved by the body and reused to synthesize new hemoglobin. The iron-free heme pigment is **bilirubin.** Because the breakdown of red cells proceeds in reticuloendothelial tissues throughout the body, small quantities of bile pigment are continually present in the blood. When the blood passes through the liver, the bilirubin is removed by the liver cells. Excretion is accomplished by combining the bilirubin with other substances, a process called *conjugation,* which requires certain specific enzymes. Most of the bilirubin is conjugated with glucuronic acid and excreted as *bilirubin glucuronide.* The **conjugated bilirubin** is much more soluble and less toxic than the unconjugated material. The bile pigment is excreted into the small bile channels between the liver cell cords; it is collected into large ducts at the periphery of the lobules that eventually unite to

Bile

form the major bile ducts. Figure 21–3 summarizes the basic anatomy of the biliary duct system.

Composition and Properties

Bile is an aqueous solution containing various dissolved substances excreted by the liver. In addition to conjugated bilirubin, it contains bile salts, lecithin, cholesterol, water, minerals, and other materials that have been detoxified by liver cells and excreted. **Cholesterol** is a lipid with a complex ring structure that is classified as a *sterol*. **Bile salts,** the major constituent of bile, are derivatives of cholesterol and certain amino acids. They function as detergents because of their molecular structure, which contains both a lipid-soluble (*hydrophobic*) and a water-soluble (*hydrophilic*) part. **Lecithin** is a phosphorous-containing lipid (*phospholipid*) that has detergent properties similar to bile salts. Bile is secreted continually and is concentrated and stored in the gallbladder. During digestion, the gallbladder contracts, squirting bile into the duodenum. Bile does not contain digestive enzymes but functions as a biologic detergent. Bile salts emulsify fat into small globules, increasing the surface area so that the fat can be acted upon more readily by pancreatic and duodenal enzymes. Digestion of fat is much less efficient in the absence of bile.

FIGURE 21–3

Anatomy of the biliary duct system. Right and left hepatic ducts form the common hepatic duct, which is joined by the cystic duct to form the common bile duct, which opens into the duodenum with the pancreatic duct through a common channel.

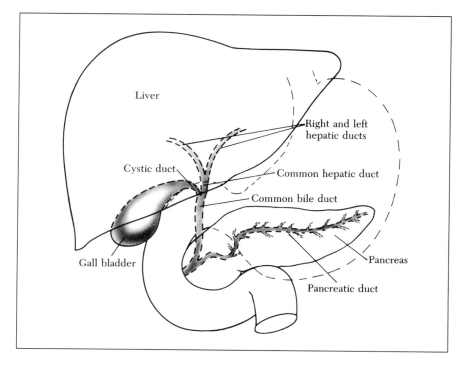

The liver is vulnerable to injury by many agents. Histologically, liver injury may be manifested by necrosis of liver cells, by accumulation of fat within the liver cell cytoplasm, or by a combination of the two. Some injurious agents primarily cause cell necrosis, whereas others chiefly induce fatty change in liver cells.

The effect of hepatic injury depends on the extent of damage induced by the injurious agent. If liver injury is mild, the liver cells will completely recover, restoring liver function to normal. Fortunately, this is the usual outcome. If the injury is extremely severe, large amounts of liver tissue are completely destroyed and not enough liver may remain to sustain life. If the patient does survive, healing of the severe injury may be associated with severe scarring (*postnecrotic scarring*) and liver function may never return to normal. Multiple episodes of relatively mild liver injury may have a cumulative effect, leading to scarring and permanent impairment of liver function. Similarly, any chronic or progressive injury may cause scarring and impairment of function.

Liver cell injury caused by drugs, chemicals, alcohol, or toxins can produce fatty change in liver cells rather than necrosis. Figure 21–4 diagrams the general causes and possible effects of various degrees of liver injury.

Clinically, the most common types of liver disease characterized by injury to liver cells are viral hepatitis, fatty liver, alcoholic hepatitis, and cirrhosis of the liver.

Within recent years, much new information has become available about the hepatitis viruses. The term *viral hepatitis* applies to several clinically similar infections. Two of these diseases, *hepatitis A* (formerly called infectious hepatitis) and *hepatitis B* (formerly called serum hepatitis) have been recognized as separate diseases since the early 1940s. Subsequently, a third type of viral hepatitis, originally designated *non-A, non-B hepatitis* and later called *hepatitis C,* was recognized as a separate entity. These three types account for most cases of viral hepatitis. Recently, two additional types of viral hepatitis have been identified. One type, called *hepatitis D* or *delta hepatitis,* is more common in third world countries than in North America. Another type, called *hepatitis E,* also is primarily found in third world countries, and only a few cases have been recognized in the United States.

Clinical Manifestations and Course

Viral **hepatitis** is a type of liver injury, and the comments regarding the course and outcome of any liver injury also apply to viral hepatitis. The clinical manifestations of viral hepatitis are quite variable. About one-third of affected subjects experience loss of appetite, feel ill, and become jaundiced. Laboratory tests reveal evidence of liver cell injury. Another third become ill, and their laboratory tests are abnormal, but they never become jaundiced. This condition is often called *anicteric hepatitis* (*ana* = without + *icterus* = jaundice). The remaining third have few symptoms and often do not seek

FIGURE 21–4

Summary of causes and effects of liver injury. Many agents can cause injury to liver cells, manifested either as fatty change, necrosis, or a combination of both. Mild injury is followed by complete recovery. Severe, chronic, or progressive injury may lead to hepatic failure or diffuse scarring with impaired hepatic function.

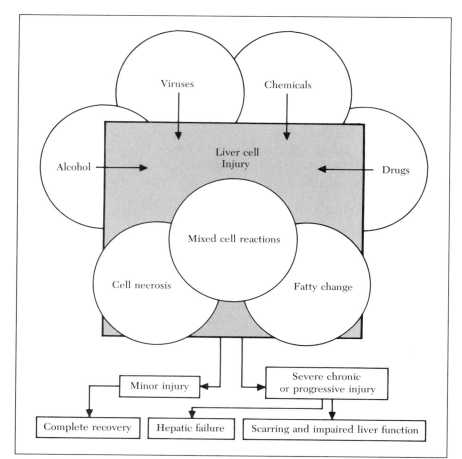

medical attention, but laboratory tests reveal liver injury. Their infection, which could easily escape detection, is sometimes called *subclinical hepatitis*. Despite the absence of symptoms, these subjects can transmit the infection to others.

Fortunately, most cases of viral hepatitis are mild, and patients recover without complications. An unfavorable outcome occurs in only a small percentage of cases. Rarely, death results from massive hepatic necrosis; if the patient survives, recovery is followed by severe liver scarring. Some persons with hepatitis B and hepatitis C infections become chronic carriers of the virus or develop chronic progressive hepatitis that eventually leads to liver failure. Table 21–1 summarizes the salient features of the three main types of viral hepatitis.

Hepatitis A

Hepatitis A virus (HAV) is an RNA-containing virus measuring 27 nm (1 nanometer, abbreviated nm, equals 1 billionth of a meter). Hepatitis A has

	Type A	Type B	Type C	
				TABLE 21–1
Transmission	Direct contact, contaminated food or water	Infected blood or secretions	Infected blood or secretions	Characteristics of type A, type B, and type C hepatitis
Incubation	2–6 weeks	6 weeks–4 months	3–12 weeks	
Immunity	50 percent of population has anti-HA antibody and is immune	5–16 percent of population has anti-HBs and is immune	Unknown	
Complications	No carriers or chronic liver disease	10 percent become carriers: may develop chronic liver disease	50 percent become carriers; many develop chronic liver disease	
Prevention of disease after exposure	Gamma globulin	Gamma globulin or hepatitis B immune globulin	Gamma globulin (possibly effective)	

a relatively short incubation period that varies from two to six weeks. The virus is excreted in oropharyngeal (nose and throat) secretions and in the stools during the late-incubation period and for about two weeks after onset of symptoms. Transmission is by direct person-to-person contact or by fecal contamination of food or water. Food- or water-borne infections frequently occur in epidemics. One epidemic of 107 cases, which occurred in a large city, was traced to a food-service employee who had contracted hepatitis A from her grandson and contaminated the food that she was preparing (Levy et al. 1975). In another epidemic, 240 persons developed hepatitis from eating raw oysters grown in virus-contaminated water (Portnoy et al. 1975).

The infection is self-limited, and there are no chronic carriers of the virus. Antibody to hepatitis A virus, which appears in the blood after recovery, provides immunity against hepatitis A virus but not against other hepatitis viruses. Hepatitis A is a common infection in the United States, and almost half the adult population have antibodies against the virus. If a susceptible person is exposed to hepatitis A, gamma globulin provides protection if administered within ten days of exposure. An inactivated hepatitis A vaccine is available. It is recommended for immunizing persons who are at relatively high risk of becoming infected, such as health care workers who have frequent contact with infected persons, and persons traveling in foreign countries where there is a high incidence of hepatitis A in the population.

Hepatitis B

Hepatitis B virus (HBV) is a DNA-containing virus measuring 42 nm, which is somewhat larger than the hepatitis A virus. It is composed of an inner core and an outer coat. The core consists of a double strand of DNA and an enzyme (*DNA polymerase*) enclosed within a protein shell. The DNA strand and its inner protein shell together are called the **hepatitis B core antigen** (abbreviated **HBcAg**). The outer coat composed of lipid and protein is called the **hepatitis B surface antigen** (abbreviated **HBsAg**). The core antigen and surface antigen together form the complete virus particle, which is often called the *Dane particle* after the pathologist who first described it.

In contrast to hepatitis A, hepatitis B has a much longer incubation period, which varies from six weeks to four months. When an individual becomes infected, the virus invades the liver and multiplies within the hepatic cells. The core of the virus is produced in the nucleus, and the surface antigen is produced in the cytoplasm. For some unexplained reason, much more surface antigen is produced within the infected cells than is necessary to coat the virus particles, and the large excess is released into the bloodstream, where it can be detected by special laboratory tests (figure 21–5). Such blood is called *surface-antigen (HBsAg) positive*. Although the laboratory tests detect only the surface antigen, HBsAg-positive blood is infectious because it also contains complete virus particles (figure 21–6).

In the course of an infection, the surface antigen first appears during the incubation period and can be detected during the first few weeks of the infection. Normally, it does not persist in the blood for more than two or three weeks. Then antibodies begin to appear, both to the core of the virus (anti-HBc) and to the surface antigen (anti-HBs). Various other antigens and antibodies also appear in the blood of persons with HBV infection. One is a soluble protein called the **hepatitis B e antigen** (**HBeAg**), which appears along with HBsAg. The corresponding antibody, anti-HBe, often appears

FIGURE 21–5

Assembly of complete virus particles from core and surface antigen, resulting in large excess of surface antigen, which can be detected in blood of infected patient.

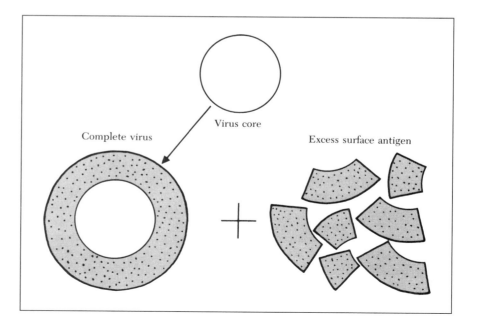

Complete virus
Virus core
Excess surface antigen

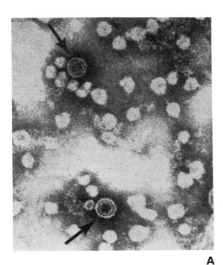
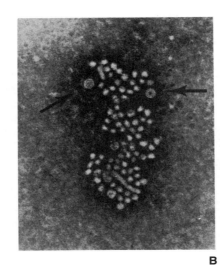

A   B

FIGURE 21–6

Electron photomicrographs of complete virus particles (*arrows*) and excess surface antigen in blood of patient with hepatitis B. **A,** Original magnification × 290,000. **B,** Original magnification × 130,000. (From: Dane, D. S.; Cameron, C. H.; and Briggs, M. 1970. Virus-like particles in serum of patients with Australia-antigen-associated hepatitis. *Lancet* 1:695–98. Used by permission.)

along with anti-HBs during recovery. About 10 percent of the population possess antibodies against the virus as a result of prior infection and are immune to reinfection.

Most infected individuals eliminate the virus from the bloodstream in a few weeks and recover completely, but about 10 percent become chronic carriers of the virus. Some of the carriers develop chronic hepatitis, which causes progressive liver damage. About 1 percent of the U.S. population are asymptomatic chronic carriers of the virus, and their blood is infectious. The carrier rate is much higher among drug abusers and male homosexuals. In the Vietnamese and some other population groups, the carrier rate may approach 20 percent.

Hepatitis B virus is not excreted in the stool. Consequently, transmission does not occur by means of contaminated food or water. Most HBV infections result from contact with the blood or secretions of HBsAg-positive individuals. Drug abusers may transmit the virus by sharing needles and syringes. Physicians, dentists, nurses, laboratory personnel, and other health professionals may become infected from contact with blood of HBsAg-positive patients. Contaminated dental instruments or instruments used for ear piercing also may transmit HBV. Because HBV is also present in saliva, vaginal secretions, and seminal fluid, infection may also be spread by close family contacts or sexual contacts. An HBsAg-positive mother may transmit the virus to her newborn infant, who usually acquires the infection from maternal blood and vaginal secretions at the time of delivery, and the infected infant may become a chronic carrier of the virus. Formerly, many cases followed blood transfusions, but this is no longer true because all blood collected for transfusion is now tested routinely for HBsAg, and antigen-positive blood is not used for transfusion.

Hepatitis B immune globulin provides some protection if administered promptly after exposure to the virus and is given routinely to newborn infants born to HBsAg-positive mothers. A vaccine is available to immunize against HBV. The vaccine induces the formation of anti-HBs and provides a high degree of immunity against HBV infection. Originally, the vaccine was recommended only for persons at risk of infection, such as health-care personnel, male homosexuals, intravenous drug abusers, and those having sexual contact with high-risk persons. Now, universal vaccination is recommended, and HBV vaccination is included in vaccination schedules recommended for newborn infants.

Hepatitis C

Some cases of hepatitis still develop after blood transfusions, and most of these cases are due neither to HAV nor to HBV but to a newly recognized virus measuring 80 nm called *hepatitis C virus* (HCV). The incubation period is longer than that of HAV infection but shorter than HBV infection. The infected persons develop antibodies against the hepatitis C virus, but antibodies may not appear for several months after infection. Anti-HCV antibody testing is used both as a diagnostic test for HCV infection and as a screening test by blood banks so that HCV antibody-positive blood is not used for transfusions. About half the infected persons become chronic carriers of the virus and many develop chronic hepatitis. There is some evidence to suggest that gamma globulin may also prevent this type of hepatitis in exposed persons.

Although hepatitis C is often considered a transfusion-associated disease, in many cases transmission is by contact with the blood or secretions of infected individuals, as in the transmission of the hepatitis B virus described earlier.

Hepatitis D (Delta Hepatitis)

This type of hepatitis is caused by a small defective RNA virus that can only infect persons who are already infected with the hepatitis B virus, either chronic carriers of HBV or those with an acute HBV infection. The delta virus is always associated with an HBV infection because the virus is unable to produce its own outer viral coat and can reproduce itself only by coating itself with HBsAg produced by HBV, thereby forming complete but hybrid virus particles composed of a delta virus core and a HBsAg outer layer. Delta hepatitis is less common than other types of viral hepatitis, and most cases in the United States are found among intravenous drug abusers who became infected by sharing contaminated needles.

Hepatitis E

Hepatitis E is caused by an RNA virus that is transmitted by the fecal-oral route, like the hepatitis A virus; most of the cases are in third world countries, where outbreaks have been traced to contaminated water supplies. Only a few cases have been reported in North America, and the infected persons acquired the disease while traveling outside the United States. A diagnostic test has been developed to detect anti-HEV antibodies as an indication of HEV infection. Gamma globulin does not provide protection against HEV infection, because gamma globulin preparations do not contain anti-HEV antibodies.

Other Hepatitis Viruses

Other viruses may at times cause a mild hepatitis. These include the **Epstein-Barr (EB) virus,** which causes infectious mononucleosis (see chapter 14), and another somewhat similar virus called **cytomegalovirus,** which may also cause an infection resembling infectious mononucleosis.

Hepatitis among Male Homosexuals

All types of viral hepatitis are common in male homosexuals and are transmitted by sexual contact. The hepatitis A virus is excreted in the stool of infected subjects and may also contaminate the anal-genital skin. Consequently, the virus is readily transmitted by anal-oral and oral-genital sexual activity. Hepatitis B virus, which is present in the blood and secretions of infected individuals, is transmitted among male homosexuals primarily by anal intercourse, and hepatitis C also may be transmitted in this way. Minor abrasions of the anal, rectal, and genital mucosa of sexual partners permits transfer of virus-infected blood and body fluids between partners. Because male homosexuals may have multiple sexual contacts, a single infected individual may transmit hepatitis to many other persons.

The following case illustrates the usual clinical and laboratory features of viral hepatitis as a result of HBV infection:

> A twenty-two-year-old man was seen by a physician because of upper abdominal discomfort, nausea, loss of appetite, and jaundice. The patient had noted that his urine had become darker in color. He was homosexual and stated that a sexual partner had had a similar illness recently. Physical examination revealed a jaundiced young man with a slightly enlarged, tender liver. There were no findings to suggest chronic liver disease. Laboratory studies revealed a slight elevation of bilirubin and abnormalities of several liver-function tests. Tests for hepatitis B surface antigen were positive. The patient was considered to have hepatitis B, probably contracted through sexual activities with a partner who either had active hepatitis or was a chronic carrier of the virus. The patient made an uneventful recovery. Hepatitis B surface antigen was no longer detected in the blood three weeks later, and antibody to hepatitis B surface antigen appeared during convalescence.

CASE 21–1

Fatty liver is a special type of liver injury in which fat accumulates in liver cells (figure 21–7). A number of injurious agents are capable of disrupting the metabolic processes within the liver cell, leading to such accumulation

Fatty Liver

FIGURE 21–7

Cut surface of fatty liver that appears pale because of excess fat.

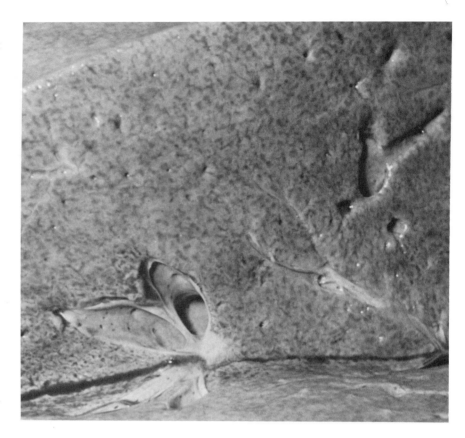

of fat (figure 21–8). In the United States, the most common cause of fatty liver is excessive alcohol ingestion. Fatty liver is relatively common in heavy drinkers and in persons who are chronic alcoholics. In addition to alcohol, a number of volatile solvents, drugs, chemicals, and some poisons can cause fatty liver, which is also encountered in a condition called *Reye's syndrome,* described later in this chapter. Heavy fat infiltration impairs liver function, but the effect is reversible and the liver cells return to normal when the injurious agent is no longer present.

Alcoholic Hepatitis

Heavy intake of alcohol not only promotes fatty change in liver cells, but causes other degenerative changes as well and may actually induce liver cell necrosis. A rather characteristic feature of severe alcoholic liver injury is the accumulation of irregularly shaped, pink deposits within the cytoplasm of the liver cells. These structures, which are called **Mallory bodies** or *alcoholic hyalin,* indicate that the cell has been irreparably damaged. Neutrophilic leukocytes also accumulate in response to the liver cell necrosis, and the injury is followed by progressive fibrous scarring throughout the liver. The term *alcoholic hepatitis* is used to refer to this type of liver injury,

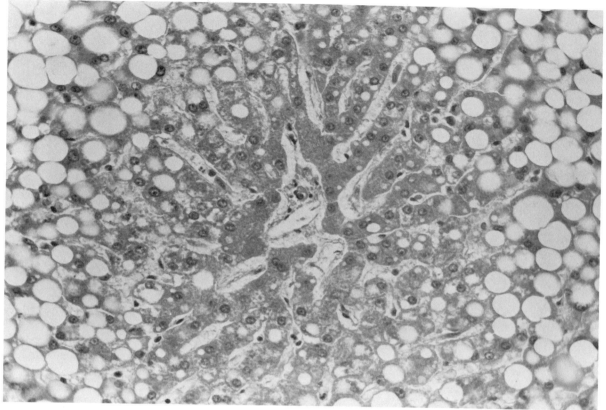

FIGURE 21–8

Photomicrograph of fatty liver. Liver cord cells in *center* of photograph appear relatively normal. Other cells contain large fat globules that appear as clear areas in photograph. (Original magnification × 100.)

which is characterized not only by fatty change, but also by liver cell degeneration with Mallory bodies, leukocyte infiltration, and fibrous scarring (figure 21–9). In this case, the term "hepatitis" refers to the inflammatory cell infiltration secondary to liver cell necrosis and does not imply an infection, as in viral hepatitis.

The term **cirrhosis of the liver** refers to diffuse scarring of the liver from any cause (figure 21–10). Any substance capable of injuring the liver may cause cirrhosis under certain conditions. The more common causes of cirrhosis are as follows:

Cirrhosis

1. Repeated bouts of alcoholic hepatitis
2. An episode of severe liver necrosis, such as after an attack of severe viral hepatitis (sometimes called *posthepatitic cirrhosis* or *postnecrotic cirrhosis*)

FIGURE 21–9

Photomicrographs showing hepatic cellular structure in alcoholic hepatitis.
A, Swollen liver cells containing Mallory bodies. *Arrow* indicates cluster of neutrophils. (Original magnification × 400.)
B, High-magnification photomicrograph of Mallory body in swollen liver cell. (Original magnification × 1000.)

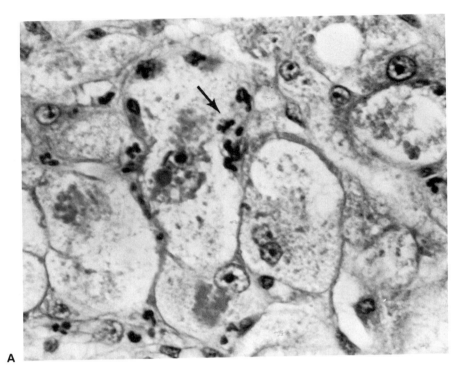

A

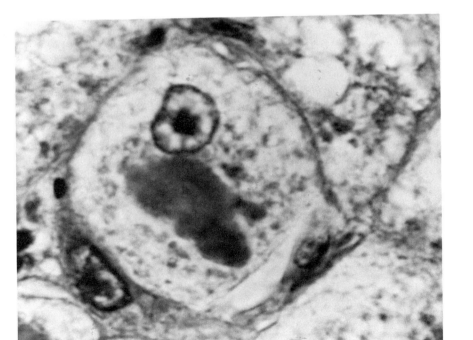

B

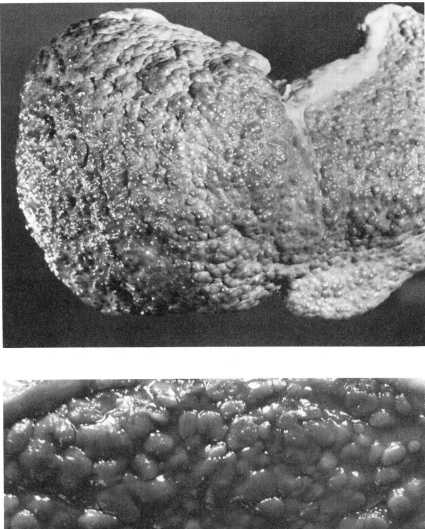

A

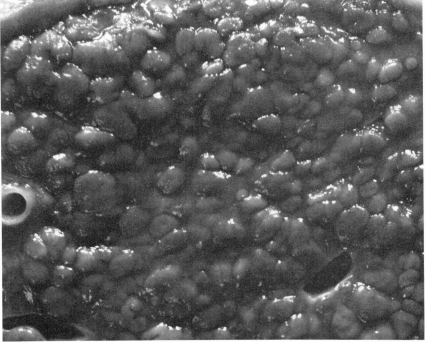

B

FIGURE 21–10

Advanced hepatic cirrhosis, illustrating elevated nodules of liver tissue surrounded by depressed areas of scar tissue. **A,** Exterior of liver. **B,** Closer view of liver in cross-section.

3. Repeated episodes of liver injury or chronic progressive liver cell damage, as occurs in some types of viral hepatitis or from various other causes

In the United States, most cases of cirrhosis of the liver are related to heavy alcohol ingestion and follow repeated episodes of alcoholic hepatitis. It is generally considered that a person must drink more than one pint of whiskey daily (or its equivalent in other alcoholic beverages) for ten to fifteen years in order to develop alcoholic cirrhosis. However, there is considerable individual variation in susceptibility to alcoholic liver injury. Occasionally, the disease develops more rapidly, and it has been seen in teenagers and young adults. Other cases of cirrhosis follow viral hepatitis or liver injury from various toxic drugs and chemicals. Sometimes, the actual cause of cirrhosis in a given patient cannot be determined.

The following clinical summary illustrates the clinical features seen in a patient who died of advanced alcoholic liver disease with cirrhosis:

CASE 21-2

A thirty-three-year-old man had been drinking heavily for many years and was in the habit of consuming about one quart of liquor per day. Recently, he had noticed weakness and loss of appetite. The physical examination revealed that he was slightly jaundiced. His liver was enlarged, and there was moderate ascites. Laboratory studies revealed a reduced serum albumin and a moderate elevation of serum bilirubin. Other tests of liver function also were abnormal. The clinical impression was cirrhosis with ascites caused by chronic alcoholism. Despite intensive therapy, the patient's condition did not improve, and he eventually died of chronic liver failure. The autopsy revealed advanced cirrhosis and active alcoholic hepatitis with many Mallory bodies in the cytoplasm of the liver cells.

Derangements of Liver Structure and Function

In cirrhosis, the liver is converted into a mass of scar tissue containing nodules of degenerating and regenerating liver cells, proliferating bile ducts, and inflammatory cells (figure 21–11). The normal architectural pattern of the liver is completely disorganized, and the intrahepatic branches of the hepatic artery and portal vein are constricted by scar tissue.

The two major functional disturbances in cirrhosis are impaired liver function and portal hypertension.

Impaired Liver Function

As a result of liver cell damage, scarring, and impairment of blood supply to the liver caused by scarring, the number of functioning liver cells is greatly reduced. Eventually, a patient with cirrhosis may die of liver failure. Clinical manifestations commonly found in men with advanced cirrhosis are testicular atrophy, loss of sex drive, and breast hypertrophy. These manifestations result from impaired liver function and appear to be the result of an excess of estrogen. Normally, men produce not only male sex hormone

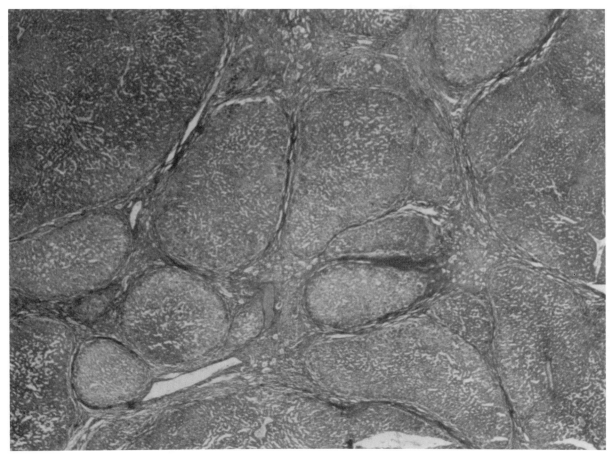

FIGURE 21–11

Low-magnification photomicrograph of cirrhotic liver illustrating nodules of liver cells circumscribed by scar tissue. Normal architectural pattern is lost. Compare with figure 21–1. (Original magnification × 25.)

(testosterone), but small amounts of estrogen as well. The estrogen is normally inactivated by the liver and exerts little effect. The cirrhotic liver, however, is unable to accomplish this function efficiently; so estrogen accumulates and produces these associated clinical manifestations.

Portal Hypertension

Normally, the portal vein blood passes through sinusoids into the hepatic veins and then into the inferior vena cava. In cirrhosis, venous return through the portal system is impaired, and the pressure in the portal vein rises because the blood flow is obstructed by scar tissue. The high pressure affects the portal capillaries, and this contributes to excessive leakage of fluid from the capillaries. Eventually, the abdomen becomes distended by fluids that accumulate within the abdominal cavity (*ascites*), (figure 21–12).

A reduced concentration of albumin in the blood also contributes to ascites because albumin is crucial to maintaining the normal colloid osmotic pressure of the blood, which is the force that tends to hold fluid in the capillaries (chapter 12). Albumin, which is produced by the liver, is reduced in cirrhosis because the cirrhotic liver is unable to manufacture this protein in sufficient quantities; consequently, the colloid osmotic pressure of the blood is lower than normal and fluid leaks from the portal capillary bed.

Because of the obstruction of portal venous return, a collateral circulation develops in an attempt to bypass the intrahepatic obstruction and deliver portal blood directly into the systemic circulation. Anastomoses develop where tributaries of portal and systemic veins are closely associated, and they shunt blood from the portal system of veins where the pressure is high into the veins of the systemic circulation where the pressure is much lower (figure 21–13). The communications that are most important clinically are the anastomoses developing between veins around the stomach and

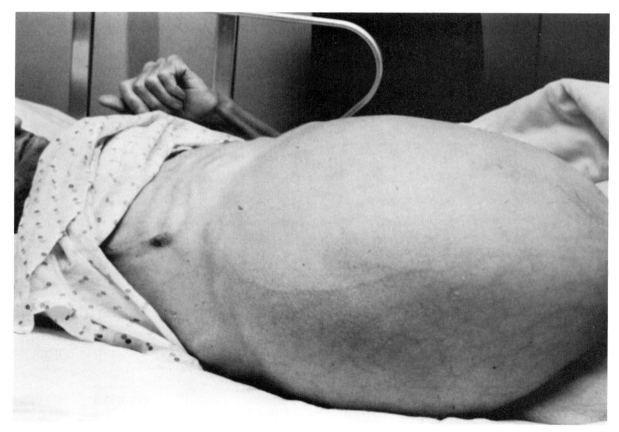

FIGURE 21–12

Severe ascites in patient with advanced cirrhosis.

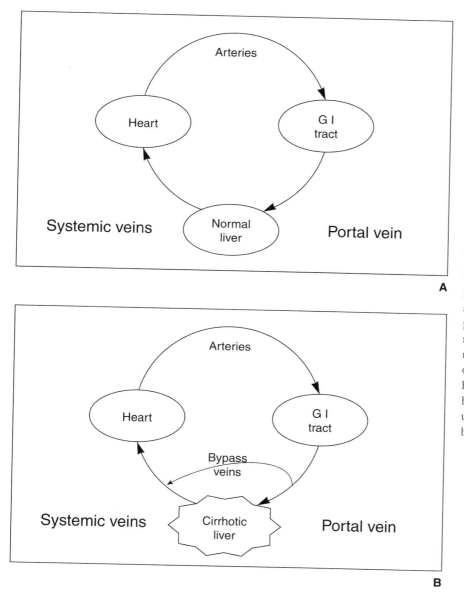

FIGURE 21–13

Comparison of normal blood-flow pathways with those in cirrhosis. **A,** Normal flow pattern. Heart pumps blood through aorta to gastrointestinal tract from which blood collects in portal vein and flows through hepatic sinusoids into hepatic veins, then into inferior vena cava, and finally back to heart to be repumped. **B,** Flow pattern in cirrhosis. Blood pumped to gastrointestinal tract is collected in portal vein, but flow through hepatic sinusoids is interrupted by intrahepatic scarring, and portal vein pressure rises. Bypass channels shunt blood into superior or inferior vena cava in order to return blood to the heart. Bypass veins cannot handle increased blood flow under increased pressure and become dilated.

spleen, which drain into the portal vein, and the esophageal veins that eventually drain into the superior vena cava by way of the intercostal veins and azygos veins (figure 21–14). The esophageal veins are not equipped to handle the increased blood flow and high pressure and therefore become dilated and form varicose veins, which are called *esophageal varices* (plural of *varix*). Esophageal varices are thin-walled vessels covered by a thin layer of esophageal epithelium (figure 21–15) and frequently rupture, leading to profuse and often fatal hemorrhage.

FIGURE 21–14

Formation of collateral venous channels (described in text) that return blood of systemic circulation when portal blood flow is impeded by cirrhosis. *Arrows* indicate direction of blood flow.

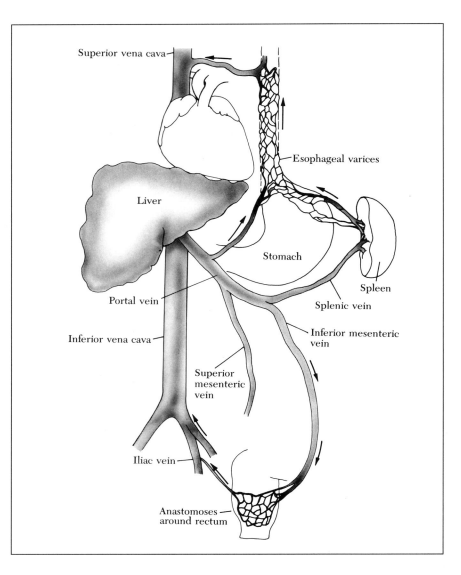

Other anastomoses develop between branches of the portal vein and the veins draining the abdominal wall that eventually flow into either the superior or the inferior vena cava. Still other anastomoses develop around the rectum between branches of the inferior mesenteric veins and the iliac veins, permitting blood to flow through the iliac veins into the inferior vena cava.

The blood flow through the collateral channels reduces the engorgement of the abdominal organs that has resulted from overdistention of the portal circulation. The elevated portal pressure also declines somewhat but does not return to normal.

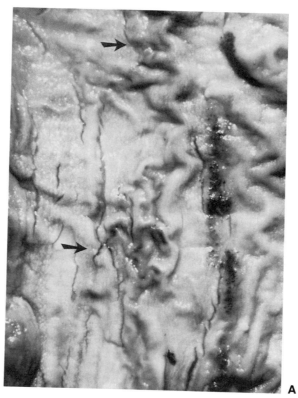

A

FIGURE 21–15
A, Mucosal surface of esophagus illustrating varices, which appear as tortuous elevations of the mucosa (*arrows*).
B, Photomicrograph of a varix. The very thin vein wall (*arrow*) is covered only by a thin layer of esophageal squamous epithelium and is very susceptible to rupture. (Original magnification × 40.)

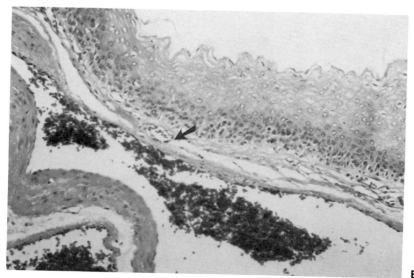

B

Procedures to Treat Manifestations of Cirrhosis

Portalsystemic Anastomoses

If a patient has developed esophageal varices and is at risk of hemorrhage, it is possible to lower the pressure in the portal system by surgically connecting the splenic vein to the renal vein side-to-side (**splenorenal shunt**) or making a side-to-side connection between the portal vein and inferior vena cava (**portacaval shunt**). A shunt decompresses the portal system by permitting portal blood to flow directly into the inferior vena cava (figure 21–16). Blood no longer is forced to circumvent the scarred liver by collateral channels. The dilated esophageal veins decrease in size, and the risk of hemorrhage from varices is greatly reduced. A more recent procedure accomplishes a portal-systemic communication to lower the pressure in the portal system without requiring an operative procedure. Under x-ray guidance, with the use of the same types of procedures described in connection

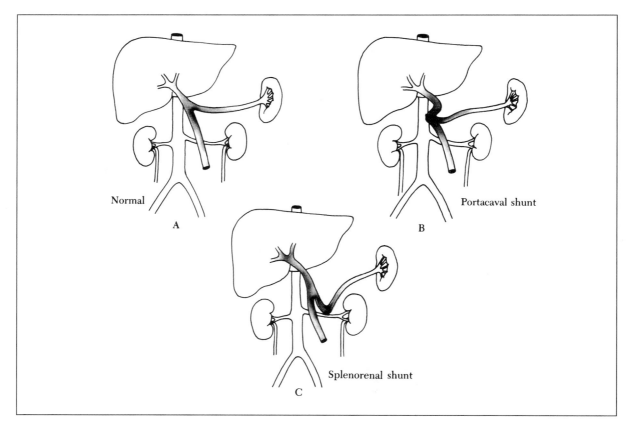

FIGURE 21–16

Operative procedures to create portalsystemic anastomosis for treatment of esophageal varices. **A,** Normal anatomic relation. **B,** Portacaval shunt. **C,** Splenorenal shunt.

with coronary angioplasty (chapter 13), a catheter is introduced into the right internal jugular vein and passed retrograde into the inferior vena cava and then into one of the hepatic veins (which drain blood from the liver into the inferior vena cava). Then a guide wire is passed through the catheter, which penetrates the hepatic vein wall, and passes through the liver tissue to connect with a large intrahepatic branch of the portal vein. The procedure creates a tract between portal vein and hepatic vein within the liver. The tract is dilated and a device (called a stent) is inserted to keep the tract open. When the procedure has been completed, much of the portal blood flows directly from a portal vein branch directly into one of the hepatic veins and then into the inferior vena cava, without flowing through the hepatic sinusoids. As a result, the high pressure in the portal vein falls toward normal.

Obliteration of Varices by Sclerosing Solution

Another way to treat varices is to obliterate them by injecting them with a sclerosing solution. The procedure is performed by first visualizing the lining of the esophagus and the location of the varices by means of an esophagoscope. The sclerosing solution is then injected directly into the dilated veins and connective tissue around the vein. The solution, which is very irritating, causes an inflammation in and around the dilated veins, which is followed by scarring and eventual obliteration of the varices. Multiple injections over a period of several months are usually required.

Shunts to Control Ascites

Severe ascites that does not respond to medical treatment is sometimes treated surgically by means of a shunt. One type of shunt, named the *LeVeen shunt* after the physician who developed the procedure, is illustrated in figure 21–17. A perforated tube is placed in the peritoneal cavity and connected to the internal jugular vein in the neck by a tube passed through the subcutaneous tissue. In this way, the ascitic fluid is shunted from the abdominal cavity back into the systemic circulation. A valve is interposed in the system to assure one-way flow. The procedure controls the ascites. However, occasional patients develop a disseminated intravascular coagulation syndrome (described in chapter 11) resulting from activation of the clotting mechanism by thromboplastin-rich tissue fluids and other components present in the ascitic fluid. This complication has limited the use of the procedure.

Reye's Syndrome

Reye's syndrome (rhymes with "eye") is a relatively uncommon acute illness that develops in infants and children after a mild viral infection and is characterized by both marked swelling of the brain with neurologic dysfunction, and accumulation of fat within the cytoplasm of liver cells associated with impaired liver function. Clinically, the illness manifests as sudden onset of vomiting and impaired consciousness, which may progress to delirium and coma. Laboratory tests reveal the disturbed liver function that is related to the accumulation of fat in the liver cells, and some patients become jaun-

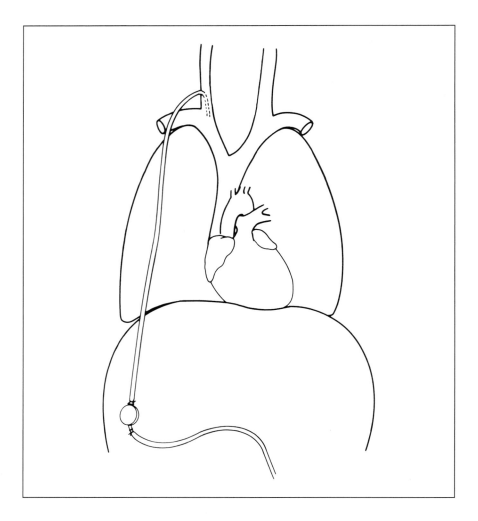

diced. In severely affected patients, the mortality rate is about 25 percent,
and some of the survivors may be left with neurologic abnormalities or psy-
chiatric disturbances. There is no specific treatment.

Current evidence suggests that Reye's syndrome is related in some way
to acetylsalicylic acid (aspirin) given to treat the fever and discomfort associated with the viral infection. The aspirin may increase the injurious effects
of the virus or interact with the virus to cause the liver and brain injury.
Therefore, acetaminophen (for example, Tylenol) is recommended to treat
symptoms of viral infections in infants and children.

Cholelithiasis

The formation of stones within the gallbladder is called **cholelithiasis**
(*chole* = bile + *lith* = stone). Gallstones are very common and are estimated
to develop in about 20 percent of the population. Most gallstones are com-

posed entirely or predominantly of cholesterol, and they form because the bile contains more cholesterol than can be held in solution by the available bile salts and lecithin (figure 21–18).

Factors Affecting the Solubility of Cholesterol in Bile

Because cholesterol is a lipid, it is not soluble in an aqueous solution such as bile but is brought into solution by bile salts and lecithin, which aggregate in clusters called **micelles.** In a micelle, the lipid-soluble (*hydrophobic*) parts of the bile salt molecules are oriented toward the center of the cluster, and the opposite water-soluble (*hydrophilic*) ends face outward. Cholesterol becomes soluble by dissolving in the hydrophobic center of the micelles, and the cholesterol-containing micelles dissolve in the bile because the peripheral hydrophilic parts of the bile salt molecules are water soluble. Lecithin participates in the formation of the micelles by fitting between the molecules of the bile salts (figure 21–19).

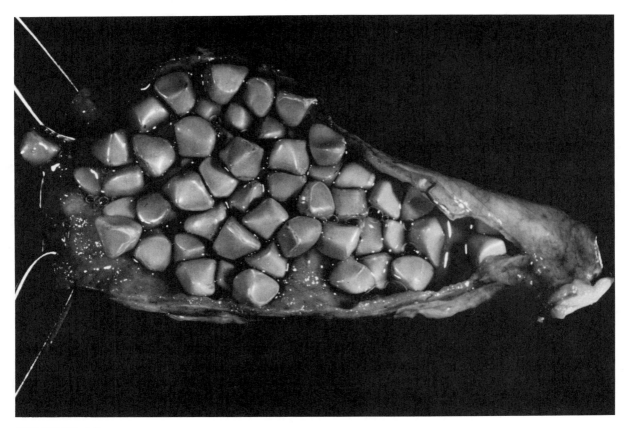

FIGURE 21–18

Opened gallbladder filled with gallstones composed of cholesterol.

FIGURE 21–19

Manner in which cholesterol dissolves in micelles composed of bile salts and lecithin. If bile salt concentration is insufficient relative to that of cholesterol, cholesterol will precipitate and form gallstones.

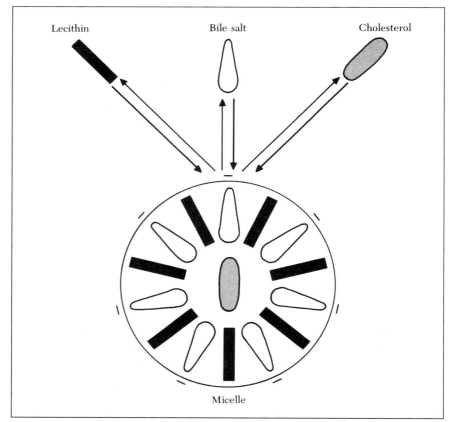

Lecithin   Bile salt   Cholesterol

Micelle

Approximately seven molecules of bile salts interspersed between lecithin molecules in a micelle are required to dissolve one molecule of cholesterol. Consequently, the solubility of cholesterol in bile depends not only upon its cholesterol content, but also on its content of bile salts and lecithin, because these substances are needed to hold the cholesterol in solution. Cholesterol remains soluble provided its concentration is not excessive in relation to the amounts of available bile salts and lecithin. If there is an excess of cholesterol relative to bile salts and lecithin, the bile becomes supersaturated with cholesterol and cholesterol crystals may precipitate. On the other hand, if there is an excess of bile salts and lecithin relative to cholesterol, the bile becomes unsaturated with cholesterol and more cholesterol can dissolve in the bile. These relations can be conceptualized by a board on a fulcrum, one end of the board being weighted by cholesterol and the other end by bile salts and lecithin. Variations in the "weight" on either end of the board cause corresponding changes in the solubility of the cholesterol in the bile (figure 21–20).

Whenever bile contains a relative excess of cholesterol, it becomes supersaturated with cholesterol and, under proper conditions, the cholesterol may

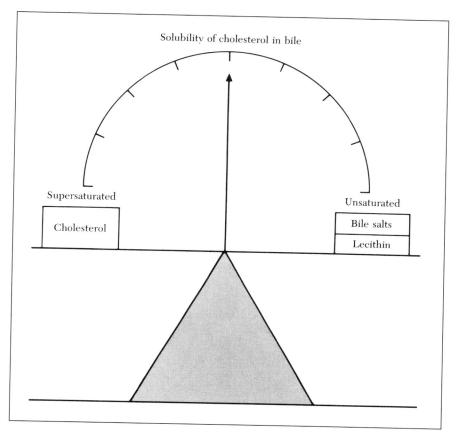

FIGURE 21–20

"Board-and-fulcrum" concept illustrating factors that affect solubility of cholesterol in bile.

precipitate to form the beginnings of gallstones. This situation may arise because of an increased excretion of cholesterol in the bile, a reduced excretion of bile salts and lecithin, or a combination of both factors. As long as the bile remains supersaturated, cholesterol crystals continue to accumulate around those that have already precipitated, and the gallstones slowly increase in size. Eventually, the gallbladder may become filled with gallstones, the end stage of a process that began several years earlier.

Some people are known to have an increased risk of forming gallstones. The incidence of gallstones is:

1. Higher in women than in men.
2. Higher in women who have borne several children than in childless women.
3. Twice as high in women who use contraceptive pills as in women who use other types of contraception.
4. Higher in obese women than in women of normal weight.

The incidence of gallstones is higher in these groups because their bile is more highly saturated with cholesterol. The incidence is higher in women than in men because estrogen promotes increased excretion of cholesterol in the bile while decreasing excretion of bile salts. The correlation of gallstones with multiple pregnancies is related to the high estrogen levels associated with pregnancy. (Estrogen levels are much higher in pregnancy than in the nonpregnant state because large amounts of estrogen are produced by the placenta.) Contraceptive pills predispose to cholelithiasis because they contain synthetic estrogens that, like natural estrogens, increase the saturation of gallbladder bile. Obesity predisposes to gallstones because extremely overweight persons excrete more cholesterol in their bile than do persons of normal weight.

Less commonly, gallstones form as a result of infection of the gallbladder. Infection predisposes to gallstones by reducing the solubility of cholesterol and other constituents in the bile.

Complications of Gallstones

Gallstones that remain in the gallbladder do not cause symptoms. Unfortunately, gallstones are sometimes extruded into the cystic duct or common bile duct when the gallbladder contracts after a fatty meal, and they may become impacted within the biliary ducts. This event causes severe abdominal pain called **biliary colic.** The pain results from spasm of the smooth muscle in the ducts combined with forceful contractions of the gallbladder that attempt to propel the stone through the ducts. Sometimes a stone can be passed through the ducts into the duodenum, but often it becomes impacted. If the stone lodges in the cystic duct, bile can neither enter nor leave the gallbladder, but flow of bile from the liver into the duodenum is not disturbed even though storage of bile in the gallbladder is no longer possible. If the gallbladder is the site of a chronic infection, the impaction of the stone may precipitate a flare-up of the infection in the gallbladder called **cholecystitis** (figure 21–21). If there is no underlying gallbladder infection, the bile trapped within the gallbladder by the impacted stone is gradually absorbed into the bloodstream, and eventually the contents of the gallbladder consist only of mucus that has been secreted by the epithelial cells lining the gallbladder.

If the stone blocks the common duct, bile can no longer be excreted into the duodenum and it accumulates in the bloodstream. This condition is called *obstructive jaundice.*

Treatment of Gallstones

The standard treatment of gallstones producing symptoms is surgical removal of the diseased gallbladder. In the past, it was necessary to perform a major surgical operation to remove the gallbladder. Now, most cholecystectomies can be performed by means of a laparoscopic procedure through a very small incision in the abdomen. It is possible, however, to dissolve cholesterol gallstones in some carefully selected patients, thereby avoiding surgery. This is accomplished by administering a bile salt (either *ursodeoxycholic acid* or

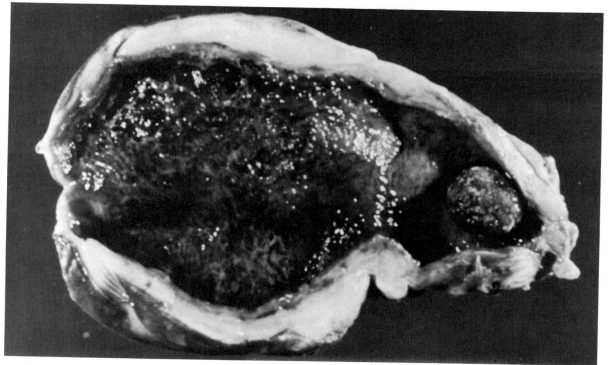

FIGURE 21–21

Inflamed thick-walled gallbladder with stone impacted in neck of gallbladder.

chenodeoxycholic acid or a combination of both), which decreases the amount of cholesterol excreted in the bile. As the cholesterol content of the bile decreases, the bile becomes more unsaturated with cholesterol and more cholesterol can be dissolved in the bile. As a result, the cholesterol contained within the gallstones becomes soluble in the unsaturated bile and the gallstones slowly dissolve. Unfortunately, even if the stones are dissolved successfully, new stones often form within the gallbladder after the treatment is discontinued. Other methods are currently being investigated for dissolving gallstones or for fragmenting the stones by sonic shock waves, employing methods like those used to fragment kidney stones (described in chapter 19).

Inflammation of the gallbladder is called **cholecystitis** (*chole* = bile + *cyst* = bladder + *itis* = inflammation). It is a relatively common disease. Chronic cholecystitis appears to predispose an individual to the development of gallstones. As previously described, impaction of a gallstone in the neck of the gallbladder or the cystic duct may precipitate an acute cholecystitis if the gallbladder is the site of a preexisting chronic inflammation.

Cholecystitis

Tumors of the Liver and Gallbladder

Primary tumors of the liver and gallbladder are uncommon. Benign hepatic **adenomas** develop occasionally in women taking contraceptive pills, but we do not know why the pills predispose to tumors in some women. *Primary carcinoma* of the liver is quite rare in the United States and Canada but is a common malignant tumor in Asian and African countries. The current evidence indicates that chronic carriers of the hepatitis B virus (HBV) not only have a relatively high incidence of chronic liver disease, but also carry an increased risk of developing a primary liver carcinoma, suggesting that chronic HBV infection predisposes both to liver injury and to liver cancer. The frequency of primary liver cancer in Asia and Africa is probably related to the high incidence of chronic HBV carriers in these populations. Failure of the body's immune defenses to destroy the infected liver cells and eliminate the virus leads to a smoldering chronic infection that may eventually lead to cirrhosis and predisposes to liver cancer. Patients with chronic HCV infections also are at risk of cirrhosis and liver cancer (figure 21–22).

In contrast to the infrequency of primary liver cancer in developed countries, the liver is a common site of *metastatic carcinoma* (figure 21–23). Carcinoma arising in the gastrointestinal tract may spread to the liver, bits of tumor being carried to the liver in the portal venous blood. Tumors from the breast, lung, and other sites also often spread to the liver. The tumor cells are carried in the blood delivered to the liver by the hepatic artery. Sometimes enlargement of the liver as the result of metastatic carcinoma may be the first sign of a malignant tumor that originated in some other part of the body. Various diagnostic procedures can be used to identify tumors in the liver. The computed tomographic (CT) scan described in chapter 1 is a very effective means of detecting cysts and tumors in the liver (figure 21–24).

Jaundice

Jaundice is a yellow discoloration of the skin and the sclerae (whites of the eyes) that results from accumulation of bile pigment (bilirubin) in the tissues and body fluids. This accumulation can have several causes. Bile pigment is derived from the breakdown of red cells, as described elsewhere in this text. The pigment is extracted from the blood by the liver cells, conjugated, and excreted into the biliary ducts. It is convenient to classify jaundice on the basis of the disturbance responsible for the retention of bile pigment. On this basis, jaundice is classified as *hemolytic, hepatocellular,* or *obstructive.* Jaundice can usually be classified correctly on the basis of certain laboratory tests in conjunction with the clinical features.

Hemolytic Jaundice

In conditions associated with accelerated breakdown of red cells, excessive bile pigment is delivered to the liver, beyond the liver's ability to conjugate and excrete the pigment. Therefore, unconjugated bile pigment accumulates in the blood. Hemolytic jaundice is sometimes seen in adults with hemolytic anemia,

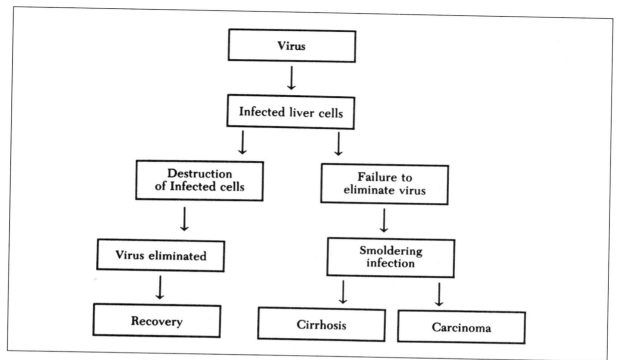

FIGURE 21–22

Possible outcomes of hepatitis B and hepatitis C infections. Failure to eliminate virus leads to chronic infection, which may be complicated by cirrhosis and liver cancer.

but it is encountered most frequently in newborn infants with hemolytic disease as a result of blood group incompatibility between mother and infant (chapter 18).

Hepatocellular Jaundice

If the liver is severely damaged, as in hepatitis or cirrhosis, conjugation of bilirubin is impaired. Moreover, the excretion of conjugated bilirubin is extremely hampered because of injury to liver cells and disruption of small bile channels that lie between liver cell cords. As a result, conjugated bilirubin leaks back into the blood through the ruptured intrahepatic bile channels.

Obstructive Jaundice

In obstructive jaundice, the extraction and conjugation of bilirubin by liver cells are not impaired, but jaundice develops because the bile duct is obstructed, preventing delivery of bile into the duodenum. Often the obstruction is caused by an impacted stone in the common duct. Carcinoma of the head of the pancreas is another common cause of common bile duct obstruction. As indicated

FIGURE 21–23

Cross-section of liver containing multiple nodules of metastatic carcinoma.

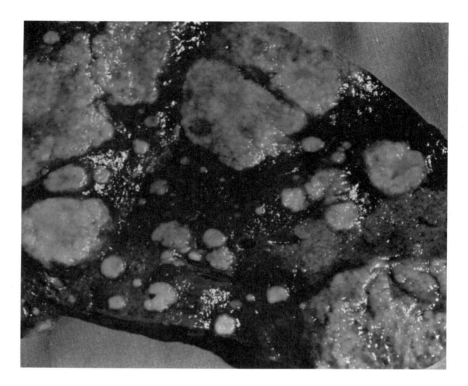

FIGURE 21–24

Computed tomographic (CT) scan of upper abdomen illustrating liver and upper abdominal organs. Large irregular area in liver (*arrows*) is caused by deposit of metastatic carcinoma.

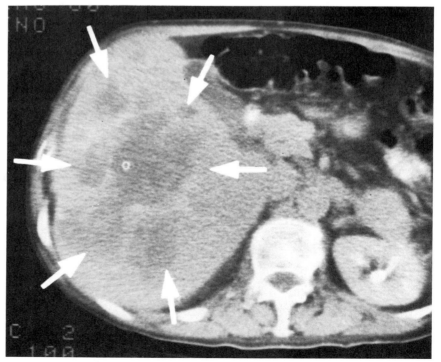

in figure 21–3, the common duct passes very close to the head of the pancreas as it enters the duodenum. Therefore, a pancreatic tumor frequently compresses and invades the common duct.

Biopsy of the Liver

Many times, the exact cause and extent of liver disease in a given patient is difficult to determine. In such cases, a biopsy of the liver can be performed by inserting a needle through the skin directly into the liver and extracting a small bit of liver tissue. This can be examined microscopically by the pathologist, and generally an exact diagnosis of the nature and severity of the liver disease can be made. This information can provide a basis for proper treatment.

Questions for Review

1. What are some of the principal functions of the liver? How does the blood supply to the liver differ from that to the other organs? Why does severe liver disease cause disturbances in blood clotting?

2. What is the difference between hemoglobin and bilirubin? How does conjugated bilirubin differ from unconjugated bilirubin? What is the difference between bilirubin and bile? What role does bile play in digestion?

3. What are the possible causes and effects of liver injury (see figure 21–4)? What is the usual outcome of a liver injury?

4. What is viral hepatitis? What are its major symptoms? How is hepatitis transmitted?

5. What is the difference between hepatitis A and hepatitis B? What is anicteric hepatitis? What is subclinical hepatitis?

6. What effect does alcohol have on the liver? What types of liver disease are associated with excessive alcohol ingestion?

7. What is cirrhosis? What liver diseases may lead to cirrhosis? Why does portal hypertension develop in patients with cirrhosis? Why does ascites develop in patients with cirrhosis? Why do esophageal varices develop?

8. What is jaundice? How is jaundice classified? Under what circumstances do gallstones cause jaundice?

9. What factors predispose to the development of gallstones?

10. What is the difference between viral hepatitis and alcoholic "hepatitis"?

Supplementary Readings

Alter, H. J. 1989. Detection of antibody to hepatitis C virus in prospectively followed transfusion recipients with acute and chronic non-A, non-B hepatitis. *New England Journal of Medicine* 321:1494–1500. Posttransfusion patients developed anti-HCV; antibody may not appear for four to five months after onset of illness.

Alter, M. J., et al. 1989. Importance of heterosexual activity in the transmission of hepatitis B and non-A, non-B hepatitis. *Journal of the American Medical Association* 262:1201–5. Heterosexual activity is an important factor in transmission.

Alter, M. J. 1993. The detection, transmission, and outcome of hepatitis C virus infection. *Infectious Agents and Disease.* 2:155–66. Hepatitis C is a major cause of acute and chronic hepatitis and cirrhosis worldwide. Most cases are associated with blood exposure, but sexual, household, or perinatal transmission occurs.

Centers for Disease Control. 1993. Hepatitis E among U.S. travelers. *Morbidity and Mortality Weekly Report* 42:1–4. Hepatitis E outbreaks in third world countries are related to contaminated water supplies. Although the infection is not established in the United States, a few cases have been reported, and cases of hepatitis E may become more frequent among residents of states at the U.S.-Mexico border. Gamma globulin does not contain anti-HEV antibodies; so gamma globulin does not provide protection against infection.

Columbo, M., et al. 1989. Prevalence of antibodies to hepatitis C virus in Italian patients with hepatocellular carcinoma. *Lancet* 2:1006–8. HCV is an important factor associated with hepatocellular carcinoma in non-A, non-B chronic hepatitis.

Dane, D. S., et al. 1970. Virus-like particles in serum of patients with Austrial-antigen-associated hepatitis. *Lancet* 1:695–98. The original article by the pathologist who described the complete virus particle.

Davis, G. L., et al. 1989. Treatment of chronic hepatitis C with recombinant interferon alfa. *New England Journal of Medicine* 321:1501–6. Interferon therapy controls disease activity in many patients with hepatitis C, but many patients relapse after cessation of treatment.

Hadler, S. C., et al. 1980. Hepatitis A in day-care centers. *New England Journal of Medicine* 302:1222–27. Child day-care centers may be an important source for spreading hepatitis A.

Isselbacher, K. J. 1977. Metabolic and hepatic effects of alcohol. *New England Journal of Medicine* 296:612–16. Describes the metabolism of alcohol by the liver and effects of alcohol on carbohydrate, protein, and fat metabolism. Describes alcohol-related disorders.

Klatskin, G. 1977. Hepatic tumors: Possible relationship to use of oral contraceptives. *Gastroenterology* 73:386–94. Describes incidence, pathology, and complications. Larger adenomas may cause serious bleeding.

Lemon, S. M. 1994. Inactivated hepatitis A vaccines (Editorial). *Journal of the American Medical Association* 271:1363–64. A formalin inactivated hepatitis A vaccine provides effective protection, which will probably last from five to ten years.

Levy, B. S., et al. 1975. A large food-borne outbreak of hepatitis A. *Journal of the American Medical Association* 234:289–94. Describes a large food-borne outbreak of hepatitis A in Minneapolis, traced to a sandwich-maker in a restaurant.

Martin, P. 1990. Hepatitis C: From laboratory to bedside. *Mayo Clinic Proceedings* 65:1372–76. Reviews diagnostic test, diagnosis, and principles of management.

Osmond, D. H., et al. 1993. Risk factors for hepatitis C virus seropositivity in heterosexual couples. *Journal of the American Medical Association* 269:361–65. Heterosexual transmission of HCV is relatively infrequent compared with transmission by blood and blood products, but it does account for a significant number of new infections in the United States annually.

Portnoy, B. L., et al. 1975. Oyster-associated hepatitis. *Journal of the American Medical Association* 233:1065–68. Describes an outbreak of hepatitis A associated with eating raw oysters from virus-contaminated water.

Redinger, R. N., and Small, D. M. 1972. Bile composition, bile salt metabolism, and gallstones. *Archives of Internal Medicine* 130:618–30. A good review article on cholelithiasis.

Steffen, R., Kane, M. A., Shapiro, C. N., et al. 1994. Epidemiology and prevention of hepatitis A in travelers. *Journal of the American Medical Association* 272:885–89. Hepatitis A vaccine (or gamma globulin if vaccine not available) is recommended for all nonimmune travelers visiting developing countries.

Vallari, D. S., Jett, B. W., Alter, H. J., et al. 1992. Serologic markers of posttransfusion hepatitis C viral infection. *Clinical Microbiology* 30:552–56. A review of antibody response to various components of HCV. Antibodies may not appear until three to four months after infection.

Wapnick, S., et al. 1977. LeVeen continuous peritoneal-jugular shunt. *Journal of the American Medical Association* 237:131–33. Describes the shunt and its effects on refractory ascites in cirrhotic patients.

Zemel, G., Katzen, B. T., Becker, G. J., et al. 1991. Percutaneous transjugular portosystemic shunt. *Journal of the American Medical Association* 266:390–93. An intrahepatic shunt between a branch of the hepatic and portal veins can decompress the portal venous pressure effectively.

See also sections in standard textbooks of medicine and surgery, as listed in General References. The sections in *Scientific American Medicine* are particularly useful.

Chapter 21 ▪ Outline Summary

Structure and Function of the Liver / 603
Important Features

Complex metabolic functions.

Double blood supply from hepatic artery and portal vein.

Liver lobule is basic structural unit.

Branches of hepatic artery, portal vein, and bile duct travel in portal tracts.

Blood flow in lobule is from portal tract to central vein.

Bile flow in canaliculi is from central vein toward portal tract.

Bile / 605
Formation and Excretion of Bilirubin
Bile pigment derived from breakdown of red blood cells in reticuloendothelial system.

Conjugation and excretion by liver.

Composition and Properties
Contains bile pigment, cholesterol, bile salts, lecithin, and other materials.

Functions as biologic detergent: no digestive enzymes.

Causes and Effects of Liver Injury / 607
Manifestations
Cell necrosis.

Fatty change.

Mixed necrosis and fatty change.

Clinical Effects
Mild injury with complete recovery.

Severe injury with hepatic failure.

Chronic or progressive injury causes scarring with impaired liver function.

Common Types of Liver Injury
Viral hepatitis.

Fatty liver.

Alcoholic hepatitis.

Cirrhosis.

Viral Hepatitis / 607
Clinical Manifestations and Course
One-third become sick and jaundiced.

One-third become sick but not jaundiced.

One-third asymptomatic but liver function abnormal.

Hepatitis A
RNA virus.

Short incubation period.

Virus in secretions and stools during early phases.

Transmitted by direct contact or contaminated food or water.

Self-limited, low mortality, no carriers.

Gamma globulin provides protection.

Hepatitis B
DNA virus.

Long incubation.

Large amount of surface antigen produced by virus can be detected in blood of carriers and infected persons.

Ten percent of infected persons become chronic carriers of virus.

High carrier rate in some populations.

Transmitted by blood or secretions of infected persons.

Gamma globulin provides some protection.

Immunizing vaccine provides protection against infection.

Hepatitis C
Transmitted like hepatitis B. May also follow blood transfusion.

Incubation period intermediate between HAV and HBV.

Many persons become chronic carriers.

Gamma globulin may provide some protection.

Hepatitis D (Delta Hepatitis)
Virus only infects persons with acute or chronic HBV infection.

Delta virus unable to produce own virus coat and uses HBsAg produced by HBV.

Other Hepatitis Viruses
Epstein-Barr (EB) virus.

Cytomegalovirus.

Hepatitis among Male Homosexuals
Spread by sexual practices.

Fatty Liver / 613
Pathogenesis
Fat accumulates in liver cells owing to liver injury.

Common in heavy drinkers and alcoholics.

Sometimes caused by other chemicals and solvents.

Impaired liver function but injury reversible.

Alcoholic Hepatitis / 614
Pathogenesis
More severe alcoholic injury.

Mallory bodies indicate severe damage to liver cells.

Leukocytes accumulate in response to injury.

Healing with scarring.

Cirrhosis / 615
Definition
Scarring in liver from any cause.

Repeated bouts of alcoholic hepatitis.

Massive liver necrosis.

Repeated episodes of liver injury.

Associated derangements of liver cell regeneration and liver function.

Manifestations
Impaired liver function.

Portal hypertension.

Bypass routes connect systemic-portal venous systems.

Risk of fatal hemorrhage from esophageal varices.

Surgical Procedures to Treat Cirrhosis

Portal-systemic anastomoses to control varices.

Splenorenal shunt.

Portacaval shunt.

LeVeen shunt to control ascites.

Tube drains ascitic fluid into jugular vein.

Materials in ascitic fluid may cause intravascular coagulation syndrome and other complications.

Reye's Syndrome / 625
Pathogenesis

Probably related to combined effect of viral illness and aspirin.

Acetaminophen recommended rather than aspirin to reduce risk.

Characteristics

Affects primarily infants and children.

Fatty liver with liver dysfunction.

Cerebral edema with neurologic dysfunction.

No specific treatment available.

Cholelithiasis and Cholecystitis / 626
Factors Influencing Solubility of Cholesterol in Bile

Cholesterol insoluble in aqueous solution.

Dissolved in micelles composed of bile salts and lecithin.

Solubility of cholesterol depends on ratio of cholesterol to bile salts and lecithin.

Supersaturated bile promotes calculi.

Complications of Gallstones

Asymptomatic in gallbladder.

Biliary colic results if stone extruded into ducts.

Common duct obstruction: obstructive jaundice.

Cystic duct obstruction: no jaundice, but acute cholecystitis may occur if preexisting infection of gallbladder.

Treatment of Gallstones

Cholecystectomy.

Chenodeoxycholic acid dissolves gallstones.

Cholecystitis

Chronic infection common.

Gallstones may predispose to infection.

Impaction of stone in neck of gallbladder may precipitate acute cholecystitis.

Tumors of the Liver and Gallbladder / 632
Incidence

Benign adenomas uncommon: occur in women taking oral contraceptives.

Primary carcinoma uncommon: occurs in patients with cirrhosis.

Metastatic carcinoma common.

Spread from gastrointestinal tract, breast, lung, or other sites.

CT scan aids in recognition.

Jaundice / 632
Classification

Hemolytic: excessive red cell breakdown.

Hepatocellular: liver cell injury.

Obstructive: common duct obstruction by tumor or stone.

Biopsy of the Liver / 635
Indications and Method

Indicated when cause of liver disease undetermined after clinical and laboratory evaluation.

Needle inserted through skin directly into liver.

Biopsy specimen examined histologically by pathologist.

The Pancreas and Diabetes Mellitus

Learning Objectives

1. Describe the pathogenesis and treatment of acute pancreatitis.
2. Describe the pathogenesis, manifestations, complications, and prognosis of pancreatic cystic fibrosis.
3. Differentiate between the two principal types of diabetes mellitus with respect to pathogenesis, incidence, manifestations, complications, and treatment.

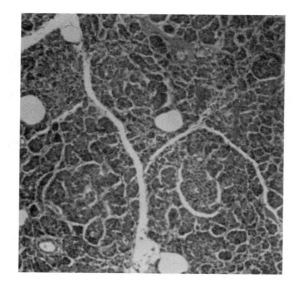

Chapter 22 ▪ Contents

The pancreas is actually two glands in one: a digestive gland and an endocrine gland. The *exocrine tissue* of the pancreas, which is concerned solely with digestion, secretes an alkaline pancreatic juice rich in digestive enzymes into the duodenum through the *pancreatic duct.* The *endocrine tissue* of the pancreas consists of multiple small clusters of cells scattered throughout the gland called the *pancreatic islets* or **islets of Langerhans,** which discharge their secretions directly into the bloodstream. Each islet is composed of several different types of cells. The three main types are alpha cells, beta cells, and delta cells. *Alpha cells* secrete a hormone called *glucagon.* The more numerous *beta cells* secrete *insulin.* Both glucagon and insulin regulate the levels of glucose in the blood but have opposing effects. Glucagon raises blood glucose; insulin lowers it. *Delta cells* produce a hormone called *somatostatin,* which inhibits secretion of both glucagon and insulin. Three other relatively rare cell types also have been described, and they produce hormones concerned primarily with regulating gastrointestinal functions. Figure 22–1 shows the anatomy and cellular structure of the pancreas.

Structure and Function of the Pancreas

Acute Pancreatitis

Acute pancreatitis is caused by escape of pancreatic juice from the ducts into the substance of the pancreas. The pancreatic digestive enzymes in the juice cause widespread destruction of pancreatic tissue and severe hemorrhage (figure 22–2). Patients with acute pancreatitis have severe abdominal pain and are seriously ill; many such patients die.

The pathogenesis of acute pancreatitis usually involves active secretion of pancreatic juice while the pancreatic duct is obstructed at its entrance into the duodenum. The build-up of obstructed secretions greatly increases the pressure within the duct system, causing the ducts to rupture and the pancreatic juice to escape. Two factors predispose to acute pancreatitis: disease of the gallbladder and excessive alcohol consumption.

Pancreatitis often develops in patients with gallstones, because in most individuals the common bile duct and common pancreatic duct usually enter the duodenum through a common channel (the *ampulla of Vater*). If a stone becomes impacted in the ampulla, it can obstruct the pancreatic duct and precipitate pancreatitis.

Patients who drink excessive amounts of alcohol also are prone to pancreatitis. Alcohol is a potent stimulus of pancreatic secretions, and it may also induce edema and spasm of the pancreatic sphincter in the ampulla of Vater. Pancreatitis develops because alcohol-induced hypersecretion combined with sphincter spasm leads to high intraductal pressure, followed by duct necrosis and escape of pancreatic juice.

Pancreatitis

Chronic Pancreatitis

Occasionally, patients develop repeated episodes of mild inflammation within the pancreas, leading to progressive destruction of pancreatic tissue. This is called *chronic pancreatitis.*

FIGURE 22–1

A, Duct system of the pan-creas. The main duct usually joins the common bile duct, as shown here, to enter the duodenum by a single open-ing at the ampulla of Vater. Sometimes the two ducts have separate openings. There is often an accessory pancreatic duct, as illus-trated, that opens separately into the duodenum. **B,** Photomicrograph of islet surrounded by exocrine pancreatic tissue. More than a million islets are scattered throughout the pancreas. Alpha cells secrete glucagon. Beta cells secrete insulin. Delta cells secrete somato-statin. (Original magnifica-tion × 400.)

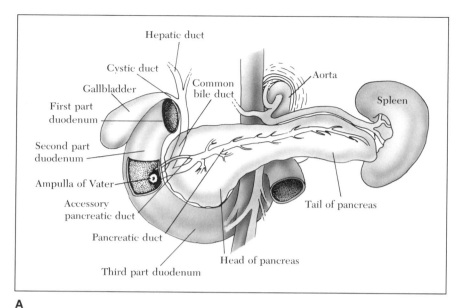

A

B

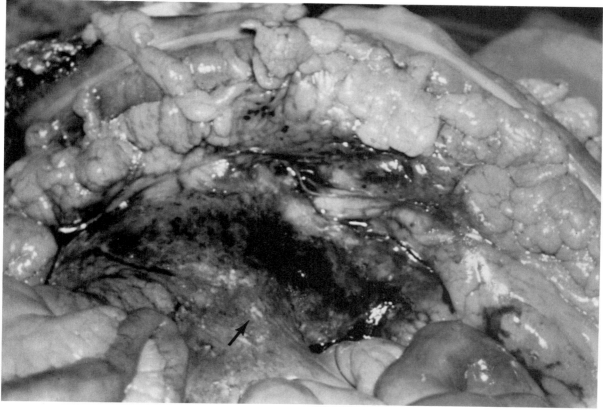

FIGURE 22–2

Acute pancreatitis. Transverse colon (*upper part of photograph*) has been elevated to reveal pancreas (*arrow*), which is inflamed and contains large areas of hemorrhage.

Cystic fibrosis is a relatively common, serious hereditary disease that is transmitted as an autosomal recessive trait and first becomes manifest in infancy and childhood. The disease has an incidence of about one per two thousand Whites but is quite rare in Blacks and other races. The abnormal gene involved in the disease results from a mutation of a normal gene called the *CF gene,* which codes for a cell-membrane–associated protein that regulates chloride transport across cell membranes. The gene has been localized to the long arm of chromosome 7, and screening tests have been developed that can detect carriers of the gene mutation responsible for most cases of cystic fibrosis. In some individuals, the disease is relatively mild and compatible with survival into adolescence or adult life. Others, with more severe disease, die in childhood. Modern treatment has improved survival but, nevertheless, more than 50 percent of patients with cystic fibrosis die before reaching the age of twenty-eight.

Cystic Fibrosis of the Pancreas

As a result of the gene mutation, there is defective transport across cell membranes of chloride, sodium, and the water molecules in which they are dissolved. Electrolyte and water secretion is deficient in the mucus secreted by the epithelial cells of the pancreas, bile ducts, mucosa of respiratory tract, and other mucus-secreting cells throughout the body. As a result, the mucus becomes abnormally thick and tends to precipitate, forming dense plugs that obstruct the pancreatic ducts, bronchi and bronchioles, and bile ducts.

The most significant structural abnormalities are usually in the pancreas. Mucous plugs in the small pancreatic ducts block the secretion of pancreatic juice, which accumulates under increased pressure within the obstructed ducts. Eventually, the ducts become cystically dilated. The pancreatic secretory cells, unable to discharge their secretions into the duodenum, undergo atrophy and are replaced by fibrous tissue, but the pancreatic islets are unaffected because they discharge their hormones directly into the bloodstream. Eventually, the pancreas becomes converted into a mass of cystically dilated ducts surrounded by dense fibrous tissue (figure 22–3). The name of the disease derives from these characteristic structural abnormalities.

In the lungs, the small bronchi and bronchioles become obstructed by the thick mucous secretions of the epithelial cells lining the respiratory tract. Bronchial obstruction predisposes to pulmonary infection, leading to bronchitis, bronchiectasis, and repeated bouts of pneumonia in the lung distal to the blocked bronchi. Eventually, the lungs are severely damaged by the repeated infections.

The function of sweat glands also is abnormal in cystic fibrosis. The sweat glands are unable to conserve sodium and chloride, and the sweat of affected individuals contains an excessively high salt concentration. This biochemical abnormality has served as the basis of a diagnostic test for cystic fibrosis called a *sweat test*. A small quantity of sweat is collected, and the sodium and chloride concentrations are determined. The salt concentration of the sweat is low in normal persons and high in persons with cystic fibrosis.

The discovery of the *CF* gene and its defective counterpart have stimulated active research efforts that may eventually lead to treatment of affected patients by "gene therapy" in which the patient's cells are supplied with normal CF genes to override the effect of the defective gene.

Diabetes Mellitus

Diabetes mellitus is a very common and important metabolic disease that results either because the pancreatic islets are incapable of secreting sufficient insulin or because the insulin is not being utilized efficiently. One of its major manifestations is an elevated level of glucose in the blood, which is called **hyperglycemia** (*hyper* = excess + *glyc* = sweet + *heme* = blood).

Diabetes is divided into two major groups, depending on whether the diabetes results from insulin deficiency or inadequate response to insulin. The former type is designated *insulin dependent* or *type I* diabetes. The latter is called *non-insulin dependent* or *type II* diabetes. Type I diabetes is sometimes called *juvenile-onset diabetes* because of its frequency in children,

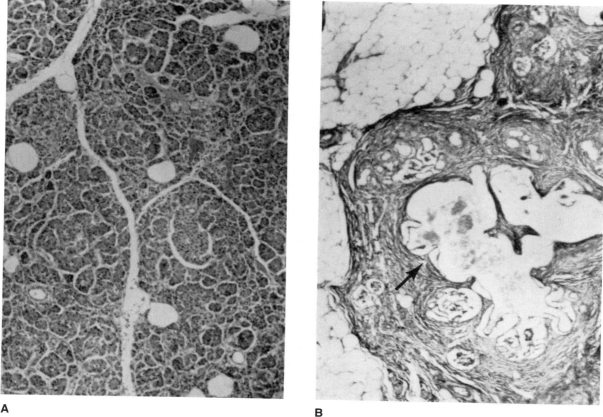

A

B

FIGURE 22–3

Low-magnification photomicrographs comparing normal pancreas (**A**) with pancreas of patient with cystic fibrosis (**B**). Duct in center of field (*arrow*) exhibits cystic dilatation. Most of pancreatic glandular tissue has undergone atrophy and has been replaced by fibrous tissue. (Original magnification × 25.)

and type II diabetes has been called *adult-onset* or *maturity-onset diabetes* because it usually develops in older adults. The two types of diabetes are not restricted to the age groups implied by this terminology, however, and these terms are used less frequently now.

Table 22–1 compares the major features of the two types.

Insulin Dependent (Type I) Diabetes

Insulin dependent diabetes usually results from damage or destruction of the pancreatic islets, leading to reduction or absence of insulin secretion. In some cases, onset of diabetes follows a viral infection, suggesting that the virus may have induced the disease by injuring or destroying the islets. Many patients with this type of diabetes have autoantibodies directed against their

TABLE 22-1

Comparison of two major
types of diabetes mellitus

	Insulin dependent (type I)	Non-Insulin dependent (type II)
Usual age of onset	Childhood Young adulthood	Middle age or later
Body build	Normal	Overweight
Plasma insulin	Absent or low	Normal or high
Complications	Ketoacidosis	Hyperosmolar coma
Response to insulin	Normal	Reduced
Response to oral antidiabetic drugs	Unresponsive	Responsive

own islet cells, indicating that an abnormal immune response may play a part in causing the disease. Type I diabetes occurs primarily in children and young adults, and affected subjects are prone to develop a condition called **diabetic ketosis** caused by lack of insulin. There is a hereditary predisposition to type I diabetes. Persons who inherit certain HLA-D types are at increased risk of acquiring this type of diabetes. (HLA types and predisposition to disease were considered in chapter 3.)

Non-Insulin Dependent (Type II) Diabetes

Non-insulin dependent diabetes is by far the more common type and is a more complex metabolic defect. The condition develops most frequently in older overweight and obese adults. The pancreatic islets secrete normal or increased amounts of insulin, but the tissues are relatively insensitive to the action of insulin and are unable to respond appropriately. (Inadequate response to insulin is called *insulin resistance.*) The reason for the impaired response to insulin is not completely understood, but it seems to be related in some way to obesity, because weight reduction restores insulin responsiveness and frequently controls the diabetes. Ketosis is not a complication of type II diabetes, but affected persons may develop another complication called **hyperosmolar coma,** which results from the marked hyperglycemia.

Although insulin resistance plays an important role in the pathogenesis of non-insulin dependent diabetes, islet cell function is not completely normal either, because the pancreas is unable to increase insulin output sufficiently to compensate for the insulin resistance.

Non-insulin dependent diabetes is a hereditary disease, in which genetic factors play an even greater role than in insulin dependent diabetes, although we do not yet know the exact mode of inheritance or the genes that predispose to this type of diabetes. Children of parents who have type II diabetes are at significant risk of also eventually becoming diabetic. In some population groups, such as the Pima Indians of Arizona, as many as 40 percent of adults are diabetic.

Actions of Insulin

Insulin has multiple effects that influence not only carbohydrate metabolism, but protein and fat metabolism as well. The chief sites of insulin action are on liver cells, muscle, and adipose tissue (fat). Insulin promotes entry of glucose into cells and favors utilization of glucose as a source of energy. In muscle and liver cells, it promotes storage of glucose as **glycogen.** In adipose tissue, insulin favors the conversion of glucose into fat (triglyceride) and storage of the newly formed triglyceride within the fat cells. Insulin also promotes entry of amino acids into the cells and stimulates protein synthesis. The main stimulus for insulin release is elevation of the level of glucose in the blood, as occurs after a meal.

Fat Metabolism and Formation of Ketone Bodies

When fat is metabolized as a source of energy, it is split first into **fatty acid** and glycerol. The fatty acid is broken down into two carbon-acetate fragments, which are combined with a large carrier molecule called *coenzyme A* (CoA). The combination is called **acetylcoenzyme A** or *acetyl-CoA.* Some of the acetyl-CoA molecules are normally converted by the liver into compounds called **ketone bodies:** acetoacetic acid, beta-hydroxybutyric acid, and acetone. *Acetoacetic acid* is formed by condensation of two acetyl-CoA molecules, with loss of coenzyme A. *Beta-hydroxybutyric acid* is formed by the addition of a hydrogen atom to an oxygen atom, which becomes converted into a hydroxyl (OH) group. The term *beta* designates the carbon atom to which the hydroxyl group is attached. The first carbon after the carboxyl (COOH) group is called the *alpha carbon,* and the second is the *beta carbon. Acetone* is formed by removal of the carboxyl group of acetoacetic acid (figure 22–4).

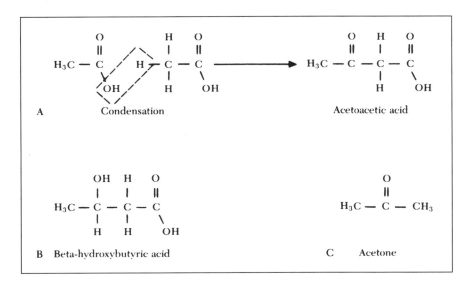

FIGURE 22–4

Structure of ketone bodies. **A,** Condensation of two acetyl-CoA molecules (illustrated as acetic acid) to form acetoacetic acid. **B,** Beta-hydroxybutyric acid, which is formed by reduction of the keto group to form a hydroxyl group. **C,** Acetone formed by dicarboxylation of acetoacetic acid.

Biochemical Disturbances in Diabetes

In diabetes mellitus, glucose is absorbed normally. However, because of lack of insulin or insulin insensitivity, it is not used normally for energy and is not stored normally as glycogen. Consequently, it accumulates in the bloodstream, resulting in a high level of blood glucose (**hyperglycemia**). The excessive glucose "spills over" in the urine and is excreted. Because glucose must be excreted in the urine in solution, the body loses excessive amounts of water and electrolytes. This may lead to disturbance in water balance and acid-base balance. (Water and electrolyte balance is discussed in chapter 24.)

Protein synthesis is also compromised, and body protein is broken down into amino acids. The liver converts these amino acids into glucose, augmenting the hyperglycemia and leading to additional losses of glucose, water, and electrolytes in the urine.

Diabetic Ketoacidosis

In insulin dependent diabetes, fat deposition in adipose tissue is impaired and body fat is mobilized as a source of energy. Large amounts of fatty acid are oxidized, producing acetyl-CoA molecules in such large quantities that they cannot be oxidized efficiently to yield energy. The excess acetyl-CoA molecules condense to form large quantities of ketone bodies, which also are produced in much greater quantities than can be metabolized. This condition is called **ketosis.** The ketone bodies accumulate in the blood and are excreted in the urine, carrying with them more water and electrolytes. The acid ketone bodies can be buffered to some extent by the bicarbonate buffer systems in the bloodstream. If the diabetes is extremely severe, however, so many ketone bodies may be produced that the buffer systems cannot maintain a normal blood pH and *diabetic acidosis* develops. The term *ketoacidosis* is often used for this type of acidosis because of its relation to overproduction of ketone bodies. Severe acidosis may lead to coma because acidosis has an adverse effect on cerebral function.

All these effects can be reversed by supplying insulin, which promotes normal utilization of glucose and storage of glycogen. The disturbances of fat and protein metabolism also are reversed by the action of insulin. Figure 22–5 summarizes the major metabolic disturbances in insulin dependent diabetes.

The following case illustrates the clinical and biochemical disturbances in severe diabetic ketoacidosis.

CASE 22–1

A middle-aged diabetic woman became unconscious while babysitting and was brought to the hospital by ambulance. Her temperature was moderately elevated. Respirations were rapid and deep. Blood pressure was normal. The patient was comatose but responded to painful stimuli. The skin was warm and dry. The remainder of the physical signs were normal. The patient's urine contained large amounts of glucose and a small amount of albumin. There was a strongly positive reaction for acetone and other ketone bodies. Blood glucose was 865 mg/dL (normal

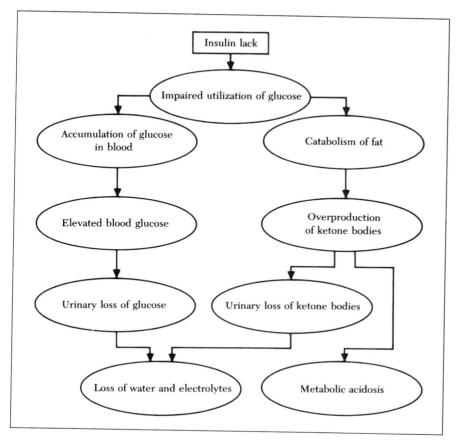

FIGURE 22–5

Major metabolic derangements in insulin-dependent diabetes.

range 70–110 mg/dL). Other laboratory studies revealed a low blood pH and reduced plasma bicarbonate of 8 mEq/L (normal range 24–28 mEq/L). The patient was considered to have severe diabetic acidosis probably precipitated by a respiratory infection. She received intensive treatment with intravenous fluids, insulin, and antibiotics. Her condition gradually improved. The following day she was conscious and oriented and was able to take fluids orally. She continued to improve and was eventually discharged from the hospital on a diabetic diet and supplementary insulin therapy.

Hyperosmolar Hyperglycemic Nonketotic Coma

Persons with non-insulin dependent diabetes mellitus may become comatose as a result of the extreme hyperosmolarity of body fluids that results from severe hyperglycemia in the absence of ketosis. (Osmotic pressure and osmolarity are considered in chapter 2 in connection with movement of materials into and out of cells.)

Although individuals with non-insulin dependent diabetes exhibit a reduced responsiveness to insulin, much less insulin is required to inhibit fat mobilization than is needed to promote entry of glucose into cells. In these subjects, the response to insulin is sufficient to prevent ketosis but inadequate to prevent hyperglycemia. Consequently, blood glucose rises, often to levels that are from ten to twenty times normal. (Normal blood glucose levels are 70–110 mg/dL.) The extreme hyperglycemia causes the osmolarity of the body fluids to rise significantly, and water moves by osmosis from the cells into the more concentrated extracellular fluids. The cells become dehydrated, which disturbs the function of neurons and causes coma. Treatment consists of supplying insulin to reduce the hyperglycemia and administering hypotonic fluids to help reduce the hyperosmolarity of the body fluids, as illustrated by the following case.

CASE 22–2

A fifty-two-year-old woman who was not previously known to be diabetic had experienced increased urinary output and thirst for the previous two weeks and had consumed large quantities of sugar-containing soft drinks. She became progressively more confused and eventually lapsed into coma. She was found by a neighbor and was brought to the hospital by ambulance. On admission she was comatose and dehydrated. Her respiratory rate was not increased. Blood pressure was normal. The urine contained a large amount of glucose but no ketone bodies. Blood pH and bicarbonate were normal. Blood glucose was 1750 mg/dL (normal range 70–110 mg/dL), and the osmolarity of the plasma was 396 mOsm/L (normal range 275–295 mOsm/L). A diagnosis of hyperosmolar nonketotic coma was made, and she was treated with large volumes of hypotonic (0.45%) saline solution and with insulin. Her condition gradually improved over the succeeding several days. Her blood glucose gradually fell toward normal and eventually reached 150 mg/dL on the fourth day. Plasma osmolarity also returned to normal as the elevated blood glucose declined.

Complications of Diabetes

Diabetics are liable to develop a number of complications that can be reduced to some extent by proper adherence to diet and other prescribed treatments. They have an *increased susceptibility to infection,* apparently related to the high levels of blood glucose. Pathogenic bacteria seem to grow more readily in the presence of elevated blood glucose levels. They may develop *diabetic coma,* as a result either of *ketoacidosis* or of the greatly *increased osmolarity* of body fluids resulting from hyperglycemia. They have a greater incidence of *arteriosclerosis* and its associated vascular complications such as strokes, heart attacks, and gangrene of the legs and feet as a result of poor circulation. The vascular problems probably result both from abnormalities in fat metabolism associated with diabetes and from the elevated blood lipids frequently found in diabetics. They are also subject to other late complications, which increase in frequency with the duration of the disease. The small blood vessels supplying the retina of the eye often undergo degenerative changes, which may eventually lead to *blindness* in some subjects. The glomerular arterioles and capillaries within the kidneys also undergo degenerative changes, which impair renal function and may result in *renal failure* (described in chapter 19). The peripheral nerves may undergo degenerative changes, called *peripheral neuritis,* which cause pain and disturbed sensation in the extremities.

Treatment of Diabetes

Treatment of diabetes consists of a diet in which carbohydrate intake is controlled. Insulin dependent diabetics also require insulin, and the dosage should be adjusted in order to control the level of blood glucose as closely as possible, because this appears to reduce late complications. Most insulin dependent diabetics require several insulin injections spaced throughout the day in order to maintain blood glucose within reasonably normal limits. Frequent measurements of blood glucose permit better regulation of insulin dosage and improve control of the diabetes. Products are available for home use that permit diabetics to monitor their own blood glucose. A drop of blood is drawn by a sterile disposable lancet, collected on a specially treated strip of paper, and inserted into an instrument that displays the glucose concentration.

Insulin pumps are a recent innovation that are sometimes useful for insulin-dependent diabetics who are difficult to treat because of their need for frequent insulin injections. An insulin pump is a small battery-operated device that can be attached to the patient's belt. A short length of tubing extends from the pump to a fine (27 gauge) needle that is inserted into the subcutaneous tissue of the abdominal wall and secured with tape. The pump is programmed to deliver a small constant infusion of insulin, supplemented by larger doses just before meals, simulating the release of insulin by the pancreas. Despite the convenience, use of an insulin pump requires very close medical supervision because complications can arise from pump malfunction or infections at the site of needle placement.

Non-insulin dependent diabetics can frequently be managed by diet and weight reduction alone; if they do not respond adequately, oral hypoglycemic drugs or insulin also may be prescribed. Oral hypoglycemic drugs act by promoting release of insulin from the pancreatic islets. They are useful only in non-insulin dependent (type II) diabetics, because the islets of insulin dependent (type I) diabetics are unable to produce insulin and therefore cannot respond to the drug.

Although oral hypoglycemic agents can lower blood glucose and control type II diabetes in many patients who do not respond adequately to diet and weight reduction, they are less effective than insulin, and many patients do not respond adequately to these agents. In other patients, oral hypoglycemic agents control blood glucose initially, but eventually they become ineffective. For these reasons, many physicians recommend that insulin rather than oral hypoglycemic drugs be used to treat type II diabetic patients who cannot be managed adequately by diet and weight reduction. Oral hypoglycemic agents are reserved for patients who are unable to use insulin because of some physical disability, such as blindness or severe arthritis, that makes self-administration of insulin impractical.

Other Causes of Hyperglycemia

Other conditions at times may lead to impaired glucose utilization and hyperglycemia, but they are much less common than true diabetes mellitus. These conditions include:

1. Chronic pancreatic disease, in which the hyperglycemia results from damage or destruction of pancreatic islets
2. Endocrine diseases associated with overproduction of pituitary or adrenal hormones, because these hormones act in various ways to raise blood glucose
3. Ingestion of many different drugs, such as diuretics or antihypertensive drugs, in which glucose utilization is impaired as a side effect of the drug
4. A few rare hereditary diseases in which carbohydrate metabolism is disturbed

Hypoglycemia

The normal pancreas continually monitors the blood glucose and automatically adjusts its output of insulin to maintain the blood glucose level within the normal range. The insulin-dependent diabetic patient, however, must adjust the dose of insulin to match the amount of carbohydrate to be metabolized. If there is insufficient insulin, the blood glucose is too high. If there is too much insulin, the blood glucose is too low, a condition called *hypoglycemia* (*hypo* = under). Two conditions predispose to hypoglycemia in a diabetic patient taking insulin. The first is a reduced intake of food, such as skipping a meal; blood glucose falls because carbohydrate intake is insufficient in relation to the amount of insulin injected. The second condition is increased activity, such as vigorous exercise, which lowers blood glucose by increasing glucose utilization. As a result, there is a relative excess of insulin. Too much insulin causes a precipitous drop in the level of glucose in the blood and initiates a chain of events called an *insulin reaction* or *insulin shock*. The adrenal medulla responds to the hypoglycemia by discharging epinephrine (adrenaline), which tends to raise blood glucose by converting liver glycogen into glucose. Epinephrine exerts widespread systemic effects as well: rapid heart rate, rise in blood pressure, constriction of cutaneous blood vessels causing the skin to appear pale, stimulation of sweat glands causing a cold sweat, and stimulation of the nervous system leading to increased excitability, anxiousness, hyperactive reflexes, and tremors.

Neurologic manifestations appear if the blood glucose continues to fall, because the nervous system requires glucose to carry out its metabolic processes and begins to malfunction when deprived of its energy source. The subject becomes confused, loses consciousness, may have convulsions, and soon lapses into a deep coma. Prolonged severe hypoglycemia may cause permanent brain damage.

If the patient is still conscious and able to swallow, the insulin reaction can be stopped by ingesting a quick-acting carbohydrate, such as a piece of candy or a glucose tablet. The diabetic patient should always have a quick-acting carbohydrate available for such emergencies. If the patient is unconscious, an injection of glucagon can be given; this raises blood glucose by mobilizing glucose from liver glycogen. A concentrated glucose solution may also be given intravenously.

Table 22–2 compares the clinical manifestations of insulin shock with those of diabetic ketoacidosis and hyperosmolar nonketotic coma, two other conditions to which the diabetic patient is predisposed.

Severe hypoglycemic reactions can also be caused by oral hypoglycemic drugs. Rarely, nondiabetic persons with emotional problems may deliberately ingest oral hypoglycemic drugs or inject themselves with insulin. They then consult a physician or enter a hospital emergency room with manifestations of severe hypoglycemia. If the possibility of self-induced hypoglycemia is suspected, special laboratory tests can determined the level of insulin in the blood. Tests can also determine whether the insulin in the patient's blood was secreted by the patient's own pancreas or is the type of insulin that is used by diabetic patients. Unfortunately, tests to identify oral hypoglycemic drugs in the blood are not readily available.

Diagnostic feature	Insulin shock	Ketoacidosis	Hyperosmolar coma
Food intake	May be insufficient	Normal or excessive	Normal or excessive
Insulin	Excessive	Insufficient	Normal or increased
Onset of symptoms	Rapid	Gradual (several days)	Gradual (several days)
Skin	Cold sweat, pale	Dry and flushed	Dry and flushed
Respirations	Normal or shallow	Slow and deep	Usually normal
Reflexes	Hyperactive	Depressed	Normal
Heart rate	Rapid	Rapid	Usually normal
Blood pressure	Normal or slightly elevated	Low	Usually normal
Glucose in urine	Absent	Large amount	Large amount
Blood glucose	Very low	High	Extremely high
Blood bicarbonate and pH	Normal	Low	Normal
Acetone in blood and urine	Absent	Present	Absent

TABLE 22–2

Differentiation of insulin shock from ketoacidosis and hyperosmolar coma

Tumors of the Pancreas

Carcinoma of the pancreas is relatively common and develops most often in the head of the pancreas. In this location, the neoplasm blocks the common bile duct, resulting in obstructive jaundice. Carcinoma elsewhere in the pancreas is usually far advanced when first detected and produces no specific symptoms.

Sometimes, benign tumors arise from the islet cells and produce symptoms as a result of overproduction of hormones. Beta cells give rise to insulin-secreting tumors that cause episodes of severe hypoglycemia similar to those experienced by a diabetic who receives too much insulin.

Questions for Review

1. What is the difference between acute and chronic pancreatitis?

2. What are the major metabolic disturbances in insulin dependent (type I) diabetes? How does insulin correct these disturbances?

3. What are the major complications of diabetes?

4. Which type of diabetes can be treated by diet alone?

5. What is meant by the following terms: *sweat test, hyperosmolar nonketotic hyperglycemic coma, ketoacidosis,* and *ketone bodies?*

6. What is cystic fibrosis of the pancreas? What are its clinical manifestations? What is its pattern of inheritance?

7. What is hypoglycemia? What are its clinical manifestations? How is it treated?

8. What are the major differences between diabetic ketoacidosis and insulin shock?

Supplementary Readings

Bantle, J. P. 1988. The dietary treatment of diabetes mellitus. *Medical Clinics of North America* 72:1285–99. Describes dietary measures needed to manage patients. Weight control essential in managing type II patients but difficult to achieve. See also other articles in this same issue dealing with various other aspects of diabetes.

Chong, G. L., and Thibodeau, S. N. 1990. A simple assay for the screening of the cystic fibrosis allele in carriers of the Phe[508] deletion mutation. *Mayo Clinic Proceedings* 65:1072–76. The major mutation accounting for about 70 percent of cystic fibrosis cases has been identified. A method for screening carriers of this mutation is described.

Diabetes Control and Complications Trial Research Group. 1993. The effect of intensive treatment on the development and progression of long-term complications in insulin-dependent diabetes mellitus. *New England Journal of Medicine* 329:977–86. Intensive therapy delays the onset and slows the progression of eye, kidney, and nervous-system complications in patients with diabetes.

Dobersen, M. J., et al. 1980. Cytotoxic autoantibodies to beta cells in the serum of patients with insulin dependent diabetes mellitus. *New England Journal of Medicine* 303:1493–98. Information supporting the autoimmune basis of diabetes in some patients.

Foster, D. W. 1994. Diabetes mellitus. In *Harrison's principles of internal medicine.* 13th ed. Ed. K. J. Isselbacher, E. Braunwald, J. D. Wilson, J. B. Martin, A. S. Fauci, and D. I. Kasper, pp. 1979–99. New York: McGraw-Hill. Reviews pathogenesis, pathophysiology, and related subjects.

Herold, K. C., and Rubenstein, A. H. 1988. Immunosuppression for insulin-dependent diabetes. *New England Journal of Medicine* 318:701–3. Type I diabetes mellitus associated with autoantibodies responds to immunosuppressive therapy. In favorable cases, remission can be maintained with continued administration of immunosuppressive agents but poses the risk of toxicity from long-term use of these agents.

Nathan, D. M. 1995. Diabetes mellitus. In *Scientific American medicine.* Ed. D. C. Dale and D. D. Federman, Section 9, Metabolism. New York: Scientific American, Inc. A comprehensive discussion of this important disease.

Pimenta, W., Korytkowski, M., Mitrakou, A., et al. 1995. Pancreatic beta-cell dysfunction as the primary genetic lesion in NIDDM. *Journal of the American Medical Association* 273:1855–61. In this group of patients with non-insulin dependent diabetes, defects in insulin secretion were demonstrated before defects in insulin sensitivity were manifest.

Rother, K. I., and Schwenk, W. F. 1994. Effect of rehydration fluid with 75 mmol/L of sodium on serum sodium concentration and serum osmolality in young patients with diabetic ketoacidosis. *Mayo Clinic Proceedings* 69:1149–53. Article describes controversies regarding the composition of rehydration fluids used to treat patients with diabetic ketoacidosis and the role of rehydration in the development of brain edema.

Thorp, F. K. 1986. Insulin pump therapy reconsidered. *Journal of the American Medical Association* 255:645–46. Rationale, applications, limitations, and complications of insulin pump therapy.

Viberti, G., Mogensen, C. E., Groop, L. C., et al. 1994. Effect of captopril on progression to clinical proteinuria in patients with insulin-dependent diabetes mellitus and microalbuminuria. *Journal of the American Medical Association* 271:275–79. The angiotensin-converting enzyme inhibitor (captopril) slows the progression of diabetic kidney disease.

Weir, G. C. 1995. Which comes first in non-insulin-dependent diabetes mellitus: Insulin resistance or beta-cell failure? Both come first. (editorial). *Journal of the American Medical Association* 273:1878–79. This type of diabetes results from a mix of genetic and environmental factors which vary among different racial and ethnic groups.

Yoon, J. W., et al. 1979. Virus induced diabetes mellitus: Isolation of a virus from the pancreas of a child with diabetic ketoacidosis. *New England Journal of Medicine* 300:1173–79. A detailed investigative study.

Chapter 22 ▪ Outline Summary

Structure and Function of the Pancreas / 641
Exocrine Function
Secretes digestive enzymes.

Endocrine Function
Islet alpha cells secrete glucagon: raise blood glucose.

Islet beta cells secrete insulin: lower blood glucose.

Islet delta cells secrete somatostatin, which inhibits insulin and glucagon secretion.

Pancreatitis / 641
Acute Pancreatitis
Pancreatic juice escapes from ducts and digests pancreas.

Serious illness with high mortality.

Chronic Pancreatitis
Mild inflammation leading to progressive destruction of pancreatic tissue.

Cystic Fibrosis of the Pancreas / 643
Incidence
One in two thousand Whites, transmitted as autosomal recessive.

Rare in Blacks and other races.

Pathogenesis
Responsible gene identified.

Tests available to identify carrier.

Cell dysfunction leads to thick mucus that plugs ducts.

Obstruction of pancreatic ducts causes atrophy and fibrosis of pancreas.

Obstruction of bronchi causes lung injury.

Obstruction of biliary ducts causes liver scarring.

Sweat Test in Cystic Fibrosis
Sweat gland function abnormal.

High concentration of sodium and chloride in sweat is basis of diagnostic test.

Diabetes Mellitus / 644
Insulin Dependent (Type I) Diabetes
As a result of damage or destruction of islets.

Insulin secretion reduced or absent.

Develops chiefly in children and young adults.

Ketosis prone.

Non-Insulin Dependent (Type II) Diabetes
More common type.

Insulin secretion normal or increased.

Tissues insensitive to insulin.

Not associated with ketosis.

Fat Metabolism and Formation of Ketone Bodies
Catabolism of fat yields acetate fragments (Acetyl-CoA).

Converted by liver into ketone bodies.

Biochemical Disturbances in Diabetes
Glucose absorbed but not utilized normally and accumulates in blood.

Excreted in urine with water and electrolytes.

Protein catabolism yields more glucose.

Ketoacidosis in insulin dependent diabetics.

Hyperosmolar nonketotic coma in non-insulin dependent diabetics.

Amount of insulin sufficient to prevent ketosis but not enough to prevent hyperglycemia.

Hyperosmolarity of extracellular fluid as a result of hyperglycemia causes cellular dehydration.

Complications of Diabetes

Increased susceptibility to infection.

Diabetic coma.

Ketoacidosis.

Hyperosmolar coma.

Arteriosclerosis.

Blindness.

Renal failure.

Peripheral neuritis.

Treatment

Diet.

Insulin required for type I diabetes.

Oral hypoglycemic drugs or insulin for type II diabetes not controlled adequately by diet alone.

Hypoglycemia / 652

Pathogenesis and Manifestations in Type I Diabetic Subjects

Excessive insulin in relation to food intake.

As glucose falls, epinephrine is released by adrenal medulla, which mobilizes glucose from hepatic glycogen and exerts widespread systemic effects.

Neurologic manifestations occur because neurons are deprived of glucose, which is required for normal function.

Prolonged hypoglycemia causes permanent brain damage.

Treatment

Give oral carbohydrate if subject is conscious and able to swallow.

Inject glucagon or intravenous glucose solution if subject is unconscious.

Other Causes of Hypoglycemia

Oral hypoglycemic drugs in type II diabetic patients.

Self-administration of oral hypoglycemic drugs or insulin by emotionally disturbed persons.

Rarely, islet cell tumor of pancreas.

Tumors of the Pancreas / 654

Carcinoma of Pancreas

Usually develops in head of pancreas.

Blockage of common bile duct causes obstructive jaundice.

Islet Cell Tumors

Beta cell tumors produce hyperinsulinism.

The Gastrointestinal Tract

Learning Objectives

1. Identify the major types of cleft lip and cleft palate deformity.
2. Explain the pathogenesis of dental caries and periodontal disease and describe prevention and treatment.
3. Name the common congenital abnormalities of the gastrointestinal tract, describe their clinical manifestations, and explain methods of diagnosis and treatment.
4. Name and describe the three most common lesions of the esophagus that lead to esophageal obstruction.
5. Explain the pathogenesis of peptic ulcer. Describe the three major complications of peptic ulcer and their treatment. Name the methods of treatment.
6. Describe the common types of chronic and acute enteritis and their clinical manifestations.
7. Differentiate between appendicitis and Meckel's diverticulitis in terms of pathogenesis, clinical manifestations, and treatment.
8. Describe the pathogenesis of diverticulitis and explain the role of diet in development of the lesion.
9. Name the causes, clinical manifestations, and complications of intestinal obstruction, carcinoma of the colon, and diverticulosis of the colon. Explain their treatment.

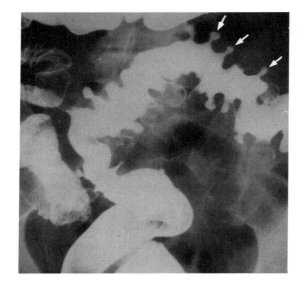

Chapter 23 ▪ Contents

The gastrointestinal tract, which is concerned with the digestion and absorption of food, comprises the oral cavity and related parts of the face, the esophagus, the stomach, the small and large intestines, and the anus.

Embryologically, the face and palate are formed by coalescence of proliferating masses of cells that merge to form the facial structures and to separate the nasal cavity from the mouth. In the upper part of the face, the areas of coalescence are located on either side of the midline in a line that passes through the upper lip and jaw and extends into each nostril. The palate is formed by two shelflike masses of tissue that grow medially and fuse in the midline to close the communication between nose and mouth. If these developmental processes are disturbed, defects may result in the upper lip and jaw (**cleft lip**) or in the palate (**cleft palate**).

Cleft lip and palate are common abnormalities that frequently occur in combination. The incidence of these abnormalities is about one per one thousand births.

Both cleft lip and cleft palate follow a *multifactorial pattern of inheritance* (described in chapter 9). The incidence is significantly higher among the children of parents who have previously given birth to an infant with a cleft lip or palate and among the children of parents who themselves have a cleft lip or palate.

Cleft lip may be unilateral or bilateral and may range in severity from a relatively minor defect in the mucosa of the lip to a large cleft extending deeply into the upper jaw. In the most severe deformity, the cleft extends completely through the upper jaw into the floor of the nose (*complete cleft*) and may also extend posteriorly into the palate (figure 23–1). Large bilateral clefts extending into the palate completely separate the hard palate from the midline tissue that forms part of the upper jaw, and the separated tissue is

Cleft Lip and Cleft Palate

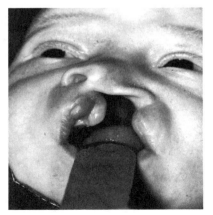

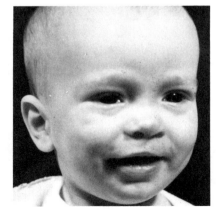

A
B

FIGURE 23–1

A, Widely cleft lip and palate in two-week-old infant. **B,** Same child at fourteen months of age after surgical correction of defect.

FIGURE 23–2

A, Complete bilateral cleft lip and cleft palate with anterior protrusion of tissues between clefts. **B,** Same child at eighteen months of age after surgical correction of defect.

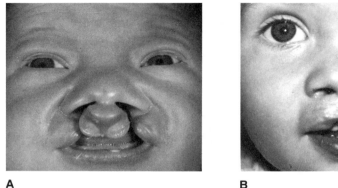

A

B

FIGURE 23–3

Types of cleft lip and palate abnormalities viewed from below. **A,** Unilateral cleft lip extending into the nose but not extending posteriorly into the palate. **B,** Bilateral cleft lip extending into the nose but not extending into the palate. **C,** Bilateral cleft lip extending into the nose and palate. **D,** Midline cleft palate. **E,** Cleft palate with unilateral cleft lip extending into the nose. **F,** Cleft palate with bilateral cleft lip extending into the nose.

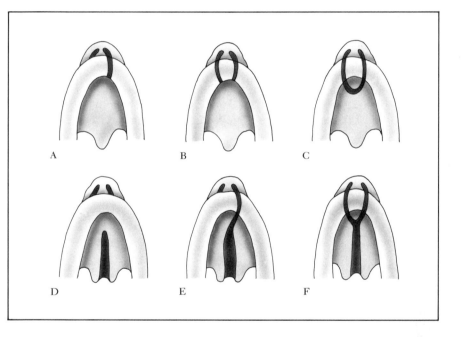

often displaced forward (figure 23–2). Midline cleft palate may occur as an isolated abnormality, but it is usually associated with unilateral or bilateral cleft lip. Figure 23–3 illustrates the various types of cleft lip and palate that are encountered clinically.

Treatment   Although cleft lip and palate frequently occur together, they are corrected surgically at different times. Generally, cleft lip is repaired very soon after birth. Repair of cleft palate is generally deferred until the child is between one and two years old. Once the cleft palate is repaired, speech therapy is begun in early childhood to correct the nasal quality that often results from abnormal palatal function.

The *teeth* are specialized structures developed in the tissues of the jaws. Each tooth consists of a solid portion called **dentine,** which forms the bulk of the tooth; an enamel *crown* covering the exposed surface of the tooth; and a central *pulp cavity* containing nerve fibers, lymphatics, and blood vessels. The *root* of the tooth, which is embedded in the jaw, is covered by a thin layer of bonelike tissue called *cementum,* and the tooth is anchored in the jaw by dense connective-tissue fibers.

There are two sets of teeth. The first set, called the *temporary* or *deciduous teeth,* consists of a total of twenty teeth (ten in each jaw) that erupt in childhood. Eventually, these temporary teeth are replaced by a second, permanent set of thirty-two teeth. When the *permanent teeth* begin to grow, they press against the roots of the temporary teeth. This causes resorption of the roots and loosening of the temporary teeth, which eventually fall out and are replaced by the permanent teeth.

Each deciduous and permanent tooth develops from a separate *tooth bud,* which is composed of two parts, one that forms the crown and a second that gives rise to the remainder of the tooth. The deciduous teeth are formed before birth and erupt during childhood. The permanent teeth do not begin to develop until after birth and erupt at various times in late childhood and adolescence. Calcium is deposited in the dentine and enamel of the tooth as it is being formed.

Missing Teeth and Extra Teeth

Absence of one or more teeth is relatively common and is often a familial trait that follows a multifactorial pattern of inheritance (figure 23–4). It results from failure of one or more tooth buds to develop. Sometimes an extra tooth bud forms, resulting in an extra tooth.

Abnormalities of Tooth Development

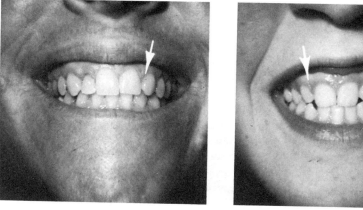

A **B**

FIGURE 23–4

Congenital absence of teeth. **A,** Mother lacks left lateral incisor (*arrow*). Left canine (cuspid) tooth is located lateral to left central incisor. Compare appearance of left side with opposite side in which all teeth are present. **B,** Daughter lacks both lateral incisors. Canine teeth (*arrows*) are adjacent to the central incisors.

Abnormalities of Tooth Enamel Caused by Tetracycline

Enamel forms within the developing teeth at specific times. If the antibiotic *tetracycline* is administered while enamel is being formed in the teeth, the antibiotic is deposited with calcium in the enamel and causes permanent yellow-gray to brown discoloration in the crowns. The antibiotic may also disturb the formation of the enamel. If a tetracycline antibiotic is taken by a pregnant woman, the drug crosses the placenta and enters the fetal circulation, where it becomes incorporated in the enamel of the developing teeth. If administered to infants and children, tetracycline is deposited in the crowns of the permanent teeth that are undergoing enamel formation at the time the antibiotic is ingested. Therefore, it is recommended that tetracycline antibiotics not be given to pregnant women or to infants and children during the time when enamel is forming in the developing permanent teeth. This period extends through infancy and childhood to about the age of eight years.

Dental Caries and Its Complications

Caries, the term for tooth decay, is a Latin word meaning *dry rot.* The condition is a decalcification of the tooth structure caused by mouth bacteria acting on bits of retained food material, such as sugar and highly refined, starchy foods. Bacterial fermentation liberates organic acids that erode the covering enamel, exposing the underlying dentine, which is attacked by the acids and invaded by mouth bacteria. The loss of tooth structure that results from the combined acid and bacterial action is called a dental **cavity.** The affected area appears discolored and is quite soft when probed with a dental instrument. Dental x-rays reveal the cavity as an area of decreased density in the affected tooth.

If the cavity is not treated and continues to enlarge, the decay eventually reaches the dental pulp. The bacteria invade the pulp and incite an inflammation that causes the throbbing pain characteristic of a toothache. Unchecked, the infection may spread to the apex of the tooth root, which is embedded in the jawbone, and from there spread to the bone surrounding the dental root. The result may be an abscess surrounding the apex of the tooth, which is called a *periapical abscess* (*peri* = around).

Prevention and Treatment

The incidence of tooth decay can be reduced by proper mouth hygiene, including frequent brushing of the teeth and use of dental floss to remove food particles that promote bacterial growth. Fluoride added to water supplies and toothpaste helps to prevent cavities by promoting formation of a more acid-resistant tooth structure that resists decay. Dental caries is treated by removing the decayed area and packing the defect with some type of dental filling material. Once infection of the pulp and dental root has occurred, more extensive treatment is required. Antibiotics may be needed if there is an acute infection or abscess at the apex of the tooth. After the infection is under control, the entire pulp cavity must be cleaned out and packed with dental filling material, a procedure called a *root canal treatment*. Sometimes the tooth cannot be salvaged and must be extracted.

Masses of bacteria and debris accumulating around the base of the teeth may incite an inflammation. Initially, the inflammation affects only the gums surrounding the roots of the teeth, which is called *gingivitis* (*gingiva* = gum). Later, the inflammation extends between the teeth and the adjacent gums, leading to the formation of small pockets of infection between the teeth and gums. This condition is called periodontal disease (*peri* = around + *dens* = tooth). If pus is discharged from the margins of the infected gums, the descriptive term *pyorrhea* (*pyo* = pus + *rhea* = flow) is often used. The infection may spread into the tooth sockets that anchor the teeth in the jawbone, causing the teeth to loosen and eventually fall out. Various methods of treatment to the gums and teeth may control or arrest the condition, which is an important cause of loss of teeth.

Periodontal Disease

An inflammation of the oral cavity is called **stomatitis** (*stoma* = mouth). It may be caused by a number of irritants and infectious agents. Common irritants are alcohol, tobacco, and hot or spicy foods. Infectious agents include the herpes virus and some other viruses, the fungus *Candida albicans* (which also causes vaginal infections), and certain bacteria that cause a type of infection called *trench mouth* or *Vincent's infection*.

Inflammation of the Oral Cavity

Carcinoma of the oral cavity, which may arise from the squamous epithelium of the lips, cheek, tongue, palate, or back of the throat, is relatively common (figure 23–5). It is treated by surgical resection or by radiation therapy.

Tumors of the Oral Cavity

The esophagus is a muscular tube extending from the pharynx to the stomach with sphincters at both upper and lower ends. The upper sphincter relaxes to allow passage of swallowed food, which is propelled down the esophagus by rhythmic peristaltic contractions. The lower esophageal sphincter (called the *gastroesophageal* or *cardiac sphincter*) relaxes when the food reaches the lower end of the esophagus and allows the food to pass into the stomach. Some of the more important conditions affecting the esophagus include

Diseases of the Esophagus

1. Failure of the lower (cardiac) sphincter to function properly
2. Tears in the lining of the esophagus from retching and vomiting
3. Esophageal obstruction as a result of carcinoma, food impaction, or stricture

FIGURE 23–5

Squamous cell carcinoma of oral mucosa (*arrow*) which appears as an irregular overgrowth of tissue arising from the mucosa of the cheek.

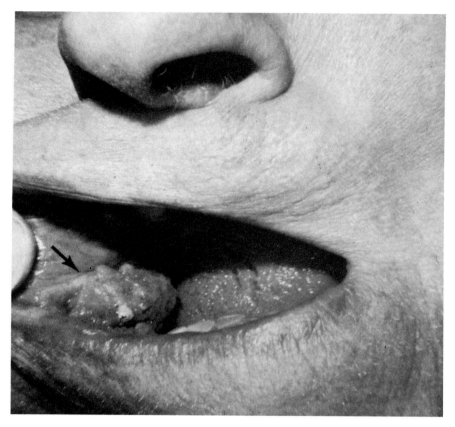

Symptoms of esophageal disease include difficulty in swallowing (*dysphagia*) together with variable degrees of substernal discomfort or pain. Complete obstruction of the esophagus leads to inability to swallow, which is often associated with regurgitation of food into the trachea, causing episodes of choking and coughing.

Cardiac Sphincter Dysfunction

The two major disturbances of cardiac sphincter dysfunction are failure of the cardiac sphincter to open properly, which is called *cardiospasm,* and inability of the sphincter to remain closed properly, which is called an *incompetent cardiac sphincter,* and leads to a condition called *reflux esophagitis.*

Cardiospasm

If the cardiac sphincter fails to open properly, food cannot pass normally into the stomach and the smooth muscle in the wall of the esophagus must contract more vigorously to force the food past the constricted sphincter. Eventually, the muscle undergoes marked hypertrophy, and the esophagus becomes dilated proximal to the constricted sphincter because of retention of food. Treatment consists of periodic stretching of the constricted sphincter by means of an instrument introduced into the esophagus or by surgically cutting the muscle fibers in the constricted area.

Incompetent Cardiac Sphincter and Its Complications

In this relatively common condition, acid gastric juice leaks back into the esophagus through the improperly closed incompetent lower esophageal sphincter. The squamous epithelial lining of the esophagus, which was not "designed" to tolerate high-acid secretions, becomes irritated and inflamed, which is called **reflux esophagitis.** In some patients the squamous mucosal lining may actually become ulcerated and scarred. Sometimes the squamous lining responds to the acidity by undergoing a change (*metaplasia*) into a more acid-resistant columnar gastric type mucosa. This condition, which is called *Barrett's esophagus* after the person who first described it, may lead to additional problems. Unfortunately, the metaplastic columnar epithelium is frequently abnormal and poses an increased risk of developing adenocarcinoma arising in the abnormal columnar epithelium. Treatment of reflux esophagitis consists of avoiding lying down soon after eating because the recumbent position promotes reflux, sleeping with the head of the bed elevated to minimize reflux, and avoiding alcoholic beverages because alcohol tends to relax the lower esophageal sphincter, which facilitates reflux.

Gastric Mucosal Tears

Retching and vomiting may cause lacerations in the mucosa of the gastroesophageal junction, where the esophagus passes through the diaphragm, or in the lining of the distal esophagus, which can lead to profuse bleeding. The repetitive, intermittent vigorous contractions of the abdominal muscles associated with vomiting raise intraabdominal pressure and forcefully jam the upper part (*cardia*) of the stomach against the opening in the diaphragm through which the esophagus passes, causing tears in the mucosa. The additional stresses resulting from vigorous contractions of the muscular walls of the stomach and esophagus associated with vomiting probably place additional stress on the mucosa, which also plays a role in causing the laceration. This vomiting-related complication most often follows the retching and vomiting related to excess alcohol intake but may follow vomiting from any cause, including self-induced vomiting to control weight.

Esophageal Obstruction

Carcinoma of the Esophagus

Carcinoma may arise anywhere in the esophagus, either from the squamous epithelium or from the columnar epithelium associated with Barrett's esophagus. The tumor gradually narrows the lumen of the esophagus, frequently infiltrates the surrounding tissues, and may invade the trachea. Necrosis of the tumor extending between the esophagus and trachea may lead to the formation of an abnormal communication between these two structures called a *tracheo-esophageal fistula* (*fistula* = tube).

Food Impaction

Obstruction of the esophagus may be caused by impaction of poorly chewed meat in the distal part of the esophagus. This is sometimes encountered in persons who are unable to chew their food properly because they have poor teeth or improperly fitting dentures or who have poor eating habits.

Stricture

A stricture is a narrowing caused by scar tissue. Reflux esophagitis with ulceration and scarring may lead to a stricture. Esophageal scarring may also result from accidentally or deliberately swallowing a corrosive chemical that causes necrosis and inflammation. Severe scarring eventually follows. A common cause of esophageal stricture in children is accidental swallowing of commercial lye solutions (used for cleaning clogged drains).

Gastritis

Inflammation of the stomach is called *gastritis,* and the inflammation may be either acute or chronic. Many patients with gastritis have few symptoms, but some experience abdominal discomfort and nausea.

Acute Gastritis

In most cases, acute gastritis is a self-limited inflammation of short duration. However, at times, the acute inflammation may be quite severe and may be complicated by ulceration of the mucosa with bleeding from the ulcerated areas. Patients in whom the acute gastritis is associated with mucosal ulceration often have more pronounced symptoms, and the ulcerated areas may bleed profusely.

There are many causes of acute gastritis, but most are caused by nonsteroidal anti-inflammatory drugs such as aspirin, ibuprofen, and naproxen. These drugs are widely used to treat symptoms of arthritis and related musculoskeletal pain problems. They act by suppressing the synthesis of prostaglandins, which are potent mediators of inflammation (as described in chapter 4). Prostaglandins, however, are produced by many different types of cells and have many different functions. Those produced by gastric epithelial cells help protect the stomach from the damaging effects of gastric acid by promoting the secretion not only of sodium bicarbonate to counteract the acid, but also of mucin to coat and protect the stomach lining. Nonsteroidal anti-inflammatory drugs reduce inflammation by inhibiting the synthesis of prostaglandin mediators of inflammation, but they also inhibit the synthesis of the prostaglandins that help protect the gastric mucosa. Consequently, the mucosa becomes more vulnerable to injury from acidic gastric juice, which may lead to acute inflammation of the mucosa and may even be followed by mucosal ulceration with bleeding.

Excess ingestion of alcoholic beverages is another common cause of acute gastritis because the alcohol is a gastric irritant and also stimulates gastric acid secretion.

Chronic Gastritis

Recent evidence indicates that many cases of chronic gastritis are related to growth (colonization) of a small, curved, gram-negative organism called *Helicobacter pylori* on the surface of the gastric mucosa. This unique organism grows in the layer of mucus covering the epithelial cells lining the stomach, where it can be identified by special bacterial stains, by culture, or by other specialized tests. The organism produces an enzyme called urease that decomposes urea, a normal by-product of protein metabolism that is present in small amounts in blood and body fluids. Decomposition of urea yields ammonia, a substance that neutralizes the gastric acid and allows the organism to flourish in an acid environment that would destroy other bacteria. *Helicobacter* also produces enzymes that can break down the layer of protective mucus that covers the epithelial surface. Presumably, the chronic gastritis is caused by the ammonia and other products produced by the organism that damage the gastric mucosa of susceptible persons.

Colonization of the gastric mucosa by *Helicobacter pylori* is very common, and not all persons who harbor the organism have chronic gastritis. Moreover, many persons harbor the organism, and the frequency of bacterial colonization increases with age. It is estimated that as many as 65 percent of persons over age sixty-five harbor the organism.

Peptic Ulcer

Peptic ulcer is a chronic ulcer that usually involves the distal stomach or proximal duodenum (figure 23–6).

Why peptic ulceration begins is not completely understood, but the immediate cause of the ulceration appears to be digestion of the mucosa by acidic gastric juice. Persons who secrete large volumes of acidic gastric juice are prone to ulcers.

The initial event is probably a small, superficial erosion of the gastric or duodenal mucosa. Gastric acid and pepsin begin to digest the deeper tissues, which have been denuded of covering epithelium. Attempts at healing in the presence of continuing digestion eventually lead to considerable scarring at the base of the ulcer. Clinically, ulcers produce pain that is usually relieved by ingestion of food or antacids that neutralize the gastric acid.

Helicobacter pylori, the same organism that is associated with chronic gastritis, also seems to play a role in the pathogenesis of both gastric and duodenal ulcers. Presumably the organism injures the mucosa and initiates the mucosal erosion that eventually develops into a chronic ulcer. The role of *Helicobacter* in causing a gastric ulcer is understandable, because this is the same organism that causes the mucosal damage leading to chronic gastritis. Its role in causing duodenal ulcers is more difficult to explain because

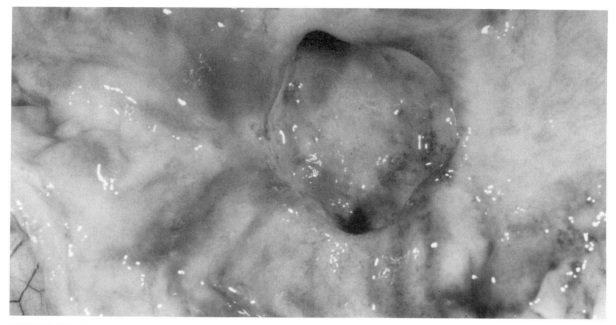

FIGURE 23–6

Large peptic ulcer of duodenum.

the organism characteristically colonizes gastric mucosa, not duodenal mucosa. Some investigators have speculated that there are small areas of gastric epithelial cells in the duodenum where the organism can grow and damage the duodenal mucosa, making it more susceptible to ulceration. An alternative explanation postulates that the organism does not damage the duodenal mucosa directly, but does so indirectly because the *Helicobacter*-induced gastritis causes the gastric mucosa to secrete excess acid, and it is the hyperacidity that causes the duodenal ulcers. According to this concept, the mucosal damage caused by the gastritis disturbs various functions of gastric mucosal cells that regulate gastric acid secretion and causes the mucosa to secrete excess acid.

Peptic ulcer has complications: hemorrhage (bleeding), perforation, and obstruction. An ulcer that erodes into a large blood vessel may cause severe *hemorrhage.* An ulcer may also erode completely through the wall of the stomach or duodenum, causing a *perforation* of the wall through which gastric and duodenal contents leak into the peritoneal cavity, resulting in a generalized inflammation of the peritoneum, the membrane that lines the abdominal cavity and covers the exterior of the abdominal organs. The inflammation is called *peritonitis.* Sometimes the scarring that follows healing of a gastric ulcer may be so severe as to cause *obstruction* of the outlet of the stomach, called the *pylorus,* preventing the stomach from emptying properly.

Peptic ulcer is generally treated by antacids, which neutralize the excess gastric acid and promote healing of the ulcer, or by drugs that block the secretion of acid by the gastric epithelial cells. Because of the strong correlation between *Helicobacter pylori* and peptic ulcers, patients with ulcers who are colonized by this organism are often treated not only with drugs to neutralize gastric acid or suppress its secretion, but also with antibiotics and other medications to eradicate *Helicobacter pylori*. Combined antiacid and antimicrobial therapy in patients with ulcers who are colonized by *Helicobacter* leads to faster healing of the ulcers and fewer recurrences than standard antiacid treatment alone.

Surgical treatment is sometimes required if medical therapy fails to heal the ulcer or if complications develop.

At one time, *carcinoma of the stomach* was the most common malignant tumor in men, but the incidence has been decreasing. The initial symptom may be only vague upper abdominal discomfort. Sometimes the first manifestation is an iron-deficiency anemia, the result of chronic blood loss from the ulcerated surface of the tumor. Gastric carcinoma is treated by resection of a large part of the stomach together with the surrounding tissues and draining lymph nodes (figure 23–7). Unfortunately, a gastric carcinoma is often far advanced by the time it causes symptoms; so long-term survival of patients with stomach carcinoma is relatively poor. Sometimes gastric carcinoma may produce symptoms similar to those of a benign peptic ulcer. At times it may be difficult for the physician to determine whether a patient has a benign peptic ulcer of the stomach or an ulcerated gastric carcinoma. The distinction can usually be made by *gastroscopy,* an examination in which a flexible *gastroscope* is passed into the stomach so that the physician can visualize the lesion and take biopsy specimens from various areas.

Carcinoma of the Stomach

The intestine may be the site of both acute and chronic inflammation. The term **enteritis** (*enteron* = bowel) is used to describe inflammation of any part of the intestinal tract. The term **colitis** denotes inflammation restricted to the colon. Inflammation of the bowel produces symptoms of crampy abdominal pain and diarrhea. If the mucosa of the bowel is ulcerated, blood may appear in the stools.

Inflammatory Disease of the Intestine

Acute Enteritis

Acute enteritis is relatively common and may be caused by many different pathogenic organisms or bacterial toxins. Clinical manifestations include nausea, vomiting, abdominal discomfort, and passage of many loose, watery stools. Usually, the enteritis is of short duration and the symptoms subside promptly.

FIGURE 23–7

Carcinoma of stomach. Stomach has been opened, revealing a large ulcerated neoplasm arising from gastric mucosa (*arrow*) and extending upward to gastroesophageal junction. Esophagus is seen in upper part of photograph.

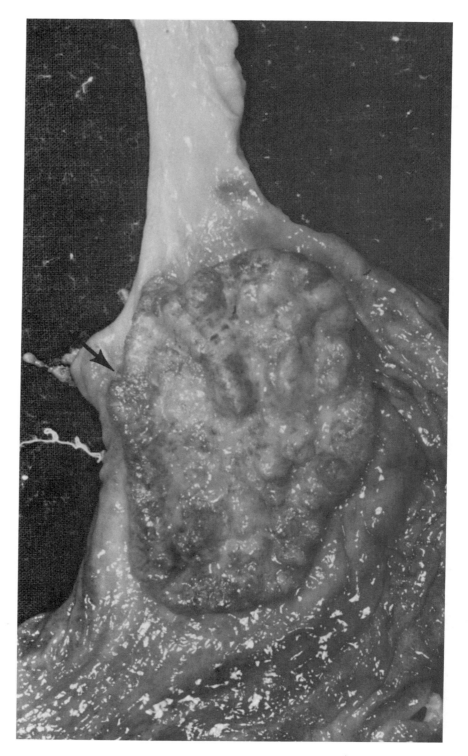

Chronic Enteritis

Chronic enteritis is less common than acute enteritis. Two major types are recognized: regional enteritis (Crohn's disease), which is localized chiefly to the distal ileum, and chronic ulcerative colitis, involving the large intestine. The causes of both types of chronic enteritis are unknown.

Regional Enteritis

Regional enteritis is a chronic inflammation primarily of the distal ileum. It is characterized by ulceration of the mucosa and marked thickening and scarring of the bowel wall (figure 23–8). The inflammation often affects scattered areas of the small bowel, leaving normal intervening areas (called "skip areas") between the areas of severe disease. Manifestations of the disease can often be controlled by various drugs, but often surgical resection of the affected part of the bowel is required.

Chronic Ulcerative Colitis

Chronic ulcerative colitis is a chronic recurrent inflammation with ulceration of the mucosa of the colon, often affecting the entire colon and rectum. Treatment depends on the severity of the disease. Some patients respond to

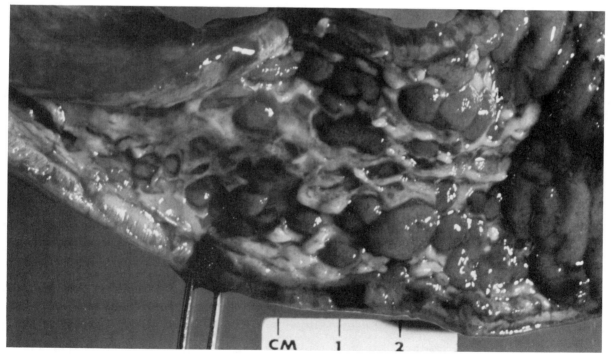

FIGURE 23–8

Regional enteritis. Mucosa is ulcerated and covered by inflammatory exudate.

antibiotics and corticosteroids, but many eventually require surgical resection of the diseased colon.

Complications of Chronic Enteritis

Patient with chronic enteritis often have serious nutritional disturbances because chronic diarrhea leads to poor absorption of food from the diseased bowel. The ulcerated areas in the bowel may bleed profusely. Sometimes the ulcerated areas undergo perforation, leading to leakage of intestinal contents into the peritoneal cavity. Occasionally, patients with regional enteritis have such severe thickening and scarring of the distal small bowel that the lumen becomes blocked, producing signs of intestinal obstruction.

Appendicitis

Appendicitis is the most common inflammatory lesion of the bowel. In many animals, the portion of the bowel represented in humans by the appendix is a large, wide-caliber intestinal segment, similar in appearance to the remainder of the colon. In humans, this segment of bowel is reduced in both size and caliber to the extent that it is a vestigial structure serving no useful function.

The high incidence of acute appendicitis is due primarily to the narrow caliber of the appendix, the base of which often becomes plugged by firm bits of fecal material. Because of the obstruction, the secretions normally produced by the epithelial cells lining the appendix drain poorly from the area distal to the blockage. The accumulated secretions create pressure within the appendiceal lumen. This compresses the blood vessels in the mucosa, impairing its viability (figure 23–9). Bacteria normally present in the appendix and colon invade the devitalized wall, causing an acute inflammation.

Clinically, appendicitis is characterized by generalized abdominal pain that soon becomes localized to the right lower part (quadrant) of the abdomen. Examination of the abdomen reveals localized tenderness over the appendix when pressure is applied to the abdomen by the fingers of the examiner. Often the patient also experiences pain when the pressure is released suddenly (*rebound tenderness*). In addition, there is usually reflex contraction of the abdominal muscles (*abdominal rigidity*) in response to the underlying inflammation. Laboratory tests reveal that the number of polymorphonuclear leukocytes in the blood also is increased as a result of the infection.

Mild cases of appendicitis may heal spontaneously. More severe inflammation may lead to rupture of the appendix and thus to peritonitis. For this reason, it is common practice to perform an exploratory operation and remove the appendix in any patient in whom appendicitis is suspected.

Meckel's Diverticulum

During embryonic development, the small intestine is connected for a time to the yolk sac of the embryo by means of a narrow tubular channel called the *vitelline duct* (*vitellus* = yolk). Normally, the duct disappears along with

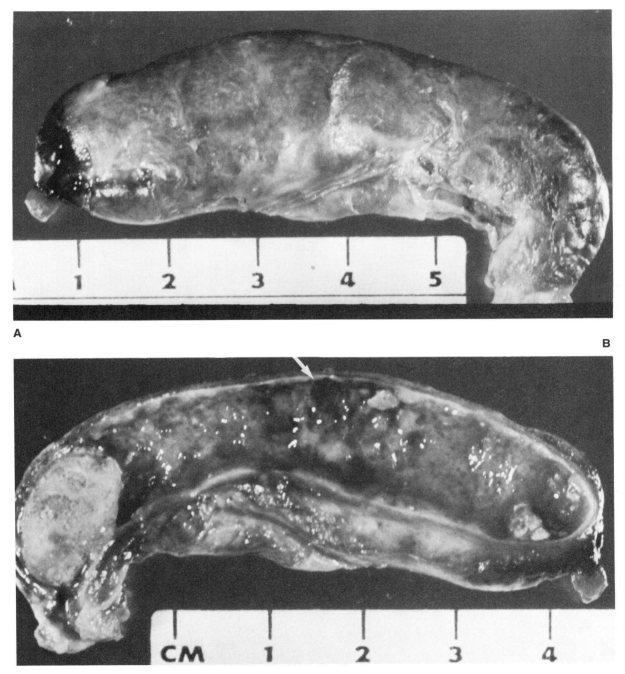

A

B

FIGURE 23–9

Acute appendicitis. **A,** Exterior of appendix is swollen, congested, and covered with inflammatory exudate.
B, Appendix bisected to reveal interior. Pus within lumen has been removed. Mucosa is congested and ulcerated
(*arrow*). Base of appendix (*left side of photograph*) is plugged by a firm mass of fecal material.

FIGURE 23–10

Meckel's diverticulum
of ileum.

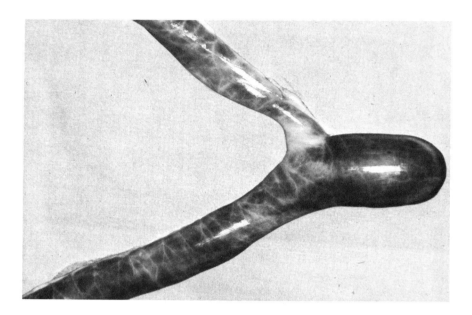

the yolk sac and no trace persists in the adult. In about 2 percent of persons, however, a remnant of the vitelline duct persists as a small tubular out-pouching from the distal ileum about twelve to eighteen inches proximal to the cecum. This structure is called a *Meckel's diverticulum* (figure 23–10). Normally, a Meckel's diverticulum has the same type of epithelial lining as that lining the small intestine, but sometimes part of the epithelial lining consists of acid-secreting gastric mucosa. Most Meckel's diverticula are asymptomatic, but sometimes the diverticulum becomes infected, causing the same symptoms and complications as an acute appendicitis. If a Meckel's diverticulum contains misplaced (ectopic) gastric mucosa, the acidic "gastric juice" secreted by the diverticulum may cause a peptic ulcer of the diverticulum, which may be complicated by bleeding or perforation, as may occur with peptic ulcers in the stomach or duodenum. Whenever an operation is performed for a suspected appendicitis or other gastrointestinal problem, the surgeon always checks to see if the patient's symptoms are caused by an inflammation or other problem in an unsuspected Meckel's diverticulum.

Disturbances of Bowel Function

Food Intolerance

Some patients manifest crampy abdominal pain, abdominal distention, *flatulence* (excessive gas in the intestinal tract), and frequent loose stools as a result of food intolerance. The two most common types are

1. Lactose intolerance
2. Intolerance to the wheat protein gluten

Lactose Intolerance

Lactose is a disaccharide found in milk and dairy products. During digestion, lactose must be split into its two component monosaccharides, glucose and galactose, before it can be absorbed. This process is accomplished by an enzyme called *lactase,* which is present on the mucosal surface of the epithelial cells in the small intestine. The enzyme is abundant in infants and young children. In many populations, however, the concentration of lactase gradually declines to very low levels during adolescence and early adult life. The enzyme is deficient in about 20 percent of adult Whites, 70 percent of American Blacks, 90 percent of American Indians, and almost all Asians.

Persons in whom lactase is deficient are unable to digest lactose. Consequently, lactose cannot be absorbed and remains within the intestinal lumen, where it raises the osmotic pressure of the intestinal contents. Because of the high intraluminal osmotic pressure, fluid is retained within the intestinal tract instead of being absorbed normally, leading to abdominal discomfort, cramps, and diarrhea. Some of the unabsorbed lactose is fermented by bacteria in the colon, yielding lactic acid and other organic acids that further raise the intraluminal osmotic pressure and contribute to the person's discomfort. The symptoms are related to ingestion of dairy products and abate promptly when intake of dairy products is reduced or discontinued.

Gluten Intolerance

Gluten, a protein found in wheat and other grains, imparts the elasticity to bread dough. Some persons become hypersensitive to this protein and develop a chronic diarrhea associated with impaired absorption of fat and other nutrients. Clinically, the condition is characterized by passage of frequent large, bulky stools containing much unabsorbed fat, associated with weight loss and vitamin deficiencies as a result of the impaired intestinal absorption. The hypersensitivity also leads to atrophy of the villi in the small intestine. This condition is called *gluten enteropathy* (*enteron* = bowel + *pathy* = disease) or *nontropical sprue.*

Diagnosis is made on the basis of the clinical features and is confirmed if biopsy of the small intestinal mucosa reveals atrophy of the intestinal villi. The specimen for biopsy is obtained by a flexible biopsy device with a small capsule on the end that is swallowed by the patient. The device is positioned in the upper jejunum and is manipulated so that a small bit of intestinal mucosa enters the capsule. Then the capsule is closed, cutting off and retaining a piece of mucosa.

Treatment by a gluten-free diet promptly cures the condition and the intestinal villi return to normal.

Irritable Bowel Syndrome

Some patients exhibit episodes of crampy abdominal discomfort, loud gurgling bowel sounds, and disturbed bowel function. Frequent loose stools sometimes alternate with periods of constipation, and excessive amounts of mucus are secreted by the colonic mucosal glands. These manifestations are frequently quite distressing to the affected individual, but no structural or biochemical abnormalities can be identified to account for the functional disturbances. This condition is often called the *irritable bowel syndrome*. Other terms for this very common condition are *spastic colitis* and *mucous colitis*. The symptoms are thought to represent a response to emotional stress, in which the emotional turmoil is manifested as disturbed bowel function.

The diagnosis of irritable bowel syndrome is one of exclusion. The physician must rule out infections as a result of pathogenic bacteria and intestinal parasites, food intolerance, and various types of chronic enteritis such as regional enteritis and chronic ulcerative colitis.

Treatment consists of measures that reduce emotional tension and improve intestinal motility. Sometimes substances that increase the bulk of the stool provide relief of symptoms.

Intestinal Infections in Homosexual Men

Some homosexual men suffer from intestinal complaints that are caused by various combinations of pathogenic bacteria, such as *Shigella* and *Salmonella* (described in chapter 6) and intestinal parasites such as *Entamoeba histolytica* and *Giardia* (described in chapter 7). Spread of the enteric infection is by anal-oral sexual practices that transfer the intestinal pathogens from the infected individual to his sexual partner. Because some homosexuals have multiple partners, the enteric infections may become quite widely distributed through the homosexual community. In some cases, the intestinal complaints may be misinterpreted as an irritable bowel syndrome if adequate diagnostic studies are not undertaken. Specific methods of treatment are available to cure these infections.

Diverticulosis and Diverticulitis of the Colon

Outpouchings of the mucosa of the colon often project through weak areas in the muscular wall of the large intestine. These outpouchings are called **diverticula** (singular, *diverticulum*), and the condition is called **diverticulosis** (figures 23–11, 23–12, and 23–13). This is an acquired condition, in contrast to a Meckel's diverticulum, which is a congenital abnormality (see figure 23–10). Diverticula, which usually occur in the distal colon, are encountered with increasing frequency in older patients. Highly refined, low-residue diets predispose to diverticula because stools are small and hard, and high intraluminal pressure must be generated by peristalsis to propel the stool through the colon. This high intracolonic pressure forces the mucosa through weak areas in the muscular wall. In contrast, people who subsist on high-residue diets have large, bulky stools that can be propelled through the colon easily at low intraluminal pressures, and diverticula occur infrequently among them.

Most diverticula are asymptomatic, but occasionally problems arise. Bits of fecal material may become trapped within these pouches and incite an inflammatory reaction called **diverticulitis.** The inflammation may be followed by considerable scarring. Occasionally, perforation of a diverticulum

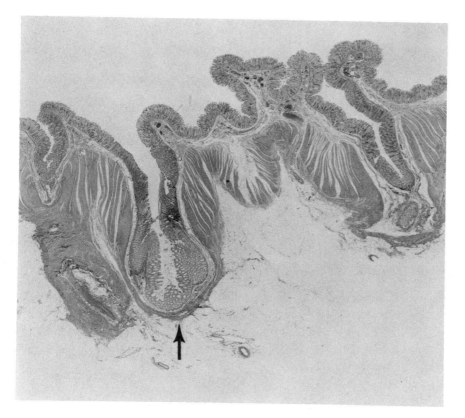

FIGURE 23–11

Low-magnification photomicrograph of colon illustrating diverticula. Mucosa of colon (*upper part of photograph*) protrudes through muscular wall (*arrow*) into the serosa of colon. (Original magnification × 10.)

may occur, leading to an abscess in the pelvis. Sometimes, blood vessels in the mucosa of the diverticulum may become ulcerated by abrasion from the fecal material, resulting in bleeding. Diverticula attended by such complications as infections, perforation, or bleeding are often treated by surgical resection of the affected segment of bowel.

Intestinal Obstruction

If the normal passage of intestinal contents through the bowel is blocked, the patient is said to have an *intestinal obstruction*. The site of the blockage may be either the small intestine (*high intestinal obstruction*) or the colon (*low intestinal obstruction*). Bowel obstruction is always serious. The severity of the symptoms depends on the location of the obstruction, its completeness, and whether there is interference with the blood supply to the blocked segment of bowel.

Obstruction of the *small intestine* causes severe, crampy pain as a result of vigorous peristalsis, reflecting the attempt of the intestine to force bowel contents past the site of obstruction. This is associated with vomiting of copious amounts of gastric and upper-intestinal secretions, resulting in loss of large

FIGURE 23–12

Diverticulosis of colon.
A, Exterior of colon, illustrating several diverticula projecting through wall of colon (*arrows*). **B,** Closer view of diverticulum.
C, Interior of colon, illustrating openings of multiple diverticula. Several of the openings are well demonstrated in the mucosa just below the clamps.

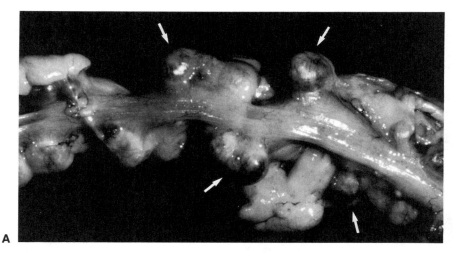

A

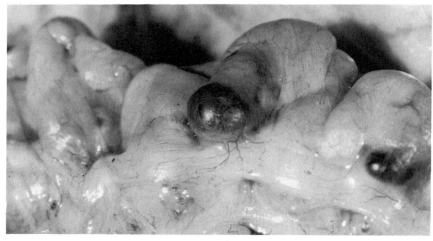

B

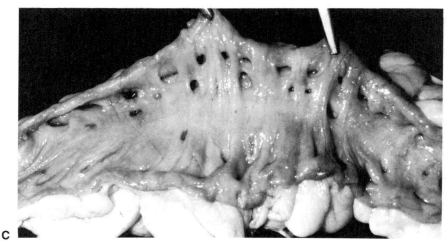

C

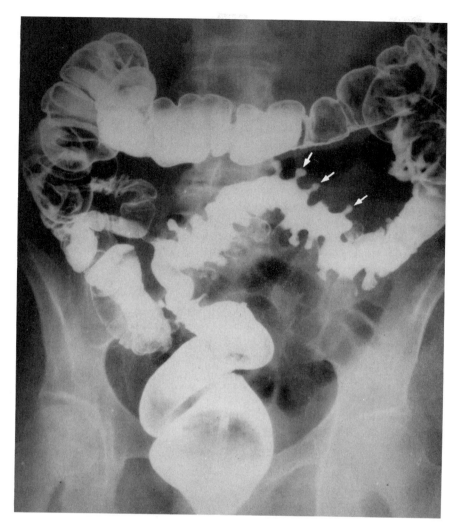

FIGURE 23–13

Diverticula of colon demonstrated by injection of barium contrast material into colon (barium enema). Diverticula filled with contrast material appear as projections from the mucosa (*arrows*).

quantities of water and electrolytes. As a consequence, the patient becomes dehydrated and develops pronounced fluid and electrolyte disturbances.

Symptoms are much less acute when the *distal colon* is obstructed. There may be mild, crampy abdominal pain and moderate distention of the abdomen. However, vomiting with associated loss of fluid and electrolytes is not as serious a problem as in high intestinal obstruction. Disturbances of fluid and electrolytes do not develop as rapidly.

The common causes of intestinal obstruction are:

1. Intestinal adhesions
2. Hernia
3. Tumor
4. Volvulus
5. Intussusception

Adhesions

Adhesive bands of connective tissue (**adhesions**) may form within the abdominal cavity after surgery (figure 23–14). Sometimes a loop of bowel becomes kinked, compressed, or twisted by an adhesive band, causing obstruction proximal to the site of the adhesion.

Hernia

A **hernia** is a protrusion of a loop of bowel through a small opening, usually in the abdominal wall. The herniated loop pushes the peritoneum ahead of it, forming the hernia sac. *Inguinal hernia* is quite common in men (figure 23–15). A loop of small bowel protrudes through a weak area in the inguinal ring and may descend downward into the scrotum. Umbilical and femoral hernias occur in both sexes. In an *umbilical hernia,* the loop of bowel protrudes into the umbilicus through a defect in the abdominal wall (figure 23–16). In a *femoral hernia,* a loop of intestine extends under the inguinal ligament along the course of the femoral vessels into the groin. If a herniated loop of bowel can be pushed back into the abdominal cavity, the hernia is said to be *reducible.* Occasionally, a herniated loop becomes stuck and cannot be reduced. This is called an *incarcerated hernia.* Sometimes the loop of bowel is so tightly constricted by the margins of the defect that allowed the herniation that the blood supply to the herniated bowel is obstructed, causing necrosis of the protruding segment of bowel. This is called a *strangulated hernia* and requires prompt surgical intervention.

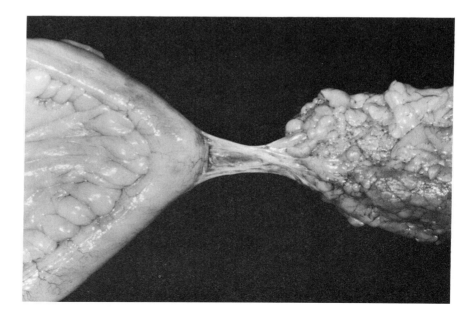

FIGURE 23–14

Fibrous adhesion between loop of small intestine (*left side of photograph*) and omentum.

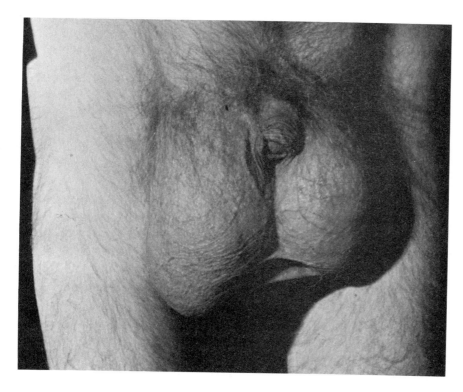

FIGURE 23–15

Large bilateral inguinal hernias extending into scrotum.

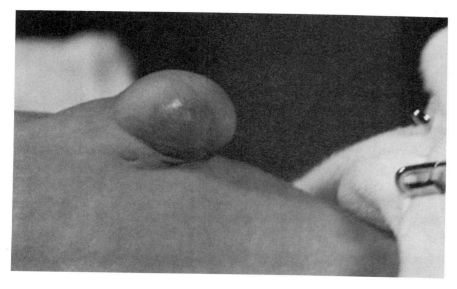

FIGURE 23–16

Large umbilical hernia in infant.

Volvulus and Intussusception

A **volvulus** is a rotary twisting of the bowel on the fold of peritoneum that suspends the bowel from the posterior wall of the abdomen, which is called the *mesentery of the bowel.* The blood supply to the twisted segment also is impaired because the blood vessels supplying the bowel travel in the mesentery, and they are compressed when the bowel and mesentery become twisted. The sigmoid colon is the usual site (figure 23–17).

An **intussusception** is a telescoping of one segment of bowel into an adjacent segment. This is a common cause of intestinal obstruction in children and usually results from vigorous peristalsis that telescopes the terminal ileum into the proximal colon through the ileocecal valve (figure 23–18). In adults, the condition is usually secondary to a benign tumor of the bowel that is supported by a narrow stalk. A tumor of this type is often called a *pedunculated tumor,* the name being derived from the stalk (*pedicle*) that supports it (*pediculus* = little foot). As the tumor is propelled by a peristaltic wave, the base of the tumor exerts traction on the bowel wall at its site of

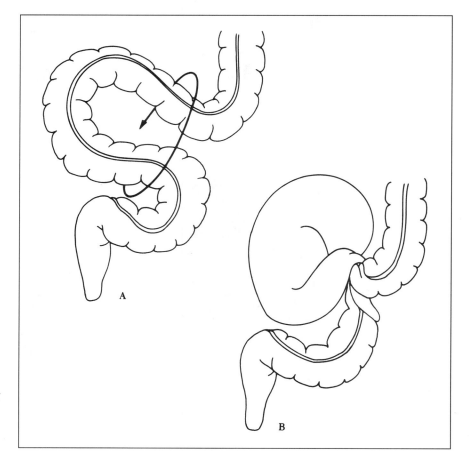

FIGURE 23–17

Pathogenesis of volvulus of sigmoid colon. **A,** Rotary twist of sigmoid colon on its mesentery. **B,** Obstruction of colon and interruption of its blood supply caused by volvulus.

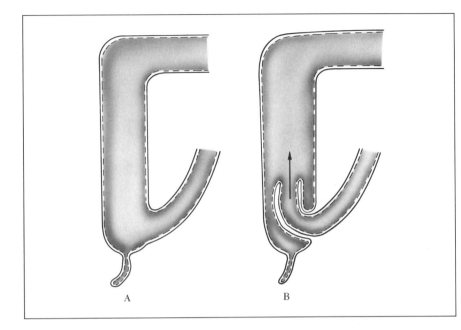

FIGURE 23–18
Pathogenesis of ileocecal intussusception. **A,** Normal anatomic relationships. **B,** Vigorous peristalsis carries distal ileum into cecum. *Dashed line* indicates mucosa.

attachment, causing the proximal segment of bowel to be pulled into the distal segment (figures 23–19 and 23–20).

Carcinoma of the colon may obstruct the distal colon and is a common cause of low intestinal obstruction.

Mesenteric Thrombosis

The blood supply to the gastrointestinal tract is derived from several large arteries arising from the aorta. The blood supply to most of the bowel is provided by the superior mesenteric artery. This vessel supplies blood to the entire small intestine and the proximal half of the colon. The arteries supplying the gastrointestinal tract may develop arteriosclerotic changes and become occluded by thrombosis in the same way as may other arteries. Thrombosis of the superior mesenteric artery leads to an extensive infarction of most of the bowel.

Tumors of the Bowel

Tumors of the small intestine are uncommon, whereas *benign pedunculated polyps* of the colon occur quite frequently. Usually they do not cause symptoms, but occasionally the tip of the polyp may become eroded and cause bleeding. Often a polyp can be removed by inserting a flexible instrument called a *colonoscope* into the bowel through the rectum and cutting the narrow stalk.

FIGURE 23–19

Pathogenesis of intussusception caused by tumor. **A,** Pedunculated tumor protrudes into lumen of bowel. **B,** Peristalsis propels tumor and produces traction on its base causing proximal segment of bowel to be telescoped into distal segment. *Dashed line* indicates mucosa.

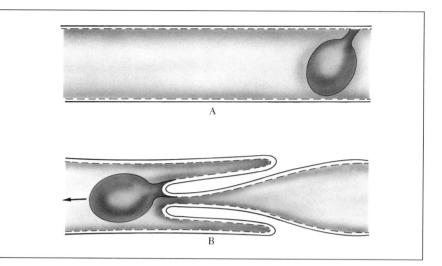

FIGURE 23–20

Intussusception of colon as a result of colon tumor. Midportion of colon is swollen owing to the telescoping of proximal segment (*left side of photograph*) into distal segment (*right side of photograph*).

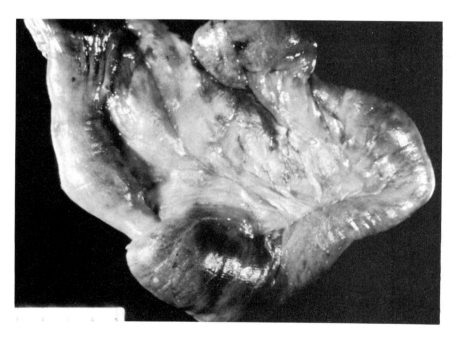

Carcinoma of the colon is a common tumor that may arise anywhere in the large intestine or rectum. Carcinoma arising in the cecum and right half of the colon generally does not cause obstruction of the bowel, because the caliber of this portion of the colon is large and the bowel contents are relatively soft. However, the tumor often becomes ulcerated and bleeds, leading to chronic iron-deficiency anemia. The patient with a carcinoma of the right half of the colon may consult his physician because of weakness and fatigue caused by the anemia, without experiencing any symptoms referable to the intestinal tract.

Carcinoma of the distal portion of the colon, which has a much smaller caliber than the proximal colon, often causes partial obstruction of the bowel and leads to symptoms of lower intestinal obstruction (figures 23–21 and 23–22).

Imperforate anus is an uncommon congenital abnormality in which the colon fails to acquire a normal anal opening (figure 23–23). There are two major types. In one type, the rectum and anus are normally formed and extend to the level of the skin, but no anal orifice is present. Often a small tract (fistula) extends from the blind end of the anal canal to terminate in the urethra, the vagina, or on the surface of the skin. Usually, this type of imperforate anus can be easily treated by excising the tissue covering the anal opening. In the second type of imperforate anus, the entire distal rectum fails to develop, and often there are associated abnormalities of the urogenital tract and skeletal system. Surgical repair of this type of abnormality is much more difficult, and results are less satisfactory.

Imperforate Anus

Hemorrhoids are varicosities of the venous plexus that drains the rectum and anus (figure 23–24). Constipation and increased straining during bowel movements predispose to their development. *Internal hemorrhoids,* which

Hemorrhoids

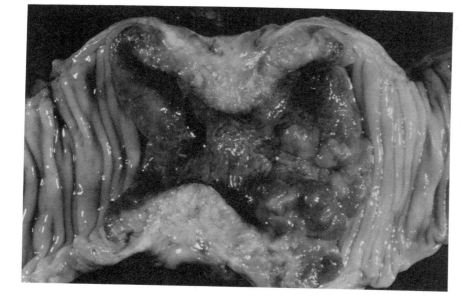

FIGURE 23–21

Large, ulcerated carcinoma that completely encircles and constricts colon. Colon has been opened to reveal the ulcerated surface of the tumor. (See also figure 10–18.)

FIGURE 23–22

Colon carcinoma demonstrated by barium enema. The tumor narrows the lumen of the colon, which appears as a filling defect in the column of barium (*arrows*).

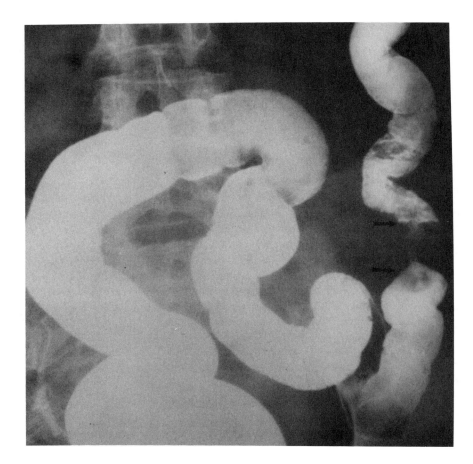

involve the veins of the lower rectum, may become eroded and bleed, may become thrombosed, or may prolapse through the anus. *External hemorrhoids* involve the veins of the anal canal and perianal skin. They sometimes become thrombosed, which causes considerable anorectal discomfort.

Symptoms of hemorrhoids can often be relieved by a high-fiber diet rich in fruits and vegetables, which promotes large, bulky stools that can be passed without excessive straining. Stool softeners and local application of rectal ointments may also provide temporary relief. Hemorrhoids can be removed surgically if they do not respond to more conservative therapy.

Diagnostic Evaluation of Gastrointestinal Disease

Unfortunately, the gastrointestinal tract cannot be examined as easily as many other parts of the body. However, it is possible to visualize the interior of the esophagus, the stomach, the duodenum, and the entire colon by *endoscopic procedures* using specially designed instruments that are inserted into the gastrointestinal tract either through the oral cavity or the anus. Endoscopy is described in chapter 1 in the section on diagnostic procedures.

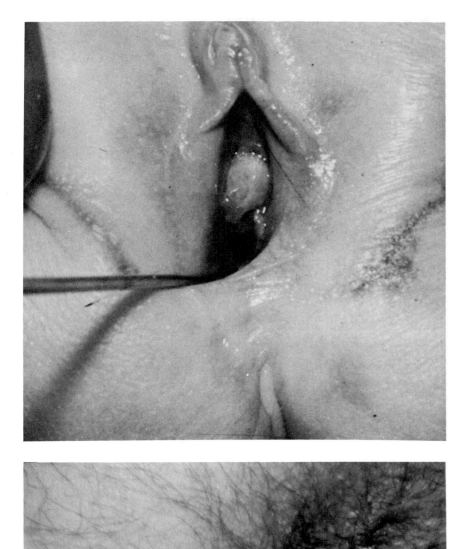

FIGURE 23–23

Imperforate anus in newborn infant. Metal probe has been placed in vagina.

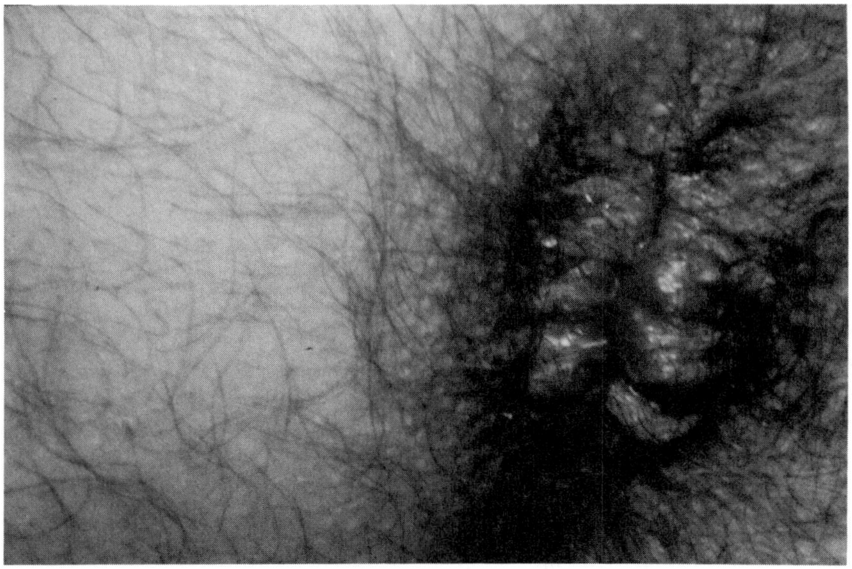

FIGURE 23–24

Large protruding hemorrhoids.

Endoscopic procedures are generally employed if the patient experiences symptoms suggesting disease of the esophagus, stomach, or colon. Abnormal areas in the mucosa can be visualized, biopsied, and examined histologically.

Areas that cannot be visualized directly can be studied by *radiologic examination*. Examination of the upper gastrointestinal tract is accomplished by having the patient ingest a radiopaque material (contrast medium), allowing the clinician to visualize the transport of the material through the intestinal tract by x-ray studies. Any areas where the motility of the bowel appears abnormal, indicating disease, can be seen on the film. This technique also allows the clinician to visualize the contours of the gastrointestinal mucosa and thereby to identify the location and extent of disease affecting the bowel mucosa, such as ulcer, stricture, tumor, or an area of chronic inflammation. The colon can be studied in a similar manner by instilling radiopaque material into the bowel through the anus, in order to outline the contours of the large intestine. This type of study is called a *barium enema* (see figures 23–13 and 23–22).

Questions for Review

1. What is a cleft palate? What is its usual mode of inheritance? How is it treated?

2. What factors effect the development of dental caries? What complications may result from dental caries? What are the causes and possible effects of periodontal disease?

3. What are some of the major causes of esophageal obstruction? What symptoms does esophageal obstruction produce?

4. What is peptic ulcer? In what parts of the gastrointestinal tract are peptic ulcers encountered? What factors contribute to the development of peptic ulcers? What are the complications of a peptic ulcer?

5. What is the difference between regional enteritis and chronic ulcerative colitis? Diverticulosis and diverticulitis?

6. What is a Meckel's diverticulum? Where is it located? What clinical manifestations can it produce?

7. What is intestinal obstruction? What symptoms does it produce? What are some of the common causes of intestinal obstruction?

8. What is the pathogenesis of acute appendicitis?

9. What symptoms and physical findings are likely to be encountered in a patient with a carcinoma of the colon? Why?

10. What is an intussusception? How is it caused? What is the difference between volvulus and intussusception?

Supplementary Readings

Almy, T. P., and Howell, D. A. 1980. Diverticular disease of the colon. *New England Journal of Medicine* 302: 324–31. Describes pathogenesis, prevalence, diagnosis, treatment, and complications. A very common condition, but most individuals are asymptomatic.

Hackford, A. W., et al. 1985. Diverticular disease of the colon: Current concepts and management. *Surgical Clinics of North America* 65:347–61. Many patients have an acute episode as initial manifestation. Discusses methods of prevention and treatment.

Marshall, B. J. 1995. *Helicobacter pylori:* The etiologic agent for peptic ulcer. *Journal of the American Medical Association* 274:1064–66. Reviews the evolution of the infection, diagnostic methods for detecting the infection, and methods of treatment. Proposes explanation for the high frequency of infection in asymptomatic persons, and suggests how the organism may cause hypersecretion of gastric acid by disturbing the function of gastric epithelial cells that regulate gastric secretion.

NIH Consensus Development Panel. 1994. *Helicobacter pylori* in peptic ulcer disease. *Journal of the American Medical Association* 272:65–68. Treatment of bacterial infection is required to treat peptic ulcers effectively.

Ransohoff, D. F. 1993. Gastroenterology. *Journal of the American Medical Association* 270:206–7. Discusses role of *Helicobacter.*

Reid, B. J., et al. 1988. Endoscopic biopsy can detect high-grade dysplasia or early adenocarcinoma in Barrett's esophagus without grossly recognizable neoplastic lesions. *Gastroenterology* 94:81–90. Patients with Barrett's esophagus are at risk of adenocarcinoma and require close follow-up with biopsies to detect dysplasia or early cancer.

Smith, P. D., et al. 1988. Intestinal infections in patients with acquired immunodeficiency syndrome (AIDS): Etiology and response to therapy. *Annals of Internal Medicine* 108:328–33. Diarrhea in AIDS patients is a result of enteric pathogens. Identification of the causative agent and specific therapy leads to improvement.

Winters, C., Jr., et al. 1987. Barrett's esophagus: A prevalent, occult complication of gastroesophageal reflux disease. *Gastroenterology* 92:118–24. A review article.

Chapter 23 ■ Outline Summary

Face and Oral Cavity / 659

Cleft Lip and Palate

Face and palate formed by coalescence of cell masses.

Maldevelopment leads to defects in lip, jaw, and palate.

Multifactorial inheritance pattern.

Treatment by surgical correction of defect.

Abnormalities of Tooth Development

Missing teeth common. Multifactorial inheritance pattern.

Tetracycline stains enamel of developing teeth and may cause abnormal tooth development.

Do not give to pregnant women.

Do not give to children under eight years of age.

Dental Caries (Tooth Decay) and Its Complications

Organic acids produced by bacterial fermentation of retained food particles erode enamel.

Combined acid and bacterial action destroy tooth structure, forming cavity.

Spread of bacteria to pulp cavity causes pulp infection and toothache.

Infection may affect apex of tooth and bone in which tooth embedded.

Treatment:

Cavities treated by removing decay and filling the defect.

Pulp infection and infection in bone at apex of tooth may require antibiotics, root canal treatment, or occasionally tooth extraction.

Periodontal Disease

An infection between roots of teeth and gums.

Spread of infection into tooth sockets may cause teeth to loosen and eventually fall out.

Various local dental treatments may control or arrest condition.

Inflammation of the Oral Cavity / 663

Stomatitis

Caused by various irritants.

Tumors of the Oral Cavity / 663

Carcinoma

Arises from squamous epithelium of oral cavity.

Treated by resection or radiation.

Diseases of the Esophagus / 663

Cardiac Sphincter Dysfunction

Cardiospasm: sphincter fails to open and obstructs food transport.

Incompetent sphincter.

Reflux of acid gastric juice causes inflammation, ulceration, scarring (reflux esophagitis).

Glandular metaplasia of squamous epithelium (Barrett's esophagus) carries increased risk of esophageal cancer.

Mucosal Tears

Retching and vomiting lacerates mucosa, which may bleed profusely.

Carcinoma of Esophagus

Squamous cell carcinoma gradually narrows lumen.

May invade trachea and cause fistula.

Food Impaction

Poorly chewed meat may block esophagus.

Occurs in persons unable to chew properly.

Stricture

Esophagus narrowed by scar.

Ingestion of corrosive chemicals causes inflammation that heals by scarring.

Gastritis / 666
Acute

Often caused by nonsteroidal anti-inflammatory drugs or alcohol.

Chronic

Often associated with *Helicobacter pylori* colonization of mucosa.

Peptic Ulcer / 667
Pathogenesis

Increased acid secretions and digestive enzymes erode gastric mucosa.

Helicobacter pylori plays role in pathogenesis.

Complications

Bleeding.

Perforation.

Pyloric obstruction by scarring.

Treatment

Administer drugs to block acid secretion or neutralize acid.

Antibiotic therapy if ulcer associated with *H. pylori*.

Surgery may be required for ulcer complications.

Carcinoma of Stomach / 669
Manifestations and Treatment

Upper abdominal discomfort.

Iron-deficiency anemia from chronic blood loss.

Diagnosis established by biopsy of tumor by means of gastroscopy.

Treated by gastric resection.

Inflammatory Disease of the Intestine / 669
Acute Enteritis

Common and self-limited.

Caused by many different organisms and bacterial toxins.

Chronic Enteritis

Regional enteritis (Crohn's disease).

Chronic inflammation with scarring affects distal ileum.

Treatment by resection.

Chronic ulcerative colitis.

Recurrent chronic inflammation of colon and rectum.

Various forms of medical treatment.

Often requires resection of colon.

Complications of Chronic Enteritis

Nutritional disturbances from chronic diarrhea.

Bleeding.

Obstruction by scarring.

Perforation.

Appendicitis / 672
Pathogenesis and Treatment

Narrow caliber of appendix favors obstruction at base.

Accumulation of secretions raises intraluminal pressure, impairing viability of wall.

Intestinal bacteria invade wall.

Inflamed appendix may perforate and cause peritonitis.

Appendectomy performed in all suspected cases.

Meckel's Diverticulum / 672
Pathogenesis

Embryonic remnant of vitelline duct.

Appears as tubular outpouching from distal ileum.

Manifestations and Treatment

Usually asymptomatic.

Inflammation of diverticulum causes symptoms similar to appendicitis.

Disturbances of Bowel Function Caused by Food Intolerance / 674
Lactose Intolerance

Many adults unable to digest lactose owing to lactase deficiency.

Unabsorbed lactose raises osmotic pressure of bowel contents, leading to retention of fluid in intestinal lumen associated with cramps and diarrhea.

Symptoms abate when dairy products discontinued.

Gluten Intolerance

Hypersensitivity to wheat protein leads to impaired intestinal absorption and atrophy of intestinal villi.

Diagnosis established by small bowel biopsy.

Treatment by gluten-free diet relieves symptoms and villi return to normal.

Irritable Bowel Syndrome / 675
Pathogenesis and Manifestations

Disturbed bowel function without structural or biochemical abnormalities.

A diagnosis of exclusion.

A manifestation of emotional stress affecting bowel function.

Symptomatic treatment reduces tension and improves intestinal motility.

Intestinal Infections in Homosexual Men / 676
Pathogenesis and Manifestations

Intestinal complaints among homosexual men caused by bacterial-parasitic infections spread by sexual practices.

May be misinterpreted as irritable bowel syndrome.

Specific treatment given after diagnostic studies completed.

Diverticulosis and Diverticulitis of Colon / 676
Pathogenesis
Outpouching of colonic mucosa through weak areas in wall.

Chronic constipation and low-residue diet predisposes.

Complications
Inflammation.

Bleeding.

Treatment
Asymptomatic diverticula do not require treatment.

Surgical resection of affected bowel if complications occur.

Intestinal Obstruction / 677
High Intestinal Obstruction
Crampy pain and vomiting.

Severe water and electrolyte disturbances develop rapidly.

Low Intestinal Obstruction
Mild crampy pain and distention.

Water and electrolyte disturbances not a major problem.

Causes
Adhesions: from previous surgery.

Hernia: protrusion of bowel through weak area in abdominal wall.

Volvulus: rotary twisting of sigmoid colon on its mesentery.

Intussusception: telescoping of one segment of bowel into adjacent segment.

As a result of vigorous peristalsis.

Caused by pedunculated tumor.

Mesenteric Thrombosis / 683
Pathogenesis
Superior mesenteric artery supplies small bowel and proximal half of colon.

Artery may become blocked by thrombus, embolus, or atheroma.

Obstruction of artery causes extensive bowel infarction.

Tumors of Bowel / 683
Small Intestine
Small bowel tumors are uncommon.

Colon
Benign polyps.

Carcinoma.

Left half of colon: tumors often obstruct colon.

Right half of colon: usually causes chronic blood loss but does not obstruct.

Imperforate Anus / 685
Manifestations and Treatment
Congenitally absent anal opening, sometimes with absent distal rectum as well.

Can be corrected surgically.

Hemorrhoids / 685
Pathogenesis
Varicose veins of hemorrhoidal venous plexus.

Constipation predisposes.

Classification
Internal hemorrhoids: may bleed or prolapse or become thrombosed.

External hemorrhoids: may become thrombosed.

Treatment
Conservative treatment preferred.

Can be treated surgically if not responsive to conservative therapy.

Diagnostic Evaluation of Gastrointestinal Tract Disease / 686
Diagnostic Methods
Endoscopy: tube inserted to visualize interior of gastrointestinal tract. Biopsies performed if indicated.

X-ray studies.

24

Water, Electrolyte, and Acid-Base Balance

Learning Objectives

1. Explain the basic concepts relating to the regulation of the concentration of electrolytes in the body. List the major ions in the intracellular and extracellular water and define units of concentration.
2. Describe the common disturbances of water balance and their pathogenesis.
3. Explain the physiologic mechanisms concerned with the control of pH.
4. Describe the pathogenesis of the four common disturbances of acid-base balance and the body's compensatory mechanisms.
5. Define the role of the kidneys and the lungs in the regulation of acid-base balance.

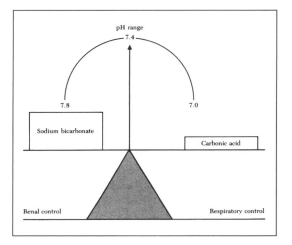

Chapter 24 ▪ Contents

About 70 percent of the body consists of water. Most is within cells as *intracellular water*. The remainder, called *extracellular water,* is within the interstitial tissues surrounding the cells and in the blood plasma. The body water contains dissolved mineral salts (**electrolytes**) that dissociate in solution, yielding positively charged ions (**cations**) and negatively charged ions (**anions**). The body fluids are electrically neutral, and the sum of the positively charged ions in solution is always balanced by the sum of the negatively charged ions. In disease, the concentrations of the individual ions may vary, but electrical neutrality is always maintained.

For purposes of description, it is convenient to give separate consideration to disturbances of body water and abnormalities in the concentrations of electrolytes. This separation is artificial, however, because all body fluids contain dissolved mineral salts. If the electrolyte concentration of the body changes, there is usually a corresponding change in body water. Conversely, changes in body water are usually associated with changes in electrolyte concentrations.

Interrelations of Intracellular and Extracellular Fluid

Fluid and electrolytes diffuse freely between the intravascular and interstitial fluids. However, the capillaries are impermeable to protein; so the interstitial fluid contains very little protein.

The fluid within the cells is separated from the interstitial fluid by the cell membrane, which is freely permeable to water but relatively impermeable to sodium and potassium ions. The principal extracellular ions are *sodium* (Na^+) and *chloride* (Cl^-), whereas the principal intracellular ions are *potassium* (K^+) and *phosphate* (PO_4^{2-}). The differences in the concentration of the ions on different sides of the cell membrane are a result of the metabolic activity of the cell.

In general, the amount of sodium in the body determines the volume of the extracellular fluid, because this is the chief extracellular cation, and the amount of potassium in the body determines the volume of the intracellular fluid, because this is the chief intracellular cation.

Units of Concentration of Electrolytes

In dealing with disturbances of electrolytes, the clinician is concerned primarily with concentrations of the various ions and with the interrelation of positively and negatively charged ions with one another, rather than with the actual number of milligrams or grams of the various salts dissolved in the plasma. Therefore, the concentrations of electrolytes are expressed in units that define their ability to combine with other ions.

The quantity that expresses "combining weight" is termed the *equivalent weight*. An equivalent weight is the molecular weight of a substance in grams divided by its valence. When one equivalent weight of a substance is dissolved in a solution to make one liter (1 L), the concentration is *one equivalent per liter.* For a monovalent substance, this is the same as a molar solution.

As an example, the equivalent weight of sodium chloride is determined by adding 23 g (molecular weight of sodium) to 35.5 g (molecular weight of chloride) and dividing by the valence (which is 1), to equal 58.5 g of sodium chloride, the equivalent weight.

In body fluids, the concentrations of electrolytes are low and are usually expressed in *milliequivalents per liter* (abbreviated mEq/L) rather than in equivalents. A milliequivalent is 1/1000 of an equivalent. Concentrations of ions expressed in milliequivalents have equal combining properties, even though their equivalent weights are not equal. For example, a milliequivalent of bicarbonate ion is equal in electrical and ionic characteristics to a milliequivalent of chloride ion, even though the molecular weight of bicarbonate is greater than that of chloride.

Regulation of Body Fluid and Electrolyte Concentration

The amount of water and electrolytes in the body represents a balance between the amounts ingested in food and fluids and the amounts excreted in the urine, through the gastrointestinal tract, in perspiration, and as water vapor excreted by the lungs. The kidneys are important in controlling the concentration of body water and electrolytes. Under the influence of adrenal cortical and posterior pituitary hormones, the kidneys regulate the internal environment of the body by selectively excreting or retaining water and electrolytes as required to maintain a uniform composition of the body fluids.

Disturbances of Water Balance

Dehydration

The most common disturbance of water balance is *dehydration,* which may be caused by inadequate water intake or excess water loss. Most cases of dehydration seen in medical practice result from excessive loss of fluid from the gastrointestinal tract as a consequence of vomiting or diarrhea. Fluid intake is usually decreased, contributing to the dehydration. Occasionally, comatose or debilitated patients become dehydrated because of inadequate intake of fluid.

Overhydration

Overhydration is less common than dehydration. Occasionally, it results from an excessively large intake of fluids by a patient in whom renal function is impaired. Sometimes overhydration is caused by excessive administration of intravenous fluids.

In general, the same conditions that produce disturbances of water balance also disturb the electrolyte composition of the body fluids. Most electrolyte disturbances result from depletion of body electrolytes. Depletions of sodium and potassium generally occur together, often because of loss of electrolytes along with water from the gastrointestinal tract as a result of vomiting or diarrhea. Large amounts of sodium and potassium may also be lost in the urine as a result of prolonged use of diuretics. *Diuretics* are substances that promote excretion of salts and water by the kidneys by impairing reabsorption of these substances from the glomerular filtrate; they are often administered to patients with heart failure, cirrhosis of the liver, and some types of kidney diseases. Loss of large amounts of electrolytes may also accompany excessive excretion of water in the urine in uncontrolled diabetes, as a result of the diuretic effect of the excreted glucose (chapter 22), or in renal tubular disease, in which the regenerating renal tubules are unable to conserve electrolytes and water (chapter 19).

Disturbances of Electrolyte Balance

The body may be considered an acid-producing machine that generates large amounts of organic and inorganic acids in consequence of normal metabolic processes. It produces various *nonvolatile acids* such as sulfuric, phosphoric, and uric acid in the breakdown of proteins. It forms *ketone bodies* in the oxidation of fat (chapter 22) and produces *lactic acid* from breakdown of glucose when oxygen supplies are insufficient. Large amounts of carbon dioxide also are formed as by-products of intracellular metabolic processes, and some of the carbon dioxide dissolves in body fluids to form *carbonic acid.*

Despite the large amounts of acid produced, the body fluids remain slightly alkaline, and their pH is maintained within the narrow range of 7.38 to 7.42. The body is able to maintain the alkalinity of body fluids because it has three regulatory mechanisms that neutralize and eliminate the acids as rapidly as they are formed:

Acid-Base Balance

1. The buffer systems of the blood
2. The lungs, which regulate the carbonic acid concentration
3. The kidneys, which control bicarbonate concentration

Buffers

The *buffer systems of the blood* are the first line of defense against change in pH. In a general sense, a buffer is anything that cushions a blow or absorbs an impact. Chemically, a buffer may be defined as a weak acid and a salt of the acid or as a weak base and its salt. Buffers minimize change in hydrogen ion concentration by converting strong (completely ionized) acids and bases into weaker (less completely dissociated) acids and bases.

The major buffer system of the blood is the *sodium bicarbonate–carbonic acid system.* This system is of major importance because both components of the buffer system are present in large amounts, and the concentration of each component can be regulated by the body. The concentration of carbonic acid (dissolved carbon dioxide) is controlled by the lungs, and the concentration of bicarbonate is controlled by the kidneys. Although the bicarbonate–carbonic acid buffer system is not the only buffer system of the body, the system is in equilibrium with the other buffer systems. Therefore, measurement of the components of this system provides an overall evaluation of the acid-base status of the patient.

Respiratory Control of Carbonic Acid

Carbonic acid represents physically dissolved carbon dioxide in plasma. This is in equilibrium with the carbon dioxide in the pulmonary alveoli. (The concentration of a gas is expressed in terms of its *partial pressure;* it is also common to speak of the partial pressure as the *tension* of gas.) Hyperventilation lowers the alveolar carbon dioxide partial pressure (tension) and leads to a rapid decrease in the concentration of carbon dioxide in the plasma. Decreased or inadequate pulmonary ventilation results in elevation of alveolar carbon dioxide tension, and this is associated with an increase in plasma carbonic acid concentration.

Control of Bicarbonate Concentration

The kidneys regulate bicarbonate concentration in the plasma by selectively reabsorbing filtered bicarbonate as necessary to meet the body's requirements. In addition, the kidneys can manufacture bicarbonate to replace the amounts lost in buffering acids produced as a consequence of normal metabolic processes. These two bicarbonate-regulating functions depend on the secretion of hydrogen ions by the renal tubules in exchange for sodium ions, which are simultaneously reabsorbed from the tubular filtrate into the circulation as illustrated in figure 24–1. Under the influence of the enzyme *carbonic anhydrase,* carbonic acid (H_2CO_3) is formed from carbon dioxide (CO_2) and water (H_2O) within the tubular epithelial cells and dissociates into hydrogen (H^+) and bicarbonate (HCO_3^-) ions. The hydrogen ions enter the tubular filtrate in exchange for sodium ions (Na^+). The bicarbonate ions enter the bloodstream along with the sodium ions that have been absorbed from the filtrate.

Relation between pH and Ratio of Buffer Components

In any buffer system, the pH depends on the ratio of the two components and not on the absolute quantities of the components. For the bicarbonate–carbonic acid buffer system, at normal body pH of 7.4, the normal ratio consists of twenty parts of sodium bicarbonate and one part of carbonic acid.

Another way of visualizing the bicarbonate–carbonic acid relation is to think of a board on a fulcrum. One side of the board is weighted by twenty parts of sodium bicarbonate, and the other side is weighted by one part of

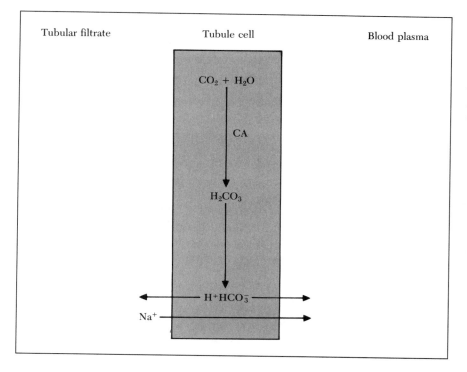

Tubular filtrate   Tubule cell   Blood plasma

$$CO_2 + H_2O$$

CA

$$H_2CO_3$$

$$H^+ HCO_3^-$$

$$Na^+$$

FIGURE 24–1

Formation and excretion of hydrogen ions by renal tubular epithelial cells in exchange for sodium. *CA* indicates carbonic anhydrase.

carbonic acid. The fulcrum is placed so that the board is exactly in balance, corresponding to a body pH of 7.4. Variations in the "weight" of either the sodium bicarbonate or the carbonic acid can be visualized as unbalancing the board, resulting in a shift of pH to a new level, either higher or lower than the normal value (figure 24–2).

A disturbance in which blood pH is shifted to the acid side of the physiologic range is called **acidosis.** It may be caused by an excess of carbonic acid or by a reduced amount of bicarbonate. A shift in the opposite direction is termed **alkalosis.** This shift may be the result of a decrease in carbon dioxide or to an excess of bicarbonate. These possibilities allow classification of acid-base disturbances into four large categories:

Disturbances of Acid-Base Balance

1. Metabolic acidosis (decrease in bicarbonate)
2. Respiratory acidosis (increase in carbonic acid)
3. Metabolic alkalosis (increase in bicarbonate)
4. Respiratory alkalosis (decrease in carbonic acid)

The term *metabolic* is applied when the disturbance lies primarily in the bicarbonate member of the buffer pair. The term *respiratory* indicates that the primary disturbance lies in the carbonic acid component of the buffer.

The various forms of acid-base disturbance are compared in table 24–1.

FIGURE 24–2

"Board-and-fulcrum" concept of normal bicarbonate–carbonic acid relations.

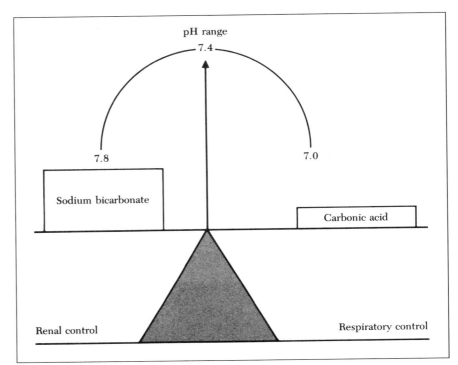

Compensatory Mechanisms Responding to Disturbances in pH

If the acid-base disturbance shifts the pH outside of the physiologic range, various control measures are activated to resist the change in pH. Compensatory mechanisms attempt to preserve the normal 20:1 ratio of bicarbonate to carbonic acid and thereby return the pH to physiologic range. For example, if the concentration of carbonic acid rises, there is a compensatory increase in bicarbonate that tends to restore the ratio of the two constituents and maintain pH in the physiologic range. Conversely, if there is a decrease in bicarbonate, compensation involves a decrease in the concentration of carbonic acid to maintain a relatively normal ratio. The body's major concern is maintaining a normal ratio of constituents to maintain a physiologic pH, even though this is accomplished by changing the absolute concentrations of the members of the buffer pair. Compensation is accomplished by both renal and respiratory methods.

For the student attempting to grasp the fundamentals of the major disturbances in acid-base balance, the "board-and-fulcrum" concept shown in figure 24–2 is frequently helpful. The "weight" of carbonic acid is controlled by respiration, and the "weight" of bicarbonate is controlled by renal excretion or conservation of bicarbonate. The student should consider two things: (1) the nature of the primary disturbance and how it will "unbalance" the

Disturbance	Primary abnormality	Compensation	Usual causes
Metabolic acidosis	Excess endogenous acid depletes bicarbonate	Hyperventilation lowers PCO_2; kidney excretes more hydrogen ions and forms more bicarbonate	Renal failure; ketosis; overproduction of lactic acid
Respiratory acidosis	Inefficient excretion of carbon dioxide by lungs	Formation of additional bicarbonate by kidneys	Chronic pulmonary disease
Metabolic alkalosis	Excess plasma bicarbonate	None	Loss of gastric juice; chloride depletion; excess corticosteroid hormones; ingestion of excessive bicarbonate or other antacids
Respiratory alkalosis	Hyperventilation lowers PCO_2	Increased excretion of bicarbonate by kidneys	Severe anxiety with hyperventilation; stimulation of respiratory center by drugs; central nervous system disease

TABLE 24–1

Comparison of common acid-base disturbances

board, and (2) the steps that the body should take to bring the board back into balance. These are the compensatory mechanisms, and they generally consist of "adding weight" or "subtracting weight" from the other member of the board. Admittedly, this is a mechanical oversimplification of a complex process, but it is a helpful learning device.

The two most common clinical disturbances of acid-base balance are metabolic acidosis and respiratory acidosis.

Metabolic Acidosis

Metabolic acidosis, a common problem in medical practice, occurs when the amount of acid generated exceeds the body's buffering capacity. The concentration of bicarbonate in the plasma falls because it is consumed in neutralizing the excess acid (figure 24–3A). Three of the more common conditions leading to metabolic acidosis are

1. Renal failure (uremia)
2. Ketosis (overproduction of ketone bodies)
3. Lactic acidosis (excessive production of lactic acid)

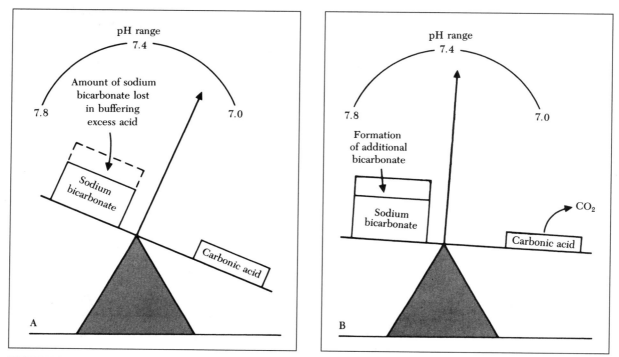

FIGURE 24-3

A, Derangement of acid-base balance in metabolic acidosis. **B,** Compensation by reduction of carbonic acid and formation of additional bicarbonate.

Uremia is the end stage of many different types of kidney disease, as described in chapter 19. Metabolic acidosis occurs because the failing kidneys are unable to efficiently excrete the various acid waste products that are produced by the body's normal metabolic processes. **Ketosis** results from overproduction of the acid ketone bodies *acetoacetic acid* and *beta-hydroxybutyric acid,* which are derived from the metabolism of fat.

Ketosis commonly occurs in untreated insulin dependent diabetes because the body is unable to utilize carbohydrate efficiently and is forced to rely on fat as a major energy source (chapter 22). Ketosis may also occur in any condition in which carbohydrate intake is inadequate, as in starvation or if persistent vomiting prevents the retention of nutrients. In such cases, the body has to metabolize adipose tissue because carbohydrate is not available as an energy source.

Lactic acidosis occurs in a number of different conditions, such as shock or severe heart failure, in which the tissues receive as inadequate supply of oxygen. The lactic acid is formed from the breakdown of glucose in the presence of an insufficient oxygen supply.

Compensatory Mechanisms

Compensation for metabolic acidosis is accomplished both by the lungs and by the kidneys (figure 24–3B). The acidosis stimulates the respiratory center in the brain stem, leading to an increase in both the rate and the depth of respiration. The hyperventilation reduces the partial pressure of carbon dioxide (PCO_2) in the alveoli, which in turn leads to a reduction in the amount of dissolved carbon dioxide and carbonic acid in the plasma. The decline in carbonic acid tends to restore the bicarbonate–carbonic acid ratio and pH toward normal. If renal function is not impaired, the kidneys also produce more bicarbonate to replenish the depleted supplies and at the same time excrete more hydrogen ions.

The following case illustrates a severe metabolic acidosis secondary to renal insufficiency. Case studies dealing with other diseases that cause metabolic acidosis are considered in chapters 19 and 22.

CASE 24–1

A sixty-five-year-old woman consulted her physician because of discomfort in the low back. Physical examination revealed moderate enlargement of both kidneys. Laboratory studies revealed a small amount of albumin in the urine and a moderate degree of anemia. Urea nitrogen was 57 mg/dL, a moderate elevation (normal range 10–20 mg/dL). A pyelogram revealed bilateral polycystic kidneys. The patient declined further treatment but was readmitted six months later because of further deterioration of her condition. She was more anemic, and the blood urea nitrogen had risen to 148 mg/dL. Blood pH was reduced to 7.2 (normal range 7.38–7.42). Plasma bicarbonate was also reduced to 10 mEq/L. The PCO_2 was 30 mm Hg, a slight decrease that was secondary to hyperventilation. The patient was considered to be in uremia with marked metabolic acidosis. She was not considered a suitable candidate for hemodialysis, and she died in the hospital ten days after admission.

Respiratory Acidosis

In *respiratory acidosis,* the primary abnormality is failure of the lungs to excrete carbon dioxide efficiently. This is usually secondary to chronic lung disease such as pulmonary emphysema, but it may occur in any situation in which pulmonary ventilation is severely impaired (chapter 15). In many instances, a respiratory infection in a patient with an underlying chronic lung disease may precipitate acute respiratory acidosis.

Retention of carbon dioxide leads to a rise in the alveolar PCO_2. Because the amount of carbon dioxide dissolved in the plasma is in equilibrium with the carbon dioxide gas in the pulmonary alveoli, a rise in alveolar PCO_2 also increases the amount of carbon dioxide dissolved in the plasma. As more carbon dioxide is dissolved, more carbonic acid is formed and the pH shifts to the acid side of the physiologic range (figure 24–4A).

Compensatory Mechanisms

The body's compensatory mechanism is the formation of additional bicarbonate by the kidneys, raising the level of bicarbonate in the plasma. This

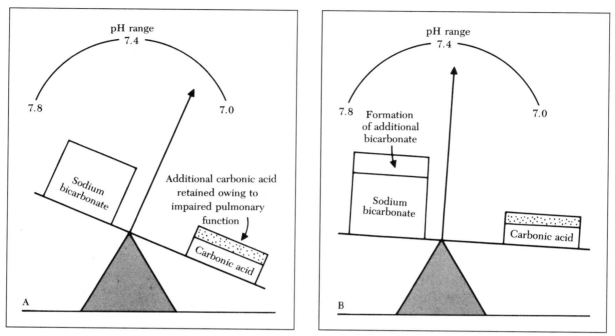

FIGURE 24–4

A, Derangement of acid-base balance in respiratory acidosis. **B,** Compensation by formation of additional bicarbonate.

tends to restore the normal ratio of the two buffer components, thereby shifting the pH back toward the physiologic range (figure 24–4B).

The following case illustrates an example of respiratory acidosis precipitated by a right lower-lobe pneumonia in an emphysematous patient.

CASE 24–2

A sixty-four-year-old man had noted progressive chronic cough and shortness of breath on exertion and repeated bouts of respiratory infection. He had become so short of breath that he was no longer able to climb stairs or do any kind of work around the house. Chest x-ray revealed hyperinflation of the lungs, compatible with pulmonary emphysema, and pulmonary function studies also showed marked impairment. Physical examination revealed a severely dyspneic man who was also slightly cyanotic. Scattered wheezes were heard throughout both lungs with a stethoscope. The temperature was slightly elevated. Chest x-ray revealed pulmonary emphysema and an area of consolidation in the right lower lobe of the lung representing a superimposed pneumonia. Arterial blood oxygen saturation was reduced; partial pressure of carbon dioxide was increased (PCO_2 50 mm Hg), and blood pH was reduced (pH 7.30). The patient was treated with antibiotic therapy and supplementary oxygen. He eventually recovered from the pneumonia and was able to leave the hospital.

Metabolic Alkalosis

Metabolic alkalosis is characterized by an increase in the concentration of plasma bicarbonate relative to the concentration of carbonic acid, which shifts the pH to the alkaline side of the physiologic range. The main causes of the metabolic alkalosis are

1. Loss of acid gastric juice
2. Chloride depletion
3. An excess of adrenal corticosteroid hormones
4. Ingestion of excessive amounts of sodium bicarbonate or other antacids

Loss of Gastric Juice

Excessive amounts of gastric juice may be lost by prolonged vomiting. Sometimes it is necessary to keep the stomach empty by continuous aspiration of gastric contents by means of a tube inserted through the nose into the stomach (*nasogastric tube*). In both situations, the loss of gastric juice causes loss of hydrogen ions. Alkalosis results because of the way that hydrochloric acid (HCl) is formed in the stomach. Within the gastric epithelial cells, carbon dioxide (CO_2) and water (H_2O) combine under the influence of the enzyme carbonic anhydrase to form carbonic acid (H_2CO_3), which dissociates into hydrogen (H^+) and bicarbonate (HCO_3^-). The hydrogen ion (H^+) is secreted along with the chloride ion (Cl^-) to form hydrochloric acid, and the remaining bicarbonate ion is absorbed into the blood plasma.

Normally, most of the acid secreted by the stomach is neutralized in the duodenum by alkaline pancreatic juice that is rich in bicarbonate ions. Consequently, the amount of bicarbonate decomposed in the duodenum when gastric juice is neutralized is equivalent to the amount of bicarbonate that is absorbed when acid was being secreted; so there is no net increase in the plasma bicarbonate concentration. However, if gastric juice is lost by vomiting or by continuous aspiration of gastric juice, the bicarbonate absorbed when acid is secreted is not "cancelled out" by loss of an equivalent amount of bicarbonate to neutralize acid in the duodenum. Consequently, the concentration of bicarbonate in the plasma rises and alkalosis occurs.

Chloride Depletion

Chloride depletion results from loss of gastrointestinal secretions caused by severe vomiting or diarrhea. It may also follow administration of some diuretics. Chloride and bicarbonate are the two chief anions in the plasma, and their concentrations vary inversely. When the plasma chloride falls, plasma bicarbonate rises so that the total concentration of anions in the extracellular fluids remains relatively constant.

Excess Adrenal Corticosteroids

An excess secretion of adrenal corticosteroids that regulate salt and water metabolism (*mineralocorticoids*) often causes not only metabolic alkalosis, but potassium depletion as well. A major site of action of corticosteroids is the distal renal tubule, where the hormone promotes absorption of sodium in exchange for potassium. An excess of mineralocorticoids increases absorption of sodium in exchange for potassium in the distal tubules, leading to excessive potassium loss and depletion of body potassium. As potassium deficiency develops, less potassium is available for exchange, and much of the sodium must be absorbed from the distal tubules in exchange for hydrogen ions rather than potassium ions. (The secretion rates of hydrogen and potassium ions vary inversely.) Each hydrogen ion secreted by the renal tubules is associated with the formation of a bicarbonate ion that diffuses into the plasma, as previously described (see figure 24–1). Consequently, plasma bicarbonate rises when hydrogen ions are secreted in excess and metabolic alkalosis results.

Ingestion of Antacids

Sometimes persons with gastric or duodenal ulcers take antacids to neutralize the excess gastric juice. If large amounts of sodium bicarbonate are ingested, some of the bicarbonate is absorbed and causes metabolic alkalosis by increasing the total amount of plasma bicarbonate. Other antacids also may cause metabolic alkalosis even though they are not absorbed from the gastrointestinal tract, because they neutralize gastric acid, which has the same effect as loss of gastric juice by vomiting or continuous aspiration of gastric juice.

Compensatory Mechanisms

Compensatory measures in metabolic alkalosis are quite inefficient. Respiratory compensation is extremely limited. If pulmonary ventilation was decreased enough to raise alveolar carbon dioxide tension, oxygenation of the blood would be inadequate. Bicarbonate excretion by the kidneys is inefficient in the presence of potassium deficiency, which frequently coexists with metabolic alkalosis. When intracellular potassium is depleted, sodium reabsorption from the distal tubule occurs primarily in exchange for hydrogen ions. The increased secretion of hydrogen ions leads to the formation of additional bicarbonate ions which diffuse into the circulation and raise the concentration of bicarbonate in the plasma. As a result, the potassium-depleted kidney not only is unable to compensate for the alkalosis, but actually accentuates it by forming excess bicarbonate. Successful treatment of metabolic alkalosis generally requires simultaneous correction of the potassium deficiency.

Respiratory Alkalosis

Respiratory alkalosis is a result of hyperventilation, which lowers the alveolar PCO_2. This in turn leads to a corresponding decrease in the amount of dissolved carbon dioxide and carbonic acid in the plasma. As a result, there is a relative excess of bicarbonate and the blood pH tends to rise (figure 24–5A). The hyperventilation that initiates this disturbance may result from stimulation of the respiratory center by drugs or may result from disease of

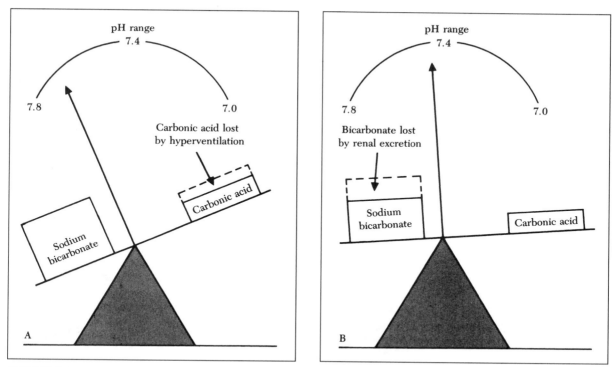

FIGURE 24–5

A, Derangement of acid-base balance in respiratory alkalosis. **B,** Compensation by excretion of bicarbonate.

the nervous system. Sometimes the hyperventilation is the result of an emotional disturbance such as severe anxiety.

Compensatory Mechanisms

Compensation is achieved by increased excretion of bicarbonate by the kidneys, which lowers the plasma bicarbonate and tends to restore the ratio of the buffer components toward normal (figure 24–5B).

Diagnostic Evaluation of Acid-Base Balance

In evaluating the acid-base status of a patient, the clinician frequently determines the concentration of the bicarbonate in the plasma as an index of the patient's overall status. This is supplemented in many cases by the determination of the blood pH and the determination of the carbonic acid in the plasma. The clinical state of the patient, as evaluated by the clinician, together with these various laboratory tests, generally permits a determination of the patient's acid-base status and serves as a guide for effective treatment.

Question for Review

1. What is the difference between intracellular fluid and extracellular fluid?

2. What is meant by the following terms: *milliequivalent, diuretic, carbonic anhydrase,* and *buffer*?

3. What is metabolic acidosis? How does it arise? What are the body's compensatory mechanisms?

4. What is respiratory acidosis? How does it arise? What are the body's compensatory mechanisms?

5. What is metabolic alkalosis? How does it arise? What are the body's compensatory mechanisms?

6. What is respiratory alkalosis? How does it arise? What are the body's compensatory mechanisms?

Supplementary Readings

Cogan, M. G. 1991. *Fluid & electrolytes: Physiology & pathophysiology.* Norwalk, Conn.: Appleton & Lange. Covers subject well.

Cohen, R. D., et al. 1983. Lactic acidosis revisited. *Diabetes* 32:181–91. Reviews sites of production of lactic acid, pathophysiology, and treatment.

Davenport, H. W. 1974. *The ABC of acid-base chemistry.* 6th ed. Chicago: University of Chicago Press. The classic monograph on this subject.

Kaehny, W. D. 1983. Respiratory acid-base disorders. *Medical Clinics of North America* 67:915–28. A review article. See also other articles on acid-base disorders in the same issue.

Lowenstein, J. 1993. *Acid and basics: A guide to understanding acid-base disorders.* New York: Oxford University Press. A concise treatment of acid-base disorders.

Narins, R. G., et al. 1982. Diagnostic strategies in disorders of fluid, electrolyte, and acid-base homeostasis. *American Journal of Medicine* 72:496–520. Discusses pathophysiology and biochemistry of acid-base and fluid-electrolyte disturbances.

Sloane, E. 1994. *Anatomy and physiology: An easy learner.* Chap. 17. Boston: Jones and Bartlett Publishers. Basic concepts in outline format. Good section on chemistry of electrolytes.

Chapter 24 ▪ Outline Summary

Interrelations of Intracellular and Extracellular Fluid / 695
Basic Concepts

Intracellular water is 70 percent of total body water.

Water contains dissolved electrolytes.

Sum of positive ions balanced by negative ions.

Disturbances of body water are associated with corresponding changes in electrolytes.

Fluids and electrolytes diffuse readily but capillaries are impermeable to protein.

Sodium (Na^+) and chloride (Cl^-) are chief extracellular ions; potassium (K^+) and phosphate (PO_4^{2-}) are principal intracellular ions.

Units of Concentration

Molecular weight of substance in grams divided by valence dissolved in one liter equals one equivalent per liter (1 Eq/L).

Units usually expressed in milliequivalents per liter (1000 mEq = 1 Eq).

Regulation of Body Fluid and Electrolyte Concentration / 696
Physiologic Concepts

Amount of water and electrolytes in body is balance between amount ingested and amount excreted.

Kidneys are major excretory organs.

Disturbance of Water Balance

Dehydration.

Inadequate intake: comatose or debilitated patients.

Excess water loss: vomiting or diarrhea.

Overhydration.

Excessive fluid intake when renal function impaired.

Excessive administration of intravenous fluids.

Disturbance of Electrolyte Balance

Depletion of electrolytes.

Vomiting or diarrhea.

Excessive use of diuretics.

Excessive diuresis in diabetic acidosis.

Renal tubular disease.

Acid-Base Balance / 697
Physiologic Concepts
Body produces large amounts of acid.

Regulatory mechanisms maintain pH.

Blood buffers: resist pH change.

Lungs: control carbonic acid concentration.

Kidneys: control bicarbonate concentration.

Disturbances of Acid-Base Balance
Metabolic acidosis.

Excess acid neutralized by bicarbonate, and bicarbonate concentration falls (uremia, ketosis, lactic acidosis).

Compensation by hyperventilation (lowers PCO_2) and increased production of bicarbonate by kidneys.

Respiratory acidosis.

Respiratory insufficiency leads to retention of CO_2 and rise in carbonic acid (H_2CO_3).

Compensation by increased production of bicarbonate by kidneys.

Metabolic alkalosis.

Increased concentration of bicarbonate as a result of various causes (loss of gastric juice, chloride depletion, excess corticosteroids, excess antacids).

Frequently coexisting potassium deficiency.

Compensation inefficient, and requires correction of coexisting potassium deficiency.

Respiratory alkalosis.

Hyperventilation lowers PCO_2, and H_2CO_3 falls.

Compensation by excretion of bicarbonate by kidneys.

Evaluation of Acid-Base Balance by the Clinician
Clinical evaluation.

Laboratory studies: pH, PCO_2, bicarbonate.

25

The Endocrine Glands

Learning Objectives

1. Explain the normal physiologic functions of the pituitary hormones, name the common endocrine disturbances, and describe the methods of treating each disturbance.

2. Describe the major disturbances of thyroid function and their clinical manifestations, and explain methods of treatment.

3. Explain the normal physiologic functions of the adrenal cortex and medulla, name the common endocrine disturbances resulting from dysfunction, and describe methods of treatment.

4. Define the causes and effects of parathyroid dysfunction, and describe methods of treatment.

5. Understand the concept of ectopic hormone production by nonendocrine tumors.

6. Name the adverse health effects of obesity. Describe the surgical procedures used in treatment of massive obesity, and explain the rationale for each procedure.

7. Explain how stress affects the endocrine system.

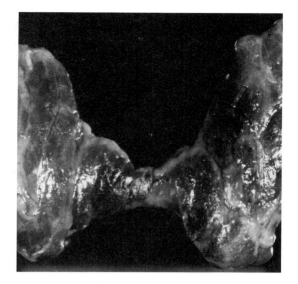

Chapter 25 ■ Contents

Endocrine glands liberate their secretions directly into the bloodstream and exert a regulatory effect on various metabolic functions.

The major endocrine glands are the pituitary, thyroid, and parathyroid glands; the adrenal cortex and medulla; the pancreatic islets; and the ovaries and the testes. However, these glands are not the only sites of hormone production. Many groups of specialized cells throughout the body also secrete hormones. Renin and erythropoietin are secreted by the kidneys; the hormones gastrin, secretin, and cholecystokinin are produced by the mucosa of the gastrointestinal tract. By convention, these hormones are considered along with the organs with which they are associated and are not generally regarded as part of the endocrine system.

The amount of hormone synthesized and released into the circulation by an endocrine gland may be regulated directly, by the level of hormone circulating in the blood, or indirectly, by the level of a substance under hormonal control, such as the concentration of glucose or sodium in the blood. The latter type of control mechanism is called a *feedback mechanism*. Most commonly, an increase in the level of hormone or hormone-regulated substance suppresses further hormone output. This is called a *negative feedback mechanism* or *feedback inhibition* and is illustrated by the control mechanisms regulating output of pituitary hormones.

A disorder of an endocrine gland may consist of either *hypersecretion* of the gland, manifested as overactivity of the target organ regulated by the gland, or *insufficient secretion,* resulting in underactivity of the organ controlled by the gland.

The clinical effects of a disturbance of endocrine gland function are determined by the degree of dysfunction of the gland and by the age and sex of the affected individual. All degrees of glandular dysfunction may be encountered, ranging from barely detectable variations from normal to extreme hypofunction or hyperfunction.

The age of the person when the endocrine disturbance becomes manifest has a pronounced effect on the clinical features. Some endocrine glands, such as the thyroid gland, affect growth and development as well as metabolic processes; so disturbed function in a child will produce a somewhat different clinical picture than will a similar disturbance in an adult.

The sex of the individual also influences the effect of disturbed endocrine function. Many hormones are concerned with the development and maintenance of sexual function and secondary sexual characteristics, and several endocrine glands produce sex hormones. Some endocrine disturbances cause alteration in sexual development in children, whereas the effects are much less pronounced in adults. Overproduction of an inappropriate sex hormone in some endocrine diseases causes masculinization (virilization) of the female or feminization of the male; conversely, overproduction of a sex hormone appropriate to the sex of the individual has little clinical effect.

The Pituitary Gland

The *pituitary gland* is a small, pea-shaped gland suspended by a narrow stalk from the hypothalamus at the base of the brain. The gland is located within a small depression at the base of the skull, just behind the optic chiasm and optic nerves. It is composed of an anterior lobe, a posterior lobe, and a small intermediate lobe that is a rudimentary structure in humans.

The *anterior lobe* is composed of cords of epithelial cells containing hormones that are synthesized and stored within this lobe. It has been conventional to classify anterior-lobe cells on the basis of the staining reaction of their cytoplasmic granules, using routine staining methods. Three cell types were recognized: **eosinophils,** which contain bright-red–staining cytoplasmic granules; **basophils,** which have abundant blue-staining granules in their cytoplasm; and **chromophobe cells,** which contain sparse, poorly stained granules. Newer, more specialized staining methods, however, have identified five different cell types, each producing its own specific hormones. Currently, these cells are more commonly designated by the hormones that they produce rather than by the staining reactions of their granules.

The anterior lobe is connected to the hypothalamus by a special system of blood vessels called a *portal system,* which begins as capillaries in the hypothalamus and extends down the pituitary stalk to terminate as capillaries around the cells of the anterior lobe. Release of the hormones stored within the cells of the anterior lobe is regulated by hormonal substances called *releasing hormones,* which are synthesized in the hypothalamus and carried to the cells of the anterior lobe in the blood flowing through the portal system.

The *posterior lobe* consists of a meshwork of nerve fibers intermixed with specialized cells resembling nerve cells. It is connected to the hypothalamus by bundles of nerve fibers extending through the pituitary stalk rather than by the portal circulation. The hormones in the posterior lobe are synthesized within the hypothalamus and are then transmitted down the nerve axons in the pituitary stalk to the posterior lobe, where they are stored. They are then released from the posterior lobe in response to nerve impulses transmitted from the hypothalamus down the pituitary stalk.

The **hypothalamus,** which controls release of hormones from both the anterior and posterior lobes, is in turn under the control of higher cortical centers; consequently pituitary secretion is to some extent influenced by emotional stimuli such as anxiety, rage, and fear and is also influenced by sensory impulses that enter the nervous system and are in turn relayed to the hypothalamus.

Pituitary Hormones

The pituitary gland secretes a total of nine separate hormones, which have multiple functions. Six are produced by the anterior lobe:

1. Growth hormone
2. Prolactin

3. Thyroid-stimulating hormone (TSH)
4. Adrenocorticotrophic hormone (ACTH)
5. Follicle-stimulating hormone (FSH)
6. Luteinizing hormone (LH)

The intermediate lobe produces melanin-stimulating hormone (MSH). The posterior lobe produces two hormones: antidiuretic hormone (ADH) and oxytocin.

Anterior-Lobe Hormones

Growth hormone, also called *somatotropin,* has multiple actions, all concerned with general tissue growth. **Prolactin** stimulates the secretion of milk by the breast that has been previously stimulated by estrogen and progesterone. **Thyroid-stimulating hormone (TSH)**, also called *thyrotropin,* stimulates the thyroid gland to secrete thyroid hormone. **Adrenal corticotrophic hormone (ACTH)**, also called *corticotropin,* stimulates the adrenal cortex to manufacture and secrete adrenocortical hormones. It exerts its main effect on the adrenal hormones that control carbohydrate metabolism (*glucocorticoids*). **Follicle-stimulating hormone (FSH)** and **luteinizing hormone (LH)** are called *gonadotropic hormones.* They regulate the growth and development of the *gonads* (ovaries and testes) and control the output of sex hormones that are responsible for the development of male and female secondary sex characteristics.

Intermediate-Lobe Hormone

Melanin-stimulating hormone (MSH) causes darkening of the skin. It is an important hormone in some lower animals but has no important function in humans.

Posterior-Lobe Hormones

Antidiuretic hormone (ADH) causes the cells of the renal collecting tubules to become more permeable to water so that more water is absorbed and a concentrated urine is excreted. Secretion of ADH is regulated by receptors in the hypothalamus that respond to variations in the osmolarity of the extracellular fluid. If the osmolarity rises, the hypothalamic neurons send impulses to the posterior lobe to stimulate release of ADH. Water is retained instead of being excreted, which dilutes the extracellular fluid and lowers its osmolarity. Conversely, if the extracellular fluids become too dilute, the hypothalamus directs the pituitary to decrease its output of ADH. More water is excreted in the urine, which causes the osmolarity of the body fluids to rise.

Oxytocin stimulates the contraction of the pregnant uterus and causes ejection of milk from the lactating breast. Oxytocin is secreted in response to stimulation of the nipples during nursing. The sensory nerve impulses are transmitted to the hypothalamus, and the hypothalamic neurons in turn send impulses to the posterior lobe that cause the release of oxytocin.

Physiologic Control of Pituitary Hormone Secretion

The level of the various trophic hormones elaborated by the pituitary is regulated by the level of circulating hormone produced by the target gland (figure 25–1). Cells in the hypothalamus measure the level of the various hormones in the blood and liberate various releasing and inhibiting hormones that control the release of pituitary hormones into the circulation. When the concentration of the hormone falls below a certain level, *releasing hormones* are elaborated. They travel by the portal venous system to the pituitary gland, causing release of the trophic hormone. This, in turn, affects the target organ.

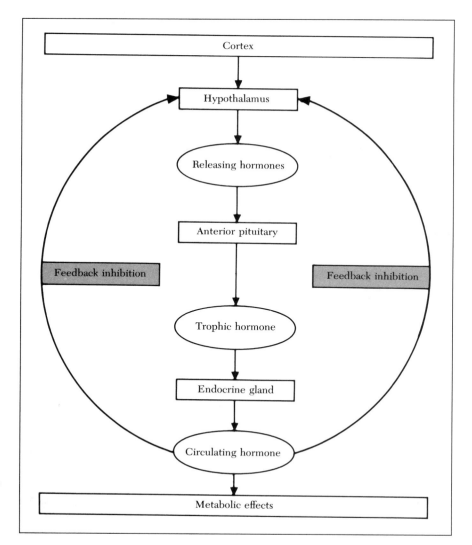

FIGURE 25–1

Normal mechanisms controlling elaboration of trophic hormones by the pituitary gland.

The level of the hormone elaborated by the target organ rises until it reaches the upper range of normal. At this point, the high level of circulating hormone "shuts off" further elaboration of trophic hormone. This mechanism maintains a relatively steady hormone output from the target organ and prevents wide fluctuations in hormonal level that might disrupt the smooth functioning of the body's hormone-regulated organ systems.

Prolactin secretion is regulated by a somewhat different mechanism from that of the other pituitary hormones. With other hormones, the main effect of hypothalamic releasing hormones is to stimulate secretion. For prolactin, however, the principal control is by an inhibitory hormone called **prolactin inhibitory factor** (**PIF**). Secretion of prolactin would continue unabated if it were not continuously suppressed. If PIF output falls for any reason, prolactin secretion rises. Secretion of PIF is regulated by hypothalamic neurons, which release a chemical mediator called **dopamine.** Therefore, drugs that alter the concentration of dopamine in the hypothalamus or block dopamine receptors also change the secretion of PIF, which in turn changes the output of prolactin. Release of prolactin is also affected by stimuli from the nipples that are relayed to the hypothalamus and act by decreasing output of PIF.

Although dopamine is the major regulator of prolactin secretion, *thyrotropin-releasing hormone* (*TRH*), which stimulates release of TSH by the pituitary, also directly stimulates release of prolactin as well.

Abnormalities in the secretion of trophic hormones may involve either single or multiple hormones and may be manifested as either a hypofunction or an overproduction of pituitary hormone.

Pituitary Hypofunction

Sometimes the anterior lobe of the pituitary gland is destroyed by a tumor or undergoes necrosis owing to a disturbance of its blood supply. In this condition, called **panhypopituitarism** (*pan* = multiple + *hypo* = decrease), the anterior lobe fails to secrete any hormones. The functions of the thyroid gland, adrenal glands, and gonads are impaired because trophic hormone stimulation is lost.

An isolated deficiency of growth hormone in a child leads to a condition called *pituitary dwarfism,* which is characterized by retarded growth and development. Normal growth and development can be restored by administering growth hormone produced by recombinant DNA technology (genetic engineering).

Diabetes insipidus is a rare disease characterized by failure of the posterior lobe of the pituitary gland to secrete ADH. Because of lack of ADH, the affected person is unable to absorb water from the renal collecting tubules and excretes a large volume of extremely dilute urine. Large amounts of water must be consumed to compensate for the excessive water loss in the urine and to prevent dehydration. Treatment consists of administering drugs having antidiuretic activity to replace the deficient ADH.

Overproduction of Growth Hormone

Sometimes an adenoma arising in the anterior lobe secretes an excess of growth hormone. The clinical features of a hormone-secreting tumor depend on the amount of hormone it produces, the size of the tumor, and the age of the subject. Overproduction of growth hormone in children and adolescents, whose epiphyses have not yet fused, causes excessive growth in the length of bones, and the subject becomes too tall. This condition is called *pituitary gigantism.* Some associated coarsening of the facial features usually occurs in response to the effect of growth hormone on the structure of the facial bones.

In adults, excessive growth hormone causes **acromegaly.** Because the epiphyses have fused, there can be no growth in height, but the growth hormone produces thickening and coarsening of bones and generalized enlargement of the viscera. Affected individuals have coarse facial features, large prominent jaws, and large spadelike hands, but they are no taller than normal (figure 25–2). The term *acromegaly* (*acron* = extremity + *megas* = large) describes one prominent feature of the disease.

In addition to the hormonal effects, manifestations related to the size and location of the tumor may also occur. The adenoma may cause enlargement of the bony cavity at the base of the skull where the pituitary is located, called the *pituitary fossa* or **sella turcica.** The tumor may also cause visual disturbances by pressing on the nearby optic nerves or tracts. Treatment consists of surgical resection or radiation therapy.

Overproduction of Prolactin

In a nonpregnant woman, excess secretion of prolactin may cause spontaneous secretion of milk from the breasts (**galactorrhea**) and cessation of menstrual periods (**amenorrhea**). Galactorrhea results from the effect of the hormone on breast tissue. Amenorrhea occurs because high levels of prolactin also inhibit secretion of pituitary gonadotropins FSH and LH, which in turn leads to cessation of ovulation and menstrual cycles. This is sometimes called the *amenorrhea-galactorrhea syndrome.* Figure 25–3 summarizes the various factors regulating prolactin secretion and the pathogenesis of this syndrome.

A prolactin-secreting pituitary adenoma is an important cause of the amenorrhea-galactorrhea syndrome. Sometimes the tumor is quite small (called a *microadenoma*) and causes few symptoms other than those related to the increased prolactin production. Larger tumors may cause enlargement of the pituitary fossa and visual disturbances like those produced by adenomas that secrete growth hormone. A prolactin-secreting pituitary adenoma can be removed surgically, but a small adenoma can often be inhibited by a drug called *bromergocriptine,* which acts by increasing output of PIF, thus suppressing growth and secretion of the adenoma.

There are other causes of hyperprolactinema. Some drugs and medications may at times raise prolactin levels, resulting in amenorrhea and galac-

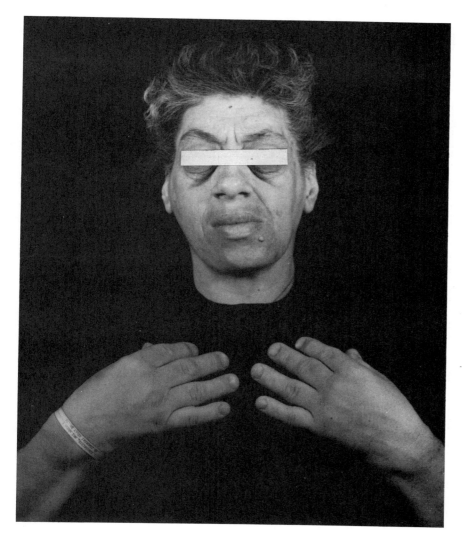

FIGURE 25–2

Appearance of subject with advanced acromegaly.

torrhea. These include estrogens, antihypertensive drugs, and drugs used to treat mental or emotional problems. The estrogens in contraceptive pills raise prolactin levels by stimulating the proliferation of prolactin-producing cells in the pituitary gland, and occasionally women taking contraceptive pills develop galactorrhea. Antihypertensive drugs, phenothiazine drugs (used to treat mental illness), and antidepressant drugs raise prolactin levels by depleting dopamine or blocking dopamine receptors in the hypothalamus. Consequently, less PIF is secreted and prolactin rises. Prolactin levels also rise in hypothyroidism because the reduced level of circulating thyroid hormone stimulates hypothalamic TRH, which in turn stimulates pituitary TSH in an attempt to increase thyroid hormone output. The increased TRH output also stimulates release of prolactin from the pituitary as a side effect.

FIGURE 25–3

Factors regulating prolactin secretion and pathogenesis of amenorrhea-galactorrhea syndrome. *PIF* indicates prolactin inhibitory factor. *TRH* indicates thyrotropin-releasing hormone.

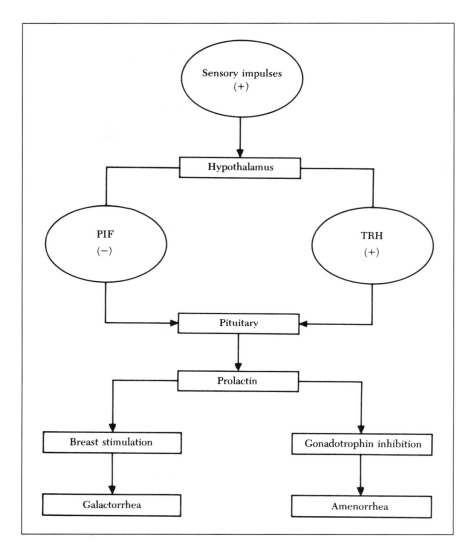

The Thyroid Gland

The *thyroid gland* consists of two lateral lobes connected by a narrow isthmus (figure 25–4A). It is located in the neck overlying the upper part of the trachea and is regulated by pituitary thyroid-stimulating hormone (TSH). The four *parathyroid glands* are located on its posterior surface.

Histologically, the thyroid gland is composed of multiple minute spherical vesicles called *thyroid follicles*. Each follicle consists of a central mass of eosinophilic protein material called **colloid,** surrounded by a layer of cuboidal epithelial cells called *follicular cells* (figure 25–4B). Under the influence of TSH, the follicular cells synthesize two hormones called *triiodothy-*

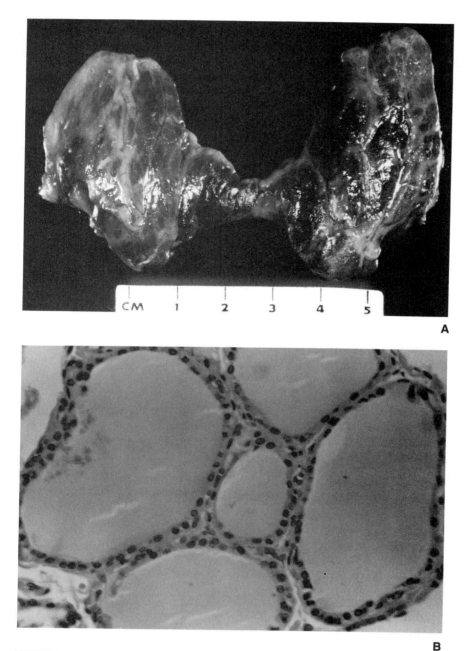

FIGURE 25–4

A, Normal thyroid gland, illustrating two lateral lobes connected by narrow isthmus. **B,** High-magnification photomicrograph of normal thyroid follicles, illustrating central masses of colloid surrounded by follicular epithelial cells. (Original magnification × 400.)

ronine (T$_3$) and *thyroxin* (T$_4$), which regulate the body's metabolic processes and are also required for the normal development of the nervous system. The term *thyroid hormone* is a general term that refers to the two metabolic hormones T$_3$ and T$_4$. Most of the thyroid hormone circulates bound to a protein called *thyroid-binding globulin* and is biologically inactive. The small amount of hormone that circulates unbound to protein is the physiologically active form of the hormone.

Specialized cells called *parafollicular cells,* which are located between the thyroid follicles, elaborate a third hormone called **calcitonin.** This hormone tends to lower blood calcium but plays a relatively minor part in regulating the level of calcium in the blood.

Actions of Thyroid Hormone

Thyroid hormone controls the rate of metabolic processes; it is also required for normal growth and development. Sometimes the thyroid gland secretes an inappropriate amount of hormone. An excess of thyroid hormone, called *hyperthyroidism,* leads to an acceleration of all bodily metabolic functions. Conversely, a decrease in the level of thyroid hormone, called *hypothyroidism,* slows metabolic processes.

Clinically, some of the most pronounced effects of excess thyroid hormone are manifested in the cardiovascular and neuromuscular systems. The heart rate is accelerated. Reflexes are hyperactive, and frequently a fine tremor of the muscles is apparent. The hormone also has conspicuous effects on emotional and intellectual functions. Individuals with excess thyroid hormone are hyperactive, emotionally labile, and often quite irritable. They may have difficulty concentrating because mental processes are accelerated excessively.

The effects of thyroid hypofunction are the reverse of those in hyperthyroidism. The hypothyroid individual is slow and lethargic. Bodily metabolic functions are subnormal. Reflexes and speech are slow and sluggish. Table 25–1 summarizes the major clinical effects resulting from abnormal levels of thyroid hormone.

Goiter

An enlargement of the thyroid gland is called a **goiter.** The gland may be uniformly enlarged, called a *diffuse goiter,* or multiple nodules of proliferating thyroid tissue may form a *nodular goiter.* An enlarged gland is called a *toxic goiter* is it produces an excessive amount of hormone and causes symptoms of hyperthyroidism. A goiter that does not increase output of hormone by the gland is called a *nontoxic goiter.*

Nontoxic Goiter
The basic cause of both nodular and diffuse nontoxic goiter is an inadequate secretion of thyroid hormone. The reduced hormone output causes the hypothalamus to elaborate releasing hormone, which in turn stimulates the

	Hyperthyroidism	Hypothyroidism
Cardiovascular effects	Rapid pulse, increased cardiac output	Slow pulse, reduced cardiac output
Metabolic effects	Increased metabolism, skin hot and flushed, weight loss	Decreased metabolism, cold skin, weight gain
Neuromuscular effects	Tremor, hyperactive reflexes	Weakness, lassitude, sluggish reflexes
Mental, emotional effects	Restlessness, irritability, emotional lability	Mental processes sluggish and retarded, personality placid and phlegmatic
Gastrointestinal effects	Diarrhea	Constipation
General somatic effects	Warm, moist skin	Cold, dry skin

TABLE 25–1

Comparison of major effects of hyperthyroidism and hypothyroidism

pituitary to liberate more TSH (figure 25–5). As a result, the gland enlarges in order to produce more hormone.

Three major factors predispose to the development of a nontoxic goiter:

1. Iodine deficiency
2. Deficiency of enzymes required for synthesis of thyroid hormone or ingestion of substances that interfere with the function of these enzymes
3. Increased hormone requirements

Iodine Deficiency   If iodine is deficient in the diet, not enough will be available to produce adequate hormone for the needs of the individual. The enlargement of the gland in response to TSH stimulation is an attempt to extract the meager amount of iodine from the blood more efficiently to make enough hormone. Iodine deficiency is rarely a cause of goiter in the United States because table salt, bread, and many other foods are fortified with iodine. Consequently, the average American diet actually contains an excess of iodine.

Enzyme Deficiency of Impaired Enzyme Function   Goiter more commonly results from a mild deficiency in a glandular enzyme that is required for hormone synthesis; the enzyme-deficient gland is unable to produce sufficient hormone without enlarging. Less commonly, the enzymes are present in normal amounts, but their functions are impaired by ingestion of drugs or other substances that interfere with the action of the enzymes. Even some "natural" foods, such as cabbage and turnips, contain small amounts of substances that interfere with thyroid-hormone synthesis, but these foods are not usually eaten in quantities sufficient to cause difficulty.

FIGURE 25–5

Pathogenesis of nontoxic
goiter.

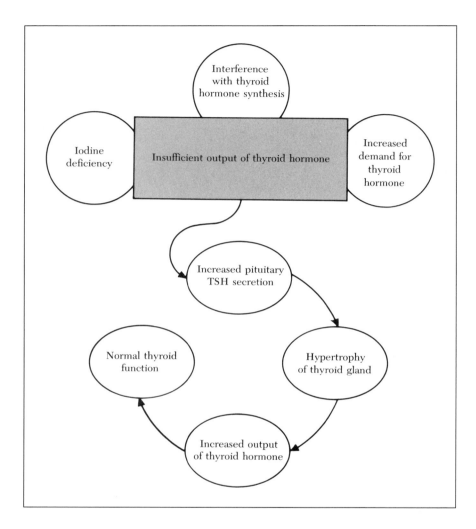

Increased Hormone Requirements   Normally, the need for thyroid hormone increases in puberty, during pregnancy, and under conditions of stress. In some individuals, the thyroid gland may be able to produce adequate hormone under normal circumstances but may be unable to increase its output in response to increased requirements without enlarging.

   Whenever hormone output is inadequate, no matter what the cause, more TSH is released in order to step up hormone production. Because hormone requirements often fluctuate, a gland may undergo successive alternating periods of enlargement and reduction in size. At first, the gland enlarges uniformly in response to TSH stimulation, and it returns to its original size when increased hormone output is no longer required. Eventually, however, the gland may respond in an irregular manner to TSH stimulation. If this occurs, the enlargement of the gland is not uniform and a nodular goiter results (figure 25–6).

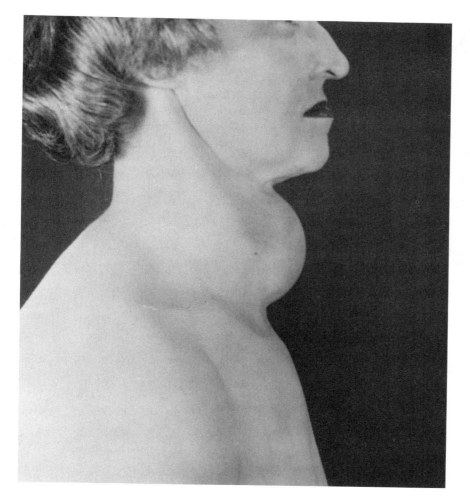

FIGURE 25–6

Large nodular goiter.

Treatment of Nontoxic Goiter   Because a nontoxic goiter results from excessive stimulation of the thyroid gland by TSH, it is usually treated by administration of thyroid hormone, which suppresses TSH output by the negative feedback mechanism. Treatment usually causes the enlarged gland to shrink because it is no longer being stimulated by TSH. A large nodular goiter may have to be removed surgically if it compresses the trachea, interferes with respiration, or obstructs the neck veins returning blood to the heart. Figure 25–7 shows a large nodular goiter obstructing the venous drainage of the head, neck, and chest.

Toxic Goiter

A goiter that secretes excess hormone causes hyperthyroidism. The gland is diffusely enlarged in most hyperthyroid patients, but the degree of enlargement is not marked (figure 25–8). The condition is called *diffuse toxic goiter* or *thyrotoxicosis.* The term *exophthalmic goiter* is sometimes also applied to

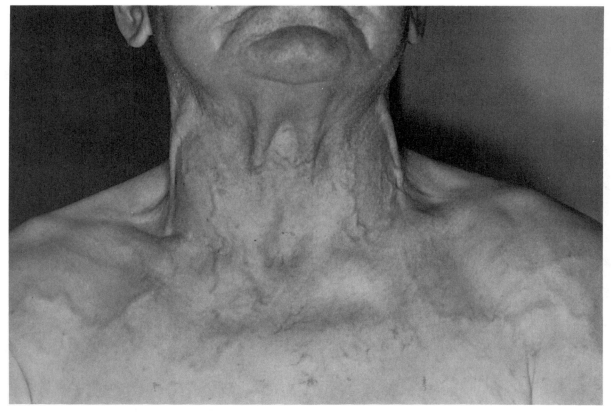

FIGURE 25–7

Nodular goiter obstructing veins draining blood from head, neck, and chest. Note large dilated veins in skin of neck and chest. Treated by thyroidectomy.

this condition because hyperthyroid persons frequently have prominent, protruding eyes (*exo* = out + *ophthalmos* = eye). The overactivity of the thyroid gland in diffuse toxic goiter is not caused by increased TSH stimulation. On the contrary, the excessive output of thyroid hormone suppresses TSH. The stimulus that provokes the gland to enlargement and hyperfunction is an antithyroid autoantibody produced by the affected individual's own lymphocytes. The antibody mimics the effects of TSH but is not subject to the control mechanisms that normally regulate TSH output. The antithyroid antibody can be detected in the blood and is termed *thyroid-stimulating immunoglobulin.*

Treatment of Toxic Goiter   At present, no method is available to block the stimulation of the thyroid gland by the TSH-like protein produced by the lymphocytes. It is possible, however, to control the hyperthyroidism. Three different methods of treatment can be used:

1. Antithyroid drugs can be administered to block synthesis of hormone by the hyperactive gland.
2. A large portion of the gland can be removed surgically, reducing the source of the hormone.
3. A large dose of radioactive iodine can be administered to be taken up by the thyroid gland. The irradiation destroys part of the gland and reduces its hormone output.

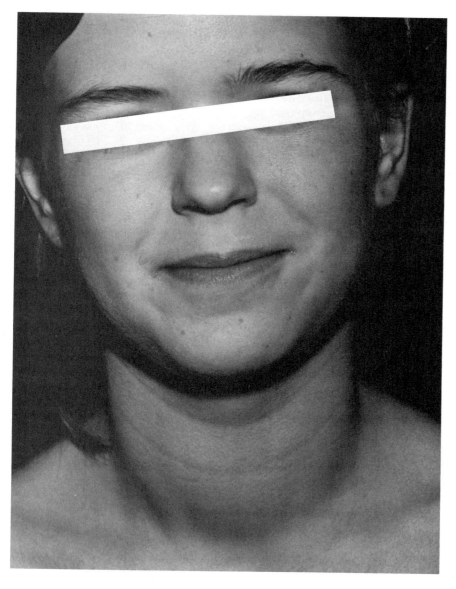

FIGURE 25–8

Small diffuse toxic goiter in young woman (case 25–1).

The following case illustrates successful treatment of a diffuse toxic goiter by means of antithyroid drugs and thyroidectomy.

CASE 25–1

A fifteen-year-old girl was referred to her physician because of recent onset of hyperactivity, rapid speech, and some prominence of the eyes (see figure 25–8). Examination revealed prominent eyes, a fine tremor, and hyperactive reflexes. Thyroid function studies indicated an elevated level of thyroid hormone in her blood, together with an increased uptake of iodine and increased synthesis of hormone as demonstrated by radioactive iodine tracer studies. The patient was considered to have a diffuse toxic goiter. She was treated initially by an antithyroid drug to control the hyperthyroidism, and a thyroidectomy was subsequently performed.

Hypothyroidism

Hypothyroidism in the Adult

Hypothyroidism in the adult is sometimes called **myxedema** (figure 25–9). It is manifested by a general slowing of the body's metabolic processes. Frequently, there are localized accumulations of mucinous material in the skin, from which the disease received its name (*myx* = mucin + *edema* = swelling). Hypothyroid individuals have low levels of circulating thyroid hormone and high levels of TSH that reflect stimulation of the gland in an unsuccessful attempt to increase hormone output. The condition is treated by supplying the deficient hormone, which results in clinical improvement, return of thyroid hormone level to normal, and fall in TSH, as illustrated by the following case.

CASE 25–2

A twenty-five-year-old woman visited her physician because of recent weight gain and menstrual irregularities. On examination, she was moderately overweight and her thyroid gland was slightly enlarged, but there were no other abnormalities. The level of thyroid hormone in her blood was reduced to 2.1 µg/dL (normal range 4.5–11.0 µg/dL), and thyroid-stimulating hormone (TSH) level was markedly increased to 310 microunits/mL (normal range 2–10 microunits/mL). She was considered to have hypothyroidism, probably the result of chronic thyroiditis (described in a subsequent section). She was treated with a thyroid hormone preparation (Synthroid). The level of thyroid hormone rose, and the elevated TSH level gradually returned to normal. She felt much better and lost some weight. Her menstrual periods became normal.

Neonatal Hypothyroidism

Hypothyroidism in the infant is called **cretinism.** This condition may be caused by failure of development of the thyroid gland, called *athyreotic cretinism* (*a* = without + *thyroid*), or to genetically determined deficiencies of enzymes necessary for thyroid-hormone synthesis, called *goiterous cretinism.* In the latter, the gland undergoes hyperplasia owing to excessive TSH stimulation, but it is incapable of producing adequate hormone because of a congenital deficiency of glandular enzymes.

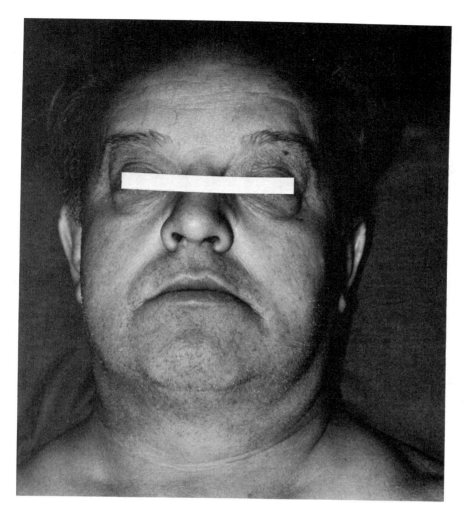

FIGURE 25–9

Appearance of patient with myxedema.

Manifestations of hypothyroidism may not be conspicuous at birth but usually become prominent during the neonatal period (figure 25–10). Thyroid hormone not only regulates metabolic processes, but is also required for normal growth. The hormone is also essential for the normal development of the nervous system, which continues for several months after birth. If neonatal hypothyroidism is recognized and treated promptly, the affected infant will usually grow and develop normally. If the condition remains undetected, the individual will remain permanently stunted in growth and mentally retarded. Screening tests for neonatal hypothyroidism can be performed on only a few drops of blood. The tests can detect the low levels of thyroid hormone and elevated levels of TSH that are characteristic of this condition. Such screening tests, which are required by law in many states, have assured early recognition and prompt treatment of affected infants.

FIGURE 25–10

Characteristic appearance of neonatal hypothyroidism (cretinism) as a result of congenital absence of thyroid gland. Treatment with thyroid hormone reversed manifestations of hypothyroidism.

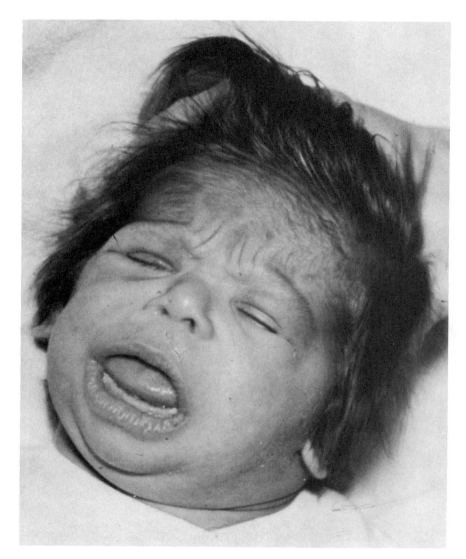

Thyroiditis

For reasons that are not well understood, some individuals develop auto-antibodies to their own thyroid tissue. The antibodies cause destruction of the thyroid, often leading to hypothyroidism. The disease is generally called *chronic thyroiditis,* and the thyroid gland is usually enlarged by a diffuse infiltration by lymphocytes and plasma cells. Normal cell structure and cell structure in chronic thyroiditis are compared in figure 25–11. The cellular infiltration is not the result of an infection but is a manifestation of the immunologic reaction between the antigen (thyroid tissue) and the antithyroid antibody. The infiltration of lymphocytes and plasma cells is a mani-

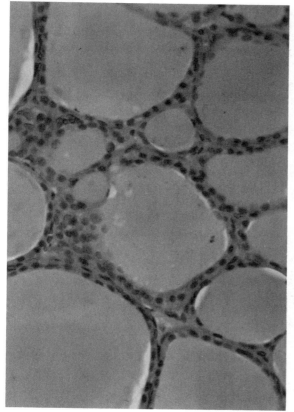
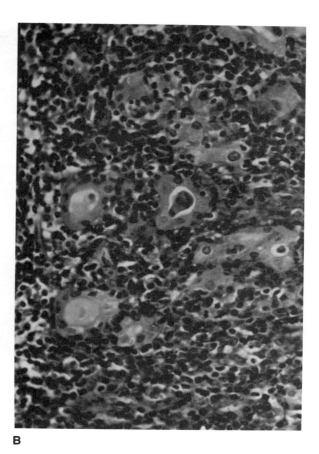

A   **B**

FIGURE 25–11

Low-magnification photomicrographs comparing cellular structure of normal thyroid gland (**A**) with that in chronic thyroiditis (**B**). Gland is heavily infiltrated by lymphocytes. Follicles are small and lack colloid. (Original magnification × 100.)

festation of the autoimmune reaction directed against thyroid tissue that is destroying the thyroid gland.

Tumors of the Thyroid

The thyroid gives rise to benign adenomas and several different types of carcinoma. Thyroid **adenomas** are well-circumscribed tumors composed of mature follicles that often contain large amounts of colloid (figure 25–12). There are three distinct types of thyroid cancer.

1. Well-differentiated carcinoma
2. Undifferentiated carcinoma
3. Medullary carcinoma

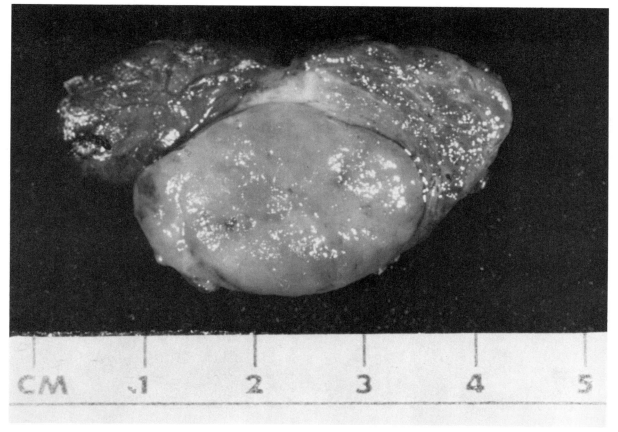

FIGURE 25–12

Benign, well-circumscribed adenoma of thyroid gland. Surrounding thyroid tissue appears normal.

Well-differentiated carcinoma usually develops in young adults and is of very low-grade malignancy. The two characteristic histologic patterns are shown in figure 25–13. *Follicular carcinoma* resembles the normal follicles of the thyroid. *Papillary carcinoma* is composed of well-differentiated papillary processes covered by mature epithelium. Treatment of both types is by surgical resection.

Undifferentiated carcinoma develops in older persons, is composed of rapidly growing bizarre tumor cells, and has a poor prognosis. Treatment is by means of surgical resection combined with radiation and chemotherapy.

Medullary carcinoma is an uncommon tumor that is derived from the calcitonin-secreting parafollicular cells of the thyroid. It has a characteristic histologic pattern. Measurement of calcitonin levels in the blood has been used as a diagnostic test for this type of thyroid cancer because the tumor cells often secrete calcitonin. Although the effect of calcitonin is to lower blood calcium, the excess hormone secretion has no significant effect on

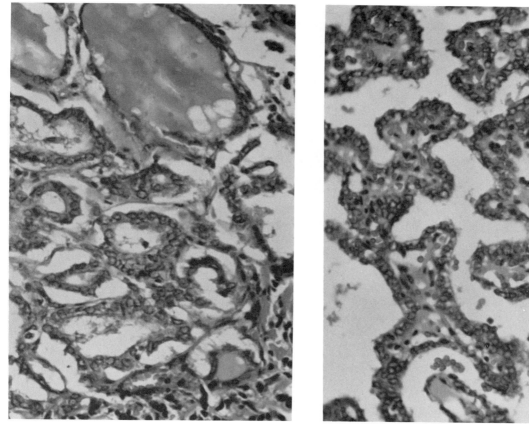

A   B

FIGURE 25–13

Low-magnification photomicrographs of well-differentiated thyroid carcinoma. **A,** Follicular carcinoma. Note formation of colloid by well-differentiated tumor cells. **B,** Papillary carcinoma. (Original magnification × 100.)

blood calcium, because the effect of the calcitonin is counteracted by an increased secretion of parathyroid hormone, preventing blood calcium from falling. (The physiologic effects of parathyroid hormone are considered in conjunction with diseases of the parathyroid glands.)

Radiation and Thyroid Tumors

The incidence of both benign and malignant tumors of the thyroid has been increasing and the increase appears related to previous thyroid radiation. In the 1930s and early 1940s, radiation therapy was used to treat enlargement of the thymus gland in infants, hypertrophied tonsils and adenoids, some fungus infections of the scalp, acne, and various other conditions of the head and neck. The treatments also exposed the thyroid gland to radiation. A small percentage of these patients developed various benign and malignant tumors of the thyroid from five to thirty years after the radiation exposure. Fortunately, most of the postradiation malignant tumors are well differentiated and of low malignancy. Because persons who have had previous radiation to the head and neck have an increased risk of thyroid tumors, they should have periodic medical examinations to assure that any thyroid tumors that develop subsequent to radiation will be recognized and treated promptly.

The Parathyroid Glands and Calcium Metabolism

The blood calcium is in equilibrium with the calcium salts present in bone. Half the blood calcium is present as calcium ions (Ca^{2+}) and is the active form. The other half is bound to blood proteins and is biologically inactive. An adequate concentration of ionized calcium is required for normal cardiac and skeletal muscle contraction, for transmission of nerve impulses, and for coagulation of the blood. A subnormal level of ionized calcium causes increased excitability of nerve and muscle cells, leading to spasm of skeletal muscles, which is called **tetany.** Conversely, a high level of ionized calcium diminishes neuromuscular excitability and leads to generalized muscular weakness.

The level of ionized calcium in the blood is regulated primarily by *parathyroid hormone,* which is secreted by four small *parathyroid glands* located on the posterior surface of the lateral lobes of the thyroid gland. The parathyroid hormone regulates the level of calcium by regulating the release of calcium from bone, the absorption of calcium from the intestine, and the rate of excretion of calcium by the kidneys. The secretion of parathyroid hormone is regulated by the level of ionized calcium in the blood rather than by a trophic hormone elaborated by the pituitary gland. If the level of ionized calcium in the blood decreases, the parathyroids secrete more hormone. If the ionized calcium level rises, parathyroid hormone secretion declines. Any abnormality in the secretion of parathyroid hormone changes the concentration of ionized calcium in the blood and will eventually alter the amount of calcium deposited in bone.

Hyperparathyroidism

Hyperparathyroidism is a relatively common problem and is usually the result of a hormone-secreting parathyroid adenoma. In response to increased output of hormone, the blood calcium rises (*hypercalcemia*) and excessive calcium is withdrawn from bone. The bones become excessively fragile and are easily broken.

Excessive amounts of calcium are excreted in the urine (*hypercalciuria*), sometimes leading to formation of calcium stones within the urinary tract. Occasionally, calcium precipitates out of the blood and becomes deposited in the kidneys, lungs, and other tissues, producing tissue injury and functional impairment. Treatment consists of surgical removal of the tumor.

Hypoparathyroidism

Hypoparathyroidism usually results from accidental removal of all four parathyroid glands during an operation for a diffuse toxic goiter or a nodular goiter in which most of the thyroid gland is removed. Blood calcium falls precipitously, which leads to increased neuromuscular excitability and tetany. Treatment consists of raising the level of blood calcium by administration of a high-calcium diet and supplementary vitamin D, which promotes absorption of calcium from the intestinal tract.

The Adrenal Glands

The *adrenals* are paired glands located above the kidneys. Each adrenal consists of two separate endocrine glands: an inner *adrenal medulla* surrounded by an outer *adrenal cortex*. The two glands secrete different hormones.

The Adrenal Cortex

The adrenal cortex secretes three major classes of steroid hormones:

1. Glucocorticoids
2. Mineralocorticoids
3. Sex hormones

Glucocorticoids
Glucocorticoids have three main actions:

1. They raise the blood glucose by decreasing glucose utilization in many tissues, except the brain, and promote fat breakdown with utilization of fatty acids rather than glucose as an energy source.
2. They inhibit protein synthesis and promote breakdown of body proteins, some of which are converted into glucose by the liver. The net effect is to deplete tissue proteins and raise blood glucose. (The adverse effect of glucocorticoids on wound healing and tissue repair is a result in part of their protein-depleting effects.)
3. They act as multiple sites to suppress the inflammatory reaction. (The use of adrenal corticosteroids to treat various types of inflammatory disease is related to the anti-inflammatory property of the glucocorticoids.)

Glucocorticoids are secreted in response to stimulation of adrenocorticotrophic hormone (ACTH), and their output is controlled by the same type of negative feedback mechanism that regulates secretion of thyroid hormone. The major glucocorticoid is **cortisol** (*hydrocortisone*).

Mineralocorticoids
Mineralocorticoids regulate electrolyte and water balance by promoting absorption of sodium and water, and excretion of potassium by the

FIGURE 25–14

Patient with Addison's disease (case 25–3), **A,** Appearance of face illustrating increased skin pigmentation. **B,** Appearance of hand (*right side of photograph*) compared with hand of normal subject. Note increased pigmentation of palms and pigmentation of skin creases.

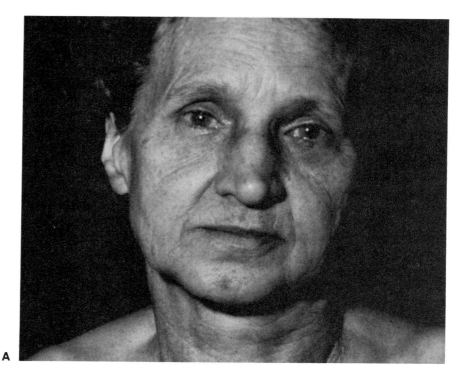

A

B

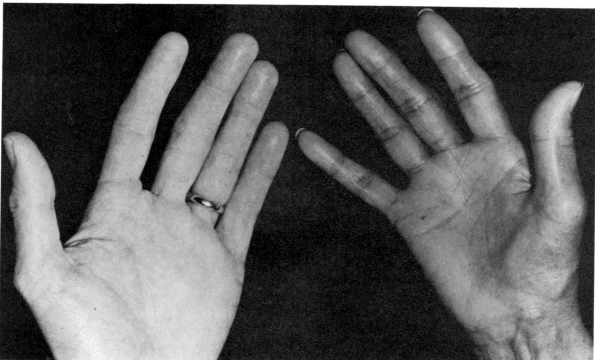

renal tubules. The major mineralocorticoid is **aldosterone,** and its secretion is regulated by more than one mechanism. Although ACTH increases aldosterone secretion to some extent, the most potent stimulus for aldosterone secretion is the *renin-angiotensin system* (described in chapter 19), which responds to a reduction in renal blood flow or blood pressure. One can think of the kidneys as "interpreting" the reduced blood flow and pressure to mean that blood volume is low; aldosterone secretion is then called for to promote retention of sodium and water, thus increasing blood volume.

Sex Hormones

Small amounts of estrogen, progesterone, and testosterone are produced by the adrenal glands of both males and females. The small amount of testosterone produced by the adrenals appears to be responsible for sex drive in the female, but otherwise production of sex hormone by the adrenals has little physiologic function under normal circumstances. In certain diseases, however, one or more of these hormones may be overproduced.

Abnormal adrenal cortical function produces abnormalities in the metabolism of carbohydrates and protein as a result of abnormal glucocorticoid secretion, as well as disturbances of salt and water metabolism caused by disturbed mineralocorticoid secretion.

Addison's Disease

Adrenal cortical hypofunction is called **Addison's disease.** It results from atrophy or destruction of both adrenal glands, leading to deficiency in both glucocorticoids and mineralocorticoids. As a result of a glucocorticoid deficiency, the blood glucose level is subnormal and may decline during fasting to such a low level that symptoms develop. The body's ability to regulate the content of sodium, potassium, and water in body fluids is disturbed as a result of the mineralocorticoid deficiency. Blood volume and blood pressure fall, as does the concentration of sodium in the blood, and blood potassium rises. The blood volume may become so reduced that the circulation can no longer be maintained efficiently.

Persons with Addison's disease also frequently exhibit increased pigmentation of the skin that is caused by an increased secretion of ACTH and MSH (figure 25–14). Both these pituitary hormones cause increased pigmentation of the skin, and cortisol normally inhibits both hormones by means of a negative feedback mechanism. In Addison's disease, secretion of cortisol is greatly diminished and consequently there is no feedback inhibition. The hyperpigmentation is a manifestation of the increased output of the hormones ACTH and MSH. Treatment of Addison's disease consists of administration of the deficient corticosteroids, as illustrated by the following case.

CASE 25-3

A sixty-six-year-old woman had noted gradual loss of energy and some weight loss over the previous two or three years. Her skin had become darker. She was in the habit of working outdoors in the summer and becoming suntanned, but recently her tan did not fade in the winter. Physical examination was unremarkable except for increased skin pigmentation. Pigmentation was also noted in the oral mucosa and in the skin creases. Laboratory studies revealed normal thyroid function. Plasma corticosteroid hormone level was reduced to 5 µg/dL (normal range 7–28 µg/dL). Plasma adrenocorticotrophic hormone (ACTH) level was markedly increased to more than 2000 pg/mL (normal less than 120 pg/mL). A diagnosis of Addison's disease was made. The very high ACTH level represented a loss of feedback inhibition with stimulation of the adrenal by the pituitary in an attempt to increase hormone output. The patient was treated with cortisone and responded satisfactorily.

Cushing's Disease

Cushing's disease results from overproduction of adrenal corticosteroid hormones. In the majority of patients, the adrenal hyperfunction is caused by a very small ACTH-secreting adenoma (called a *microadenoma*) arising in the anterior lobe of the pituitary gland, which induces secondary adrenal cortical hyperplasia and hypersecretion of adrenal corticosteroids. Less commonly, it is caused by a corticosteroid-hormone–secreting tumor of one adrenal gland. The glucocorticoid excess causes disturbances of carbohydrate, protein, and fat metabolism. The blood glucose rises. Protein synthesis is impaired and body proteins are broken down. The disturbed fat metabolism causes a redistribution of body fat, which tends to accumulate on the trunk while the extremities remain thin and appear wasted owing to muscle atrophy. The face appears full and rounded, which is sometimes called a "moon face." Salt and water are retained because of the increased output of mineralocorticoids, leading to an increase in blood volume and a rise in blood pressure.

Large amounts of adrenal corticosteroids are sometimes administered along with other drugs to patients with acute leukemia in order to induce a remission and to help suppress the immune response in patients who have received a kidney or other organ transplant. The large doses of corticosteroids produce the same clinical manifestations as those encountered in Cushing's disease. The condition is often called *Cushing's syndrome* to distinguish it from the condition caused by a pituitary or adrenal tumor. The manifestations subside spontaneously when the dosage of corticosteroid is reduced or the drug is discontinued.

Treatment of Cushing's Disease

The treatment of Cushing's disease depends on its cause. If it is a result of a pituitary microadenoma, the usual method of treatment is surgical resection of the tumor. The pituitary gland is relatively difficult to approach surgically through the cranial cavity. However, it can be approached from below through the nasal cavity, roof of the nose, and sphenoid sinus. Specialized instruments can be used to enter the pituitary fossa in this way, and a microadenoma can be visualized and resected. (A similar approach is used to resect prolactin-secreting pituitary microadenomas, which are described in a foregoing section.) Cushing's disease secondary to an adrenal tumor is treated by resection of the tumor.

Successful treatment is followed by regression of the clinical manifestations of the disease (figures 25–15 and 25–16).

Overproduction of Adrenal Sex Hormones

Adrenal gland dysfunction associated with abnormal production of sex hormone is uncommon. This may result from *congenital hyperplasia* of the adrenal gland or from an adrenal *sex-hormone–producing tumor.*

Congenital adrenal hyperplasia is the result of a congenital deficiency of certain enzymes required for the synthesis of various steroid hormones. In the normal biosynthesis of hormones by the adrenal cortex, cholesterol is initially converted into an intermediate compound (*pregnenolone*), which is a precursor of the other steroids produced in the adrenal (figure 25–17). The chief metabolic pathways are concerned with the conversion of the intermediate compound into *aldosterone,* the major mineralocorticoid (pathway 1), and into the *glucocorticoid cortisol* (pathway 2). A third minor metabolic pathway leads to the production of *adrenal androgens* (pathway 3).

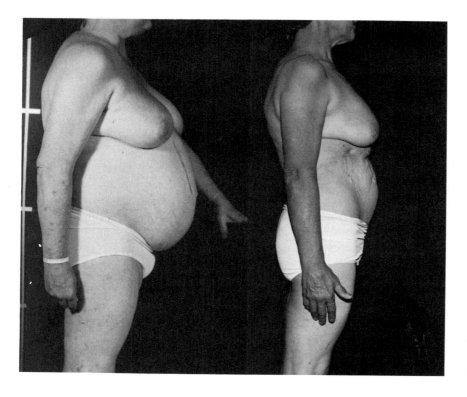

FIGURE 25–15

Cushing's disease before and after treatment. *Left,* Before treatment, illustrating obesity of trunk with thin extremities. *Right,* After treatment, illustrating normal body configuration.

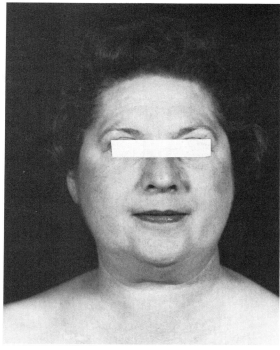

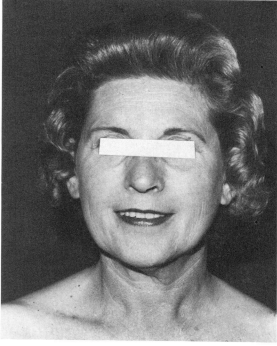

A

B

FIGURE 25–16

Cushing's disease before and after treatment. **A,** Full, rounded face ("moon face") prior to treatment. **B,** Normal facial appearance after treatment.

Biosynthesis of hormones in the major pathways (1 and 2) requires a series of additions of hydroxyl groups to the steroid molecules, and the enzymes that catalyze these reactions are called *hydroxylases*. If certain hydroxylases are absent or deficient, synthesis of aldosterone and cortisol will be impaired. This leads to increased ACTH secretion (because the pituitary interprets the low steroid levels in the blood as a signal to produce more ACTH). ACTH stimulation produces hyperplasia of the adrenal glands and increased synthesis of precursor compounds. However, because an enzymatic block affects the major pathways of steroid production, biosynthesis is shifted in the direction of androgenic steroids (pathway 3). Consequently, the major steroid output from the adrenals consists of androgenic compounds.

The clinical disorder produced by these enzymatic defects is often called the **adrenogenital syndrome.** There are several clinical varieties of this syndrome, depending on which of the hydroxylase enzymes is deficient and the extent of the deficiency. All have the common feature of producing premature sexual development, called *precocious puberty*. In the female, sex-

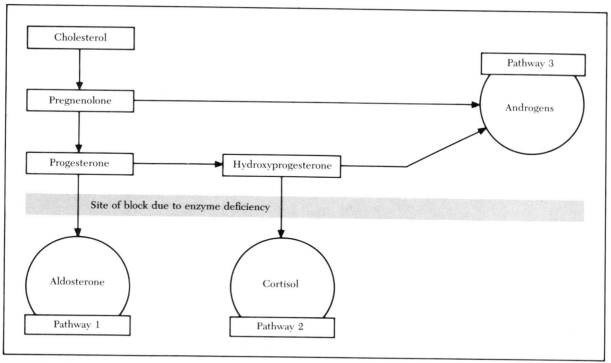

FIGURE 25–17

Biosynthesis of adrenal cortical hormones. *Shaded area* indicates site of enzymatic block leading to overproduction of adrenal androgens.

ual development is masculine because of the effect of the androgens. The age at which the hormonal effects become manifest depends on the degree of the enzyme deficiency. *Congenital virilization* may be noted at birth (figure 25–18). If the deficiency is less severe, symptoms may not appear until the child is older.

Adrenal tumors that elaborate sex hormones are rare. When such a tumor develops, however, either androgen or estrogen may be produced. The clinical features depend on the age of the individual when the tumor becomes manifest and on the sex of the affected person. In a child, the tumor produces precocious puberty, and the character of the sexual development depends on the type of hormone elaborated. In adults, an estrogen-producing neoplasm elicits no hormonal symptoms in women but induces feminization in men. An androgen-secreting tumor masculinizes a woman but causes no hormonal symptoms in a man.

The adrenal medulla produces two similar hormones called **norepinephrine** (noradrenaline) and **epinephrine** (adrenaline), which belong to a

The Adrenal Medulla

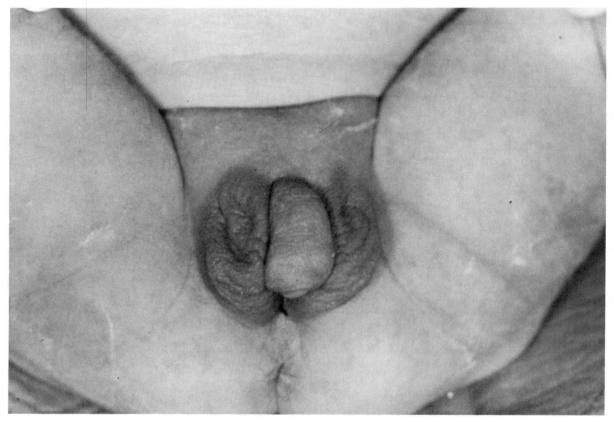

FIGURE 25–18

Masculinization of external genitalia of infant girl. Enlarged clitoris resembles penis. Vulvar labia are wrinkled and resemble scrotum.

class of compounds called **catecholamines.** The hormone-producing cells of the medulla are arranged in small groups surrounded by a rich network of capillaries. The cell cytoplasm is filled with fine granules that become dark brown when treated with chromium salts, and the cells are termed *chromaffin cells* because of this staining affinity.

The catecholamines produced by the chromaffin cells are stored within the cells and are released in response to nerve impulses transmitted to the medulla by the sympathetic nervous system. Any emotional stress, such as anger, fear, or anxiety, activates the sympathetic nervous system and causes the adrenal medulla to release its hormones. The liberated catecholamines cause a rapid heart rate, rise in blood pressure, and other effects that prepare the individual to cope with the stress of an emergency.

Tumors of the Adrenal Medulla

Rarely, a benign tumor called a **pheochromocytoma** arises from the chromaffin cells of the medulla. The tumor derives its unusual name from the staining reaction of the tumor cells to chromium salts, which is similar to that of the normal chromaffin cells from which the tumor arose (*pheo* = dark + *chromo* = color + *cyte* = cell + *oma* = tumor). A pheochromocytoma often secretes large amounts of catecholamines and produces severe effects on the heart and vascular system. The tumor may discharge catecholamines intermittently and induce periodic episodes of high blood pressure and increased heart rate. At times the blood pressure may rise so severely that a cerebral blood vessel ruptures, causing a cerebral hemorrhage. In other cases, the increased output of catecholamines by the tumor is continuous and causes a sustained high blood pressure. Treatment consists of surgical removal of the tumor.

The Pancreatic Islets

In addition to manufacturing digestive enzymes, the pancreas functions as an endocrine gland. Scattered throughout the pancreas are more than a million small clusters of cells called the *pancreatic islets* or *islets of Langerhans,* which produce three different hormones: insulin, glucagon, and somatostatin. Diseases of the islets were considered in conjunction with diseases of the pancreas (chapter 22).

The Gonads

The gonads have two functions: the production of germ cells, either eggs or sperm, and the production of sex hormones responsible for the development of secondary sexual characteristics. (This function is controlled by the gonadotrophic hormones of the pituitary gland.)

Occasionally, sex-hormone–secreting tumors develop in the ovary or testis. They may secrete sex hormone appropriate to the sex of the individual or, paradoxically, sex hormone characteristic of the opposite sex. No endocrine symptoms result from a tumor that produces the "proper" sex hormone; however, elaboration of the inappropriate sex hormone by the tumor causes masculinization in the female or feminization in the male. Sex-hormone–secreting tumors of the gonads are usually benign, and the disorder can be cured by surgical excision.

Hormone Production by Nonendocrine Tumors

Sometimes nonendocrine tumors secrete hormones that produce the same clinical manifestations as those of tumors arising from endocrine glands. Such hormones are called *ectopic hormones* (*ecto* = outside) because they are formed outside the endocrine glands, which are the normal sites of hormone production. An ectopic hormone is a protein that is either identical with the true hormone produced by the endocrine gland or has such a close resemblance that it mimics the action of the true hormone. Many different ectopic hormones have been identified including: ACTH, TSH, MSH, gonadotropins, ADH, parathyroid hormone, and insulin. Most hormone-producing nonendocrine tumors are malignant, and the majority have been elaborated by carcinomas of lung, pancreas, or kidneys or by malignant connective-tissue tumors.

Stress and the Endocrine System

The body is an integrated collection of cells organized into complex organ systems and regulated by a wide variety of control mechanisms, all designed to maintain a stable internal environment in which the cells can function efficiently. The maintenance of a steady state by the body's internal control systems is called *homeostasis,* and anything that disturbs the body's well-ordered internal environment brings into play regulatory mechanisms that attempt to reestablish the steady state under which the body functions most effectively. In a general sense, stress is any event that disturbs this stable internal environment. The event may be physical trauma, such as an injury or surgical operation, prolonged exposure to cold, vigorous exercise, pain, or a strong emotional stimulus such as anxiety or fear. Any of these events call forth a response that helps the body cope with the stress. There are two distinct but overlapping responses to stress, and the type of response generated depends both on the intensity and on the duration of the stress. The acute, short-term response is mediated by the sympathetic nervous system and the adrenal medulla, and the chronic, longer-term response includes the participation of several endocrine glands, with the adrenal cortex playing the major role. Both the acute and the chronic responses are initiated in the hypothalamus, which directs both the autonomic nervous system and many endocrine glands, and the hypothalamus in turn receives input from higher cortical centers.

The acute stress response is the well-known fear-fight-flight reaction triggered by the sympathetic nervous system. Norepinephrine released from sympathetic nerve endings, supplemented by norepinephrine and epinephrine released from the adrenal medulla in response to sympathetic nerve impulses, prepares the body to deal with the acute situation. Blood glucose rises as liver glycogen is broken down into glucose and released into the bloodstream. Peripheral vessels constrict, diverting more blood to the brain, heart, and skeletal muscles. The blood pressure rises, and the heart beats more forcefully. All of these systemic effects are of short duration, and gradually subside when the stressful event is no longer present.

In contrast, long-term stress of any type, either physical or emotional, initiates a slower but more complex chain of events. Hypothalamic releasing hormones, acting through the pituitary gland, cause the adrenal cortex to increase its output of cortical hormones; they also increase the output of growth hormone and thyroid hormone while suppressing the output of gonadotropic hormones. Excess cortisol production has pronounced effects on glucose, protein, and fat metabolism, as described earlier in connection with Cushing's disease. The cortisol excess also dampens the inflammatory response and reduces the responsiveness of the immune system. In addition, cortisol excess tends to raise blood pressure by making the peripheral arterioles more responsive to the vasoconstrictor effect of norepinephrine released from sympathetic nerve endings. Increased aldosterone output promotes retention of salt and water, which also tends to raise blood pressure by increasing intravascular fluid volume.

The stress-related fall in gonadotropin output impairs gonadal function, which has widespread physiologic effects, and in women may lead to stress-related cessation of menstrual periods. Stress-related amenorrhea has well-defined adverse effects on the skeletal system, as described in chapter 27.

The increased output of thyroid hormone speeds up metabolic processes in order to allow the body to deal more effectively with the stress, as does increased output of growth hormone, which also stimulates the body's metabolic processes.

Unfortunately, chronic stress takes its toll on the body and, over the long term, may predispose to illness. Excessive demands are placed on the cardiovascular system, which may contribute to heart disease, and the chronic corticosteroid excess places undue demand on the vascular system, as well as on other organ systems. Perhaps even more important, the chronic corticosteroid excess may increase our susceptibility to many types of illnesses by reducing our ability to generate an effective inflammatory reaction and by reducing the responsiveness of our immune system.

Stress initiates many physiologic responses that are designed to help protect us from harm, but chronic, unrelieved stress can cause us harm, and stress-relieving activities can help protect us from its long-term injurious effects.

Causes of Obesity

Obesity

Fat is the storage form of energy. Any caloric intake that exceeds requirements is stored as adipose tissue and weight is gained. Each excess pound of body weight represents the storage of approximately 3500 calories. Weight is lost if caloric intake is reduced below the amount required for normal metabolic processes. It is sometimes said that obesity is caused by a malfunction of the endocrine glands. In the vast majority of cases, obesity is the result of overeating and can be "cured" by reduction in food intake. In rare instances, hypothyroidism contributes to obesity by reducing the body's metabolic rate. *Cushing's disease* caused by adrenal cortical hyperfunction may be associated with increased deposition of fat and an abnormal distribution of body fat. These are uncommon situations. Most obese individuals have no detectable endocrine or metabolic disturbances.

Health Consequences of Obesity

Overweight persons have a higher incidence of diabetes, hypertension, cardiovascular disease, and several other diseases than do persons of normal weight. Therefore, a significant degree of overweight is undesirable, and extreme obesity is a major health hazard. Obese persons have a mortality rate almost twice that of normal individuals. The excess fat is harmful to the cardiovascular system in three ways:

1. Blood volume and cardiac output must increase to nourish the excess adipose tissue, which overworks the heart.
2. Obese persons are prone to develop high blood pressure, which places a further strain on the heart and blood vessels.
3. Blood lipids are often elevated, which predisposes to arteriosclerosis of the coronary arteries.

Other systems also are adversely affected. Large masses of adipose tissue may impair normal pulmonary ventilation, producing various types of respiratory difficulty and increased susceptibility to pulmonary infection. An otherwise relatively minor respiratory illness may, in an obese person, be a catastrophe because of the increased demands placed upon already overtaxed cardiovascular and respiratory systems.

The high incidence of diabetes in obese persons is the result of an impaired ability to utilize insulin efficiently (chapter 22). Musculoskeletal disabilities are frequent because the excess weight places undue stress on the bones, joints, and ligaments. Finally, the obese individual is at a serious disadvantage if an operation is required. The operative procedure carries a higher risk and postoperative complications are more frequent. Any surgical procedure is technically much more difficult in an obese person, and wound healing is delayed. The adipose tissue, which has a relatively poor blood supply, heals poorly and is also quite vulnerable to infection, resulting in an increased incidence of postoperative wound infections.

Treatment of Obesity

Obesity virtually always results from overeating and can be abolished by reducing food intake. However, the results of treatment of dieting have been surprisingly poor because obese individuals are either unwilling or unable to reduce their caloric intake.

Because of the limited success of treating obesity by diet, various other measures have been proposed. Drugs that suppress appetite have been used, but many of these drugs have undesirable side effects. As a last resort, massive obesity is sometimes treated by various surgical operations.

One of the first weight-reduction operations was called an **ileal bypass.** In this procedure, the ileum was divided about 18 cm proximal to the ileocecal valve, and the jejunum was divided about 30 cm distal to the duodenojejunal junction. Then the proximal jejunum and distal ileum were sutured together, bypassing the remaining part of the small intestine. The proximal (jejunal) end of the bypassed segment was closed. The distal end was connected to an opening made in the sigmoid colon, which permitted intestinal secretions to drain from the bypassed segment into the colon (figure 25–19). Weight was lost because absorption of nutrients from the greatly shortened small intestine was very poor, which had the same effect as restricting food intake. Unfortunately, this drastic procedure was associated with so many late complications resulting from inadequate absorption of nutrients that it had to be abandoned. Intestinal bypass was replaced by other types of operations that controlled food intake by reducing the capacity of the stomach. Several different types of surgical procedures have been used, and they are often grouped together under the general term of "stomach stapling operations." One of these operations is called a **gastric bypass,** and there are several variations of this procedure. In the procedure illustrated in figure 25–20, a line of staples is placed across the upper part of the stomach. This divides the stomach into two compartments: a very small upper compartment and a much larger lower compartment that is continuous with the duodenum. A loop of jejunum is connected to a small opening made in the upper gastric compartment so that the food from the upper compartment empties directly into the jejunum. The main part of the stomach no longer receives food, but gastric secretions can drain into the duodenum normally. The upper compartment of the stomach is so small that it soon becomes overdistended with food when the individual starts to eat. The subject feels "stuffed" and has to stop eating. Weight is lost by enforced reduction of food intake. Unfortunately, some gastric bypass procedures lead to late complications in many patients: anemia caused by poor absorption of iron and vitamin B_{12} and weakening of bones (osteoporosis) as a result of inadequate calcium intake and absorption.

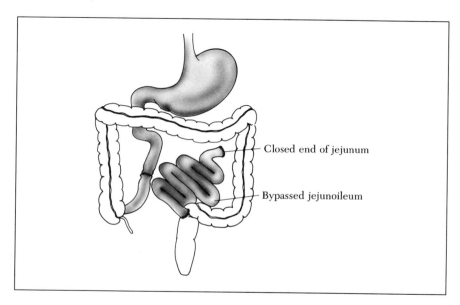

Closed end of jejunum

Bypassed jejunoileum

FIGURE 25–19

Ileal bypass procedure.

FIGURE 25–20

Principle of gastric bypass. Small upper compartment empties into jejunum through surgically created opening. Larger lower compartment no longer receives food but empties into duodenum normally.

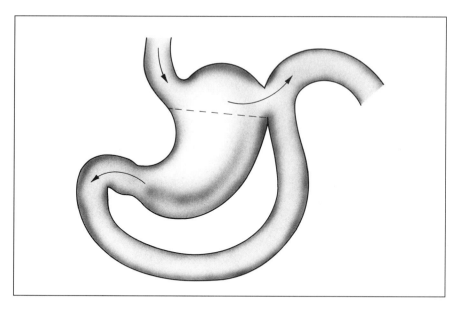

Questions for Review

1. What are the major hormones produced by the pituitary gland? What factors regulate secretion of pituitary hormones?

2. What is the effect of overproduction of growth hormone?

3. What factors regulate the rate of production of thyroid hormone? What are the major effects of an abnormal output of thyroid hormone? What is the difference between cretinism and myxedema?

4. Why does the thyroid gland become enlarged as a result of iodine deficiency?

5. What is the difference between thyrotoxicosis and thyroiditis?

6. What are the main classes of hormones elaborated by the adrenal cortex? What diseases result from adrenal cortical dysfunction?

7. What factors regulate the output of parathyroid hormone? What are the possible effects of parathyroid dysfunction?

8. What is the usual cause of obesity? What are the complications of obesity?

9. What factors regulate the release of prolactin? What are the clinical effects of hyperprolactinemia? What are the causes of hyperprolactinemia?

10. What is Addison's disease? What is the cause of the skin pigmentation?

Supplementary Readings

Abboud, C. F. 1986. Laboratory diagnosis of hypopituitarism. *Mayo Clinic Proceedings* 61:35–48. Reviews the endocrine manifestations of hypopituitarism and useful diagnostic tests.

Amino, N. 1988. Autoimmunity and hypothyroidism. *Clinics in Endocrinology and Metabolism* 2:591–671. A review.

Berkow, R., ed. 1992. *The Merck Manual of Diagnosis and Therapy.* 16th ed. Rahway, N.J.: Merck and Co., Inc. Section on endocrine disorders, pp. 1055–1134.

Bjorntrop, P. 1980. Results of conservative therapy for obesity. *American Journal of Clinical Nutrition* 33: 370–75. Extremely obese patients respond very poorly to dietary treatment.

Carpenter, P. C. 1986. Cushing's syndrome: Update of diagnosis and management. *Mayo Clinic Proceedings* 61:49–58. Describes the various types of Cushing's syndromes and diagnostic difficulties. Reviews current methods of diagnosis and treatment.

Crowley, L. V., et al. 1984. Late effects of gastric bypass for obesity. *American Journal of Gastroenterology* 79:850–60. Many patients developed iron and vitamin B_{12} deficiencies and osteoporosis as late complications of gastric bypass. Hematopoietic complications can usually be prevented and are relatively easy to treat, but musculoskeletal complications are more difficult to prevent and treat.

Drenick, E. J., et al. 1980. Excessive mortality and causes of death in morbidly obese men. *Journal of the American Medical Association* 243:443–45. A good review article.

Greenspan, F. S. 1977. Radiation exposure and thyroid cancer. *Journal of the American Medical Association* 237:2089–91. Radiation exposure is carcinogenic.

Jordan, R. M., et al. 1987. Recent advances in diagnosis and treatment of pituitary tumors. *Advances in Internal Medicine* 32:299–323. A review.

Melmed, S., et al. 1986. Pituitary tumors secreting growth hormone and prolactin. *Annals of Internal Medicine* 105:238–53. Discusses pathophysiology and principles of therapy.

Mitchell, M. L., et al. 1978. Screening for congenital hypothyroidism, *Journal of the American Medical Association* 239:2348–51. Effective screening methods can identify congenital hypothyroidism, permitting effective treatment.

Molitich, M. E. ed. 1987. Pituitary tumors (symposium). *Endocrinology and Metabolism Clinics of North America* 16:475–805. Entire issue deals with various aspects of pathophysiology, diagnosis, and treatment.

Randall, R. V., et al. 1983. Transsphenoidal microsurgical treatment of prolactin producing pituitary adenomas. *Mayo Clinic Proceedings* 58:108–21. Reviews Mayo Clinic experience.

Seaward, B. L. 1994. *Managing stress: Principles and strategies for health and well-being.* Boston: Jones and Bartlett Publishers. Discusses pathophysiology of stress and methods for coping.

Samaan, N. A. 1977. Hormone production in nonendocrine tumors. *CA: A Cancer Journal for Clinicians* 27:149–59. Describes the various hormones produced by nonendocrine tumors and why this phenomenon occurs.

Vance, M. L., et al. 1987. Prolactinomas. *Endocrinology and Metabolic Clinics of North America* 16:731–53. A relatively common pituitary tumor. Describes diagnostic approaches and treatment methods.

Wass, J. A. H., et al. 1986. The treatment of acromegaly. *Clinics in Endocrinology and Metabolism* 15:683–707. Describes current medical and surgical methods. See also several articles on growth hormone deficiency and excess in the same issue.

See also sections of textbooks of medicine, surgery, and endocrinology listed in General References.

Chapter 25 ■ Outline Summary

Pituitary Gland / 714
Structure

Arises from base of brain. Located in pituitary fossa just behind optic chiasm.

Anterior lobe connected to hypothalamus by portal blood vessels.

Posterior lobe connected to hypothalamus by nerve fibers extending down stalk.

Intermediate lobe is rudimentary structure.

Pituitary Hormones

Anterior lobe:

Growth hormone: stimulates tissue growth.

Prolactin: stimulates secretion of milk.

TSH: stimulates thyroid.

ACTH: stimulates adrenal cortex.

FSH: gonadotropic hormone.

LH: gonadotropic hormone.

Posterior lobe:

ADH: causes more concentrated urine.

Oxytocin: stimulates uterine contractions and milk secretion.

Physiologic Control of Pituitary Hormone Secretion

Trophic hormones are regulated by level of hormone produced by target gland.

A self-regulating mechanism to maintain uniform hormone output.

Prolactin secretion differs.

Tonic inhibition by hypothalamic PIF.

TSH stimulates release of prolactin as well as thyroid hormones.

Clinical Disturbances of Pituitary Hormone Secretion

Hypofunction:

Panhypopituitarism: failure of secretion of all hormones. Secondary hypofunction of all target organs.

Pituitary dwarfism: deficiency of growth hormone.

Diabetes insipidus: lack of ADH causes excretion of large volume of extremely dilute urine.

Overproduction of growth hormone: caused by pituitary adenoma.

Causes gigantism in child.

Causes acromegaly in adult.

May cause visual disturbances caused by tumor encroachment on optic chiasm.

Overproduction of prolactin:

Causes amenorrhea and galactorrhea.

Often the result of small pituitary adenoma.

May be the result of other factors affecting hypothalamic function.

Thyroid Gland / 720

Structure

Bilobed gland in neck regulated by TSH.

Composed of thyroid follicles which produce and store hormone.

Parafollicular cells produce calcitonin.

Actions of Thyroid Hormone

Controls metabolic functions.

Abnormal secretion causes hypothyroidism or hyperthyroidism.

Goiter

Nontoxic goiter:

Caused by inadequate hormone output, iodine deficiency, enzyme deficiency, inefficient enzyme function, or increased hormone requirements.

Gland enlarges to increase hormone output.

Treated by supplying hormone: gland decreases in size.

Toxic goiter:

Caused by antithyroid antibody that stimulates gland.

Treated by antithyroid drugs, thyroidectomy, or radioiodine.

Hypothyroidism

In adult: causes metabolic slowing. Treated by thyroid hormone.

In infant: causes impaired growth and central nervous system development as well as hypometabolism. Early diagnosis and treatment required to assure normal development.

Thyroiditis

Autoantibody destroys thyroid tissue and causes hypothyroidism.

Term refers to immunologic reaction, not true infection.

Tumors of Thyroid

Benign adenomas.

Carcinoma.

Well-differentiated follicular and papillary carcinoma—good prognosis. Treated by surgical resection.

Poorly differentiated carcinoma—rapidly growing with poor prognosis. Treatment by surgery, radiation, and chemotherapy.

Medullary carcinoma—rare. Secretes calcitonin.

Radiation and thyroid tumors.

Radiation increases incidence of benign and malignant thyroid tumors after latent period of five to thirty years.

Most tumors well differentiated and easily treated.

Persons who received head or neck radiation should have periodic follow-up examinations.

Parathyroid Glands and Calcium Metabolism / 734

Physiologic Concepts

Blood calcium in equilibrium with calcium in bone.

Ionized fraction is physiologically active form.

Calcium level regulated by parathyroid glands.

Reduced calcium causes tetany. Elevated level reduces neuromuscular excitability.

Hyperparathyroidism

Usually the result of parathyroid adenoma.

Hypercalcemia and hypercalcuria.

Formation of renal calculi and calcium deposition in tissues.

Decalcification of bone.

Treated by removal of tumor.

Hypoparathyroidism

Usually the result of accidental removal of parathyroids during thyroid surgery.

Hypocalcemia causes tetany.

Treated by supplementary oral calcium and vitamin D to raise calcium levels.

Adrenal Glands / 735
Hormones of Adrenal Cortex

Glucocorticoids: control carbohydrate metabolism.

Mineralocorticoids: control mineral metabolism.

Sex hormones: minor component.

Abnormalities of Adrenal Cortical Function

Addison's disease:

Glucocorticoid deficiency: hypoglycemia.

Mineralocorticoid deficiency: fall in blood volume and blood pressure.

Hyperpigmentation: caused by increased ACTH and MSH (loss of feedback inhibition).

Treated by supplying deficient corticosteroids.

Cushing's disease:

Glucocorticoid excess: disturbed carbohydrate, fat, and protein metabolism.

Mineralocorticoid excess: increased blood volume and blood pressure.

Treatment depends on cause: removal of pituitary microadenoma or adrenal adenoma or removal of hyperplastic adrenal glands.

Overproduction of adrenal sex hormones:

Congenital adrenal hyperplasia: disturbed biosynthesis of hormones caused by enzyme deficiency.

Sex-hormone–producing tumors.

The Adrenal Medulla / 741

Produces catecholamines (epinephrine and norepinephrine), which stimulate sympathetic nervous system.

Adrenal medullary tumors secrete catecholamines.

Produce pronounced cardiovascular effects.

May cause cerebral hemorrhage from high blood pressure.

Treated by removal of tumor.

Pancreatic Islets / 743

See chapter 22.

The Gonads / 743
Function

Production of sex hormones: controlled by FSH and LH.

Production of germ cells.

Tumors

May secrete sex hormones.

Treated by surgical resection.

Hormone Production by Nonendocrine Tumors / 743
Ectopic Hormones

Identical with or closely resemble normal hormones. Usually produced by malignant tumors.

Stress and the Endocrine System / 744

Stress is any event that disturbs homeostasis.

Both acute and chronic responses to stress.

Acute response: fear-fight-flight response mediated by sympathetic nervous system and adrenal medulla.

Chronic response: primarily involves adrenal cortex but other endocrines involved.

Chronic stress alters body metabolism, taxes cardiovascular system, impairs inflammatory and immune responses, and predisposes to illness.

Obesity / 745
Pathogenesis

Caloric intake exceeds requirements.

Usually not a result of endocrine disturbance.

Health Consequences

Cardiovascular disease.

Musculoskeletal problems.

Diabetes.

Impaired pulmonary function.

Operation carries high risk.

Treatment

Medical: diet often ineffective in marked obesity.

Surgical:

Ileal bypass: many complications; infrequently done.

Gastric bypass: fewer complications.

The Nervous System

Learning Objectives

1. Describe the normal structure and basic functions of the brain, meninges, and cerebro-spinal fluid as they relate to neurologic disease.

2. Define muscle tone and voluntary motor activity and relate these concepts to the two forms of muscle paralysis.

3. Explain the pathogenesis and clinical manifestations of closure defects of the central nervous system. Name the techniques used for prenatal diagnosis.

4. Describe the pathogenesis and manifestations of hydrocephalus and relate them to treatment measures.

5. Name the causes, manifestations, and treatment of transient ischemic attacks.

6. Differentiate between the two principal types of stroke in regard to pathogenesis, prognosis, and treatment.

7. Describe the pathogenesis, manifestations, and treatment of congenital cerebral aneurysms.

8. Name the types of tumors that affect the central nervous system and explain their origin, pathogenesis, clinical manifestations, and treatment.

9. Explain the pathogenesis, major clinical manifestations, and general principles of treatment of Parkinson's disease, meningitis, multiple sclerosis, and Guillain Barré syndrome.

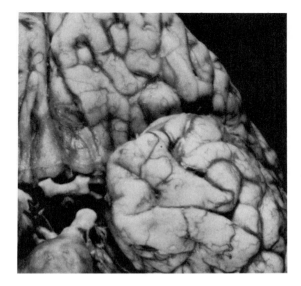

Chapter 26 ■ Contents

The central nervous system (CNS) consists of the brain and spinal cord, surrounded by several membranes called **meninges.** The firm, fibrous outer membrane is called the **dura.** The thin inner membrane, which adheres to the surface of the brain and spinal cord, is called the **pia.** The middle membrane, interposed between the pia and dura, is called the **arachnoid.** The space between the arachnoid and the underlying pia is called the **sub-arachnoid space.** It contains cerebrospinal fluid (CSF) together with fine strands of arachnoidal connective tissue that extend through the space and attach to the tips of the gyri.

The *brain* is divided into the *cerebrum, brain stem,* and *cerebellum.* The brain is hollow, containing four interconnected cavities called **ventricles.** Arterial blood is supplied to the brain by large blood vessels entering the base of the skull. These arteries join to form a circle of vessels (the *circle of Willis*) at the base of the brain. Branches from the circle extend outward to supply all parts of the brain. Venous blood is returned from the brain into large venous sinuses in the dura, which eventually drain into the jugular veins.

The brain and spinal cord are surrounded by cerebrospinal fluid and are encased within protective bony structures: the *cranium* and the *vertebral column.* The bony case protects the soft and rather fragile nervous tissue, and the cerebrospinal fluid acts as a hydrostatic cushion to insulate the brain from shocks and blows.

The nerve tissue of the brain and spinal cord is composed of nerve cells called **neurons** and supporting cells called **neuroglia** (described in chapter 2). Each individual neuron has a central body and one or more long processes extending from the cell body to transmit the impulses. According to traditional concepts, a process that transmits impulses toward the cell body is called a *dendrite* and one conducting impulses away from the cell body is called an *axon.* Often, the noncommittal term *nerve fiber* is used when describing cell processes, because the term can be applied to any nerve process without regard to its direction of impulse transmission. Most nerve fibers are covered by a fatty insulating *myelin sheath.*

Neurons are frequently arranged in chains; the neurons interconnect with other neurons to transmit impulses, but they are not in direct contact with one another. They are separated by minute gaps called *synapses.* The transmission of a nerve impulse across a synapse is by means of a chemical called a *neurotransmitter* that is released from the end of an axon and activates receptors on the dendrite or cell body of the adjacent neuron. There are several types of neurotransmitters, and each type of neuron has its own specific type of neurotransmitter. Some of the more important neurotransmitters are acetylcholine, norepinephrine, and dopamine, which is closely related to norepinephrine.

When a nerve fiber leaves the central nervous system, it becomes invested by elongated spindle cells called *Schwann cells,* which wrap around the fiber. These cells produce the myelin that insulates the fiber. (The myelin surrounding fibers *within* the central nervous system is produced by **oligo-dendroglia.**)

Structure and Function

A nerve that transmits impulses into the nervous system is called a *sensory nerve* or *afferent nerve* (*ad* = to + *ferre* = carry). A *motor nerve* or *efferent nerve* (*e* = away) conducts impulses from brain or spinal cord to muscle. The gray matter of the brain and cord is composed primarily of nerve cells and their processes. The *white matter* consists mostly of bundles of nerve fibers covered by fatty myelin sheaths.

The nervous system may be regarded as a giant switchboard, receiving sensory impulses and relaying this information to brain and spinal cord centers concerned with perception of sensation and with motor activity. The cerebral cortex receives sensory input and initiates voluntary motor activity. In the depths of each cerebral hemisphere are masses of gray matter: the *thalami* and the *basal ganglia* (*basal nuclei*). The paired thalami, which form the lateral walls of the third ventricle, function as relay stations that receive sensory impulses from lower levels and transmit them to the cortex. The basal ganglia in each hemisphere, which consist of the caudate nucleus and lenticular nucleus, are connected to another important group of neurons in the brain stem that are called the *substantia nigra* (meaning literally black substance), so named because the neuron cell bodies contain melanin pigment and the neuron collections appear gray black in color. Passing between the basal ganglia and the thalamus in each hemisphere is a large compact bundle of nerve fibers called the *internal capsule,* which carries impulses to and from the cortex.

The brain stem contains neurons that are involved in multiple functions not under direct cortical control; it also carries the bundles of nerve fibers that pass to higher and lower levels within the central nervous system. The cerebellum regulates muscle tone, coordination, posture, and balance.

The spinal cord is the continuation of the brain stem. Its central gray matter receives sensory input from spinal nerves entering the cord, and motor neurons exit from the cord to innervate muscles. Spinal sensory and motor neurons are involved in many reflex functions not under cortical control, but spinal motor neurons are also activated by motor impulses originating from cortical neurons. The spinal motor neurons in turn discharge impulses to the skeletal muscles that they supply, causing them to contract.

The fiber tracts conveying sensory impulses to the cortex and those conveying motor impulses from the cortex cross within the brain stem to the opposite side as they transmit impulses to their destination. Consequently, the right hemisphere registers sensation from the left half of the body and innervates the muscles on the left side. Conversely, the left hemisphere receives sensation from the right side of the body and activates muscles on the right side.

Development of the Nervous System

In the embryo, the central nervous system first appears as a thickened band of surface cells (ectoderm) called the *neural plate.* Its lateral margins become elevated to form *neural folds,* and the two folds then fuse to form a hollow tube called the **neural tube.** Fusion begins in the middle of the developing tube and progresses toward both ends until a completely closed tube is formed by the end of the fourth week of embryonic development. Three expansions called the *forebrain, midbrain* and *hindbrain* develop from one end of the neural tube (figure 26–1). The other end remains narrow and becomes the spinal cord.

The *cerebral hemispheres* develop as lateral outgrowths from the forebrain and soon overgrow the remaining parts of the brain. The remainder of the forebrain becomes the *diencephalon,* which is located between the

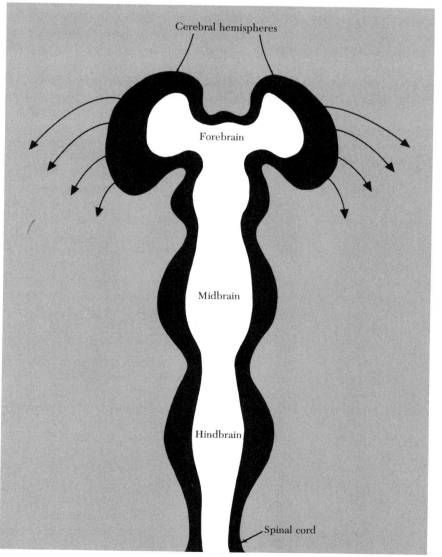

FIGURE 26–1

Early prenatal development of the brain.

cerebral hemispheres (*dia* = between + *encephalon* = brain). The *midbrain* persists as a small area connecting forebrain and hindbrain. The hindbrain gives rise to parts of the brain called the *pons, medulla,* and *cerebellum.* The diencephalon, midbrain, pons, and medulla together form the *brain stem.* The central cavity within the neural tube develops into the *ventricular system* of the adult brain. The embryonic cells (mesoderm) surrounding the developing neural tube give rise to the cranial cavity, vertebral bodies, and adjacent tissues.

Muscle Tone and Voluntary Muscle Contraction

A skeletal muscle contracts in response to impulses discharged from motor neurons in the spinal cord or from corresponding neurons of the cranial nerves in the brain stem. These neurons are often called the *lower motor neurons.* Voluntary motor activity is controlled by nerve impulses originating in motor neurons in the cerebral cortex, sometimes called *upper motor neurons.* Voluntary motor activity is controlled by two separate motor systems. One system, called the *pyramidal system,* controls voluntary motor functions, and the other system, called the *extrapyramidal system,* regulates muscle groups concerned primarily with balance, posture, and coordination.

The axons of the pyramidal system motor neurons descend in fiber tracts called the *pyramidal tracts* or *corticospinal tracts.* The corticospinal tracts cross in the brain stem, and their axons synapse with lower motor neurons in the brain stem and spinal cord, activating the lower motor neurons and causing them to discharge an impulse. Acetylcholine is the neurotransmitter released by the axon terminals of both the corticospinal tract neurons and the brain-stem–spinal motor neurons with which they synapse.

The nerve fibers of the extrapyramidal tract neurons also cross and descend to synapse with the same lower motor neurons that receive impulses from the pyramidal tract neurons, but the extrapyramidal system is a much more complex multineuron pathway. It has multiple connections with neurons in the cerebellum, basal ganglia, substantia nigra, and other groups of brain stem neurons.

The pyramidal system and the extrapyramidal system function together as a single system under cortical control to produce the smooth integrated functions of muscle groups involved in voluntary motor activity. Malfunction of the extrapyramidal system leads to loss of coordinated motor functions. The muscles do not function smoothly, and the malfunction also gives rise to abnormal uncontrollable muscular movements.

Muscle tone refers to the firmness of a muscle and its resistance to stretching. A muscle lacking tone is limp and offers no resistance when stretched. Conversely, a muscle with excess tone, if firm, resists stretching, and is said to be *spastic.* Muscle tone results from reflex contraction of muscle in response to stretching. Specialized receptors located in the muscle are activated, and afferent impulses are conveyed to the lower motor neuron, causing reflex discharge of motor impulses that stimulate the muscle to contract and resist the stretching force. Muscle tone is also influenced by impulses discharged from higher centers in the nervous system, which vary the responsiveness of the stretch receptors when stimulated.

A muscle that is no longer subject to voluntary control is said to be *para-lyzed*. There are two different types of paralysis:

1. *Flaccid paralysis,* caused by disease of the lower motor neurons or their fibers
2. *Spastic paralysis,* which results from disease affecting the cortical motor neurons or their fibers

Spastic paralysis occurs more frequently than flaccid paralysis because cortical neurons are more often damaged by disease than are spinal motor neurons.

Flaccid Paralysis

If the lower motor neuron in the spinal cord is destroyed by a disease such as poliomyelitis or if the peripheral nerve supplying the muscle (which contains the nerve fibers of the spinal neurons) is interrupted, the reflex arc responsible for muscle tone is interrupted. Muscle tone is abolished because the muscle is deprived of its innervation. The muscle becomes limp and undergoes severe atrophy.

Spastic Paralysis

If cortical motor neurons or their fibers that travel in the motor pathways are interrupted, as in a stroke, voluntary control of the muscles supplied by the affected neurons is lost because the pyramidal tract pathway is interrupted. However, because the reflex arc that maintains muscle tone is not disturbed, and thus the muscle retains its innervation, significant atrophy of the muscle does not occur. Generally, muscle tone is in fact increased because extrapyramidal motor impulses descending from the cortex tend to inhibit muscle tone, and this inhibitory effect is lost after an upper motor neuron injury.

The brain is well protected from moderate trauma. However, a severe blow may injure the brain, and sometimes the skull also is fractured (figure 26–2). Injury to the brain may be manifested by loss of consciousness and various neurologic disturbances. The injured brain becomes swollen and often shows evidence of pinpoint hemorrhages caused by disruption of small intracerebral blood vessels. Usually the brain injury is located immediately adjacent to the site of the blow, but sometimes the brain injury is caused by violent contact of the displaced brain against the cranial cavity on the side opposite the injury. For example, the force of a blow to the back of the head may displace the brain forward, injuring the front of the brain where it strikes against the front of the bony cranial cavity (figure 26–3).

FIGURE 26–2

Skull x-ray illustrating large skull fracture (*arrows*) associated with extensive injury to underlying brain.

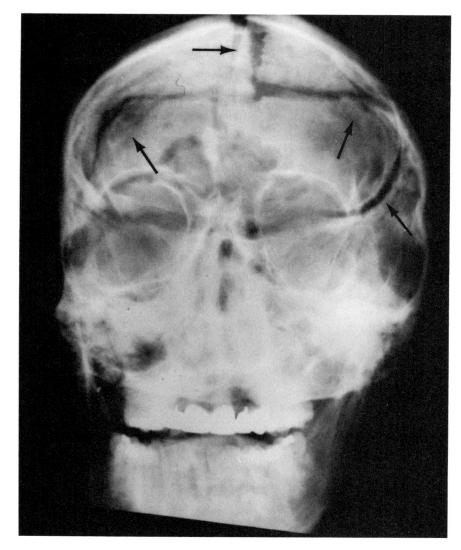

Sometimes large blood vessels over the surface of the brain are torn by the force of the injury, and blood accumulates between the skull and the underlying brain. The escaping blood may accumulate in any of several locations:

1. Between the outer layer of dura and the cranial bones (*epidural hemorrhage*)
2. Between the dura and the arachnoid (*subdural hemorrhage*)
3. Between the arachnoid and the pia (*subarachnoid hemorrhage*)

An epidural or subdural collection of blood (a *hematoma*) may compress the underlying brain and impair its functions.

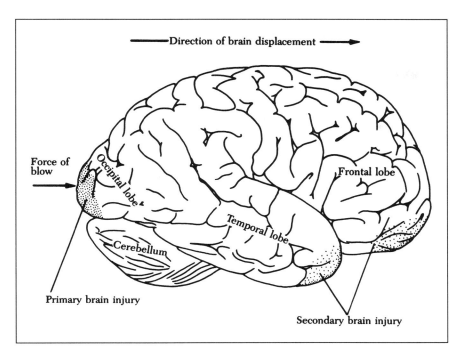

←——————Direction of brain displacement ——————→

Force of blow

Occipital lobe

Frontal lobe

Temporal lobe

Cerebellum

Primary brain injury

Secondary brain injury

FIGURE 26–3

Mechanism of injury to frontal and temporal poles of brain caused by blow to back of head.

Unfortunately, the rigid cranial cavity, which normally serves a protective function, is a disadvantage if the brain is seriously injured. The brain often swells at the site of injury, and the unyielding cranial cavity restricts the swelling and compresses the swollen brain, leading to high intracranial pressure. The elevated pressure adversely affects cerebral function and may also interfere with the blood supply to the brain by compressing cerebral blood vessels.

Neural Tube Defects

Failure of either end of the neural tube to close properly leads to serious congenital malformations called *neural tube defects,* which involve not only the nervous system but the surrounding tissues as well. A closure defect involving the end of the tube destined to form the cerebral hemispheres (called the *cephalic* end) leads to a condition called **anencephaly** (*ana* = without + *encephalon* = brain). If the opposite end of the tube (the *caudal* end) is involved, **spina bifida** results. These are the two most common congenital malformations of the nervous system. The combined incidence of these malformations is about two per one thousand births in the United States and even higher in some other countries. The malformations follow a multifactorial pattern of inheritance (described in chapter 9) and tend to recur in subsequent pregnancies. If parents have already given birth to an offspring with a neural tube defect, the risk of recurrence in a subsequent pregnancy is approximately one in twenty. The risk is one in ten when the parents have had two affected infants.

Recent evidence indicates that a deficiency of folic acid during the early part of pregnancy when the neural tube is forming plays an important role in causing neural tube defects. Intake of 0.4 mg (400 μg) of folic acid daily beginning before conception and during the early part of pregnancy can reduce by one-half the frequency of neural tube defects. As already mentioned, however, these defects follow a multifactorial inheritance pattern, and the folic acid deficiency functions along with genetic factors to cause the neural tube defect. Consumption of folic acid will reduce the frequency of neural tube defects but will not eliminate the problem, and a woman who has previously given birth to an infant with a neural tube defect still has a greater than normal risk of having an infant with a neural tube defect in a subsequent pregnancy.

Anencephaly

Anencephaly occurs most commonly in female infants and is incompatible with postnatal life.

Because the cephalic end of the neural tube fails to close, the exposed neural tissue undergoes secondary degenerative changes that convert it into a mass of vascular connective tissue intermixed with masses of degenerated brain and choroid plexus. The anencephalic infant has a striking appearance (figure 26–4). The brain is absent, as are the soft tissues of the scalp and the bones making up the vertex of the skull. The exposed base of the skull is covered only by a vascular membrane. The base of the cranial cavity is abnormally formed, and the orbits are shallow, causing the eyes to bulge outward. The trunk is short, the shoulders are broad, and the neck is absent; so the head arises directly from the trunk and cannot be flexed.

Sometimes the closure defect affects not only the brain, but also the part of the neural tube that forms the upper part of the spinal cord. When this occurs, the vertebral arches are absent, as well as the vertex of the skull, and the unclosed spinal cord lies exposed within the wide-open spinal canal.

The following case illustrates some of the obstetric problems associated with anencephaly.

CASE 26–1

A female anencephalic infant was born to a twenty-eight-year-old woman who was pregnant for the first time. The fetal heartbeat could be heard by the obstetrician throughout the last part of the pregnancy. When the patient's abdomen was examined near term, the obstetrician became concerned about the possibility of anencephaly because of inability to feel the fetal head. An x-ray film taken of the patient's abdomen confirmed the clinical impression, because only the base of the fetal skull could be seen in the x-ray film. The bones of the cranial vault were absent. The rest of the fetal skeleton appeared normally formed. The patient was delivered at term with some difficulty because the anencephalic head was unable to flex normally as it passed through the mother's pelvis, and the infant was delivered face first. The infant survived for several hours after delivery. The autopsy revealed complete absence of the cerebral hemispheres, the cerebellum, and most of the brain stem.

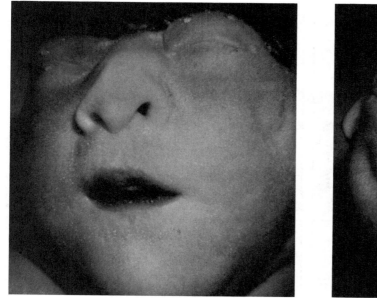

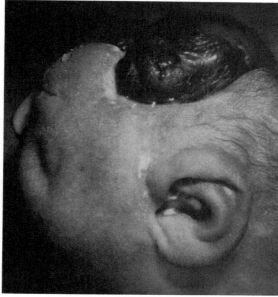

A

B

FIGURE 26–4

Characteristic appearance of anencephalic infant. Most of brain, top of skull, and scalp are absent. Maldevelopment of base of skull causes protrusion of eyes. **A,** Frontal view. **B,** Lateral view.

Spina Bifida

Malformations of the opposite (caudal) end of the neural tube and related vertebral arches are generally considered together under the term **spina bifida.** This term means literally *split spine* and refers to the characteristic failure of fusion of the vertebral arches common to all types of spina bifida (figure 26–5). Failure of fusion of vertebral arches in the lower lumbar region occurring as an isolated abnormality is called *occult spina bifida* (figure 26–5A); this type produces no clinical symptoms. The more severe types of spina bifida, sometimes called collectively *cystic spina bifida,* are characterized by a saclike protrusion of meninges or meninges and nerve tissue through the defect in the vertebral arches. The malformation is called a **meningocele** if the protrusion consists only of meninges (figure 26–5B) and is called a **meningomyelocele** (*myelo* = cord) if parts of the spinal cord or nerve roots also are included in the sac (figure 26–5C).

In meningomyelocele, there is often a severe neurologic deficit below the level of the sac because the nerve tissue is actually incorporated into the wall of the sac and is disorganized so that the conduction of nerve impulses is impaired or completely interrupted. In the most severe (and fortunately rare) form of spina bifida, the caudal end of the neural tube completely fails to close. The distal end of the spinal cord is represented by a flattened mass

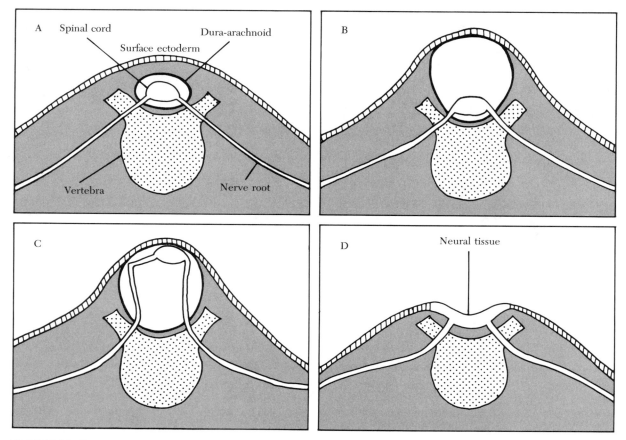

FIGURE 26–5

Various types of spina bifida. **A,** Occult spina bifida. Failure of formation of vertebral arches. No protrusion of meninges. **B,** Meningocele. Meninges protrude through the defect in the vertebral arches. Cord and nerve trunks are not present in the sac. **C,** Meningomyelocele. Protrusion of both meninges and nerve tissue. The spinal cord and nerve trunks are frequently incorporated into the wall of the sac. **D,** Failure of the neural tube to form and separate from the surface ectoderm. The neural tissue is continuous with the adjacent skin.

of nerve tissue that is continuous with the adjacent skin (figure 26–5D). The larger meningomyelocele sacs often are covered not by skin but merely by a thin, easily ruptured membrane composed only of meninges (figure 26–6).

Treatment of Spina Bifida

Occult spina bifida is asymptomatic and no treatment is required. A meningocele usually can be repaired without difficulty by excising the sac and closing the spinal dura, and the results are usually very satisfactory. Unfortunately, a large meningomyelocele is much more difficult to treat and results are much less satisfactory. Because spinal cord and nerve roots are often incorporated in the sac, there is frequently some loss of sensation and

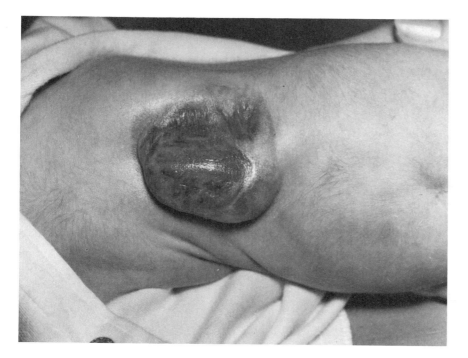

FIGURE 26–6

Large thoracic meningomye-locele covered only by a thin membrane. This condition was associated with neuro-logic disturbances resulting from incorporation of neural tissue into the wall of the sac.

motor power in the lower extremeties. Bowel and bladder function also may be impaired, leading to stasis of urine in the bladder and predisposing to urinary tract infections. These unfortunate individuals are managed best by a team of specialists in a medical center specializing in the care of patients with severe disabilities of this type. Many patients can be treated successfully and are able to lead happy and productive lives despite their disability.

The following case illustrates some of the problems encountered by the physician in the care of infants and children with large meningomyeloceles:

> A female infant was born with a very large meningomyelocele associated with complete loss of sensation and motor power below the level of the protruding sac (figure 26–7). Because of the severe neurologic deficit, she was not considered a suitable candidate for surgical treatment, and she was discharged to a boarding home for care. She was returned to the hospital six months later because the surface of the sac had become eroded, permitting the cerebrospinal fluid to leak from the sac. The hole in the sac had also allowed bacteria to gain access to the spinal canal, causing a meningitis that proved fatal despite supportive treatment and antibiotics.

CASE 26–2

Prenatal Detection of Neural Tube Defects

It is usually possible to identify a fetus with a neural tube defect prior to birth by means of **amniocentesis** (described in chapter 9) and determination of

FIGURE 26–7

Very large meningomyelocele that was associated with severe neurologic deficit. Perforation of the sac was followed by meningitis.

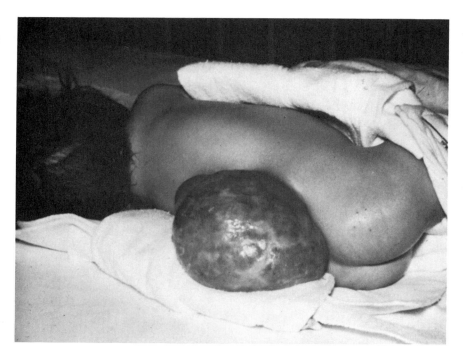

the concentration of a substance called *alpha fetoprotein* (AFP) in the amnionic fluid. This procedure is generally recommended if the mother has previously given birth to an infant with a neural tube defect because there is an increased likelihood of this abnormality in subsequent pregnancies.

Alpha fetoprotein is produced in the fetal liver beginning early in pregnancy and can be readily detected in the fetal blood. The concentration in fetal blood is highest at about thirteen weeks and then gradually declines. A small amount of AFP normally diffuses from the fetal blood into the amnionic fluid. High amnionic fluid AFP levels are encountered when the fetus is anencephalic or has a cystic spina bifida in which the defect is covered only by a thin membrane, because AFP can more easily diffuse from the fetal blood and cerebrospinal fluid through the defect directly into the amnionic fluid. Consequently, AFP levels are much higher than in a normal pregnancy.

Hydrocephalus

Cerebrospinal fluid serves as a protective cushion around the brain and spinal cord. The fluid is secreted by the choroid plexuses of the ventricles. It flows from the lateral ventricles into the third ventricle, through the cerebral aqueduct (*aqueduct of Sylvius*) into the fourth ventricle, and then out into the subarachnoid space through three small openings in the roof of the fourth ventricle. The fluid circulates around the cord and over the convexity of the brain and is resorbed into the large venous sinuses in the dura. Secretion of cerebrospinal fluid continues even if the flow of fluid through the ventricular system is blocked. Obstruction to the normal circulation of spinal fluid distends the ventricles proximal to the site of obstruction, with associated compression atrophy of brain tissue around the dilated ventricles (figure 26–8). This condition, which is called **hydrocephalus,** may be either congenital or acquired.

Congenital Hydrocephalus

Congenital hydrocephalus is usually caused by a congenital abnormality in the ventricular system, either a congenital obstruction or abnormal formation of the cerebral aqueduct or a failure of the openings in the roof of the fourth ventricle to form normally. This leads to marked distention of the ventricular system. Because the distention develops before the skull bones have fused, the head enlarges greatly and the brain undergoes pronounced atrophy secondary to compression by the dilated ventricles. Hydrocephalus may occur in the fetus prior to birth, and the head may become so large that it is unable to enter the maternal pelvis during labor. More often, the hydrocephalus develops insidiously after birth.

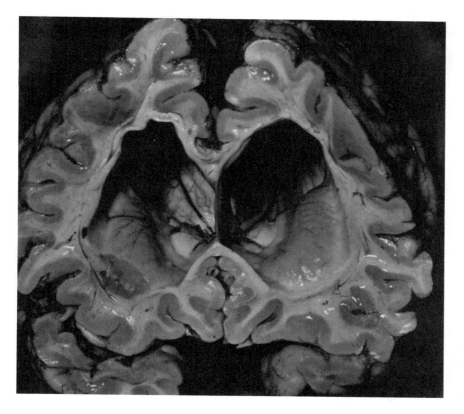

FIGURE 26–8

Cross-section of brain revealing marked dilatation of ventricles in patient with hydrocephalus.

Acquired Hydrocephalus

Acquired hydrocephalus is most commonly caused by obstruction of the circulation of the cerebrospinal fluid in the region of the fourth ventricle by fibrous adhesions, which sometimes form after a bacterial infection of the meninges (**meningitis**) and block the outflow of fluid from the fourth ventricle, or by blockage of the ventricular system secondary to a brain tumor (figure 26–9). Acquired hydrocephalus develops after the skull

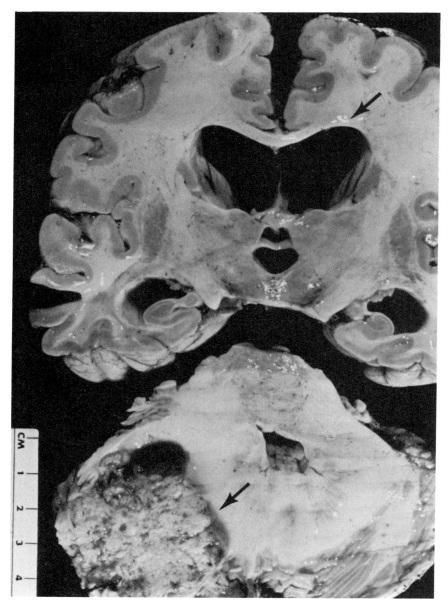

FIGURE 26–9

Hydrocephalus caused by metastatic carcinoma in cerebellum. Upper section of brain illustrates dilatation of ventricular system, best seen in the lateral ventricles (*upper arrow*). Lower section illustrates tumor in cerebellar hemisphere (lower arrow), which has compressed fourth ventricle, impeding outflow of cerebrospinal fluid.

bones fuse, and the skull cannot enlarge as in the congenital form of hydrocephalus.

Treatment of Hydrocephalus

Hydrocephalus can often be treated successfully by inserting a plastic tube into one of the dilated ventricles and rerouting (*shunting*) the fluid into another part of the body where it can be absorbed or excreted. A common method of treatment consists of making a small opening in the skull to allow insertion of a plastic tube through the cerebral hemisphere directly into one of the dilated lateral ventricles. The other end of the tube is passed through the subcutaneous tissue behind the ear and into the neck. It is then inserted into the jugular vein and threaded down the vein so that its tip is positioned in the right atrium. Reflux of blood from the atrium back into the cerebral ventricles is prevented by means of a one-way valve inserted in the tube. The shunt decreases the pressure within the dilated ventricles and arrests further damage to the brain resulting from overdistention of the ventricles (figure 26–10). Another commonly used shunt procedure directs the fluid into the peritoneal cavity. The plastic shunt tube is passed through the subcutaneous tissue of the neck, chest, and upper abdomen and is introduced into the abdominal cavity through a small incision in the peritoneum.

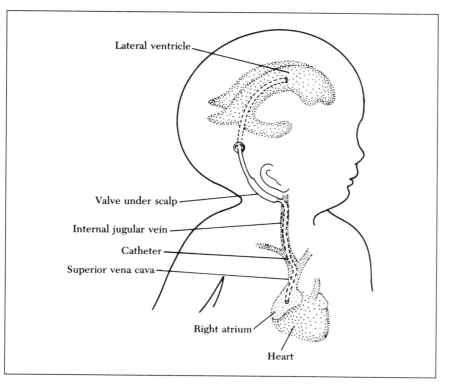

FIGURE 26–10

Principle of shunting fluid from dilated ventricle to right atrium, one method of treating hydrocephalus.

Case 26–3 illustrates some of the obstetric and pediatric problems encountered when hydrocephalus occurs in the fetus prior to delivery.

CASE 26–3

A twenty-four-year-old woman who was pregnant for the first time noted marked enlargement of her abdomen during the last part of pregnancy. X-ray examination of the abdomen revealed a hydrocephalic infant having a head diameter that was larger than the diameter of the mother's pelvis, indicating that delivery could not be accomplished vaginally. At term, an elective cesarean section was performed, and the infant was evaluated soon after delivery by a neurosurgeon. A shunt was performed in order to control the progressing hydrocephalus. The shunt prevented further enlargement of the head, and the infant did reasonably well after this operation.

Stroke

The term **stroke** is used to designate any injury to brain tissue resulting from disturbance of blood supply to the brain. Sometimes, a stroke occurs because a cerebral artery is narrowed or thrombosed owing to arteriosclerosis. In some cases, an arteriosclerotic vessel ruptures, with consequent cerebral hemorrhage, or a cerebral artery is blocked by an embolus.

Cerebral Thrombosis

In *cerebral thrombosis,* which is more common than cerebral hemorrhage, the brain tissue in the area of distribution of the blocked vessel becomes necrotic and degenerates (figure 26–11). The myelin sheath material breaks down, and the debris resulting from necrosis of brain tissue is eventually cleaned up by phagocytes, leaving a cystic cavity. Because the end stage of an infarct of the brain is cystic, in contrast with the appearance of infarcts in other tissues, the term **encephalomalacia** (*encephalon* = brain + *malacia* = softening) is often used to describe this kind of lesion (figure 26–12).

Stroke Caused by Arteriosclerosis of Extracranial Arteries

A stroke may also be caused by sclerosis of one of the major arteries arising from the aorta to supply the brain, before the vessel enters the cranial cavity. A commonly affected site is at the origin of the internal carotid artery in the neck, where atheromatous plaques may narrow the lumen and reduce cerebral blood flow. The plaques may also become ulcerated, and thrombi may form on the roughened surfaces. Bits of arteriosclerotic debris or thrombus material may break loose from the plaque and be carried into the intercerebral circulation, where they may block small cerebral arteries. Rarely, the internal carotid artery may become completely blocked by a thrombus that has formed on the roughened surface of the artery, leading to a large cerebral infarction. Figure 26–13 illustrates the possible effects of arteriosclerosis of the internal carotid artery in the neck.

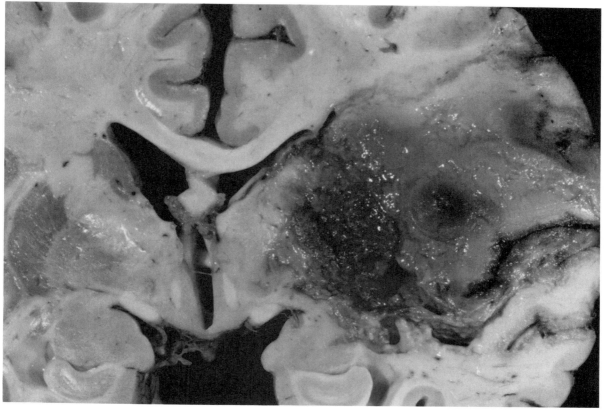

FIGURE 26–11

Large, recent infarct of cerebral hemisphere caused by occlusion of middle cerebral artery.

Diagnosis of Extracranial Vascular Disease

Cerebral blood flow can be studied by injecting a radiopaque dye into the carotid and vertebral arteries that arise from the arch of the aorta to supply the brain. In this procedure, called a *cerebral angiogram,* the course of the dye is followed by serial x-ray studies, using methods similar to those used to visualize the coronary arteries (figure 26–14). Arteriosclerotic plaques that occlude the carotid artery and impede cerebral blood flow can be removed surgically by making an incision in the carotid artery and dissecting out the arteriosclerotic lining and plaque, thereby opening up the artery (figure 26–15). The procedure is called a *carotid endarterectomy* (*endo* = within + artery + *tome* = incision).

Cerebral Hemorrhage

A *cerebral hemorrhage* is a much more serious type of stroke to which persons who have high blood pressure are prone. Blood from the rup-

FIGURE 26–12

Small, older infarct of cerebral cortex that is undergoing cystic breakdown (encephalomalacia).

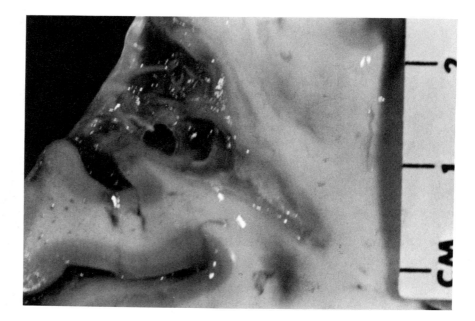

tured vessel escapes into the brain under high pressure and causes extensive damage to brain tissue. A large cerebral hemorrhage is frequently fatal (figure 26–16).

It is possible to distinguish a cerebral infarct from a cerebral hemorrhage by a specialized x-ray study called a computed tomographic (CT) scan (described in chapter 1). A CT scan can localize abnormal areas in the brain and determine their density. A cerebral hemorrhage appears as a dense area within the brain because blood is denser than normal brain tissue (figure 26–17). In contrast, an infarct is often swollen by edema and appears less dense than normal brain tissue.

Manifestations of Stroke

The clinical effects of a stroke depend on the location of the brain damage and the amount of brain tissue injured. Small infarcts may cause little functional disturbance and are usually followed by prompt recovery with little or no residual disability. Unfortunately, many strokes result from occlusions of the middle cerebral artery or one of its major branches or from a hemorrhage in a part of the brain supplied by the artery. Frequently the injury is extensive and causes partial paralysis by disrupting the nerve fibers that carry impulses to the spinal motor neurons and motor neurons of the cranial nerves (*lower motor neurons*). Nerve fibers carrying sensory impulses to the cortex are often damaged as well, leading to various sensory disturbances.

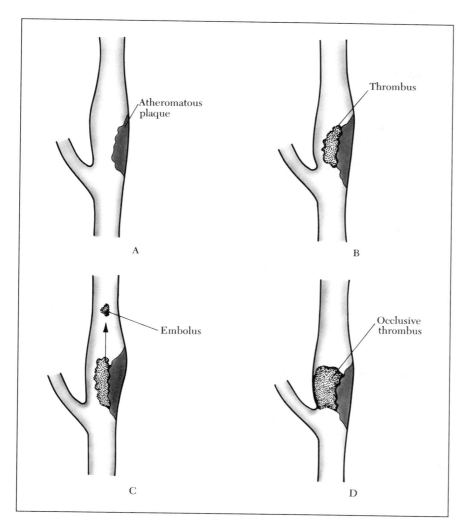

FIGURE 26–13
Effects of atherosclerosis
of carotid artery in neck.
A, Atheromatous plaque
narrows lumen, and surface
frequently becomes ulcer-
ated. **B,** Formation of thrombus on ulcerated surface of
plaque, further narrowing
vessel. **C,** Thrombus material
dislodged from plaque to
form emboli, which are carried to brain. **D,** Complete
occlusion of artery by thrombus. (Escourolle and Poirier.
*Manuel élémentaire de neu-
ropathologie.* Masson S. A.,
Paris, 1977. English transla-
tion: W. B. Saunders.
Philadelphia, 1978.)

As mentioned earlier, sensory and motor fiber tracts cross in the brain
stem as they ascend or descend; so the motor neurons from the right cerebral hemisphere supply the left side of the body, and sensory impulses
received by this hemisphere come from the left side of the body. Conversely,
the left hemisphere controls the right half of the body and receives sensory
input from the right side. Consequently, a stroke involving one cerebral
hemisphere often leads to weakness or paralysis on the opposite side, called
hemiplegia (*hemi* = half + *plege* = stroke) or *hemiparesis* (*paresis* = weakness), and often to some sensory impairment on the paralyzed side as well.
Speech also may be affected, but usually the affected individual does not
lose consciousness.

FIGURE 26–14

Angiogram revealing narrowing of carotid artery in neck (*arrows*).

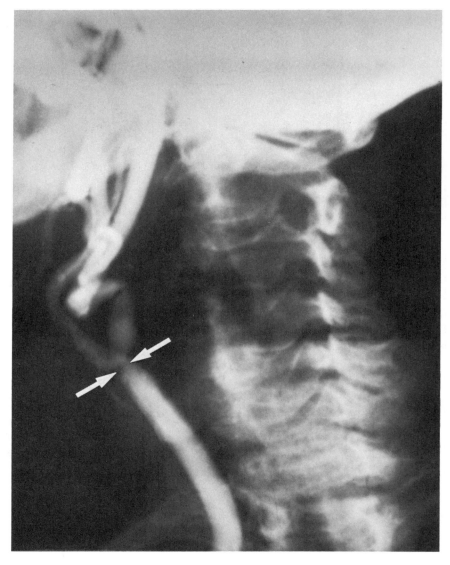

Rehabilitation of the Stroke Patient

Many patients who suffer a major stroke are partially paralyzed, and some may have speech impairment as well. Rehabilitation, which is begun as soon as possible, helps the patient achieve several goals:

1. To regain the ability to walk
2. To relearn self-care activities, such as washing, combing the hair, and eating, that may have been impaired by the stroke

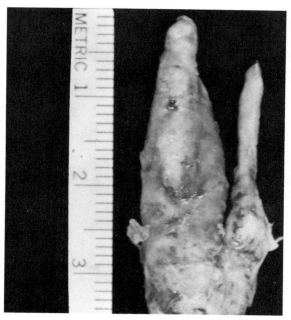

A

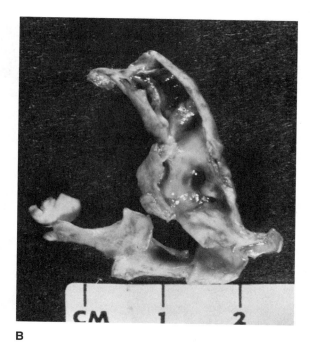

B

FIGURE 26-15

Carotid endarterectomy. **A,** Resected atherosclerotic plaque material has the contour of the common carotid artery and its two major branches, where it formed. **B,** Opened endarterectomy specimen revealing rough internal surface with areas of ulceration and hemorrhage in the atheromatous plaque.

3. To prevent stiffness and limitation of motion in the joints of the paralyzed limbs.
4. To make an emotional adjustment to the disability

These goals are achieved primarily by a program of exercises and relearning. If speech is impaired, speech therapy also is started. Many patients can learn to walk again, although in some cases a leg brace and cane may be required. It is more difficult to regain useful function in a paralyzed upper limb.

The term **transient ischemic attack,** often abbreviated to TIA, refers to brief episodes of neurologic dysfunction such as temporary paralysis of an arm or leg, loss of speech, or disturbances of vision. The episodes, which tend to occur in elderly persons, last from a few minutes to a few hours and clear completely. They are usually caused by bits of thrombus or arteriosclerotic debris that break loose from an ulcerated plaque in the internal

Transient Ischemic Attack

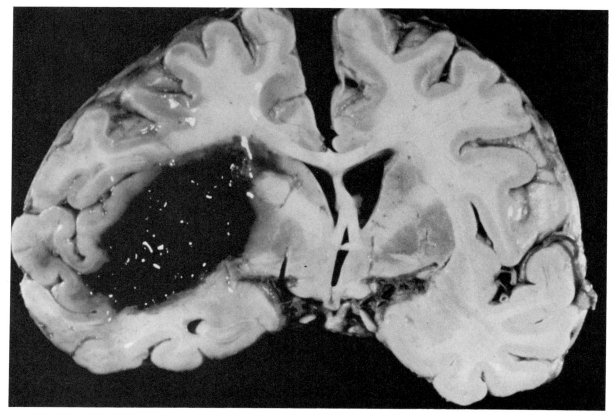

FIGURE 26–16

Cross-section of brain illustrating large intracerebral hemorrhage that has compressed and displaced the cerebral ventricles.

carotid artery and obstruct a small cerebral artery. The episodes are brief because the obstructing debris or small clot becomes fragmented and dissolved, and the circulation through the blocked vessel is restored before permanent damage to brain tissue occurs.

About one-third of patients with transient ischemic attacks eventually suffer a major stroke, but the majority experience no further difficulties. Treatment consists either of surgical resection of the ulcerated plaque in the carotid artery by means of a *carotid endarterectomy* or administration of drugs that decrease the likelihood that thrombi will form on the ulcerated plaques, thereby reducing the risk of embolization.

Cerebral Aneurysm

Occasionally, **aneurysms** occur in the large cerebral arteries at the base of the brain. The most common type, a *congenital cerebral aneurysm,* results from a congenital defect in the muscular tissue of the vessel wall, usually

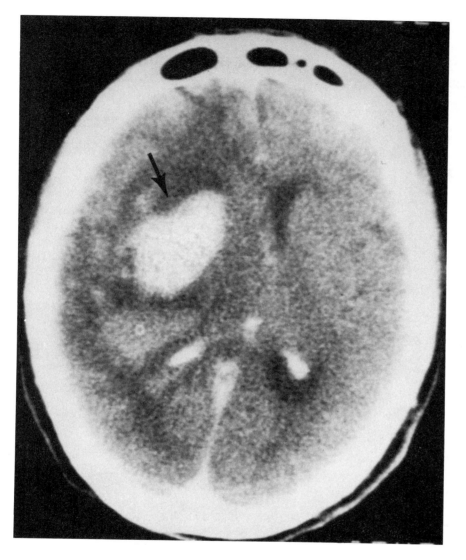

FIGURE 26–17

Computed tomographic (CT) scan of patient with cerebral hemorrhage (*arrow*), which appears white because blood is denser than brain tissue.

at the point where the artery branches. Because of the congenital weakness, the lining of the arterial wall (*intima*) eventually protrudes through the defect at the point of branching, leading to the formation of a saclike outpouching (figure 26–18).

Although the weakness of the vessel wall is congenital, the actual aneurysm does not develop until young adulthood or middle age. Congenital aneurysms are hazardous because they may rupture, producing severe and sometimes fatal hemorrhage within the cranial cavity (figure 26–19). Persons with high blood pressure are especially prone to this complication. The initial symptoms of a ruptured aneurysm are severe headache and a stiff

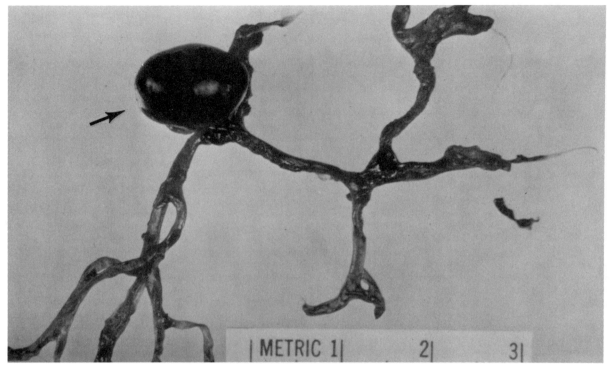

FIGURE 26–18

Dissection of vessels from brain of patient with large congenital cerebral aneurysm (*arrow*).

neck. The headache results from the increased intracranial pressure caused by the sudden escape of blood into the subarachnoid space. The stiff neck occurs because the escaping blood irritates the meninges, setting off reflex contraction of the neck muscles.

The location of the aneurysm can be determined by a *cerebral angiogram*. Radiopaque material (contrast medium) is injected into the arteries supplying the brain and fills the aneurysm sac, defining both its size and position (figure 26–20). Treatment usually consists of occluding (closing off) the aneurysm by applying a small metal clip to the narrow neck of the sac at its attachment to the arterial wall.

Rarely, one of the large cerebral arteries undergoes aneurysmal dilatation as a result of arteriosclerosis. This is termed an *arteriosclerotic aneurysm*. The aneurysm may compress the adjacent brain tissue but usually does not rupture (figure 26–21).

Infections of the Nervous System

Many different organisms can infect the nervous system, including bacteria, viruses, and fungi. An infection that predominantly affects the meninges surrounding the brain and spinal cord is called a **meningitis.** An infection of

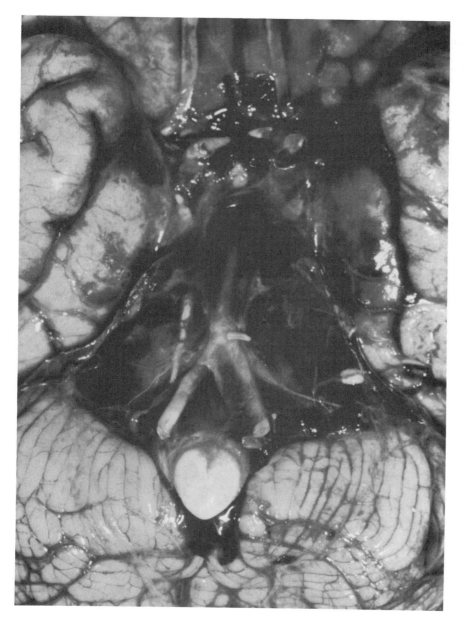

FIGURE 26–19

Undersurface of brain, illustrating subarachnoid hemorrhage secondary to ruptured cerebral aneurysm.

the brain tissue is called an **encephalitis.** If both brain and meninges are affected, the term *meningoencephalitis* is often used. An infection of the spinal cord is called a **myelitis.**

The manifestations of an infection of the central nervous system are those of any systemic infection: elevated temperature and other nonspecific symptoms. In addition, there are manifestations of meningeal irritation, consisting

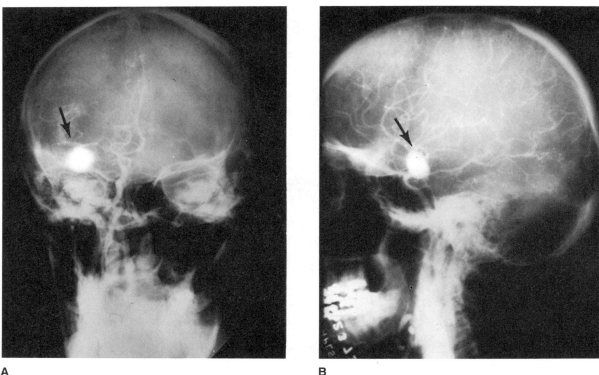

A   **B**

FIGURE 26–20

Cerebral aneurysm (*arrow*) demonstrated by angiogram. **A,** Front view. **B,** Side view.

of a headache and a stiff neck. Involvement of brain tissue is associated with alteration of consciousness and neurologic symptoms resulting from dysfunction of localized areas within the brain.

Diagnosis of a central nervous system infection is established by examination of the spinal fluid, which contains a large number of leukocytes and an elevated protein concentration if infection is present. In bacterial infections, the leukocytes are primarily neutrophils, whereas lymphocytes predominate in viral infections. In bacterial and fungus infections, the organism responsible for the infection can often be identified in stained smears prepared from the spinal fluid and by culture of the spinal fluid.

Meningitis Caused by Bacteria and Fungi

Three organisms are responsible for most cases of bacterial meningitis: *Hemophilus influenzae,* the *meningococcus,* and the *pneumococcus.* Hemophilus infections occur predominantly in children. Meningococcal infections occur primarily in young adults and often become epidemic where people live in close quarters, such as college dormitories and army camps. Pneu-

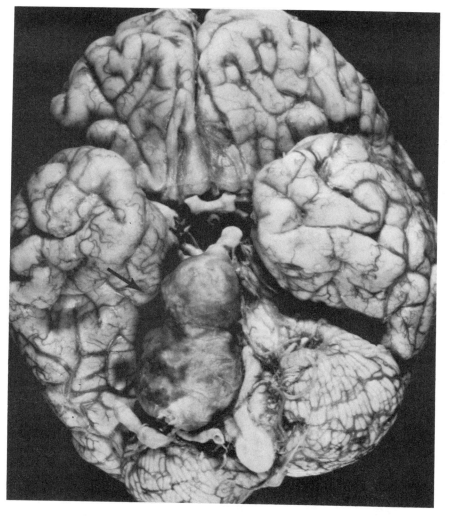

FIGURE 26–21

Large arteriosclerotic aneurysm (*arrow*) that compressed and distorted brain stem.

mococcal meningitides occur sporadically in older adults. Other bacteria may occasionally cause meningitis, especially in persons whose immunologic defenses have been weakened by disease or immunosuppressive therapy or under conditions in which bacteria are introduced directly into the nervous system.

Bacterial meningitis is often preceded by a mild upper respiratory infection, during which small numbers of bacteria gain access to the bloodstream. They are carried to the meninges, where they localize and initiate an acute infection (figure 26–22). Occasionally, the pathogens may spread directly to the meninges from a sinus or middle-ear infection or they may be introduced into the nervous system directly from a serious head injury such as a gunshot wound or severe skull fracture.

FIGURE 26–22

Bacterial meningitis, illustrating purulent exudate in the meninges. Exudate is most noticeable over the pons (*middle of photograph*) and cerebellum.

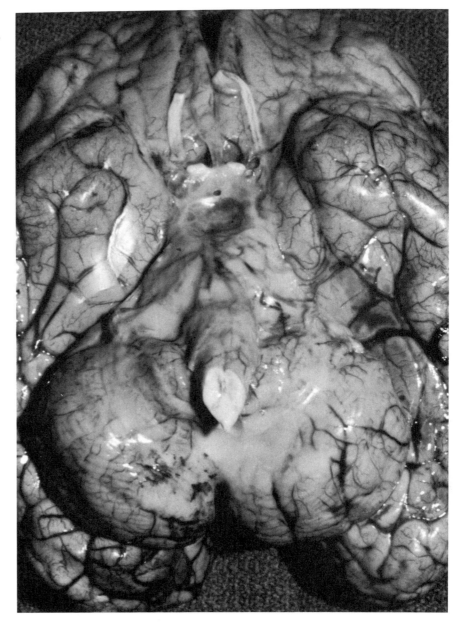

Meningitides caused by the tubercle bacillus or pathogenic fungi are uncommon and tend to be chronic rather than acute. *Tuberculous meningitis* results from spread of bacteria from a primary infection in the lung (chapter 15). *Fungus meningitis* also is usually secondary to a fungal infection of the lung, and many of the cases develop in immunocompromised persons. The most common type of fungal meningitis is that caused by the *Cryptococcus neoformans* (chapter 6).

Bacterial and fungal infections are treated with appropriate antibiotics.

Viral Infections

Many viruses can infect the nervous system, including the measles and mumps viruses, herpes virus, various intestinal and respiratory viruses, and a group of viruses called *arboviruses*. A viral infection may affect either the meninges or the brain tissue. The virus of poliomyelitis tends to primarily affect the gray matter of the spinal cord.

Viral Meningitis
A viral infection restricted to the meninges is often called *aseptic meningitis* to distinguish it from the *suppurative* (pus-producing) meningitis caused by pathogenic bacteria. The affected individual has an elevated temperature, a headache, and a stiff neck but does not usually appear seriously ill and recovers completely.

Viral Encephalitis
Viral encephalitis is a much more serious infection than viral meningitis. Some cases are fatal, and patients who recover may be left with some neurologic disability. One important group of viruses, responsible for many cases of encephalitis, causes infections of various animals; these are transmitted to human beings by infected mosquitoes. These viruses are called *arboviruses,* a contraction of the term *arthropod* (mosquito) *borne.*

Several different types of arboviral encephalitis are recognized. In the United States: *western equine encephalitis* occurs primarily in the West, and *eastern equine encephalitis* in the eastern part of the country. As the names imply, the viruses also cause encephalitis in horses (*equus* = horse). Two other types of encephalitis, called *St. Louis encephalitis* and *California encephalitis,* are not limited to the areas implied by their names but are quite widely distributed.

The arboviruses generally produce epidemics during summer and fall when the mosquito (vector) that transmits the disease is active. Encephalitis caused by other arboviruses occurs in other countries but is uncommon in the United States and Canada. Another important cause of encephalitis is the herpes simplex virus, which may cause a severe destructive inflammation; affected patients are frequently left with serious neurologic disabilities.

Unfortunately, there is no specific treatment for most cases of viral encephalitis. Some antiviral drugs may be effective in herpes simplex encephalitis if administered early in the course of the disease. (Antiviral drugs were considered in chapter 6.)

Poliomyelitis
Poliomyelitis was formerly a very important and serious disease that caused much disability and many deaths. The virus enters the body through the gas-

trointestinal tract, localizing in the gray matter of the spinal cord and sometimes also in the cell bodies of cranial nerves in the brain stem. Destruction of motor neurons leads to paralysis of the muscles supplied by the affected neurons. The name of the disease refers to the affinity of the virus for the gray matter of the cord (*polios* = gray). Fortunately, widespread vaccination has almost completely eliminated this disease in the developed countries of the world.

Slow Virus Infections of the Nervous System

Most viral infections of the central nervous system, such as those caused by the arboviruses, have a short incubation period and an acute onset of symptoms. A few, however, have a very long incubation period of months or years and an insidious onset of clinical manifestations. These unusual viral infections are called *slow virus infections* to distinguish them from the more conventional viral infections of the nervous system. Although they are relatively rare, they have received considerable attention because of their unusual characteristics.

Creutzfeldt-Jakob Disease

Named after the physicians who described it, Creutzfeldt-Jakob disease is a very unusual disease caused by a very unusual infectious agent. The disease occurs sporadically but can also be transmitted like an infectious disease, from contact with the infected tissues of a person with the disease.

The infectious agent is unusually resistant to inactivation by heat, by many disinfectants, and by ultraviolet light, but it can be destroyed by autoclaving or by household bleach. Creutzfeldt-Jakob disease was originally considered to be a slow virus infection caused by an unusual virus, but current evidence indicates that the disease is caused by an unusual protein particle called a *prion,* which is a contracted term for *proteinaceous infectious particle.* The protein aggregates to form rodlike particles called *prion rods* that can be isolated from the brain tissue of persons with the disease. In some way that we do not yet understand, the protein disrupts the functions of brain cells, causing them to degenerate, producing the manifestations of the disease.

The sporadic cases, which occur in older adults (as does Alzheimer's disease, described in the next section), are caused by a spontaneous mutation of a normal gene located on the short arm of chromosome 20. Although we do not yet know the function of the normal gene, we know that a mutation of this gene codes for the prion protein that is responsible for the disease.

Clinically, Creutzfeldt-Jakob disease is characterized by rapidly progressive mental deterioration (*dementia*) associated with neurologic disturbances. The disease is usually fatal within six months after onset of symptoms. Histologically, the brains of affected persons contain a large number of vacuoles within the neurons, which causes the affected brain tissue to have a spongy appearance. The affected neurons degenerate, and astrocytes proliferate in response to the neuron loss, but there is no inflammatory reaction. Unfortunately, no treatment is available for this devastating disease.

The cases of Creutzfeldt-Jakob disease caused by contact with infected tissues have been traced to prion-contaminated biologic products or tissues. Human growth hormone, formerly prepared from pituitary glands obtained at autopsy, was sometimes contaminated with prions. This is no longer a potential source of infection because growth hormone is now produced by recombinant DNA technology. Other infections have followed corneal, tissue, or organ transplants obtained from persons with unsuspected Creutzfeldt-Jakob disease.

Alzheimer's disease is a chronic progressive disease that affects primarily middle-aged and elderly persons. The disease is characterized by progressive failure of recent memory; difficulties in thinking, reasoning, and judgment; and is often associated with emotional disturbances such as depression, anxiety, and irritability.

Alzheimer's Disease

The brains of affected patients exhibit progressive loss of neurons with atrophy of cerebral cortex and two rather characteristic histologic changes: *neurofibrillary tangles* and *senile plaques*. Neurofibrillary tangles result from degenerative changes affecting the thin, delicate, wirelike neurofilaments, which are located within the cytoplasm of the neurons. They become converted into thick, tangled, ropy masses encircling or displacing the nuclei of nerve cells and are demonstrated by special stains containing silver compounds (figure 26–23A). Senile plaques are masses of broken, thickened nerve filaments that stain intensely with silver-containing stains and that surround a core of acellular protein material, called *amyloid protein,* with distinct staining properties (figure 26–23B). In general, there is a correlation between the degree of intellectual deterioration and the severity of the histopathologic changes. The brains of patients with advanced Alzheimer's disease contain large numbers of senile plaques and neurofibrillary tangles, whereas those with mild disease have less-striking changes.

A number of biochemical abnormalities also have been described in the brains of patients with Alzheimer's disease. One of the more important is a decrease in the concentration of acetylcholine and an acetylcholine-synthesizing enzyme (choline acetyl transferase) in the brain.

Unfortunately, we do not yet understand the basic cause of Alzheimer's disease even though we can recognize the associated anatomic and biochemical changes. Undoubtedly, these changes are the result of some underlying disturbance in brain metabolism. Further research in this field should help us understand the pathogenesis of the disease and perhaps point the way to effective treatment.

The diagnosis of Alzheimer's disease is made by excluding other conditions that can impair brain function, such as chronic infections of the nervous system or multiple strokes. Unfortunately, there is no specific treatment that can arrest the relentless progression of the disease.

FIGURE 26–23

Alzheimer's disease.
A, Thickened neurofilaments encircle and obscure nucleus of nerve cell (*arrow*) forming neurofibrillary tangle. Compare with normal nucleus of cell in lower right-hand corner. (Silver stain, original magnification × 400.) **B,** Three senile plaques, composed of broken masses of thickened neurofilaments. (Silver stain, original magnification × 100.)

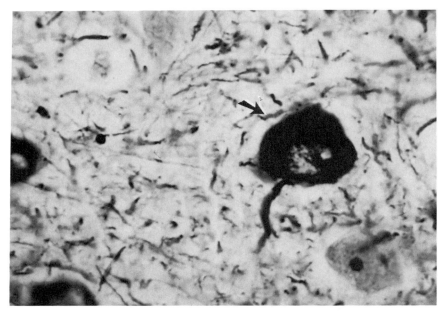

A

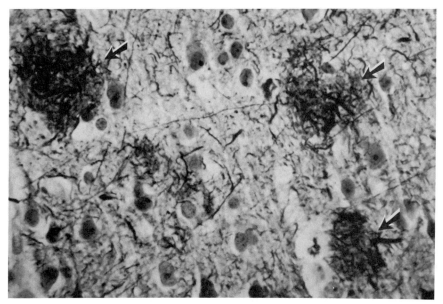

B

Multiple sclerosis is a chronic disease of unknown etiology characterized by the development of focal areas of degeneration of the myelin sheaths of the nerve fibers in the brain and spinal cord. The lesions develop in a random manner throughout the brain and spinal cord. The areas of demyelination eventually heal by forming masses of glial scar tissue (figure 26–24). The name of the disease is derived from the characteristic *multiple* areas of involvement that heal by *sclerosis* (another name for scarring). The glial scarring in this disease is produced by a type of neuroglial cell called an **astrocyte** and differs somewhat from the usual fibrous scar produced by connective-tissue cells. The discrete areas of myelin loss with glial scarring are called *multiple sclerosis plaques.* They are readily demonstrated within the nervous systems of affected persons by means of magnetic resonance imaging (MRI, described in chapter 1). This diagnostic procedure is extremely useful for evaluating patients with neurologic disease in whom multiple sclerosis is suspected (figure 26–25).

Multiple Sclerosis

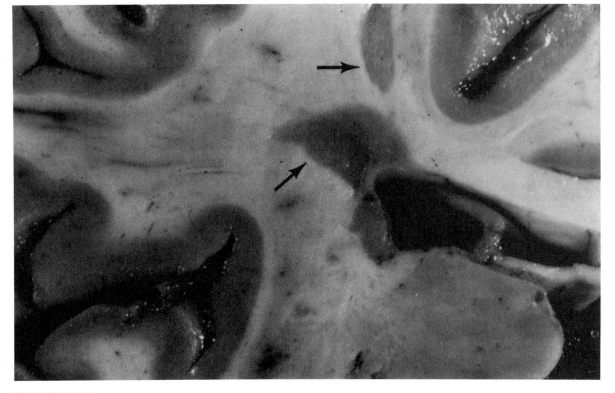

FIGURE 26–24

Cross-section of brain illustrating areas of glial scarring (*arrows*) adjacent to ventricle in multiple sclerosis. The demyelinated areas appear much darker than the adjacent normal white matter because of loss of myelin.

FIGURE 26–25

Multiple sclerosis demonstrated by magnetic resonance imaging (MRI). Ventricular system is well demonstrated in the center of the photograph. Dense white areas adjacent to posterior horns of the ventricles and scattered throughout the brain lateral to the ventricles (*arrows*) are multiple sclerosis plaques.

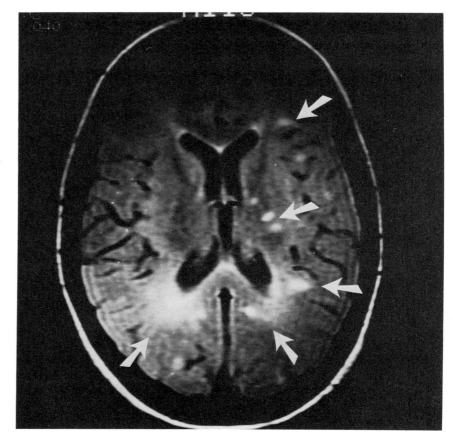

Multiple sclerosis is a disease of young adults. Onset of symptoms before age fifteen or after age forty is rare. Clinically, the disease is characterized by periodic episodes of acute neurologic disturbances, the nature depending on the location of the demyelination. Each episode is followed by a period of recovery and remission. The course of the disease is prolonged and quite unpredictable, with repeated acute episodes followed by remissions extending over many years. Eventually, the neurologic disabilities become permanent as a consequence of multiple areas of glial scarring, which impair conduction of nerve impulses in the brain and spinal cord. There is no specific treatment that can arrest the progression of the disease. A number of measures, however, are available to relieve symptoms and minimize the neurologic disabilities.

Although the cause of multiple sclerosis is unknown, much evidence suggests that the disease may be caused by a viral infection that stimulates an abnormal immune response directed against myelin sheath proteins in a genetically predisposed individual. According to this concept, multiple sclerosis may be considered an autoimmune disease.

The striking geographic variation in its prevalence suggests that the disease is infectious. The incidence is quite low in tropical areas, ranging from five to ten cases per 100,000 population. It is ten times as high in temperate zones. Moreover, exposure to the presumed infectious agent that predisposes to the development of multiple sclerosis occurs at an early age, which would be consistent with some type of viral infection having a long incubation period. There is also a genetic susceptibility to multiple sclerosis that appears to be related to multiple genes, including genes that code for the individual's HLA antigens. (The relation of HLA antigens to disease susceptibility is considered in chapter 3.) As an example, a specific HLA antigen designated HLA-DR2 is present in 60 percent of patients with multiple sclerosis but in only about 25 percent of control subjects, which is a highly significant difference. The incidence of multiple sclerosis is higher than usual in persons with a family history of the disease, probably because some of the family members may have inherited some of the same HLA and other susceptibility genes as those possessed by the affected individual. Apparently, persons having specific HLA types react to a viral infection by an abnormal immune response that is manifested by focal demyelination of nerve tissue.

Parkinson's Disease

Parkinson's disease is a chronic disabling disease characterized by rigidity of voluntary muscles and tremor of fingers and extremities. The disease results from a progressive loss of neurons in the substantia nigra of the midbrain. The axons of these neurons synapse with neurons in the basal ganglia, where they release the neurotransmitter dopamine, and this is one of the important connections of the extrapyramidal motor system. As a result of the progressive neuron loss in the substantia nigra, fewer fibers are available to release dopamine in the basal ganglia, and the concentration of dopamine in the basal ganglia falls. The muscular rigidity, increased muscle tone, and abnormal repetitive involuntary movements, which are common manifestations of the disease, result from the deranged function of the extrapyramidal system.

In most cases, the cause of Parkinson's disease is unknown. Some cases develop subsequent to viral infections of the nervous system (encephalitis) that damage the dopamine-producing extrapyramidal circuits, or to the use of illicit or toxic drugs that damage these neurons. Parkinson-like extrapyramidal symptoms may also develop after the administration of some of the drugs used to treat mental and emotional illnesses. These drug inhibit the action of dopamine on brain neurons, and generally the effects subside when the drugs are discontinued.

The manifestations of the disease can be relieved by a drug called *L-dopa,* which is converted within the brain into dopamine. The drug therapy alleviates symptoms because it raises the concentration of dopamine in the basal ganglia, thereby supplying the neurotransmitter that is deficient. Various other drugs also have been used successfully to control the manifestations of Parkinson's disease. Treatment, however, does not arrest the progressive neuron loss in the substantia nigra, nor does it stop the progression of the disease.

A new experimental approach to treatment is to transplant dopamine-producing cells into the brains of affected patients, using cells from the adrenal medulla or from fetal brain tissue. Some results have been promising. Many research studies on experimental animals are investigating the best way to establish a population of functional dopamine-producing cells within the brain and eventually find a "cure" for Parkinson's disease.

Degenerative Diseases of Motor Neurons

A group of diseases of unknown cause affecting middle aged and older adults is characterized by degeneration of motor neurons in the cortex, of cranial nerve neurons in the brain stem, and of spinal motor neurons. A small proportion of these cases are familial and follow an autosomal dominant inheritance pattern. Most cases, however, occur sporadically, and no hereditary background can be identified. Many of these diseases receive specific names, depending on which neuron groups are affected most severely, and the clinical manifestations of the neuron degeneration depend on what part of the nervous system suffers the greatest degenerative changes. In general, the symptoms are rapidly progressive muscular weakness leading to severe incapacitation and breathing difficulties resulting from weakness or paralysis of respiratory muscles. Death usually results from respiratory failure, often complicated by superimposed pulmonary infections. Unfortunately, there is no way to arrest the relentless progression of these devastating diseases.

One of the best known of these neuronal degenerative diseases is called *amyotrophic lateral sclerosis,* better known as Lou Gehrig's disease. The disease affects not only cortical motor neurons (upper motor neurons), but also cranial nerve and spinal motor neurons (lower motor neurons). The loss of lower motor neuron function leads to weakness and eventual flaccid paralysis of muscles. The degeneration of the cortical neurons is followed by secondary degeneration of the corticospinal tracts that descend to synapse with the lower motor neurons in the spinal cord.

Tumors of the Nervous System

Tumors of the nervous system may arise from three sites:

1. The peripheral nerves
2. The meninges
3. Cells within the brain or spinal cord

Tumors of the Peripheral Nerves

Tumors of peripheral nerves arise from the Schwann cells that invest the nerve fibers. Such tumors may be solitary or multiple, benign or malignant.

Most solitary Schwann cell tumors are benign. They form discrete, well-circumscribed nodules attached to larger nerve trunks and usually can be dissected easily from the adjacent nerve (see chapter 10, figure 10–2). This type of tumor is often called a *neuroma,* although the terms *Schwannoma* or *neurofibroma* also are used.

Sometimes a neuroma arises from one of the cranial nerves at the base of the brain or from one of the spinal nerves within the spinal canal. A tumor in either of these locations is much more difficult to remove. One of the more common locations for an intracerebral neuroma is the vestibulo-cochlear nerve (cranial nerve VIII), which is often called by its older name of acoustic nerve. The nerve exits the brain at the junction between the pons, medulla, and cerebellum. The tumor arising from this nerve is usually called an *acoustic neuroma.* Frequently, the tumor compresses the adjacent brain and the nearby cranial nerves as it grows, and it may also erode the adjacent temporal bone. Clinically, the tumor causes ringing in the ear (*tinnitus*) on the affected side. Compression of the nerve causes partial hearing loss on the affected side, and symptoms related to pressure on the adjacent cranial nerves and the brain stem also may be present. Although the tumor is benign, its inaccessibility makes surgical removal difficult.

Multiple tumors of the peripheral nerves occur in a hereditary disease called *multiple neurofibromatosis* or *von Recklinghausen's disease,* an uncommon condition transmitted as a Mendelian dominant trait. In this condition, the skin is disfigured by multiple tumors that grow from the cutaneous nerves and appear as variously sized nodules covering the entire body (figure 26–26). The nodules are usually associated with localized light-brown patches of hyperpigmented skin. The neoplastic proliferations involve all the components of the nerves, nerve fibers as well as Schwann cells. Multiple tumors also arise from the more deeply placed nerves supplying the internal organs. Sometimes, in localized areas, the cellular proliferation extends diffusely through the skin and subcutaneous tissue instead of forming discrete tumors. This causes the skin to become so greatly thickened that it hangs in large, disfiguring folds. In addition to being disfigured, the affected individual is at risk of having one or more of the tumors undergo malignant change. A malignant tumor of this type is called a *Schwann cell sarcoma* and occurs in about 10 to 15 percent of persons with this disease. There is no specific treatment for this disease. Large tumors that encroach on vital organs or are cosmetically disfiguring can be removed surgically. A Schwann cell sarcoma is treated by wide surgical excision, in the same way as is any malignant tumor.

Tumors of the Brain

Malignant tumors arising in the breast, colon, lung, or other sites frequently metastasize to the brain. *Primary brain tumors* are less common than metastatic tumors. They may arise from the meninges, from the glial supporting tissues of the brain, from the cells lining the ventricular system, or rarely from other tissues such as the blood vessels within the brain. Neuromas may also arise from the cranial nerves, as described in the foregoing section. Tumors do not develop from neurons, because adult nerve cells are no longer capable of cell division.

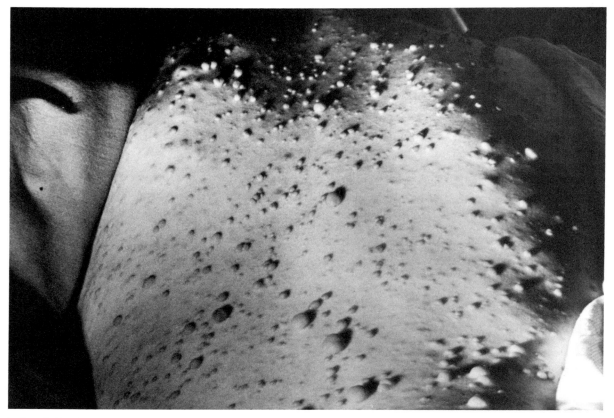

FIGURE 26–26

Multiple skin tumors in a patient with multiple neurofibromatosis (von Recklinghausen's disease).

A tumor of meninges is called a **meningioma.** This is a well-circumscribed benign tumor arising from arachnoid cells and is firmly adherent to the dura. The tumor causes symptoms as a result of compression of the underlying brain and can be removed successfully if it is located in an accessible location.

Any tumor of neuroglial origin is called a **glioma.** These tumors are further classified according to the type of glial supporting cell from which the neoplasm arises. The most common type arises from astrocytes and is called an *astrocytoma*. A special name, *glioblastoma multiforme,* is applied to a highly undifferentiated, rapidly growing astrocytoma. The name describes the primitive appearance of the neoplastic astrocytes (*blast* = primitive cell) and their great variability in shape and appearance (*multiform* = having many shapes). Gliomas arise less frequently from other supporting cells. One arising from oligodendroglia is called an *oligodendroglioma*. Two other types of tumors are often considered along with the gliomas. One is an uncommon malignant tumor arising from primitive cells in the cerebellum of young children, which is called a *medulloblastoma.* The other is a tumor arising from the cells lining the ventricular system. These cells are called ependymal cells, and the tumor is called an *ependymoma.*

Lymphomas also may arise within the central nervous system, and they are relatively common tumors in patients with AIDS.

Primary central nervous system tumors do not normally spread outside the nervous system, but many carry a poor prognosis because they often lie deep within the brain. Treatment consists of surgical resection of as much of the tumor as possible. In selected cases, surgery is followed by radiation and sometimes by anticancer chemotherapy as well. Primary lymphomas respond poorly to treatment, although radiotherapy may control the tumor for a time.

The symptoms of a brain tumor depend on the size and location of the neoplasm. Headache is a common initial manifestation because the increased volume within the cranial cavity caused by the tumor raises the intracranial pressure. Growth of the tumor also disrupts nerve cells and fiber tracts within the brain, leading to various neurologic disturbances.

Tumors of the Spinal Cord

The types of tumors that affect the brain may also occur in the spinal cord. Ependymomas may arise from the thin filament of tissue extending from the caudal end of the spinal cord, which is called the filum terminale. In addition, metastatic tumors within the vertebral bodies or **multiple myeloma,** a tumor of plasma cells within the bone marrow (described in chapter 10), may extend from the vertebrae to compress or invade the adjacent spinal cord. If this occurs, sensation and motor function below the level of cord injury may be partially or completely lost.

Peripheral Nerve Disorders

Peripheral nerves and nerve roots may undergo demyelination and varying degrees of axon degeneration. Clinical manifestations depend on the degree of nerve degeneration and on which nerves are affected. Involvement of a single nerve is usually secondary to injury or external compression. Involvement of multiple nerves, called **polyneuritis** or *peripheral neuritis,* is usually a manifestation of systemic disease. A special type of autoimmune polyneuritis with characteristic clinical manifestations is called the *Guillain Barré syndrome* or *idiopathic polyneuritis.* Tumors of peripheral nerves were discussed in the foregoing section.

Peripheral Nerve Injury

A peripheral nerve may be damaged in association with a deep laceration, a fracture, or a crushing injury. A common cause of a more chronic type of nerve injury is external compression by a fibrous band or ligament. This condition is often called a *nerve-entrapment neuropathy.* The median nerve that supplies sensory and motor fibers to the hand is often involved. The nerve is usually compressed on the anterior surface of the wrist, within the confined space between the wrist bones and the overlying ligaments that cross the wrist joint and stabilize the positions of the flexor tendons. The nerve compression causes pain and **paresthesias** (abnormal sensations such as burning, numbness, and tingling) in the index and middle fingers, together with decreased sensation in the part of the hand supplied by the nerve. The small muscles of the hand at the base of the thumb, which are supplied by the nerve, may also undergo atrophy. Sometimes symptoms can be relieved by conservative measures such as injecting a corticosteroid mixed with a local anesthetic into the confined space (called the *carpal tunnel*) in which the nerve is compressed. In many cases, however, it is necessary to relieve the compression surgically by resecting the part of the ligament that compresses the nerve.

Polyneuritis (Peripheral Neuritis)

Polyneuritis, also called *peripheral neuritis,* is characterized by progressive muscular weakness, numbness and tingling, tenderness, and pain in the parts of the body supplied by the peripheral nerves (called the *distribution* of the nerves). Often the muscles supplied by the involved nerves also exhibit some degree of atrophy. Usually the weakness and sensory disturbances affect the distal parts of the limbs, whereas strength and sensation remain relatively normal in the proximal parts of the extremities. This "glove and stocking" pattern of sensory and motor dysfunction is quite characteristic of polyneuritis. Most cases result from systemic diseases such as longstanding diabetes or various collagen diseases or from occupational exposure to toxic drugs, heavy metals, or industrial compounds. Alcoholism is another common cause of peripheral neuritis, which is probably related to a coexisting deficiency of B vitamins. Treatment of the underlying disease may produce some symptomatic improvement.

Guillain Barré Syndrome (Idiopathic Polyneuritis)

Guillain Barré syndrome, or *idiopathic polyneuritis,* is characterized by widespread patchy demyelination of nerves and nerve roots with mild inflammatory changes and sometimes by axon degeneration as well. Onset is usually a few weeks after a mild respiratory infection or following a viral infection such as measles or mumps; some cases have followed immunizations. The illness appears to be a type of autoimmune reaction to myelin that is triggered by a preceding viral infection.

Clinically, the disease is characterized by muscular weakness that usually begins in the legs and often spreads rapidly to affect the muscles of the trunk and upper extremities. Sensory disturbances are infrequent. Severe respiratory distress may occur if the nerves supplying the intercostal muscles are involved. Cranial-nerve involvement causes difficulty in swallowing and other neurologic disturbances related to cranial-nerve dysfunction. The muscular weakness generally progresses for one to two weeks, remains stationary for a time, and then gradually improves. The patient usually recovers rapidly if the nerve injury is limited to demyelination. Recovery may take several months, however, if the nerve axons are damaged, and some weakness may persist. The spinal fluid characteristically contains an increased concentration of protein without an increase in white cells, a valuable diagnostic test. The high protein concentration is apparently secondary to the inflammatory and degenerative changes within the spinal nerve roots in the subarachnoid space. There is no specific treatment, although corticosteroids are frequently used because of the apparent immunologic nature of the disease. A mechanical ventilator may be necessary temporarily if respiration is impaired.

The nervous system is often involved in persons infected with the human immunodeficiency virus (AIDS virus, described in chapter 8). In one large group of patients with AIDS-related complex or AIDS, 39 percent had some type of neurologic disturbance. Neurologic manifestations of AIDS virus infections fall into three large categories:

Neurologic Manifestations of Human Immunodeficiency Virus Infections

1. Infections of the nervous system directly caused by the AIDS virus
2. Infections of the nervous system caused by opportunistic pathogens
3. AIDS-related tumors of the nervous system

AIDS Virus Infections of the Nervous System

Although the AIDS virus causes its major damage by infecting and destroying helper T lymphocytes, the virus also infects monocytes that can transport the virus into the brain, where it can injure the nervous system. In some patients, the infection may be manifested as an acute viral meningitis occurring soon after the initial infection with the AIDS virus. In others, the infection causes a more chronic progressive degeneration of the brain with symptoms similar to those of Alzheimer's disease, which is called *AIDS-related dementia* or *AIDS encephalopathy* (*encephalon* = brain + *pathy* = disease). Polyneuritis involving either cranial or spinal nerves also may occur in some patients as a result of infection by the AIDS virus.

Opportunistic Infections of the Nervous System

Many of the opportunistic viruses, bacteria, fungi, and parasites that afflict AIDS patients can cause a primary infection of the nervous system. The clinical manifestations depend on the location of the infection within the nervous system and the amount of neurologic damage caused by the pathogen. Some of the more common opportunistic infections of the nervous system are those caused by the herpes virus, cytomegalovirus, the fungus *Cryptococcus neoformans* (chapter 6), and the protozoan parasite *Toxoplasma gondii* (chapter 7). Some of these infections respond to appropriate antibiotics and chemotherapeutic agents.

AIDS-Related Tumors

Persons with AIDS are at risk of various malignant tumors, especially Kaposi's sarcoma and lymphoma, and these tumors may metastasize to the nervous system as well as to other sites within the body. AIDS patients may also develop primary lymphomas of the nervous system. These tumors carry a very poor prognosis and do not respond well to treatment.

Questions for Review

1. Briefly describe the organization of the central nervous system. Describe the function and circulation of cerebrospinal fluid. What is meant by the following terms: *upper motor neuron lesion, lower motor neuron lesion, flaccid paralysis,* and *spastic paralysis?*

2. What are some of the possible effects of a severe blow to the head?

3. What is a stroke? What are the common causes of a stroke? What is an encephalomalacia? What is a congenital aneurysm of the circle of Willis?

4. What are the common causes of hydrocephalus? How does a brain tumor cause hydrocephalus?

5. What is a neural tube defect? How can it be recognized prior to birth?

6. What is meant by the following terms: *arachnoid, subdural hemorrhage, anencephaly,* and *meningioma?*

7. What is a transient ischemic attack? How is it treated?

8. Describe the common tumors of the nervous system. What are their clinical manifestations?

9. What is the difference between a polyneuritis (peripheral neuritis) and Guillain Barré syndrome?

10. Compare Creutzfeldt-Jakob disease and Alzheimer's disease.

11. Describe the role of magnetic resonance imaging in the diagnosis of multiple sclerosis.

12. Describe the effects of human immunodeficiency virus infections on the nervous system.

Supplementary Readings

Ahlskog, J. E. 1993. Cerebral transplantation for Parkinson's disease: Current progress and future prospects. *Mayo Clinic Proceedings* 68:578–91. Reviews current status and discusses how genetic engineering and other technics may ultimately ameliorate the manifestations of Parkinson's disease.

Barnett, H. J. M., Barnes, R. W., and Robertson, J. T. 1992. The uncertainties surrounding carotid endarterectomy. *Journal of the American Medical Association* 268:3120–21. Patients with significant stenosis do better with endarterectomy than with medical management.

Brown, R. D., et al. 1994. Transient ischemic attack and minor ischemic stroke: An algorithm for evaluation and treatment. *Mayo Clinic Proceedings* 69:1027–39. Describes initial diagnostic studies and selection of patients for possible hospitalization and anticoagulation therapy.

Centers for Disease Control and Prevention. 1993. Recommendations for use of folic acid to reduce the number of spina bifida cases and other neural tube defects. *Journal of the American Medical Association* 269:1233–38. All women of childbearing age should consume 0.4 mg of folic acid per day to reduce their risk of having a pregnancy affected with a neural tube defect.

Kannel, W. B., et al. 1981. Systolic blood pressure, arterial rigidity, and risk of stroke. *Journal of the American Medical Association* 248:1225–29. Elevation of systolic blood pressure carries an increased risk of stroke.

Kokmen, E. 1984. Dementia: Alzheimer's type. *Mayo Clinic Proceedings* 59:35–42. A clearly written review discussing clinical features, structural and biochemical abnormalities, theories as to etiology, principles of diagnosis, and management.

Lemire, R. J. 1988. Neural tube defects. *Journal of the American Medical Association* 259:558–62. Discusses common defects, predisposing factors, and incidence.

Levy, R. M., et al. 1985. Neurological manifestations of acquired immunodeficiency syndrome (AIDS): Experience at USCF and review of the literature. *Journal of Neurosurgery* 62:475–95. A review of the neurologic manifestations of AIDS virus infection in 352 homosexual patients with AIDS or generalized lymphadenopathy.

McKhann, G., et al. 1984. Clinical diagnosis of Alzheimer's disease. *Neurology* 34:939–44. Criteria for diagnosis and approaches for excluding other neurologic diseases simulating Alzheimer's. Discusses the diagnostic usefulness of laboratory tests such as CT and MRI.

Matchar, D. B. 1990. Decision-making in the face of uncertainty: The case of carotid endarterectomy. *Mayo Clinic Proceedings* 65:756–60. Excellent discussion of risks, benefits of therapeutic procedures, and biases. The wish to do everything possible for the patient must not lead to misguided actions.

Mayberg, M. R., and Winn, H. R. 1995. Endarterectomy for asymptomatic carotid artery stenosis: Resolving the controversy (Editorial). *Journal of the American Medical Association* 273:1459–61. Carotid endarterectomy helps prevent strokes in a selected group of subjects. MRI procedures may replace carotid ultrasound and angiography as the primary diagnostic procedures used to identify carotid artery stenosis.

Ojemann, R. G. 1981. Management of unruptured intracranial aneurysm (Editorial). *New England Journal of Medicine* 304:725–26. From approximately 3 to 4 percent of patients each year with asymptomatic aneurysm will experience cerebral hemorrhage as the result of rupture. The larger the aneurysm, the greater the likelihood of rupture. Aneurysm larger than 7 mm should be treated surgically.

Zervas, N. 1978. Subarachnoid hemorrhage (Editorial). *New England Journal of Medicine* 299:147–48. Operative management preferred for unruptured cerebral aneurysms. Incidence of ruptured cerebral aneurysm is about 1:10,000 persons per year.

See also sections in standard textbooks of medicine, pathology, and neurology listed in the General References.

Chapter 26 ■ Outline Summary

Structure and Function of the Brain and Nervous System / 755
The Meninges
Dura: fibrous outer covering.

Pia: inner membrane adherent to brain and cord.

Arachnoid: middle membrane interposed between other two. Contains cerebrospinal fluid and blood vessels.

The Brain
Divided into cerebrum, cerebellum, and brain stem.

Surrounded by cerebrospinal fluid secreted by choroid plexus.

Ventricles: hollow interior cavities.

Blood supply from arterial circle (circle of Willis) at base of brain.

Venous blood returns into venous sinuses in dura.

Voluntary Muscles
Muscle tone caused by reflex arcs.

Voluntary motor activity controlled by cortical neurons.

Development of the Nervous System / 756
Early Development
Neural plate becomes tube.

Forebrain forms cerebral hemispheres and diencephalon.

Midbrain and hindbrain form remainder of adult brain.

Mesoderm surrounding neural tube forms cranial cavity, vertebral bodies, and surrounding structures.

Muscle Paralysis / 759
Flaccid Paralysis
Destruction of motor neurons by disease.

Peripheral-nerve destruction.

Spastic Paralysis
Injury to cortical neurons stops voluntary control.

Reflex arc unaffected.

Tone increased and atrophy does not develop.

Closure Defects / 761
Anencephaly
Failure of normal development of brain and cranial cavity.

Multifactorial inheritance.

Spina Bifida
Several types: differ in severity.

Most severe type associated with meningomyelocele.

Prenatal Determination of Neural Tube Defect

Alpha fetoprotein leaks from fetal blood into amnionic fluid through open neural tube defect; high levels found in amnionic fluid.

Perform amniocentesis and measure alpha fetoprotein.

Hydrocephalus / 766

Formation and Absorption of Cerebrospinal Fluid

Secreted by choroid plexuses.

Flows through ventricles and exits through openings in roof of fourth ventricle.

Circulates around brain and spinal cord.

Absorbed into venous sinuses in dura.

Congenital Hydrocephalus

Caused by congenital obstruction of aqueduct or absence of openings in roof of fourth ventricle.

Head enlarges as ventricles dilate because cranial structures have not fused.

Acquired Hydrocephalus

Obstruction of cerebrospinal fluid by tumor or adhesions blocking opening in fourth ventricle.

Ventricles dilate but head does not enlarge because cranial structures are fused.

Treatment of Hydrocephalus

Shunt cerebrospinal fluid into venous system by tube extending from ventricles into jugular vein or peritoneal cavity.

Pressure in ventricles falls and enlargement of ventricles is arrested.

Stroke / 770

Encephalomalacia

Thrombus or embolus in vessel leads to breakdown of brain tissue.

Cystic cavity forms.

May be caused by atherosclerosis of internal carotid artery in neck.

Thrombi form on ulcerated plaque.

Atheromatous debris or thrombi from plaque form emboli carried to brain.

Rarely, artery is completely occluded in neck.

Condition of artery in neck can be determined by x-ray studies using radiopaque material.

Treated by carotid endarterectomy.

Hemorrhage

Ruptured artery in brain discharges blood under high pressure.

Hypertension predisposes.

Can be distinguished from encephalomalacia by CT scan.

Manifestations of Stroke

Depend on location and size.

Paralysis or sensory loss or both on opposite side of body.

Rehabilitation of the Stroke Patient

A program of graduated exercises and relearning.

Most patients can learn to walk; useful function of upper limbs less likely.

Transient Ischemic Attack (TIA) / 775

Manifestations and Treatment

Brief episodes of neurologic dysfunction.

Dysfunction usually a result of embolization of material from plaque in carotid artery in neck.

Treated by endarterectomy or medical therapy.

Cerebral Aneurysm / 776

Congenital Aneurysm of Circle of Willis

Congenital weakness in arterial wall allows lining (intima) to protrude.

Weakness is congenital but aneurysm develops in adult life.

Hypertension predisposes.

Rupture causes subarachnoid hemorrhage.

Treated by occluding aneurysm surgically.

Arteriosclerotic Aneurysm

Arteriosclerotic cerebral artery dilates and compresses adjacent brain.

Rupture very uncommon.

Infections of the Nervous System / 778

Manifestations

Systemic infection: fever, nonspecific symptoms.

Meningeal irritation: headache, stiff neck.

Infection of brain: alteration of consciousness, focal neurologic symptoms.

Abnormalities of spinal fluid: neutrophil increase in bacterial infection. Lymphocyte increase in virus infection.

Bacterial and Fungal Meningitis

Usually caused by *Hemophilus influenzae*, pneumococcus, meningococcus.

Bacteria carried to meninges in bloodstream. Less commonly spread from sinuses or middle ear or introduced after cerebral injury.

Tuberculous and fungus infections less common.

Usually spread from lung.

Viral Infections

Meningitis: usually mild illness with complete recovery.

Encephalitis: more serious disease with occasional deaths and late complications.

Many cases caused by arboviruses that infect animals and are transferred to humans by mosquitoes.

Herpes virus may cause severe destructive inflammation.

No specific treatment for most cases. Antiviral chemotherapy may be useful in some cases of herpes infection.

Poliomyelitis:

Affects gray matter of spinal cord; damages motor neurons, causing paralysis.

Largely eradicated in developed countries by widespread immunization.

Slow Virus Infections

Uncommon diseases.

Long incubation period and insidious onset.

Creutzfeldt-Jakob Disease / 784

Caused by small protein particle (prion) produced as a result of gene mutation.

Causes dementia and neurologic dysfunction.

Most cases sporadic, but transmissible by contaminated biologic products or infected transplanted cornea or organs.

Invariably fatal. No treatment available.

Alzheimer's Disease / 785
Characteristics

Affects chiefly middle-aged and elderly.

Progressive mental deterioration and emotional disturbances.

Relentless progression. No treatment available.

Anatomic and Biochemical Features

Reflect unknown disturbance in brain metabolism.

Thickening of neuron neurofilaments forming neurofibrillary tangles.

Clusters of thick, broken neurofilaments form senile plaques.

Brain enzyme deficiencies.

Multiple Sclerosis / 787
Pathogenesis and Manifestations

Probably autoimmune disease in genetically predisposed individual.

Random foci of demyelination followed by glial scarring.

Neurologic symptoms depend on location of plaques.

MRI useful diagnostic test to demonstrate plaques in CNS.

Parkinson's Disease / 789
Manifestations and Pathogenesis

Rigidity of muscles and tremor.

As a result of decreased concentration of dopamine in central nervous system.

Symptoms relieved by L-dopa, which is converted into dopamine in brain.

Degenerative Diseases of Motor Neurons / 790

Affect both upper and lower motor neurons.

Cause weakness, paralysis, respiratory problems.

Some cases are familial.

No specific treatment.

Tumors of Nervous System / 790
Peripheral Nerve Tumors

Usually solitary: arise from Schwann cells.

Neuromas of cranial nerves often involve acoustic nerve and are difficult to remove surgically.

Multiple nerve tumors occur in multiple neurofibromatosis.

Transmitted as Mendelian dominant trait.

Disfiguring skin nodules, thickened patches of skin, and focal hyperpigmentation of skin.

Sarcoma arises from preexisting tumors in 10 to 15 percent of cases.

Brain Tumors

Metastatic tumors common.

Meningioma: from arachnoid cells. Good prognosis.

Gliomas: including ependymoma and medulloblastoma. Many carry poor prognosis because of deep location in brain. Treatment by surgery, radiation, chemotherapy.

Spinal Cord Tumors

Same types of tumors that arise in brain.

Tumors involving vertebral bodies may invade or compress cord.

Peripheral Nerve Disorders / 793
Peripheral Nerve Injury

Traumatic injury: associated with lacerations, fractures, crush injury.

Nerve entrapment neuropathy.

External compression by fibrous band.

Median nerve commonly involved.

May require surgical release if no response to conservative treatment.

Polyneuritis (Peripheral Neuritis)

Sensory and motor dysfunction in "glove and stocking" distribution. Proximal sensation and motor function preserved.

As a result of systemic disease, toxins, alcoholism.

Treatment of underlying disease may lead to improvement.

Guillain Barré Syndrome (Idiopathic Polyneuritis)

Patchy demyelination of nerves and nerve roots with mild inflammation and sometimes axon degeneration.

An autoimmune reaction to myelin triggered by preceding viral infection.

Progressive weakness usually followed by complete recovery. No specific treatment.

Neurologic Manifestations of Human Immunodeficiency Virus Infection / 795

As a Result of HIV Infection of Nervous System

Acute viral meningitis.

AIDS encephalopathy—chronic and progressive.

Polyneuritis.

Caused by Opportunistic Infections of Nervous System

Many pathogenic organisms can infect nervous system directly.

Manifestations depend on location of infection and extent of damage to nervous system.

Herpes, cytomegalovirus, *Cryptococcus neoformans,* and *Toxoplasma gondii* are commonly implicated organisms.

AIDS-Related Tumors

Kaposi's sarcoma, lymphoma, or other malignant tumors may metastasize to nervous system.

Primary lymphoma of brain may occur.

Tumors respond poorly to treatment.

27

The Musculoskeletal System

Learning Objectives

1. Name the common congenital abnormalities of the skeletal system.
2. List the three major types of arthritis, describe their pathogenesis and clinical manifestations, and explain the methods of treatment.
3. Describe the causes and effects of osteoporosis and name the methods of treatment.
4. Describe the structure of the intervertebral disks and explain their function. Describe the clinical manifestations of a herniated disk.
5. Compare the pathogenesis and clinical manifestations of muscular atrophy and muscular dystrophy. Name and describe the common types of each.
6. Describe the pathogenesis, manifestations, and treatment of myasthenia gravis.

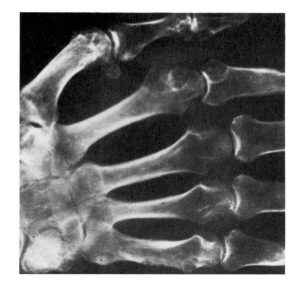

Chapter 27 ▪ Contents

The skeleton is the rigid supporting structure of the body. All bones have the same basic structure. They are composed of an outer layer of *compact bone,* the cortex, and an inner, spongy layer in which the bone is arranged in a loose meshed latticework of thin strands called *bone trabeculae.* The spaces between the trabeculae contain the bone marrow, which consists of fat and blood-forming tissue.

Individual bones vary in size and appearance. They may be long, short, flat, or irregular in shape. The typical long bone, such as is found in the upper and lower limbs, has a tubular shape with expanded ends. The *shaft* is the long cylindrical part, and the expanded ends of the shaft are called the *epiphyses.* The center of the shaft is hollowed out to form the *marrow cavity,* which is filled with fat and bone marrow. This type of construction provides considerable strength without excessive weight.

Bone is a specialized type of connective tissue. It is composed of a dense connective-tissue framework that is impregnated with calcium phosphate salts along with smaller amounts of calcium carbonate and other minerals. Bone is not a static structure. It is continually being broken down and reformed, and calcium salts in bone and calcium ions in the blood and body fluid are continuously interchanged.

In general, the strength and thickness of the bones depends on the activities of the individual. A person accustomed to strenuous physical labor has thicker, heavier bones than one who is normally engaged in light, sedentary activities. If an extremity is immobilized and is not allowed to bear weight, as after a fracture, the immobilized bone undergoes significant thinning and decalcification, called *disuse atrophy.*

The bones of the skeleton are connected by *joints.* There are three types: fibrous joints, cartilaginous joints, and synovial joints. In a *fibrous joint,* such as occurs between the bones of the skull, the bones are firmly joined by fibrous tissue to form a firm union called a *suture line.* In a *cartilaginous joint,* such as occurs between adjacent vertebral bodies in the spine and between the pubic bones of the pelvis (*symphysis pubis*), the ends of the bones are joined by fibrocartilage. Joints of this type have very little mobility. A *synovial joint* is a movable joint. The ends of the bones that move against one another are covered by smooth hyaline cartilage, which is called the *articular cartilage (articulare* = to connect). The ends of the bones are held together by dense fibrous bands (*ligaments*). The joint capsule is lined by a thin synovial membrane (the *synovium*), which secretes a small amount of mucinous fluid to lubricate the joint. Figure 27–1 illustrates the structure of a typical movable joint. Figure 27–2 illustrates the histologic appearance of the articular cartilage and underlying layer of bone. In joint disease, these structures are altered by inflammation or degeneration, leading to derangement in the functions of the joints.

Bone Formation

There are two types of bone formation, which are fundamentally similar. In one type, called **intramembranous bone formation,** the embryonic

FIGURE 27–1

Structure of a typical movable joint.

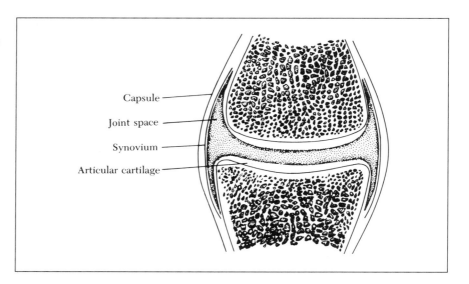

FIGURE 27–2

Low-magnification photomicrograph of cellular structure of normal articular surface, illustrating articular cartilage at *top of photograph,* junction of bone and cartilage in *middle of photograph,* and normal bone with fatty bone marrow at *bottom of photograph.* (Original magnification × 40.)

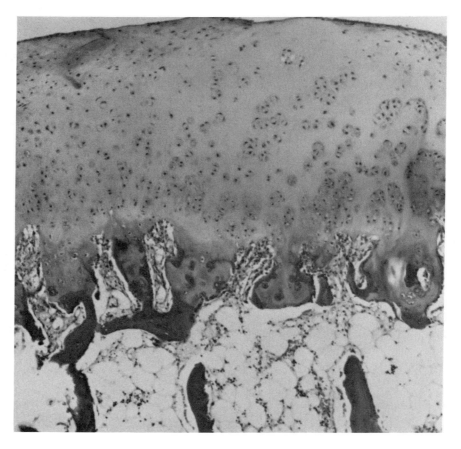

connective-tissue cells (mesodermal cells) are transformed directly into bone-forming cells (osteoblasts). The osteoblasts secrete a collagenous material called *osteoid,* which then becomes calcified to form bone. The bones of the vertex of the skull, the facial bones, and a few other bones are formed in this manner. Most of the skeletal system, however, is formed by a process called **endochondral bone formation** (*endo* = within + *chondral* = cartilage). In endochondral bone formation, the mesodermal cells differentiate first into cartilage cells, and the bones are formed initially as cartilage models. The cartilage is then absorbed and replaced by bone. Conversion of cartilage into bone is accomplished by vascular bone-forming mesoderm, which invades the cartilage. The areas of active bone formation are termed *centers of ossification.*

Bones that have been preformed in cartilage undergo ossification at specific times throughout fetal and postnatal life. The time of appearance of the various centers of ossification is characteristic for each bone. In the long bones, ossification begins first in the shaft; later, centers of ossification form at the ends (*epiphyses*) of the bone. The actively growing zone of cartilage between the shaft and the epiphysis of a long bone is called the *epiphyseal plate.*

Bone Growth

Bone grows in both length and thickness and is continually remodeled as it grows by absorption of bone in some areas and formation of new bone in others. Bone grows thicker by adding to its external surface newly formed bone that is produced by the **periosteum,** a layer of specialized connective-tissue cells surrounding the bone. The periosteal cells differentiate into osteoblasts, which in turn produce bone. Growth in the length of bone is the result of proliferation of cartilage at the epiphyseal plate, which is converted into bone. Growth in bone length continues into adolescence. Eventually, epiphyseal growth ceases, and the cartilagenous epiphyseal plate becomes converted into bone—called *closure of the epiphyses* Thereafter, no further growth in length of bone is possible.

Abnormal Bone Formation

The two most important genetically determined diseases of the skeletal system that result from abnormal bone formation are achondroplasia and osteogenesis imperfecta.

In **achondroplasia,** endochondral bone formation is faulty. The abnormality, which is transmitted as a Mendelian dominant trait, is characterized by disturbed endochondral bone formation at the epiphyseal lines of the long bones. The disturbance impairs growth of the extremities, causing a type of dwarfism in which the limbs are disproportionately short in relation

Congenital Malformations

to the trunk (*achondroplastic dwarfism*). The head is also abnormally formed because of disturbed endochondral ossification of the bones forming the base of the skull, and there is usually also an exaggerated curvature (*lordosis*) of the lumbar spine (figure 27–3).

Osteogenesis imperfecta (meaning literally "imperfect bone formation") is characterized by the formation of very thin and delicate bones that are easily broken under very minimal stress. In the most severe cases, the infant is born with multiple fractures. Some fractures occur before birth, having been sustained as a result of the very minor stresses resulting from the movements of the fetus within the uterus; other fractures occur during delivery. The intrauterine fractures of the extremities usually heal in poor alignment, causing the limbs to appear bent and disproportionately short (figure 27–4). In milder forms of the disease, the abnormal fragility of the bone may not become apparent until childhood or adolescence.

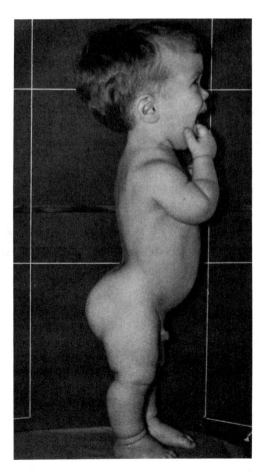

FIGURE 27–3

Characteristic appearance of child with achondroplasia, illustrating the disproportionate shortening of the extremities, large head, and severe lumbar lordosis (swayback).

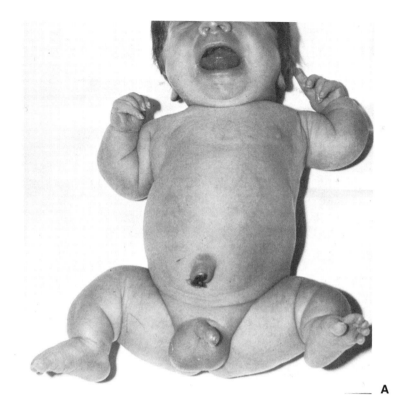

A

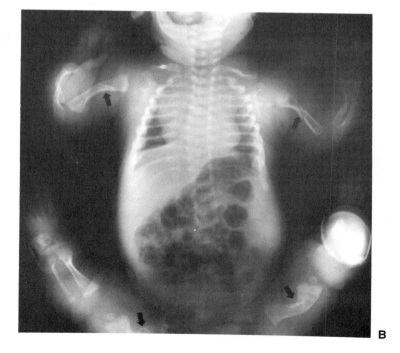

B

FIGURE 27–4

Severe form of osteogenesis imperfecta in newborn infant. **A,** Shortening and bowing of limbs resulting from multiple intrauterine fractures that have healed in poor alignment. **B,** X-ray film showing multiple fractures of ribs and limb bones, some showing poor alignment and evidence of healing. *Arrows* indicate the locations of four fractures.

Malformation of Fingers and Toes

Abnormalities of the fingers and toes are relatively common and generally can be corrected surgically. The fingers and toes may fail to separate normally during development (*syndactyly*), leading to the formation of spade-like hands and feet (figure 27–5A). In other instances, extra digits are formed (*polydactyly,* figure 27–5B).

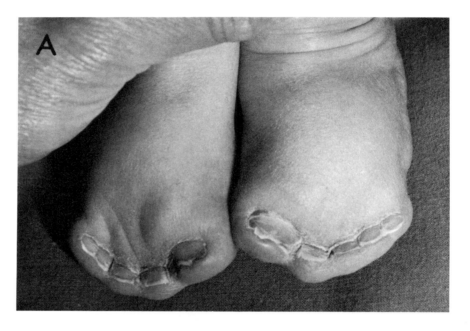

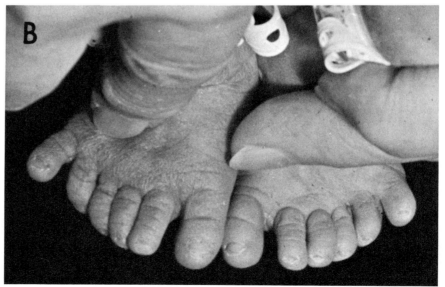

FIGURE 27–5

Common malformations of fingers and toes. **A,** Failure of separation of digits. **B,** Extra digits.

Congenital Clubfoot (Talipes)

Clubfoot is a relatively common congenital abnormality, having an incidence of about one in one thousand infants. The malformation is characterized by an abnormal position of the foot that prevents normal weight-bearing, the affected individual tending to walk on the ankle rather than on the sole of the foot (*talus* = ankle + *pes* = foot). Figure 27–6 illustrates the most common type of clubfoot deformity called *talipes equinovarus*, in which the foot is turned inward at the ankle (*varus position*) and fixed in tiptoe (*equinus*) position. Less commonly, the foot is rotated outward (*valgus position*) and fixed so that the weight is born on the heel (*calcaneus position*). Talipes follows a multifactorial pattern of inheritance (chapter 9). Any intrauterine fetal position that causes the foot to assume an abnormal position may cause the foot to develop abnormally if the fetus is genetically predisposed to this malformation. Talipes is treated by manipulating the foot into a normal position and maintaining the corrected position with casts or splints.

Congenital Dislocation of the Hip

Congenital dislocation of the hip has an incidence of about one in fifteen hundred infants, and it occurs most commonly in females. In this malfor-

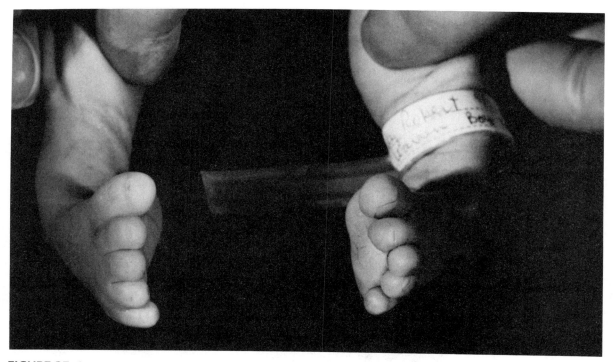

FIGURE 27–6

Common type of congenital clubfoot (talipes equinovarus) in newborn infant.

mation, the hip-joint socket (*acetabulum*) on the affected side is shallow, its upper rim is less well developed than normal, and the ligaments holding the head of the femur in the socket are relatively lax. As a consequence, the head of the femur fails to maintain its normal position and becomes displaced upward and backward out of the shallow socket (figure 27–7). Like clubfoot, congenital hip dislocation results from the interaction of genetic factors in conjunction with an abnormal intrauterine fetal position. The depth of the hip socket and the laxity of the ligaments are genetically determined. Ligamentous laxity is also related to the sex of the infant, being greater in female infants (which accounts for the more frequent occurrence of congenital hip dislocation in females). If, in addition, the fetus assumes a position that causes the foot and leg to be rotated externally, the thigh also is rotated externally, which tends to displace the head of the femur out of its socket. Some types of *breech positions* (fetal buttocks rather than head in the lower part of the uterus and the lower extremities with knees extended pressed against the fetal abdomen and chest) predispose to hip dislocation in a genetically susceptible infant.

Congenital dislocation of the hip can frequently be treated effectively by manipulating the displaced femoral head into the acetabulum and maintaining the head within the socket by means of some device that maintains the leg and thigh in proper position, such as a splint or plaster cast.

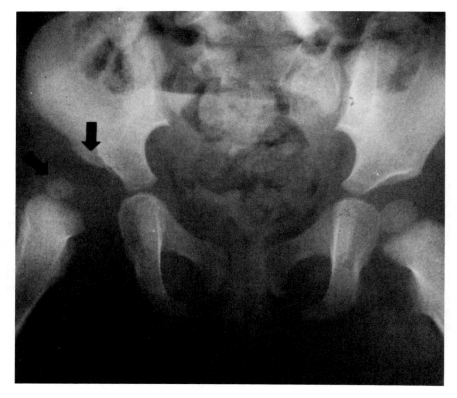

FIGURE 27–7

Congenital dislocation of right hip in an eighteen-month-old child. Radiograph shows that right hip socket (*left*) is shallow, and its upper end (*upper arrow*) is less well developed than normal, permitting the head of the femur (*lower arrow*) to be displaced upward out tó the hip-joint socket. The dislocated head is also less well developed than normal.

Arthritis is one of the most common and disabling diseases of the skeletal system. Although there are many different kinds of arthritis, the three most common are:

1. Rheumatoid arthritis
2. Osteoarthritis
3. Gout

Table 27–1 compares the major features of these conditions.

Rheumatoid Arthritis

Rheumatoid arthritis is a systemic disease affecting the connective tissues throughout the body, but the most pronounced clinical manifestations are in the joints. Clinically, the disease is seen as a chronic, disabling, and often deforming arthritis affecting several joints. Rheumatoid arthritis is encountered most frequently in young and middle-aged women; it usually affects the small joints of the hands and feet. In the joints, the arthritis produces a

	Rheumatoid arthritis	Osteoarthritis	Gout	
Age and sex of usual patient	Young and middle-aged, female	Adult, elderly, both sexes	Middle-aged, male	**TABLE 27–1** Comparison of major features of common types of arthritis
Major characteristic	Systemic disease with major effects in joints; causes chronic synovitis	"Wear and tear" degeneration of articular cartilage	Disturbance of purine metabolism; acute episodes caused by crystals of uric acid in joints	
Secondary effects of disease	Ingrowth of inflammatory tissue over cartilage destroys cartilage, leads to destruction of joint space; deformities common	Overgrowth of bone; thickening of periarticular soft tissues	Deposits of uric acid in joints with damage to joints (gouty arthritis); soft tissue tophi	
Joints usually affected	Small joints of hands and feet	Major weight-bearing joints	Small joints; joint at base of great toe often affected	
Special features	Autoantibody against gamma globulin (rheumatoid factor)	No systemic symptoms or biochemical abnormalities	High blood level of uric acid	

chronic inflammation and thickening of the synovial membrane. The inflammatory tissue extends over the surface of the articular cartilage, destroying the cartilage (figure 27–8). The severe damage to the articular surfaces makes the joint unstable; this in turn leads to deviation or displacement of the bones owing to the pull of the surrounding ligaments and tendons (figure 27–9). Fibrous adhesions often develop within the joint, and the ends of the adjacent bones may become completely fused. The end result of these various structural derangements is often severe disability and conspicuous deformity of the affected joints (figure 27–10).

The blood of patients with rheumatoid arthritis often contains a substance called *rheumatoid factor,* which is an autoantibody directed against the individual's own gamma globulin. Immune complexes composed of gamma globulin and autoantibody form within the joints, which activates complement and attracts the inflammatory cells that damage the joints. Because of the systemic nature of the disease and the presence of autoantibodies, rheumatoid arthritis is often classified as one of the autoimmune diseases (chapter 5).

As with some other autoimmune diseases, there is a genetic susceptibility to rheumatoid arthritis that is related to the individual's HLA antigens. About half the persons with rheumatoid arthritis have the HLA antigen designated HLA-DR4, which is present in only about 20 percent of control subjects, and this is considered a highly significant difference.

Rheumatoid arthritis tends to fluctuate in severity. Periods in which the disease is active may alternate with periods in which it is inactive. Although there is no cure for rheumatoid arthritis, a number of measures can be used to control the disease and minimize its attending disability and deformity.

The primary objectives of treatment are reduction of joint inflammation and pain, maximal preservation of joint function, and prevention of joint deformity (if possible). Treatment consists of rest periods for several hours every day while the disease is active, use of splints to support inflamed joints and reduce deformities caused by muscle spasm, and use of crutches and braces to aid weight-bearing. The affected joints are exercised gently in order to preserve joint mobility and muscle strength. Anti-inflammatory drugs such as aspirin are prescribed to reduce inflammation within the joints. In selected cases, corticosteroids are administered orally or injected into the affected joints. If the patient does not respond to conservative therapy, more powerful drugs may be required to control the disease. Sometimes cytotoxic immunosuppressive drugs (chapter 5) must be administered to control the destructive inflammatory process within the joints. If severe joint deformities develop, several different surgical procedures can be performed to improve joint function. These measures include excision of thickened inflamed synovium, surgical correction of joint dislocations, or even complete reconstruction of damaged joints.

Osteoarthritis

In contrast to rheumatoid arthritis (a systemic disease), **osteoarthritis** is a result of "wear and tear" degeneration of one or more of the major weight-

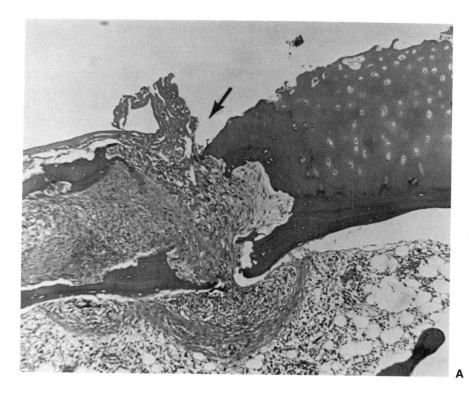

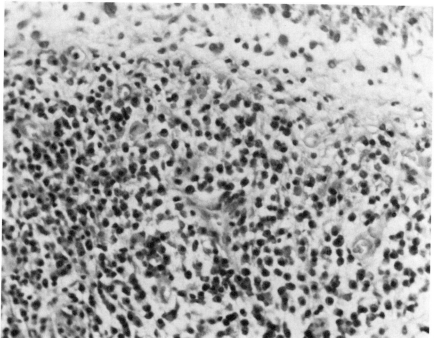

FIGURE 27–8

Rheumatoid arthritis. **A,** Low-magnification photomicrograph illustrating destruction of articular cartilage by inflammatory reaction (*arrow*) extending from synovial surface. (Original magnification × 25). **B,** Photomicrograph of chronic inflammatory reaction in synovium. (Original magnification × 100.)

FIGURE 27–9

Rheumatoid arthritis.
A, Early manifestations, illustrating swelling of knuckle joints (metacarpophalangeal joints) as a result of inflammation.
B, More advanced changes, illustrating joint deformities and ulnar deviation of fingers.

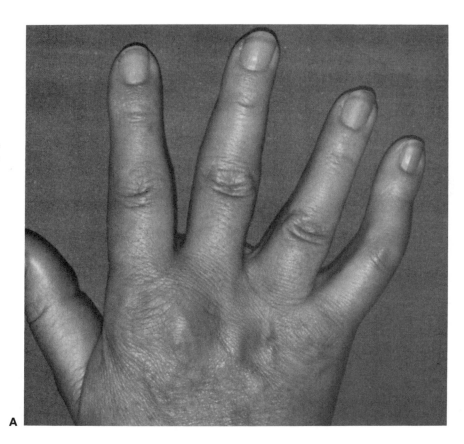

A

B

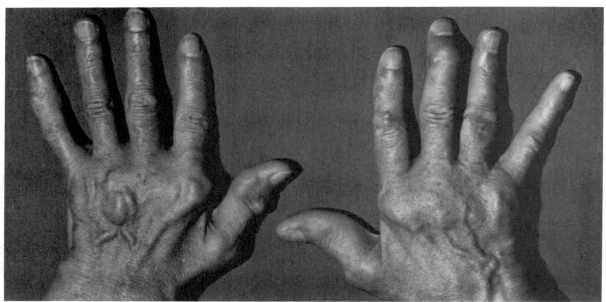

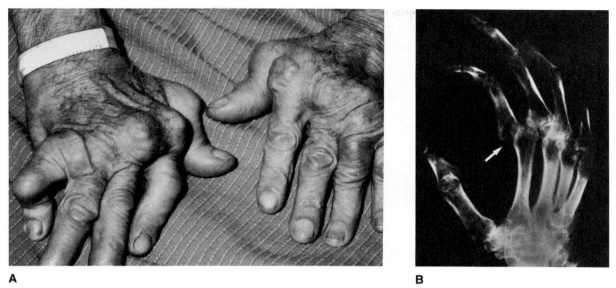

A   **B**

FIGURE 27–10

A, Advanced joint deformities caused by rheumatoid arthritis. **B,** Radiograph illustrating destruction of articular surfaces and anterior dislocation of base of index finger (*arrow*) as a result of joint instability.

bearing joints (*osteo* = bone + *arthro* = joint + *itis* = inflammation). The disease is seen in older adults and may be considered a manifestation of the normal aging process. The primary change in osteoarthritis is degeneration of the articular cartilage, leading to roughening of the articular surfaces of the bones (figure 27–11). As a consequence, the bones grate against one another when the joint moves, instead of gliding smoothly. Degeneration of the cartilage sometimes leaves large areas of underlying bone exposed. Secondary overgrowth of bone frequently occurs in response to the trauma of weight-bearing (figure 27–12), and some thickening of the synovium and adjacent soft tissues also is common.

Clinically, persons with osteoarthritis experience stiffness, creaking, and some pain on motion of the joints, but disability is usually not severe and the joints are not destroyed. However, occasional patients may experience considerable pain and disability from advanced arthritis affecting one or both hip joints. In such cases, it is possible to remove the affected femoral head and articular surface of the hip bone surgically and to replace them with an artificial hip joint. The procedure is called a *total hip joint replacement* (figure 27–13). Similar types of joint replacement procedures have been performed on the knee joint and some other joints as well. Joint replacement operations can provide excellent pain relief and greatly improved joint function in many patients.

FIGURE 27–11

A, Knee joint, illustrating smooth articular surfaces of femoral condyles.
B, Osteoarthritis of knee, illustrating loss of articular cartilage (*left arrow*) and nodular overgrowth of bone (*right arrows*).

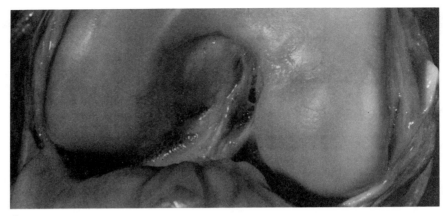

A

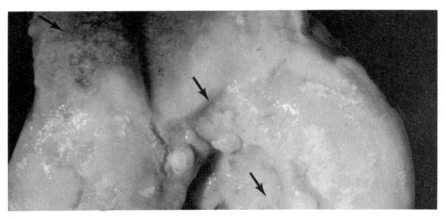

B

Gout

Gout is a disorder of purine metabolism. Purines are double-ring nitrogen compounds in the nucleotides that are joined together to form large nucleic acid molecules. Breakdown of purines within the body yields a relatively insoluble end-product called *uric acid.*

The underlying metabolic defect in gout is unknown, but it leads to excessive accumulation of uric acid in the body, and is generally associated with a higher-than-normal level of uric acid in the blood, which is called *hyperuricemia.* Clinically, the person afflicted with gout experiences periodic episodes of extremely painful arthritis in a single joint, often the joint at the base of the great toe (figure 27–14A). The acute episodes are caused by crystallization of uric acid within the joint; the crystals incite an acute inflammatory reaction. Large, lumpy masses of uric acid crystals, called *gouty tophi,* are often deposited in the soft tissues around the joints and in other

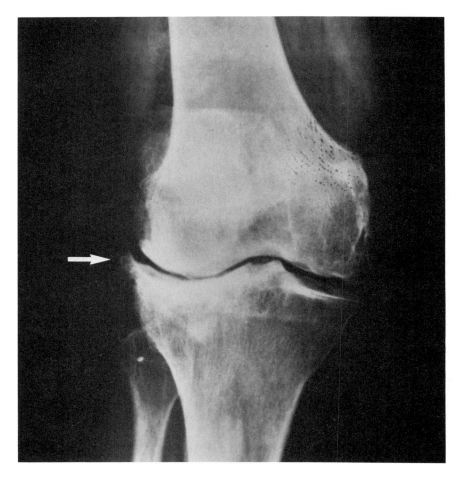

FIGURE 27–12

Osteoarthritis. Radiograph illustrates increased bone density of femoral condyle (*left side of photograph*) and adjacent tibia, with over-growth of bone at margin of tibia (*arrow*).

locations (figure 27–14B). In untreated patients, masses of uric acid crystals eventually become deposited in and around the articular surfaces of the joints, injuring the joint surfaces; this is called *gouty arthritis* (figure 27–15). Uric acid stones may form within the kidney and lower urinary tract owing to crystallization of uric acid in the urine. Uric acid may also precipitate within the distal renal tubules and collecting tubules as the uric-acid–laden tubular filtrate flows through the kidneys. The precipitates obstruct and damage the renal tubules, which is following by scarring and impaired renal function, a condition called *urate nephropathy*.

Gout is treated by administering drugs that reduce the concentration of uric acid in the blood by interfering with the formation of uric acid within the body or by promoting the excretion of uric acid by the kidneys. Patients are usually advised to avoid foods rich in nucleoproteins, such as liver, kidney, and pancreas (sweetbreads), because they tend to raise uric acid levels. Heavy intake of alcohol also should be avoided because alcohol

FIGURE 27–13

A, Femoral head that was removed surgically and replaced by artificial hip joint. Note irregularity of head and overgrowth of bone at margin of femoral head (*arrow*). **B,** X-ray illustrating total hip replacement. Opposite hip joint also shows arthritic changes.

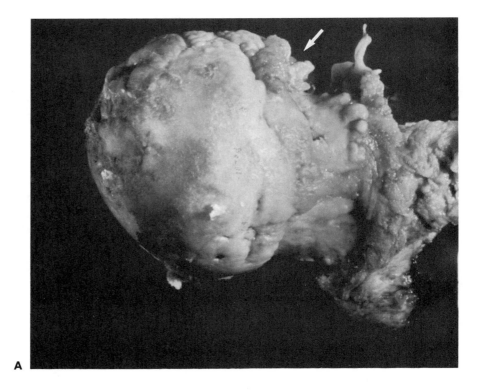

A

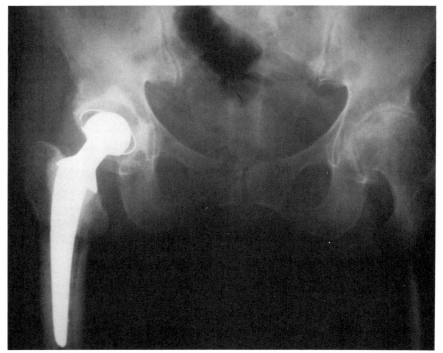

B

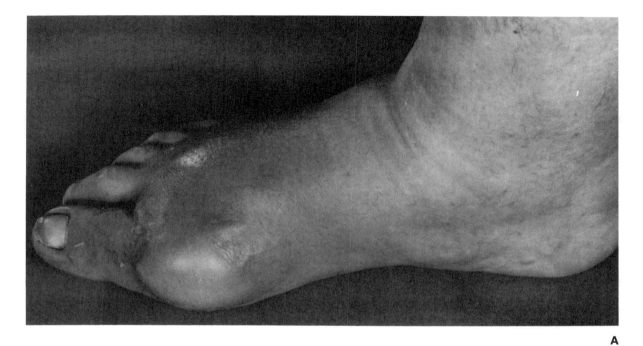

A

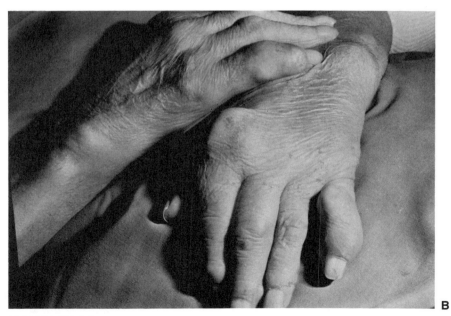

B

FIGURE 27–14

A, Acute gout affecting right great toe. (Photograph courtesy of Dr. Jeffrey Felt.) **B,** Deformities of hands caused by accumulation of uric acid crystals (tophi) in and around finger joints.

FIGURE 27–15

Radiograph of right hand of patient with gouty arthritis illustrates area of bone destruction caused by masses of uric acid crystals (*arrow*).

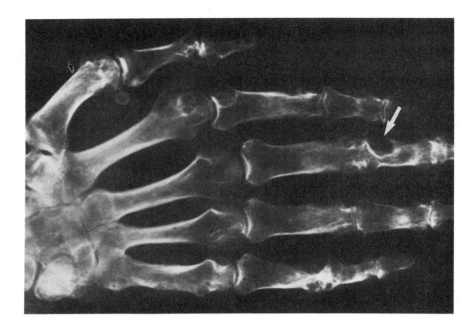

indirectly impairs excretion of uric acid by the renal tubules, causing the blood uric acid level to rise.

Some conditions other than gout also may raise blood uric acid, and at times the level may be so high that the uric acid precipitates from the blood, causing the same type of acute symptoms as those of gout. Patients with kidney failure may have high blood uric acid because the diseased kidneys are unable to excrete the uric acid efficiently, and some diuretics also may impair renal uric acid excretion. Hyperuricemia may be a problem in leukemic patients who have a greatly increased number of white blood cells, especially after treatment with drugs that destroy the leukemic cells and release large amounts of nucleoprotein from the disrupted cells. The breakdown of the nucleoprotein yields a large amount of uric acid derived from the purine-containing nucleotides in the nucleoprotein. In these conditions, there is no underlying metabolic defect in purine metabolism. The hyperuricemia results either from inadequate renal excretion of uric acid or from excessive nucleoprotein breakdown.

Fracture

A **fracture** is a break in bone. In a *simple fracture,* the bone is broken into only two pieces. The term *comminuted fracture* is used when the bone is shattered into several pieces. A *compound fracture* is one in which the overlying skin has been broken. A compound fracture is more serious than the other types because of the possibility that bacteria may invade the fracture site and cause secondary infection of bone (*osteomyelitis*).

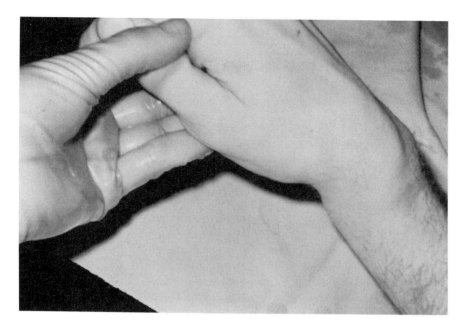

FIGURE 27–16

Displaced fracture of distal radius and ulna. Treatment by reduction of fracture and plaster cast.

After a fracture, the ends of the broken bone may remain aligned or they may be *displaced* out of position (figure 27–16). The term *reduction of a fracture* refers to realigning the ends of the broken bone so that the bone will heal in its normal anatomic position. Sometimes this can be accomplished by manipulating the injured extremity to realign the ends of the bone and then immobilizing it in a plaster cast. However, a surgical operation must sometimes be performed to reduce the fracture and hold it in position by means of a metal plate and screws or a similar device. This procedure is called an *open reduction*. Sometimes a bone may become so weakened by disease such as metastatic tumor that it breaks after minimal stress (for example, coughing or sneezing). A fracture of this type through a diseased area in bone is called a *pathologic fracture*.

Osteomyelitis is an infection of bone and adjacent marrow cavity (*osteo* = bone + *myelos* = marrow + *itis* = inflammation) that is usually the result of staphylococci or various gram-negative bacteria. The infecting organisms gain access to bone in two ways:

Osteomyelitis

1. They may be transported to bone from a distant site by way of the bloodstream, which is called *hematogenous osteomyelitis*.
2. Bacteria may be implanted directly in the bone from various causes.

Hematogenous Osteomyelitis

Hematogenous osteomyelitis is more common in children than in adults. The bacteria are usually carried to the bone from a skin infection, such as a boil, from a kidney infection, or from some other distant site. In children, the organisms tend to lodge in the growing end of the bone on the diaphyseal side of the epiphyseal plate, where they proliferate and incite an acute inflammation. Local injury to bone near its very vascular growing end seems to favor localization of bacteria in the bone, probably because a small hemorrhage forms secondary to the injury, and the collection of blood provides conditions favorable for the growth of bacteria.

Once the infection is established, it tends to spread through the bone. In children, the epiphyseal cartilage generally prevents the infection from spreading into the adjacent joint. The infection may spread through the cortex, however, and pus may accumulate under the periosteum, stripping the periosteum away from the underlying cortex. Because much of the blood supply to the cortex comes from the periosteum, the part of the cortex deprived of its blood supply may undergo necrosis. Spread of the infection within the bone may also compress blood vessels that nourish bone, thereby further compromising the blood supply to the infected bone. In adults, in whom hematogenous osteomyelitis is less frequent, the periosteum is more firmly applied to the cortex than it is in children, tending to prevent pus from accumulating under the periosteum. However, the infection may instead spread to the end of the bone and break into the joint, causing a secondary infection in the adjacent joint. This condition is called *septic arthritis*.

New bone formation proceeds concurrently with the inflammatory process, as the body attempts to repair the damage and localize the infection. Initial x-rays taken soon after the onset of the infection may show only swelling of the soft tissues surrounding the bone but no radiologic abnormalities in the affected bone at the site of infection. After the infection has been present for a time, however, evidence of bone destruction and new bone formation can be seen in the x-ray films.

Hematogenous osteomyelitis sometimes occurs in adults. Intravenous drug abusers are at risk because they often inject drugs with unclean needles and syringes that are contaminated with bacteria. Although hematogenous osteomyelitis may affect any bone, the infection frequently localizes in the vertebral bodies rather than in the long bones. Probably the stresses and trauma associated with weight-bearing predisposes to localization in the spine.

Osteomyelitis as a Result of Direct Implantation of Bacteria

Various conditions may expose bone to direct infection, including compound fractures, gunshot wounds, or other severe injuries affecting bone. Various surgical procedures performed on bone, such as open reduction and internal fixation of fractures or total joint replacement, may also be complicated by osteomyelitis. Chronic ulcers of the feet, which sometimes develop in diabetic patients, may expose the small bones of the feet to chronic infection.

Clinical Manifestations and Treatment

Usually, osteomyelitis is manifested as an acute febrile illness associated with localized pain, tenderness, and swelling over the affected bone. Sometimes, however, the manifestations are less acute, and the inflammation is manifested only as chronic pain and localized tenderness over the affected bone. X-rays taken after the inflammation is well established show characteristic changes.

Osteomyelitis is treated by a prolonged course of antibiotic therapy. In some patients, the infection may become chronic and may recur periodically. Chronic osteomyelitis is much more difficult to treat. In addition to intensive antibiotic treatment, surgical procedures may be required to remove infected degenerated bone and drain collections of pus in the bone.

Pathogenic fungi, tubercle bacilli, and various unusual opportunistic organisms may at times cause osteomyelitis, especially in immunocompromised adults. The infections are treated by appropriate antibiotics supplemented by various surgical procedures, if needed.

Bone is often affected by metastatic tumors. Carcinoma of breast or prostate, as well as many other tumors, frequently metastasizes to bone (figures 27–17 and 27–18). Occasionally, the skeletal system may be so heavily infiltrated by tumor that hematopoietic cells within the marrow are crowded out, leading to anemia, leukopenia, and thrombocytopenia (chapter 14). Nodular

Tumors of Bone

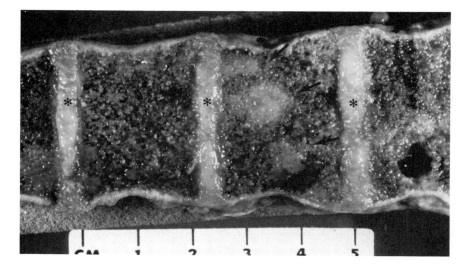

FIGURE 27–17

Cross-section of vertebral bodies illustrating deposits of metastatic carcinoma (*arrows*) from primary carcinoma in breast. Note intervertebral disks (*) between adjacent vertebral bodies.

FIGURE 27–18

Metastatic carcinoma in humerus. Primary tumor was in the kidney. Bone destruction by metastatic tumor is indicated by marked irregularity in contour of head and neck of humerus (*arrow*).

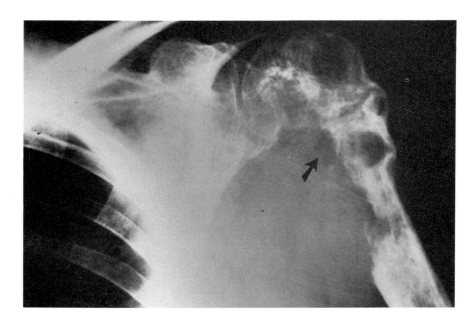

deposits of neoplastic plasma cells are frequently present throughout the skeletal system in **multiple myeloma** (chapter 10). Benign cysts and benign tumors of bone are encountered occasionally, but primary malignant tumors of bone are unusual. A malignant tumor of cartilage is called a *chondrosarcoma* (figure 27–19). One arising from bone-forming cells is called an *osteosarcoma*.

Osteoporosis

Osteoporosis, literally meaning "porous bones," is a generalized thinning and demineralization of the entire skeletal system. Most cases are found in postmenopausal women, beginning in their fifties, and a significant degree of osteoporosis is said to be present in approximately one-fourth of all women in their sixties. Osteoporosis develops whenever bone resorption exceeds bone production. The incidence is high in postmenopausal women because the loss of ovarian function results in a deficiency of estrogen, which plays an indirect role in bone formation. Loss of estrogen reduces the rate of bone formation while the normal process of bone resorption continues, resulting in slowly progressive thinning of the bones. Osteoporosis also develops in elderly men, but it develops at a much later age and is usually less severe than in women.

The osteoporotic bones are quite fragile and susceptible to fracture. Fractures of vertebral bodies are frequent, either from the stress of weight-bearing or after minor exertion (figure 27–20). Such fractures produce back pain and tenderness and are often characterized by collapse of the anterior portions of the vertebral bodies (*compression fractures*). Collapse of vertebral

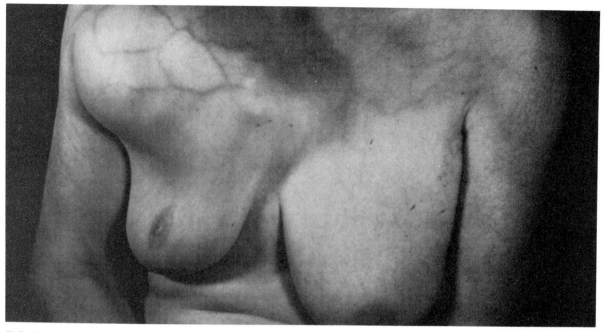

FIGURE 27–19

Large, well-differentiated cartilaginous tumor (chondrosarcoma) arising from chest wall.

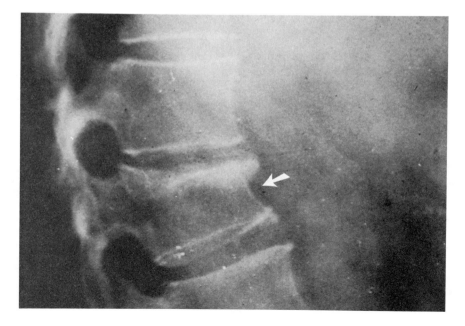

FIGURE 27–20

Osteoporosis with compression fracture of vertebral body. Vertebral bodies are less dense than normal, and the front of one vertebral body has collapsed (*arrow*). Compare the compression fracture in this vertebral body with the vertebra above in which anterior and posterior surfaces are the same height.

bodies may compress the spinal nerve roots passing through the intervertebral foramina, causing pain to radiate along the course of the compressed nerve.

Some loss of bone density is a normal part of the aging process, but excessive bone loss can be retarded by regular exercise, which helps maintain bone density, and a high calcium diet along with calcium supplements if adequate calcium intake cannot be maintained from the diet. Some physicians also recommend supplementary estrogens for postmenopausal women, believing that the advantages of the hormone in preventing osteoporosis outweigh the slightly increased risk of endometrial carcinoma associated with estrogen administration. Once marked osteoporosis has developed and fractures occur, it is difficult to restore bone density. Treatment consists of measures to retard further bone loss by exercise, supplementary calcium intake, and supplementary estrogens for postmenopausal women and measures to control pain and disability caused by fractures. Administration of sodium fluoride along with supplementary calcium will stimulate bone formation and may be useful in some patients.

Significant loss of bone density may also occur in women athletes who engage in prolonged, intense physical activity, such as runners and gymnasts. The high level of physical activity triggers the hypothalamus and pituitary gland to increase adrenal corticosteroid output as an adaptation to the exercise-induced stress. This event, however, is also associated with a fall in the pituitary gonadotropic hormones that stimulate ovarian function. The ovaries, no longer adequately stimulated by pituitary gonadotropins, fail to produce adequate estrogen, which leads to cessation of menses called *exercise-induced amenorrhea*. In addition, the estrogen-deficient athlete is also at risk of the same type of estrogen-deficiency osteoporosis that develops in postmenopausal women and is subject to the same osteoporosis-related complications.

Osteoporosis related to exercise-induced amenorrhea can be prevented by reducing the level of physical activity enough to reestablish normal menstrual cycles. Alternatively, the athlete who elects to continue the same level of exercise can reduce her risk of osteoporosis by taking supplementary estrogen and progesterone hormones to replace the missing ovarian hormones and by taking calcium supplements.

New x-ray and radioisotope methods are now available that make a quantitative assessment of a patient's bone density and compare the results with normal ranges established for persons of the same age and sex. Those patients whose bones are losing mineral content to a greater extent or more rapidly than normal are at high risk of fractures and other complications related to osteoporosis. They should be treated vigorously in an attempt to retard further bone demineralization.

Avascular Necrosis

Occasionally, the growing cartilaginous ends of bone (epiphyses) in children and adolescents undergo necrosis and degeneration, owing to interference with the blood supply to the epiphysis. This condition is termed **avascular**

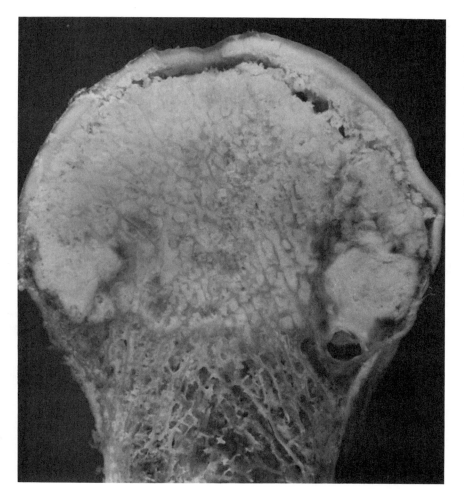

FIGURE 27–21
Avascular necrosis of femoral head. Articular cartilage has separated from underlying abnormal bone, which appears dense and lacks normal structural pattern. In contrast, bone of femoral neck (*lower part of photograph*) appears normal. Treated by removal of femoral head and replacement with artificial hip joint.

necrosis. Sometimes it follows an injury, but in most cases the reason for the vascular disturbance is unknown. Common sites of avascular necrosis are the femoral head (figure 27–21), the tibial tubercle, the articular surface of the femoral condyle, and occasionally the small bones of the ankle and foot. Symptoms consist of pain and disability related to motion of the affected joint. Avascular necrosis may also occur in adults if the blood supply to a bone is interrupted for any reason, as, for example, if the circulation to the femoral head is disrupted as a result of a hip fracture or dislocation.

The vertebral column forms the central axis of the body. It consists of a series of vertebrae joined by *intervertebral disks* and fibrous *ligaments*. The vertebral column has four curves. The *cervical* and *lumbar curves* arch forward. Those

Structure and Function of the Spine

in the *thoracic* and *sacral* regions bend in the opposite direction (figure 27–22A).

A typical vertebra has a large cylindrical *body* and a bony *arch* that encloses the spinal canal and protects the spinal cord. The parts of the arch that extend posteriorly from the body are called the *pedicles,* and the parts that roof the spinal canal are called the *laminae* (singular, *lamina*). A single midline *spinous process* projects posteriorly from the bony arch, and paired *transverse processes* extend laterally (figure 27–22B).

When the vertebrae are viewed from the side, the superior and inferior margins of the vertebral pedicles appear concave. Small disklike articular surfaces called *articular processes* are present on the upper and lower surfaces of each vertebral arch, and the vertebral bodies articulate with each other by means of small *synovial joints.* The spaces between the concave surfaces of the pedicles of adjacent vertebrae form oval openings called *intervertebral*

FIGURE 27–22

A, Side view of vertebral column illustrating normal curves. Vertebrae are numbered. **B,** Structure of a typical vertebra viewed from above. The vertebral arch extends posteriorly from the vertebral body. The spinous process projects posteriorly from the arch, and the transverse processes project laterally. The articular processes of adjacent vertebrae articulate with each other by means of small synovial joints. **C,** Side view of two vertebrae illustrating the intervertebral disk, articular processes, and intervertebral foramen.

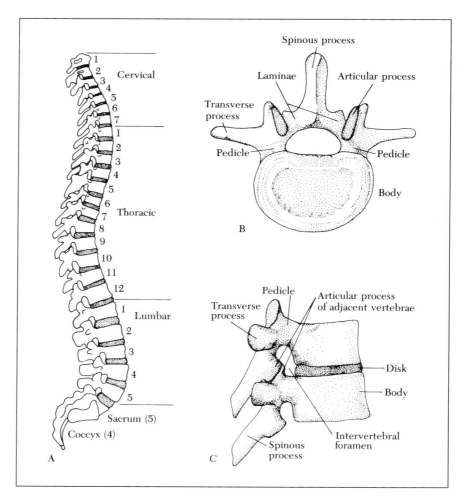

foramina (singular, *foramen*), through which the spinal nerves leave the spinal canal (figure 27–22C).

The **intervertebral disks,** interposed between adjacent vertebral bodies, consist of a peripheral fibrous ring, the *annulus fibrosus,* and a soft central *nucleus pulposus* (figure 27–23A). The **annulus fibrosus** ("fibrous ring") is structured as a ring of interlacing connective-tissue bundles firmly adherent to adjacent vertebral bodies. Longitudinal bands of connective tissue called the *anterior* and *posterior longitudinal ligaments* run the entire length of the vertebral column to reinforce the annulus. The **nucleus pulposus** ("pulpy nucleus") consists of a gelatinous material containing a carbohydrate substance called a *mucopolysaccharide* and about 80 percent water. Because of its very high water content, it is relatively incompressible.

The position of the nucleus pulposus within the disk changes slightly during flexion and extension of the spine. During flexion, as when one bends forward to pick up an object on the ground, compression forces are concentrated on the anterior parts of the vertebral bodies and cause the nucleus to shift slightly posteriorly, moving away from the compressing force. Conversely, when compression forces are concentrated on the posterior part of the vertebral bodies during extension, the nucleus pulposus tends to shift anteriorly. Slight lateral movements of the nucleus also occur during lateral flexion of the spine. The intervertebral disks function somewhat like shock absorbers. Pressure applied to the disks is distributed evenly around the annulus by the soft nucleus pulposus, absorbing the forces of compression to some extent and preventing direct impact between adjacent vertebral bodies.

Intervertebral Disk Disease

With age, the intervertebral disks undergo a progressive wear-and-tear degeneration of both the nucleus and the annulus. The nucleus becomes more dense because its water content is reduced, and the annulus becomes

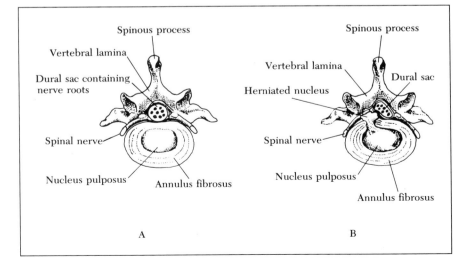

A

B

FIGURE 27–23

Cross-section through the lumbar spine at the level of the intervertebral disk. **A,** Normal relations of intervertebral disk to spinal canal, dura, and spinal nerves. **B,** Posterolateral protrusion of nucleus pulposus, impinging on the dural sac and spinal nerve.

weakened and thinned. When marked compression force is applied to the anterior part of the disk during flexion of the spine, the nucleus is forced posteriorly against the weakened annulus and part of the nucleus may be forced into the spinal canal through a weak area or tear in the annulus (figure 27–23B). Generally, a disk protrusion occurs in the lumbosacral region, because this is the part of the vertebral column where the disks are subject to the greatest mechanical compression during lifting. The disk usually protrudes in a posterolateral direction because the dense posterior longitudinal ligament reinforces the annulus in the midline, preventing a direct posterior protrusion.

Symptoms of disk protrusion, sometimes called a "slipped disk," consist of sudden onset of acute back pain after an episode of lifting. Frequently, the pain is also felt in the leg and thigh on the side of the protrusion. This occurs because the extruded disk material often impinges on lumbosacral nerve roots, causing pain to radiate along the course of the nerve compressed by the protruded nucleus pulposus. Treatment consists of bed rest and measures to minimize pain and disability, such as administration of aspirin or other pain-relieving medications, local application of heat, and use of muscle-relaxing drugs to relieve spasm of the back muscles that occurs after a disk protrusion and contributes to the disability. Protruded disk material may be resorbed, and the tear in the annulus may be repaired by fibrous tissue. Sometimes, however, surgical removal of the protruded disk material may be required. It is also possible to dissolve the protruding disk material by injecting an enzyme solution (papain) into the disk under x-ray guidance. Initially, there was considerable enthusiasm for this nonoperative procedure. Some of the long-term results have been disappointing, however, and there have been several serious complications related to escape of the enzyme solution into the spinal canal. As a result, interest in this method has declined.

The protrusion of the disk material into the spinal canal can be demonstrated by means of a special radiologic procedure called a **myelogram.** Radiopaque material is introduced into the dural sac surrounding the cord and nerve roots in order to outline the contour of the dural sac (figure 27–24A). The extruded disk material can be recognized in the x-ray film as a filling defect in the column of radiopaque material where the disk material indents the dural sac. CT and MRI scans, noninvasive radiologic examinations described in chapter 1, also have been used successfully to demonstrate disk protrusion, thereby avoiding the need for a myelogram in some cases (figure 27–24B and C).

Structure and Function of Skeletal Muscle

Muscle cells are highly specialized contractile cells. Three different types of muscle are recognized: smooth muscle, skeletal muscle, and cardiac muscle. *Smooth muscle* is found in the walls of the gastrointestinal tract, biliary tract, urogenital system, respiratory tract, and blood vessels. *Skeletal muscle* is attached to the skeleton by tendons and ligaments; it functions in voluntary muscular activity. *Cardiac muscle* closely resembles skeletal muscle but has certain special features related to its function of producing rhythmic contractions of the heart. Lesions of smooth muscles are rare, and disorders of cardiac muscle are considered in chapter 15. A discussion of skeletal muscle, the great bulk of muscle within the body, follows.

Contraction of Skeletal Muscle

Skeletal muscles are long, straplike fibers that measure as much as 5 cm in length. The cytoplasm (sarcoplasm) contains multiple nuclei located just beneath the cell membrane (sarcolemma). Filling the cytoplasm are long threadlike myofibrils composed of the contractile myofilaments actin and myosin. The cytoplasm also contains many energy-rich organic compounds, ions, and enzymes required for the metabolic activity of the muscle cell.

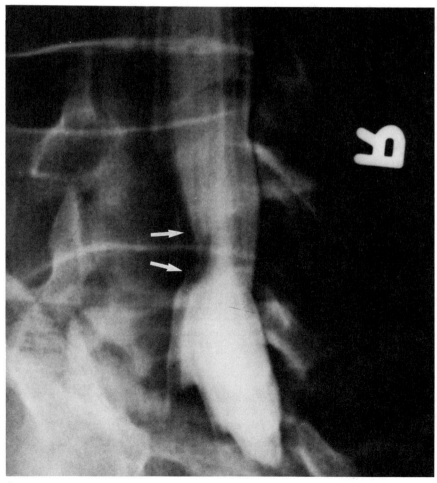

A

FIGURE 27–24

Clinical demonstration of herniated nucleus pulposus ("slipped disk"). **A,** Myelogram. Dural sac has been filled with radiopaque contrast material. Indentation of dural sac (*arrows*) results from herniated nucleus pulposus protruding into spinal canal. **B, C** (*see next page*).

FIGURE 27–24B

CT scan of lumbar region. Protruding nucleus pulposus (*arrow*) is located adjacent to the dural sac and fills intervertebral foramen. Compare with appearance of normal intervertebral foramen on the opposite side.

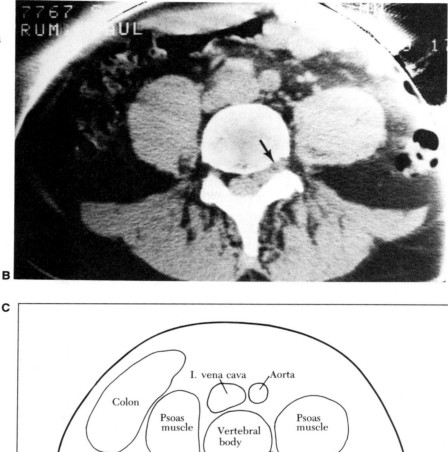

B

C

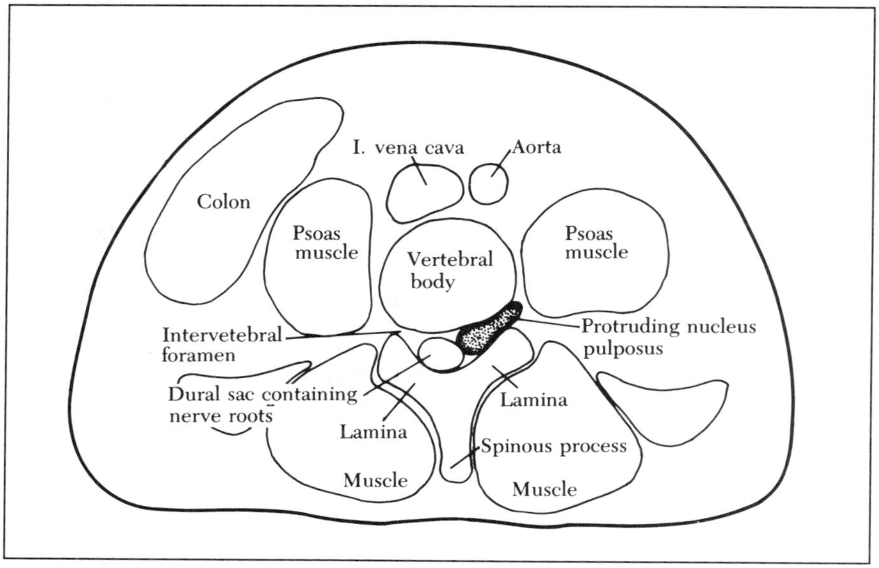

FIGURE 27–24C

Schematic of anatomic structures and lesion as demonstrated on CT scan.

Muscle cells contract in response to motor nerve impulses conveyed to the muscle. The area of communication between the nerve endings and the muscle cell is called the *myoneural junction*. The actual stimulation of the muscle cell is the result of a chemical called **acetylcholine,** which is released from the nerve endings at the myoneural junction and interacts with acetylcholine receptors on the surface of the muscle fibers. The chemical mediator acetylcholine initiates the biochemical chain of events that causes the actin and myosin filaments to slide together, which leads to shortening of the muscle fiber. The duration of the chemical mediator is quite brief because this substance is rapidly broken down by the enzyme *cholinesterase,* which is present in muscle.

Factors Affecting Muscular Structure and Function

The normal structural and functional integrity of skeletal muscle depends on an intact nerve supply, normal transmission of impulses across the myoneural junction, and normal metabolic processes within the muscle cell.

As considered in chapter 26, skeletal muscles that are not used or muscles deprived of their nerve supply undergo marked atrophy. Conversely, when additional work is required of the muscles, they undergo hypertrophy in response to the increased demands.

Muscle cells contain a highly complex metabolic machinery capable of translating nerve impulses into muscle contractions. Any disturbance in the metabolism of the muscle cell leads to a disturbance in the function of the cell. The intracellular metabolic processes are also influenced by the endocrine glands that regulate the rate of metabolism within the muscle cell and affect the concentration of the various ions required for normal muscle contraction.

Diseases of skeletal muscle are uncommon. The principal disorders consist of inflammatory lesions, muscular atrophy, degeneration (dystrophy) of muscle, and disturbance of impulse conduction at the myoneural junction.

Localized Myositis

Inflammation of Muscle (Myositis)

Small areas of inflammation in skeletal muscle are encountered in many systemic diseases and have no major clinical significance. Inflammation of muscle may also follow injury or muscular overexertion. The inflammation is secondary to necrosis and disruption of muscle cells and is associated with swelling and tenderness of the affected muscle. The inflammation gradually subsides as the muscle injury heals.

Generalized Myositis

Generalized inflammation of skeletal muscle (*polymyositis*) is an uncommon but serious systemic disease of unknown etiology, characterized by widespread degeneration and inflammation of skeletal muscle. One type of polymyositis, associated with swelling and inflammation of the skin, is called *dermatomyositis.* These disorders are often classified as connective-tissue (collagen) diseases (chapter 5) because of the necrosis of connective-tissue fibers in the affected muscles and because these diseases are presumed to have an immunologic basis.

Muscular Atrophy and Muscular Dystrophy

A group of relatively rare diseases is characterized by progressive atrophy or degeneration of skeletal muscle. Many are hereditary. Various clinical syndromes are recognized, depending on the muscle groups affected, the patterns of inheritance, and the rate of progression of the disease. In general, the diseases are characterized by progressive muscular weakness and gradually increasing disability, eventually terminating in death from paralysis of the respiratory muscles or superimposed respiratory infection.

It is customary to classify these diseases into two large categories: the *muscular atrophy* group and the *muscular dystrophy* group.

In the progressive muscular atrophy group of diseases, the muscular weakness and atrophy are secondary to progressive degeneration of motor nerve cells in the cerebral cortex, brain stem, and spinal cord, described in chapter 26 (degenerative disease of motor neurons). The clinical manifestations are related to the location of the degenerating nerve cells within the central nervous system and the rate at which the neuronal degeneration progresses.

In the muscular dystrophy group, the nerve supply to the muscles is unaffected. The basic disturbance is an abnormality in the muscle fibers that causes them to degenerate. The most common and severe type is called *Duchenne muscular dystrophy,* and a milder form of muscular dystrophy is called *Becker muscular dystrophy.* Both forms result from the mutation of a large gene on the X chromosome, and the disease is transmitted as an X-linked trait to male children of women who carry the defective gene. The normal gene codes for a muscle protein called *dystrophin,* which is located on the inner surface of the sarcolemma, where it plays a role in maintaining the structure and functions of the muscle fibers.

As a result of the gene mutation, dystrophin is absent in the muscle fibers of persons afflicted with Duchenne muscular dystrophy and is apparently responsible for the manifestations of the disease, which appear first during early childhood and progress rapidly, leading to death in late adolescence or early adulthood. The muscles primarily affected are those of the lower extremities, trunk, hips, and shoulder girdle. Often the extent of atrophy is masked because the muscles are infiltrated by fat and fibrous tissue as they atrophy. The fat infiltration may at times be so extreme that the affected muscles appear hypertrophied, leading to the paradox of profound muscular weakness in an individual whose muscles appear very well developed. The apparent hypertrophy is an illusion, which is why the term *pseudohypertrophic* is applied to this type of muscular dystrophy.

The less-severe Becker muscular dystrophy also is caused by a mutation of the same dystrophin-producing gene that causes Duchenne muscular dystrophy. Dystrophin is produced by the mutated gene but is either abnormal or produced in insufficient amounts.

Although the various types of muscular atrophy and muscular dystrophy are uncommon, they are of major concern not only to the patient, but to the family because of the hereditary nature of many of these illnesses. Unfortunately, there is no way at present to arrest the relentless progression of the disease. Recent advances in gene therapy may eventually allow insertion of replacement genes in muscle fibers that will code for the synthesis of the missing or defective dystrophin protein and thereby ameliorate the manifestations of these devastating diseases.

Myasthenia gravis is a chronic disease characterized by abnormal fatigability of the voluntary muscles as a result of an abnormality at the myoneural junction. Fatigue develops rapidly when the muscles are used and subsides when they are rested. Often, the dysfunction is most conspicuous in the small muscles of the face and in the muscles concerned with eye movement (*extraocular muscles*). Myasthenia gravis appears to be an autoimmune disease. The blood of affected patients contains an autoantibody directed against acetylcholine receptors on the surface of the muscle fibers at the myoneural junction. The manifestations of the disease occur because the antibody damages and greatly reduces the number of receptors available to interact with the acetylcholine liberated from motor nerve endings.

Symptoms can be relieved by drugs that inhibit the action of the enzyme cholinesterase. This prolongs the action of the chemical mediator acetylcholine so that it can continue to stimulate the reduced numbers of receptors for a longer time. Many patients with myasthenia gravis have either a tumor or a benign hyperplasia of the thymus gland, which is probably also caused by a disturbance of the immune system.

Myasthenia Gravis

Questions for Review

1. Describe the structure of the typical movable joint (see figure 27–1).

2. What are the three most common types of arthritis? What are their distinguishing features (see table 27–1)?

3. What is the difference between a simple fracture and a compound fracture? What are the complications of a compound fracture? What is a comminuted fracture? A pathologic fracture?

4. What is osteoporosis? Why does it develop? What symptoms and complications result from osteoporosis?

5. What is a "slipped disk"? Why does it occur? Why does it sometimes produce pain radiating down the leg? How is it treated?

6. What is meant by the following terms: *osteoporosis, multiple myeloma, nucleus pulposus,* and *rheumatoid factor?*

7. What are the types of muscle cells?

8. What is meant by the following terms: *myoneural junction, acetylcholine,* and *myositis?*

9. What is the difference between muscular atrophy and muscular dystrophy? What are the most common types of atrophic disease of the muscles? Of dystrophic disease?

10. What is myasthenia gravis? What is its relation to the immune system? How is it treated?

Supplementary Readings

Drachman, D. B. 1978. Myasthenia gravis. *New England Journal of Medicine* 298:136–42. Concepts of pathogenesis and treatment.

Drinkwater, B. L., Nilson, K., Ott, S., and Chesnut, C. H. 1986. Bone mineral density after resumption of menses in amenorrheic athletes. *Journal of the American Medical Association* 256:380–82. Bone mass may not be completely restored.

Khosla, S., and Riggs, L. 1995. Treatment options for osteoporosis. *Mayo Clinic Proceedings* 70:978–82. Osteoporosis is a major public health problem. Various treatment approaches are described, based on the rapidity of bone loss and the stage of the disease.

Loucks, A. B., Mortola, J. F., and Girton, S. S. C. 1990. Alterations in the hypothalamic-pituitary-ovarian and the hypothalamic-pituitary-adrenal axis in athletic women. *Journal of Clinical Endocrinology and Metabolism* 68:402–11. Describes pathophysiology of exercise-induced amenorrhea.

Lufkin, E. G., et al. 1988. Estrogen-replacement therapy: Current recommendations. *Mayo Clinic Proceedings* 63:453–60. Estrogen-replacement therapy is effective for the prevention and treatment of postmenopausal osteoporosis and alleviates menopausal symptoms. Benefits must be weighed against the risks of endometrial hyperplasia, carcinoma, breast tenderness, hypertension, and inconvenience of menstrual bleeding. Approaches to eliminate side effects and complications discussed.

McCarthy, D. J. 1993. *Arthritis and allied conditions.* 12th ed. Philadelphia: Lea & Febiger. A standard text.

See also sections in textbooks of medicine, surgery, and pathology listed in General References.

Chapter 27 ▪ Outline Summary

Skeletal System / 803
Structure and Function
Rigid supporting framework.

Impregnated with calcium salts.

Bone continually being broken down and reformed.

Density of bones depends on activity.

Bones connected by joints.

Movable joints are covered by articular cartilage, lubricated by synovial fluid.

Ligamentous joint capsule lined by synovium.

Bone Formation
Intramembranous bone formation: mesoderm converted directly into bone.

Endochondral bone formation: cartilage model becomes converted into bone.

Bone Growth
Growth in length from epiphysis.

Growth in thickness from periosteum.

Congenital Abnormalities
Achondroplasia:

Faulty endochondral bone formation impairs growth of extremities and disturbs formation of skull bones.

Causes dwarfism with disproportionately short limbs.

Osteogenesis imperfecta:

Thin and delicate bones, easily broken.

Infant may be born with multiple fractures.

Malformations of digits:

Extra digits (polydactyly): easily removed.

Fused digits: more difficult to correct.

Congenital clubfoot (talipes):

Multifactorial inheritance.

Talipes equinovarus most common type.

Treated by casts and splints.

Congenital dislocation of hip:

Multifactorial inheritance: more common in females.

Shallow acetabulum causes femoral head to be displaced out of socket.

Breech position favors development.

Treated by manipulation and casts.

Rheumatoid Arthritis
A systemic disease of chiefly small joints.

More common in women.

Inflammatory tissue from synovium destroys joint.

Dislocation occurs owing to joint instability.

Autoantibodies to gamma globulin demonstrated in many patients.

Osteoarthritis
"Wear and tear" degeneration of joints.

Affects major weight-bearing joints.

Usually little disability.

Severe disability can be treated by joint replacement.

Gout
Disorder of nucleoprotein metabolism.

Deposition of uric acid in and around joints.

Frequent acute episodes caused by precipitation of uric acid crystals in joint fluid.

Diet and drugs control disease by lowering uric acid.

Fractures

Simple: bone broken into two pieces.

Comminuted: bone shattered.

Compound: overlying skin broken with potential for infection.

Pathologic: secondary to disease such as metastatic carcinoma.

Treatment by reduction and casts or internal fixation.

Osteomyelitis

Hematogenous: predominantly in children.

Occurs at ends of bone.

Spread of infection may strip periosteum from cortex and devitalize bone.

Infection may spread into joint in adults.

Infection in drug abusers tends to localize in vertebral bodies.

As a result of direct implantation: after trauma or surgical procedures.

Manifestations and treatment:

Febrile illness with localizing manifestations.

X-rays reveal changes in bone.

Treatment by antibiotics supplemented by surgical procedures if needed.

Bone Tumors

Metastatic tumors: relatively common.

Multiple myeloma: plasma cell neoplasm.

Benign cysts and tumors: occur occasionally.

Primary malignant bone tumors: relatively rare.

Osteoporosis

Generalized thinning of bone.

Most common in postmenopausal women.

Treatment by high-calcium diet, estrogens in women.

Avascular Necrosis

Necrosis and degeneration at ends of bone.

Probably caused by disturbance in blood supply as a result of injury.

Causes local pain and disability.

Structure and Function of the Spine / 827
Structure

Fibrocartilaginous cushions interposed between adjacent vertebral bodies.

Function

Spine forms central axis of body.

Disks function as shock absorbers.

Intervertebral Disk Disease / 829
Pathogenesis

Disk wears out with age.

Nucleus pulposus may be extruded through tear in annulus fibrosus and impinge on nerve roots.

Sudden onset of back pain radiating down leg.

Diagnosis and Treatment

Protrusion can be demonstrated by myelogram or CT scan.

Disk material may be absorbed but often must be removed surgically.

Skeletal Muscle / 830
Contraction of Skeletal Muscle

Caused by presence of myofibrils.

Communication between nerve and muscle at myoneural junction.

Nerve stimulation liberates acetycholine, which interacts with receptors on muscle fibers and initiates contraction.

Inflammation of Muscle

Localized myositis follows injury or overexertion.

Generalized myositis: a systemic disease.

Hereditary Diseases Characterized by Muscle Atrophy and Degeneration

Progressive muscular atrophy: nerve cell degeneration with secondary muscle atrophy.

Muscular dystrophy: primary degeneration of muscle.

Myasthenia Gravis

Abnormal fatigability of voluntary muscles.

Autoantibodies formed against acetylcholine receptors on muscle.

Symptoms relieved by drugs that prolong action of acetylcholine.

General References

Anatomy and Physiology

Marieb, E. N. 1992. *Human anatomy and physiology,* 2d ed. Redwood City, Calif.: Benjamin/Cummings.

Tortora, G. J., and Grabowski, S. R. 1993. *Principles of anatomy and physiology.* New York: Harper-Collins.

Cardiology

Braunwald, E., ed. 1992. *Heart disease: A textbook of cardiovascular medicine,* 4th ed. Philadelphia: Saunders.

Grossman, W., ed. 1991. *Cardiac catheterization and angiography,* 4th ed. Philadelphia: Lea & Febiger.

Endocrinology

DeGroot, L. J., Besser, M., Burger, H. G., et al. 1995. *Endocrinology,* 3d ed. Philadelphia: Saunders.

Hershman, J. M. 1988. *Endocrine pathophysiology: A patient oriented approach,* 3d ed. Baltimore: Lea & Febiger.

Gastroenterology

Schiff, L., ed. 1993. *Diseases of the liver,* 7th ed. Philadelphia: Lippincott.

Sleisenger, M. H., Fordtran, J. S., Scharschmidt, B. F., and Feldman, M., eds. 1993. *Gastrointestinal disease,* 5th ed. Philadelphia: Saunders.

Genetics

Scriver, C. R., Stanbury, J. B., Wyngaarden, J. B., and Fredrickson, D. S., eds. 1995. *The metabolic basis of inherited diseases,* 7th ed. New York: McGraw-Hill. A standard reference.

Gynecology and Obstetrics

Boston Women's Health Book Collective Staff. 1992. *The new our bodies, ourselves.* New York: Simon and Schuster.

Hacker, N. F. 1992. *Essentials of obstetrics and gynecology.* Philadelphia: Saunders.

Hatcher, R. A. 1994. *Contraceptive technology* 1994–1996. New York: Irvington Publishers.

Hematology

Beutler, E., Lichtman, M. A., Coller, B. S., and Kipps, T. J., eds. 1995. *Williams hematology,* 5th ed. New York: McGraw-Hill.

Immunology

Stites, D. P., Terr, A. I., and Parslow, T. G., eds. 1994. *Basic and clinical immunology,* 8th ed. Norwalk, Conn.: Appleton & Lange.

Internal Medicine

Maxwell, M. H., and Kleeman, C. R. 1994. *Clinical disorders of fluid and electrolyte metabolism,* 5th ed. New York: McGraw-Hill.

Rubenstein, E., ed. 1994. *Scientific American medicine.* New York: Scientific American, Inc. Updated monthly.

Schroeder, S. A., et al., eds. 1995. *Current medical diagnosis and treatment,* 34th ed. Norwalk, Conn.: Appleton & Lange.

Microbiology

Brooks, G. F., Butel, J. S., and Ornston, L. N. 1991. *Medical microbiology,* 19th ed. Los Altos, Calif.: Lange. Revised biennially.

Oncology

DeVita, V. T., Hellman, S., and Rosenberg, S. A., eds. 1993. *Cancer: Principles and practice of oncology,* 4th ed. Philadelphia: Saunders.

Haskell, C. M. 1995. *Cancer treatment,* 4th ed. Philadelphia: Saunders.

Orthopedics

McCarthy, D. J. 1993. *Arthritis and allied conditions,* 12th ed. Philadelphia: Lea & Febiger.

Pathology

Cotran, R. S., Kumar, V., and Robbins, S. I. 1994. *Robbins pathologic basis of disease,* 5th ed. Philadelphia: Saunders.

Keeling, J. W., ed. 1993. *Fetal and neonatal pathology,* 2d ed. London: Springer-Verlag.

Rosai, J. 1995. *Surgical pathology,* 8th ed. St. Louis: Mosby. Two volumes.

Pediatrics

Taeusch, H. W., Ballard, R. A., Avery, M. E., and Schaeffer, A. J. 1993. *Shaeffer's and Avery's diseases of the newborn,* 6th ed. Philadelphia: Saunders.

Behrman, R. E., Behrman, R. E., Kliegman, R. M., and Arvin, A. M., eds. 1991. *Nelson textbook of pediatrics,* 14th ed. Philadelphia: Saunders.

Pharmacology

Katzung, B. G., ed. 1994. *Basic and clinical pharmacology,* 6th ed. Norwalk, Conn.: Appleton & Lange.

PDR: *Physicians desk reference,* 49th ed. 1995. Oradell, N.J.: Medical Economics Co.

Physiology

Brobeck, J. R., ed. 1991. *Best and Taylor's physiological basic of medical practice,* 12th ed. Baltimore: Williams & Wilkins.

Guyton, A. C. 1996. *Textbook of medical physiology,* 8th ed. Philadelphia: Saunders.

Vander, A. J., Sherman, J. H., and Luciano, D. S. 1994. *Human physiology,* 6th ed. New York: McGraw-Hill.

Radiology and Nuclear Medicine

Hendee, W. R. 1992. *Medical radiation physics: Roentgenology, nuclear medicine and ultrasound,* 3d ed. Chicago: Year Book Medical Publishers.

Surgery

Davis, J. H., Foster, R. S., and Gamelli, R. C. 1991. *Clinical surgery.* 2d ed. St. Louis: Mosby.

Sabiston, D. C., ed. 1991. *Textbook of surgery,* 14th ed. Philadelphia: Saunders. Two volumes.

Urology

Brenner, B. M., ed. 1991. *The kidney,* 4th ed. Philadelphia: Saunders. Two volumes.

Pitts, R. F. 1974. *Physiology of the kidney and body fluids: An introductory text,* 3d ed. Chicago: Year Book Medical Publishers.

Schrier, R. W., ed. 1992. *Renal and electrolyte disorders,* 3d ed. Boston: Little, Brown.

Walsh, P. C., ed. 1992. *Campbell's urology,* 6th ed. Philadelphia: Saunders.

Glossary

Common Prefixes and Suffixes

Prefixes

a, an—without

ab—from, away from

ad—toward

ante—before

bi—twice, two

circum—around

co—together

contra—against, opposed

de—down, from, away

dis—apart

dys—abnormal, difficult

endo—within

epi—upon

exo—outside

extra—outside

hemi—half

hetero—different

homo—same

hyper—above, beyond, excessive

hypo—below, under, deficient

infra—beneath

inter—between

intra—within

meta—after, beyond

para—beside

peri—around

post—behind, after

pre—before

pro—before

sub—beneath

supra—above

syn—together

Suffixes

—blast applied to formative cells (e.g., osteoblast)

—cyte applied to adult cells (e.g., osteocyte)

—itis inflammation of

—oid like

—ology study of

—oma a swelling or tumor

An Approximate Guide to Pronunciation

a as in lad

ā as in late

ä as in calm

e as in met

ē as in meet

i as in pill

ī as in pile

o as in rob

ō as in robe

u as in shut

ū as in chute

oi as in joy

ōō as in fool

ou as in loud

Note: Pronunciations given are those most commonly used in clinical practice.

A

ABO hemolytic disease A mild hemolytic disease in group A or B infants or group O mothers, as a result of maternal anti-A and anti-B antibodies.

abscess (ab'sess) A localized accumulation of pus in tissues.

acetone (as'e-tōn) An organic compound (ketone) derived from the ketone bodies acetoacetic acid and beta-hydroxybutyric acid.

acetylcholine (as-et-il-kōˈēn) A chemical secreted by nerve endings that activates neurons or muscle cells.

ac'etylcoen'zyme A (acetyl-CoA) A combination of a two-carbon acetate fragment with a complex organic compound called coenzyme A.

achondroplasia (a-kon-dro-pla'zi-yuh) A congenital disturbance of endochondral bone formation that causes a type of dwarfism.

acido'sis A disturbance in acid-base balance of the body in which body fluids have a lower pH than normal.

acinus (as'in-us) A functional unit of the lung consisting of a cluster of respiratory bronchioles, alveolar ducts, and alveoli derived from a single terminal bronchiole.

acromegaly (ak'ro-meg'al-ē) A condition resulting from excessive secretion of growth hormone in the adult.

ACTH See *adrenocorticotrophic hormone.*

Addison's disease A disease caused by chronic adrenal cortical hypofunction.

adenoma (ad-en-ō'muh) A benign tumor arising from glands.

aden'osine triphos'phate (ATP) A high-energy phosphate compound that liberates energy to power numerous cellular metabolic processes.

ADH See *antidiuretic hormone.*

adhesions (ad-hē'shuns) Bands of fibrous tissue that form subsequent to an inflammation, and bind adjacent tissues together.

adjuvant chemotherapy (ad'jōō-vent) Anticancer chemotherapy administered after surgical resection of a tumor in an attempt to destroy any small undetected foci of metastatic tumor before they become clinically detectable.

adrenaline (ad-ren'a-lin) Another name for epinephrine, one of the hormones of the adrenal medulla.

adrenocorticotrophic hormone (ACTH) (ad-rēn'o-cor'tico-trō'fik) A hormone secreted by the anterior lobe of the pituitary that stimulates the adrenal cortex to manufacture and secrete adrenal cortical hormones.

adrenogenital syndrome (ad-rēn'ō-jen'i-tul) Clinical disorder of adrenal function characterized by overproduction of adrenal sex hormones.

AIDS An infection caused by the human immunodeficiency virus. The virus attacks and destroys helper T lymphocytes, which compromises cell-mediated immunity, leading to increased susceptibility to infection and some tumors.

aldos'terone A steroid hormone produced by the adrenal cortex that regulates the rate of sodium absorption from the renal tubules.

alkalo'sis A disturbance in the body's acid-base balance in which the pH of the extracellular fluids is shifted toward the alkaline side of normal. See also *acidosis.*

alkylating agent (al'kil-ā-ting) An anticancer drug that disrupts cell function by binding DNA chains together so that they cannot separate.

allele (äh'lēl) One of several related genes that may occupy the same locus on a homologous chromosome.

allergen (al'ler-jen) A substance capable of inducing an allergic reaction in a predisposed individual.

allergy A tendency to form specific IgE antibody to antigens that do not affect most persons.

alpha cells (al'fuh) Glucagon-secreting cells of the pancreatic islets.

alpha fetoprotein (al'fuh fē'tō-prō'tēn) Protein produced by fetal liver early in gestation. Sometimes produced by tumor cells. Level is elevated in amnionic fluid when fetus has neural tube defect.

alveolus (alvē'olus) One of the terminal air sacs of the lung.

Alzheimer's disease (ahls'-hīm-er) A degenerative disease of the nervous system with characteristic structural abnormalities within neurons.

amenorrhea (äh-men-ō-rē'äh) Absence of menses.

amniocentesis (am'ni-ō-sen-tē'sis) Removal of amnionic fluid, usually accomplished by inserting a needle through the mother's abdominal and uterine walls into the amnionic cavity.

am'nion The thin, transparent inner membrane that surrounds the embryo in the uterus during pregnancy.

amnionic fluid (am-nē-on'ik) Fluid within the amnionic cavity surrounding the developing organism.

amnionic sac (am-nē-on'ik) The fluid-filled sac surrounding the embryo. One of the fetal membranes.

anaerobic (an-air-o'bik) Not requiring oxygen for growth.

anastomosis (ä-nas-ta-mō'sis) A communication between two blood vessels or other tubular structures. Also refers to a surgical connection of two hollow tubular structures, such as the divided ends of the intestine or a blood vessel (*surgical anastomosis*).

anemia (an-ē'mē-uh) A decrease in hemoglobin or red cells or both.

anencephaly (an-en-seff'uh-lē) A congenital malformation: absence of brain, cranial vault, and scalp as a result of defective closure of the neural tube.

aneurysm (an'ūr-izm) A dilatation of a structure, such as the aorta, a cerebral artery, or a part of the ventricular wall. (See *ventricular aneurysm*).

angina pectoris (an-jī'nuh pek'tōr-is) Precordial pain experienced on exertion owing to inadequate blood supply to the heart muscle.

angiogram (an'jē-ō-gram) Same as *arteriogram.*

angiotensin (an-jē-o-ten'sin) A product formed from interaction of renin with a blood protein (*renin substrate*) that raises blood pressure and stimulates the adrenal cortex to secrete aldosterone.

anion (an'ī-on) An ion carrying a negative charge.

annulus fibrosus (an'ū-lus) The dense peripheral ring of fibrocartilage making up the intervertebral disk.

antibiotic sensitivity test A laboratory test to determine the ability of antibiotics to inhibit bacterial growth.

antibody A globulin manufactured by plasma cells in response to contact with a foreign antigen.

anticoagulant drugs Drugs that inhibit the process of blood coagulation.

antidiuretic hormone (ADH) (an-ti-dī-u-ret'tik) Posterior lobe pituitary hormone that regulates urine concentration by altering the permeability of the renal collecting tubules.

an'tigen Any substance that can stimulate the formation of an antibody.

antimetabolite (an-ti-met-ab'o-līte) A substance that competes with or replaces another substance (metabolite) required for cell growth or multiplication.

aplastic anemia (ā-plas'tik) An anemia caused by bone marrow failure.

arachnoid (ar-ak'noyd) The middle of the three meninges that cover the brain.

areola (a-rē'o-la) The pigmented area surrounding the nipple.

arrhythmia (a-rith'mi-uh) An irregularity of the heartbeat.

arteriogram (är-tēr'ē-ō-gram) An x-ray technique for studying the caliber of blood vessels by injection of radiopaque material into the vessel.

arteriolosclerosis (är-tēr-ē-ólo-skler-ō'-sis) One type of arteriosclerosis characterized by thickening and degeneration of small arterioles.

arteriosclerosis (är-tēr'ē-ō-skler-ō'sis) A general term for degenerative change in the wall of an artery, often associated with narrowing of its lumen.

arteriosclerotic aneurysm (an'ur-izm) A ballooning of the aorta or a large artery as a result of weakening of the wall secondary to atherosclerosis.

arthritis (ärth-rī'tis) An inflammation of a joint. Term is also used to refer to a degenerative process in joints, as in osteoarthritis.

arthropod (är'thrō-pod) Invertebrate animal with jointed limbs and segmented body, such as insect and spider. Important arthropods that parasitize humans include the crab louse and the organism causing scabies.

articular Pertaining to a joint.

articula'tion The junction between two or more bones in the skeleton.

asbestos body (as-bes'tus) An asbestos fiber coated with protein and iron that is found in lungs and sputum of patients with asbestosis.

asbestosis (as-bes-tō'sis) A type of pneumoconiosis caused by inhalation of asbestos fibers.

Ascaris (as'kar-is) A large parasitic roundworm that infests humans.

ascites (a-si'tēz) Accumulation of fluid in the abdominal cavity.

as'trocyte A large stellate cell having highly branched processes. Forms the structural framework of the nervous system. One of the neuroglial cells.

atelectasis (ah-tel-ek'tuh-sis) Collapse of the lung, either caused by bronchial obstruction (*obstructive atelectasis*) or external compression (*compression atelectasis*).

atheroma (ah-ther-ō'muh) A mass of lipids and debris that accumulates in the intima lining of an artery and narrows its lumen.

ath'erosclero'sis A thickening of the lining (*intima*) of blood vessels caused by accumulation of lipids, with secondary scarring and calcification.

athyreotic (ā-thī-rē'ā'tik) Lacking a thyroid gland, as in one type of cretinism caused by failure of gland development.

atopic (ā-top'ik) Having a genetic predisposition to certain allergic conditions such as hay fever and asthma.

atrioventricular (AV) valve (a'trē-o-ven-trik'ū-lar) The flaplike heart valve located between the atrium and ventricle.

atrophy (ah'trō'fē) A reduction in size of a structure caused by decreased function, inadequate hormonal stimulation, or reduced blood supply.

autoantibody (aw'tō-an'ti-bod-ē) An antibody formed against one's own cells or tissue components.

autoimmune disease A disease associated with formation of cell-mediated or humoral immunity against the subject's own cells or tissue components.

autosome (aw'tō-sōm) A chromosome other than a sex chromosome.

avascular necrosis of bone (ā-vas'kēw-lär nek-rō'sis) Bone necrosis caused by interruption of its blood supply.

B

bacterial endocarditis An inflammation of the endocardium. Term usually refers to an inflammation of the heart valves.

Barr body The inactivated X chromosome that is applied to the nuclear membrane in the female. Sex chromatin body.

Barrett's esophagus A condition in which the epithelial lining of the esophagus changes from squamous to columnar type, usually as a result of reflux esophagitis.

base A solution containing an excess of hydroxyl ions and having a pH greater than 7.0.

basement membrane A thin layer of acellular material upon which epithelium rests.

bas'ophil A white blood cell that contains numerous variable-sized granules that stain intensely purple with basic dyes. (See also *eosinophil*.)

beta cells (bā'tuh) Insulin-secreting cells of the pancreatic islets.

bile A secretion of the liver containing bile salts, cholesterol, and other substances.

bile canaliculus (kan-al-ik'u-lus) Small terminal bile channel located between liver cords.

bile salts Derivatives of bile acids present in bile that act as emulsifiers to promote fat digestion and absorption.

bil'iary colic Abdominal pain that results when a gallstone enters the biliary duct system.

bilirubin (bil-i-rū'bin) One of the bile pigments derived from breakdown of hemoglobin.

biopsy (bī'op-sē) Removal of a small sample of tissue for examination and diagnosis by a pathologist.

blas'tocyst A stage of development of the fertilized ovum (*zygote*) in which a central cavity accumulates within the cluster of developing cells.

blastomycosis (blast-ō-mī-kō'sis) A systemic fungus infection caused by the fungus *Blastomyces dermatiditis*.

blighted twin A twin that fails to develop normally.

B lymphocyte A lymphocyte that differentiates into plasma cells and is associated with humoral immunity.

body stalk The structure connecting the embryo to the chorion. Eventually develops into the umbilical cord.

Bowman's capsule The cuplike expanded end of the nephron that surrounds the tuft of glomerular capillaries.

bradykinin (brā-kē-kī'nin) A chemical mediator of inflammation derived from components in the blood plasma.

bronchiectasis (bron-kē-ek'tuh-sis) Dilatation of bronchi caused by weakening of their walls as a result of infection.

bronchiole (bron'ke-ōl) One of the small terminal subdivisions of the branched bronchial tree.

bronchus One of the large subdivisions of the trachea.

buffer A substance that minimizes change in pH of a solution when an acid or base is added.

C

calcito'nin A hormone that lowers blood calcium, produced by the interfollicular cells of the thyroid gland.

cal'culus A stone formed within the body, as in the kidney or gallbladder.

capsid (kap'sid) The protein covering the central nucleic acid core of a virus.

capsomere (kap'sō-mēr) One of the subunits that make up the protein shell (*capsid*) of a virus.

carbox'yl group The acid (COOH) group of organic molecules.

carcinoembryonic antigen (CEA) (kär'sin-ō-em-bry-on'ik) A tumor-associated antigen that resembles the antigen secreted by the cells of the fetal gastrointestinal tract.

carcinoma (kär'sin-ōma) A malignant tumor derived from epithelial cells.

cardiac catheterization A specialized technique to determine the blood flow through the chambers of the heart, and to detect abnormal communications between cardiac chambers.

cardiomyopathy (kar-dē-o-my-op'-a'thē) A general term for any noninflammatory disease of heart muscle.

cardiospasm (kär'-dē-o-spazm) Spasm of the lower gastroesophageal (cardiac) sphincter.

caries (ka'rēz) Tooth decay.

catecholamines (kat-eh-kōl'uh-mēnz) The adrenal medullary hormones *epinephrine* and *norepinephrine*.

cation (kat'ī-on) An ion that carries a positive charge.

cavity (dental) A loss of tooth structure casued by the combined action of mouth bacteria and organic acids derived from bacterial fermentation of retained food particles.

cell-mediated immunity Immunity associated with population of sensitized lymphocytes.

cellulitis (sell-ū-lī'tis) An acute spreading inflammation affecting the skin or deeper tissues.

cen'trioles Short cylindrical structures located adjacent to the nucleus that participate in the formation of spindle fibers during cell division.

cen'tromere The structure that joins each pair of chromatids formed by chromosome duplication.

cen'trosome The region of the cell cytoplasm that contains the two centrioles.

chenodeoxycholic acid (kēn'-ō-dē-ox'ī-ko'lik) A bile salt that is administered orally to promote dissolution of cholesterol gallstones by reducing the saturation of the bile with cholesterol.

Chlamydia (klä-mi'dē-uh) Small gram-negative organisms that are deficient in certain enzymes and must function as intracellular parasites.

cholecystitis (ko'lē-sis-tī'-tis) An inflammation of the gallbladder.

cholelithiasis (kō'lē-lith-ī'uh-sis) Formation of gallstones.

cholesterol (kō-les'ter-ol) A complex compound (*sterol*) containing several ring structures.

cholines'terase An enzyme that hydrolyzes acetylcholine.

chordae tendineae (kor'dā ten-din'ē-ā) Fibrous cords that extend from the free margins of the atrioventricular valves to attach to the papillary muscles.

choriocarcinoma (kōr'rē-ō-kär-sin-ō'muh) A malignant proliferation of trophoblastic tissue.

chorion (kō'ri-on) The layer of trophoblast and associated mesoderm that surrounds the developing embryo.

chorionic vesicle The chorion with its villi and enclosed amnion, yolk sac, and developing embryo.

chorionic villi Fingerlike columns of cells extending from the chorion that anchor the chorionic vesicle in the endometrium.

chromatid (krō'mä-tid) One of two newly formed chromosomes held together by the centromere.

cirrhosis of the liver (si-rō'sis) A disease characterized by diffuse intrahepatic scarring and liver cell degeneration.

clearance test (klēr'ans) A test of renal function that measures the ability of kidneys to remove (clear) a substance from the blood and excrete it in the urine.

cleft lip Defect in the upper lip of variable degree, as a result of a developmental disturbance.

cleft palate Defect in hard palate allowing communication between oral cavity and nasal cavity, as a result by a developmental disturbance.

Clostridium (klä-strid'ē-yum) Anaerobic spore-forming rod-shaped bacterium.

clubfoot Congenital malposition of foot. In most common type, foot is turned inward at ankle and heel is elevated.

Coccidioides immitis (kok-sid-ē-oy'dēz im'mi-tis) A highly pathogenic fungus causing the disease coccidioidomycosis.

coccidioidomycosis (kok-sid-ē-oy'dō-mī-kō'sis) A disease caused by the pathogenic fungus *Coccidioides immitis.*

colitis (kō-lī'tis) Inflammation of the colon, such as chronic ulcerative colitis.

collateral circulation An accessory circulation capable of delivering blood to a tissue when the main circulation is blocked, as by a thrombus or embolus.

colloid An eosinophilic protein material present within the thyroid follicles.

colposcope (kol'pos-kōp) A binocular magnifying instrument used to view the cervix and endocervical canal.

coma Loss of consciousness, resulting from various causes.

communicable disease A disease transmitted from person to person.

computed tomographic (CT) scan (tō-mo-graf'ik) An x-ray technique producing detailed cross-sectional images of the body by means of x-ray tube and detectors connected to a computer. Sometimes called a CAT scan.

condyloma (kon-di-lō'ma) A warty tumor-like overgrowth in the squamous epithelium of the anorectal or genital tract, caused by a virus that is spread by sexual contact.

congen'ital Present at birth.

congenital cerebral aneurysm (an'ū-rizm) A saclike protrusion of the inner layer (*intima*) of a cerebral artery through a congenital defect in its muscular wall.

congenital polycystic kidney disease A hereditary condition characterized by formation of multiple, progressively enlarging cysts throughout both kidneys which gradually destroy renal function.

conjoined twins Identical twins that are joined to one another and often share organs in common. Siamese twins.

conjugated bilirubin A more soluble form of bilirubin produced by the addition of two molecules of glucuronic acid to the bilirubin molecule.

consumption coagulopathy See *disseminated intravascular coagulation syndrome.*

cortex The outer layer of an organ. See also *medulla.*

corticotropin (kōr-tik-kō-trō'pin) Another name for adrenal corticotrophic hormone (ACTH).

cortisol (kōr'ti-sol) The major glucocorticoid.

Corynebacterium (kōr-rī'nē-bak-te'rī-yum) An aerobic nonspore-forming gram-positive rod-shaped bacterium.

cotyledon (co-ti-lē'don) A unit of the placenta visible grossly on the maternal surface as an irregularly shaped lobe circumscribed by a depressed area.

crab louse A parasite of the pubic area; causes intense itching.

carnial fossa One of the depressions in the base of the skull, which is terraced to receive the undersurface of the brain.

creatinine (krē-at'in-ēn) A waste product derived from the breakdown of a compound present in muscle (phosphocreatine) that is excreted in the urine.

cretinism (krē'tin-izm) Hypothyroidism in the infant.

crossover Interchange of genetic material between homologous chromosomes during synapse and meiosis.

cul-de-sac (kul'de-sak) A blind pouch or cavity. The term is commonly applied to the rectouterine pouch, a peritoneum-covered recess located between the posterior fornix of the vagina and the rectum.

cyano'sis A blue tinge of the skin and mucous membranes that results from an excessively large amount of reduced hemoglobin in the blood when blood oxygenation is insufficient.

cystic fibrosis Hereditary disease characterized by glandular dysfunction, eventually leading to serious disturbances of pancreatic, hepatic, and pulmonary function.

cystitis (sis-tī'tis) Inflammation of the bladder.

cytokine A general term for any protein secreted by cells that functions as an intercellular messenger and influences cells of the immune system. Cytokines are secreted by macrophages and monocytes (monokines), lymphocytes (lymphokines), and other cells.

cytomegalovirus (sī-tō-meg'u-lō-vī-rus) One of the herpes viruses. Causes an infectious mononucleosis-like syndrome in adults; may cause congenital malformation in fetus.

cytopathogenic (sī-tō-path-ō-jen'ik) Pertaining to cell necrosis and degeneration.

cytotoxic (sī-tō-tok'sik) Producing cell necrosis or destruction.

D

D and C Dilatation and curettage of the uterus. A scraping out of the uterine lining, often performed as a diagnostic or therapeutic procedure.

daughter cell A cell resulting from division of a single cell (called the *parent cell*).

decidua (de-sid'ū-ah) The endometrium of pregnancy.

deciduous (de-sid'ū-us) Pertaining to anything that is cast off at maturity, as for example the first set of teeth.

delta cells (del'tuh) Somatostatin-secreting cells of the pancreatic islets.

Delta hepatitis A type of hepatitis caused by a defective virus that can infect only persons already infected with the hepatitis B virus.

dentine (den'tēn) Bony structure of the tooth.

deoxyribonucleic acid (DNA) The nucleic acid present in the chromosomes of the nuclei of cells that carries genetic information.

dermatomyositis (der-ma'to-mī-ō-sī'tis) A systemic disease characterized by inflammation and scarring of both skin and muscle.

dermatophyte (der-mat'o-fīt) A fungus that causes a superficial infection of the skin.

dermoid cyst (derm'oyd) A common type of benign cystic teratoma that commonly arises in the ovary.

DES Abbreviation for *diethylstilbestrol*, a nonsteroidal estrogen.

desensitization A method of inducing a diminished response to allergens by inducing the formation of specific IgG and IgA antibodies.

diabetes insipidus (dī-u-bē'tēz in-sip'id-us) A condition resulting from a deficiency of antidiuretic hormone, characterized by excretion of a large volume of very dilute urine.

diabetes mellitus (dī-u-bē'tēz mel'lit-is) A metabolic disease characterized by hyperglycemia and caused by insufficient insulin secretion or inefficient utilization of insulin.

diagno'sis The determination of the nature and cause of a patient's illness.

dial'ysis The diffusion of dissolved substances and water across a semipermeable membrane.

diaphragm (di'ä-fram) A partition separating one thing from another, applied to the dome-shaped partition between the thoracic and abdominal cavities. The term is also applied to a contraceptive device placed over the cervix prior to intercourse.

diethylstilbestrol (DES) (dī-ethyl-stilbes'trol) A nonsteroidal estrogen capable of inducing abnormalities in the genital tract of women whose mothers took the drug in pregnancy.

diffusion The process whereby particles of liquid, gas, or solids spread from a region of higher concentration to a region of lower concentration.

dissecting aneurysm (an'ur-izm) A dissection of blood into the wall of the aorta secondary to degeneration of the arterial wall with an associated tear of the lining (*intima*) of the artery.

disseminated intravascular coagulation syndrome A disturbance of blood coagulation as a result of activation of the coagulation mechanism and simultaneous clot lysis.

diverticulitis (dī-vur-tik-u-lī'tis) An inflammation of a diverticulum.

diverticulosis (dī-vur-tik-u-lō'sis) A condition characterized by an outpouching of the colonic mucosa through weak areas in the muscular wall.

diverticulum (dī-vur-tik'u-lum) An outpouching from an organ, as from the mucosa of the colon, which projects through the muscular wall.

dominant gene A gene that expresses a trait in the heterozygous state.

dopamine (dō'puh-mēn) Chemical mediator released by hypothalamic neurons.

Down syndrome A congenital syndrome usually caused by an extra chromosome 21.

dura (dū'rä) The outer covering of the brain and spinal cord.

dysfunctional uterine bleeding (DUB) Irregular uterine bleeding caused by disturbance of the normal cyclic interaction of estrogen and progesterone on the endometrium.

dysmenorrhea (dis-men-ō-rhē'uh) Painful menstruation.

dysplasia (dis-plā'sē-yuh) Abnormal maturation of cells.

dyspnea (disp'nē-uh) Difficult or labored breathing.

dys'trophy A disorder that results from defective or faulty growth of a structure or organ. See *vulvar dystrophy*.

E

ecchymosis (ek-im-ō'sis) A black-and-blue spot caused by extravasation of blood into the skin.

ectoderm (ek'tō-derm) The outer germ layer in the embryo that gives rise to specific organs and tissues.

ectop'ic (ek-top'ik) Out of its normal position, as in an extrauterine pregnancy (*ectopic pregnancy*).

ectopic pregnancy A pregnancy outside the endometrial cavity.

edema (e-dē′muh) Accumulation of an excess of fluid in the interstitial tissues.

electrocardiogram (ē lek-trō-kär′dē-ō-gram) A technique for measuring the serial changes in the electrical activity of the heart during the various phases of the cardiac cycle. (Often called ECG or EKG.)

electrolyte (ē-lek′trō-līt) A compound that in solution dissociates into positive and negative ions.

embolism (em′bō-lizm) A condition in which a plug composed of a detached clot, mass of bacteria, or other foreign material (*embolus*) occludes a blood vessel.

embryo (em′brē-ō) The developing human organism from the third through the seventh weeks of gestation.

emphysema (em-fuh-sē′muh) A disease characterized by enlargement and distention of the pulmonary air spaces distal to the terminal bronchioles.

enamel Dense outer covering of the exposed surface of the tooth.

encephalitis (en-sef-äl-ī′tis) An inflammation of the brain.

encephalomalacia (en-seff′uh-lō-mu-lā′shuh) Cystic lesion of degenerated brain tissue as a result of obstruction of cerebral blood supply. Same as cerebral infarct.

endarterectomy (end-är-ter-ek′tō-mē) Surgical resection of arteriosclerotic lining of an artery to increase its caliber and improve blood flow through the vessel.

endemic disease (en-dem′ik) A communicable disease in which small numbers of cases are continually present in a population.

endochondral bone formation (en-dō-kon′drul) Formation of bone as, first, a cartilage model that is then reabsorbed and converted into bone.

endometrial cyst (en-dō-mē′trē-ul) An ovarian cyst lined by endometrium and filled with old blood and debris. A manifestation of endometriosis.

endometriosis (en-dō-mē trē-ō′sis) Presence of endometrial tissue in abnormal locations, such as in the ovary or pelvis.

endoplas′mic reticulum A mass of hollow tubular channels within the cytoplasm of the cell, frequently bordered by ribosomes.

endoscopy (en-däs′kō-pē) An examination of the interior of the body by means of various lighted tubular instruments.

endothelium (en-dō-thē′lē-um) The internal lining of blood vessels and interior of heart.

Entameba histolytica (en-tuh-mē′buh his-tō-lit′ti-kä) A protozoan parasite causing amebiasis.

enteritis (en-ter-ī′tis) Inflammation of the intestine.

entoderm (en′tō-derm) The inner germ layer of the embryo that gives rise to specific organs and tissues.

eosinophil (ē-ō-sin′o-fil) A leukocyte whose cytoplasm is filled with large, uniform granules that stain intensely red with acid dyes. See also *basophil.*

epidemic disease (ep-i-dem′ik) A communicable disease affecting concurrently large numbers of persons in a population.

epidural space (ep-i-dū′rul) Potential space between the dura and overlying cranial bones.

epinephrine (ep-in-ef′rin) One of the compounds (catecholamines) secreted by the adrenal medulla.

Epstein-Barr virus A virus that causes infectious mononucleosis.

erythroblast (e-rith′rō-blast) A precursor cell in the bone marrow that gives rise to red blood cells.

erythropoiesis (er-ith′rō-poy-ē′sis) Production of red blood cells.

erythropoietin (er-ith-rō-poy′e-tin) A humoral substance made by the kidneys that regulates hematopoiesis.

esophageal varices (var′i-sēz) Dilated (varicose) veins of the esophagus, which are often present in patients with cirrhosis of the liver.

etiology (ē-tē-ol′ō-jē) The cause, especially the cause of a disease.

exchange transfusion Partial replacement of blood of infant with hemolytic disease by blood lacking the antigen responsible for hemolytic disease, as when transfusing Rh-negative blood to an Rh-positive infant. Performed to reduce intensity of hemolytic jaundice.

exon The part of a chromosomal DNA chain that codes for a specific protein or enzyme.

exudate (ex′yū-dāt) The fluid, leukocytes, and debris that accumulate as a result of an inflammation.

F

fatty acid A long, straight-chain carbon compound that contains a terminal carboxyl group, which enters into the formation of a triglyceride.

feedback mechanism A mechanism whereby the output of a hormone by a target gland controls the release of the regulatory hormone that stimulates the target gland.

fe′tus The unborn offspring after eight weeks' gestation.

fibrillation (fi-bril-lā′shun) Uncoordinated quivering of cardiac muscle that prevents normal contraction of the heart muscle.

fibrin The meshwork of protein threads that form during the clotting of the blood.

fibrin monomer (mä′nō-mer) A derivative of fibrinogen that polymerizes to form the fibrin clot during blood coagulation.

fibrinogen (fī-brin′ō-jen) A precursor in plasma converted into fibrin by thrombin during blood coagulation.

fibrinolysin (fi′brin-ol′is-in) A component of blood plasma capable of dissolving fibrin clots.

filtration membrane The thin membrane covering the filtration slit between pedicels of the podocytes that cover the glomerular capillaries of the kidneys.

filtration slits The narrow spaces between the pedicels of the podocytes that cover the glomerular capillaries of the kidneys.

flagellum (fla-jel′um) A whiplike process that propels an organism or sperm.

follicle-stimulating hormone (FSH) One of the gonadotropic hormones secreted by the anterior lobe of the pituitary, which regulates growth and function of the gonads (ovary and testis).

foot processes The highly branched cytoplasmic processes of the podocytes covering the glomerular capillaries of the kidneys.

fracture (frak-tūr) A broken bone.

free biliru′bin The relatively insoluble bile pigment formed from breakdown of hemoglobin by reticuloendothelial cells.

frozen section A method of rapid diagnosis of tumors used by the pathologist; tissue is frozen solid, cut into thin sections, stained, and examined microscopically.

FSH Follicle-stimulating hormone, one of the gonadotrophic hormones.

G

galactorrhea (gă-lak-tō-rē'yuh) Secretion of milk by breast not associated with pregnancy or normal lactation.

gam'etogen'esis The development of mature eggs and sperm from precursor cells.

gamma globulin (gam'ah glob'ŭ-lin) A protein antibody found in the blood.

gangrene (gang-grēn') Term has two different meanings. Refers to (1) infection caused by gas-forming anaerobic bacteria (*gas gangrene*) or (2) necrosis of an extremity caused by interruption of its blood supply (*ischemic gangrene*).

gastric bypass An operation to treat massive obesity in which the capacity of the stomach is reduced.

gene (jēn) A unit of heredity located at a definite position (*locus*) on a chromosome.

gene product A protein or enzyme specified (coded) by a gene.

gene splicing Same as recombinant DNA technology.

gene therapy Treating cells by inserting a gene into the cell to accomplish a specific purpose, such as supplying a missing enzyme in a subject with a genetic disease.

genetic code (jen-et'ik kōd) The information carried by the codons of DNA molecules in chromosomes.

genetic engineering Same as recombinant DNA technology.

germ disk A three-layered cluster of cells that will eventually give rise to an embryo.

germ layers The three layers of cells derived from the inner cell mass, each layer destined to form specific organs and tissues in the embryo.

Giardia (jē-ä'dē-uh) A small pear-shaped parasite that causes an acute inflammation of the small intestine.

glioma (glē-ō'muh) Any brain tumor arising from glial (supporting) cells of the brain.

glomerulonephritis (glo-mărŭ-lō-nef-rī'tis) An inflammation of the glomeruli caused by either antigen-antibody complexes trapped in the glomeruli or to antiglomerular basement membrane antibodies.

glomerulosclerosis (glo-mēr'ŭ-lō-sklerrō'sis) Diffuse and nodular thickening of glomerular basement membranes, a common occurrence in patients with long-standing diabetes mellitus.

glu'cagon A hormone produced by the alpha cells of the pancreatic islets that raises blood sugar.

glu'cocorticoid An adrenal cortical hormone that regulates carbohydrate metabolism.

glycogen (glī'kō-jen) A storage form of glucose present chiefly in liver and muscle.

goiter (goy'ter) Any enlargement of the thyroid gland.

Golgi apparatus (gol'jē) A group of membrane-lined sacs found in the cytoplasm of the cell near the nucleus.

gonad (gō'nad) A general term referring to either the ovary or the testis.

gonadotrop'in A hormone produced by the anterior lobe of the pituitary gland that controls the function of the gonads.

gout A disorder of nucleoprotein metabolism characterized by elevated uric acid and deposition of uric acid in and around joints.

granulosa cells (gran-u-lō'suh) Cells lining the ovarian follicles.

granulosa cell tumor (gran-u-lō'suh) A tumor arising from granulosa cells, usually associated with excess production of estrogen.

Guillain Barré syndrome (gil'yän bär rā') A type of polyneuritis resulting from an autoimmune reaction to myelin.

gynecomastia (gī-ne-ko-mas'ti-uh) Excessive development of the male breast.

H

haplotype (hap'lō-tīp) A set of HLA genes on one chromosome that is transmitted as a set.

heart block Delay or complete interruption of impulse transmission from the atria to the ventricles.

hematoma (hēm-uh-tō'muh) A large collection of blood in the tissues, such as might occur if coagulation factors are deficient.

heme (hēm) An iron porphyrin complex. Part of the hemoglobin molecule.

hemiplegia (hēm'i-plē'ji-uh) Paralysis of one side of the body.

hemizy'gous A term applied to genes located on the X chromosome in the male.

hemodialysis (hēm-ō-dī-al'i-sis) A dialysis procedure by which waste products are removed from the blood of patients in chronic renal failure, usually by means of an artificial kidney machine.

hemolysis (hēm-ol'i-sis) Destruction of red blood cells with escape of hemoglobin into the surrounding medium.

hemolytic anemia An anemia caused by increased blood destruction.

hemolytic disease of the newborn A hemolytic anemia resulting from maternal sensitization and antibody formation to fetal blood group antigens, leading to destruction of fetal cells.

hemophilia (hē-mō-fil'e-yuh) A sex-linked coagulation disturbance characterized by a deficiency of antihemophilic globulin.

hemorrhoids (hem'or-oyds) Varicosities of anal and rectal veins.

he'mosid'erin One of the storage forms of iron.

heparin An anticoagulant obtained from the liver.

hepatitis (hep-ah-tī'tis) Inflammation of the liver.

hepatitis B core antigen The antigen contained in the core of the hepatitis B virus.

hepatitis B_e antigen One of the antigens associated with the hepatitis B virus.

hepatitis B surface antigen The coating of the hepatitis B virus that is also found in great excess in the blood of infected patients.

hernia (her'nē-yuh) A protrusion of a loop of bowel through a narrow opening, usually in the abdominal wall.

herniated intervertebral disk (inter-ver'tē-bral) Protrusion of the nucleus pulposus through a tear in the annulus.

heterophile antibody (het'er-o-file') A type of antibody, capable of agglutinating sheep red cells, that is formed in patients with infectious mononucleosis.

heterozygous (het'er-o-zī'gus) Having two different alleles at given gene loci on the homologous pair of chromosomes.

high-density lipoprotein (HDL) cholesterol (li-pō-prō'tēn kō-les'ter-ul) The fraction of cholesterol carried by high-density lipoprotein, which is correlated with protection against atherosclerosis.

histocompatibility complex A cluster of genes on chromosome 6 that determines antigens on the surface of cells.

histol'ogy The study of the microscopic structure of organs and tissues.

Histoplasma capsulatum (his'tō-plas'-muh kap-sōō-lā'tum) A highly pathogenic fungus causing the disease histoplasmosis.

histoplasmosis (his'tō-plas-mō'sis) An infection caused by the fungus *Histoplasma capsulatum.*

HLA antigens A shortened form for *human leukocyte antigens.* Antigens on the surface of cells determined by genes of the major histocompatibility complex.

HLA system The genes of the histocompatibility complex and the antigens that they determine on the surface of cells.

Hodgkin's disease One type of lymphoma.

homol'ogous chromosomes A matched pair of chromosomes, one derived from each parent.

homozygous (hō-mo-zī'gus) Possessing identical alleles at a given locus on each of a pair of homologous chromosomes.

host Individual infected with a disease-producing organism.

human chorionic gonadotropin (HGC) (kŏr-ē-on'ik gō-na-dō-trō'pin) A hormone made by the placenta in pregnancy having actions similar to pituitary gonadotropins. Same hormone is made by neoplastic cells in some types of malignant testicular tumors.

human placental lactogen (HPL) (lak'tō-jen) One of the hormones produced by the placenta that has properties similar to pituitary growth hormone.

humoral immunity Immunity associated with formation of antibodies produced by plasma cells.

hydatidiform mole (hī-da-tid'i-form mōl) A neoplastic proliferation of trophoblast associated with formation of large cystic villi.

hydroceph'alus Dilatation of the ventricular system caused by pressure arising from accumulation of cerebrospinal fluid within the ventricles.

hydronephrosis (hydro-nef-rō'sis) A dilatation of the urinary drainage tract proximal to the site of an obstruction.

hydrostat'ic pressure Pressure that filters fluid from the blood through the capillary endothelium.

hydrothorax (hī-drō-thor'ax) Accumulation of fluid in the pleural cavity.

hydroureter A dilatation of the ureter secondary to obstruction of the urinary drainage system, often associated with coexisting dilatation of the renal pelvis and calyces (*hydronephrosis*).

hypercholesterolemia (hī'per-ko-les'ter-ol-ē'mi-uh) Excessive concentration of cholesterol in the blood.

hyperglycemia (hī-per-glī-sē'mi-uh) Excessively high blood glucose concentration.

hyperglyceridemia (hī-per-glis'er-id-ē'mi-uh) An elevated concentration of triglycerides in the blood.

hyperosmolar coma (hī-per-oz-mō'lär) Coma resulting from neurologic dysfunction caused by hyperosmolarity of body fluids as a consequence of severe hyperglycemia.

hyperplasia (hī-per-plā'sēē-uh) An increase in the number of cells.

hypersensitivity A state of abnormal reactivity to a foreign material.

hypertension High blood pressure.

hyperton'ic Having an osmotic pressure (*osmolarity*) greater than that of body fluids.

hyper'trophy An enlargement or overgrowth of an organ caused by an increase in size of its constituent cells.

hyphae (hī'fāy) Filamentous branching structures formed by fungi.

hypoglycemia (hī-pō-glī-sē'mē-ah) Less than normal concentration of glucose in the blood.

hy'pothal'amus A portion of the brain stem that forms the floor of the third ventricle. It contains clusters of nerve cells that regulate various body functions.

hypoton'ic Having an osmotic pressure (*osmolarity*) less than that of body fluids.

I

ileal bypass A surgical procedure performed on the small intestine to promote weight loss.

immunity Resistance to disease.

immunoglobulin (im'mū-nō-glob'u-lin) An antibody protein.

immunotherapy (im'mū-nō-ther'uh-pē) Treatment given to retard growth of a disseminated malignant tumor by stimulating to body's own immune defenses.

imperforate anus (im-per'for-āt) Congenital absence of anal opening, often associated with absence of distal rectum as well.

im'potence Inability of the male to achieve an erection.

inclusion bodies Spherical structures in the nucleus or cytoplasm of virus-infected cells.

infarct (in'färkt) Necrosis of tissue caused by interruption of its blood supply.

infection Inflammation caused by a disease-producing organism.

inflamma'tion A reaction produced by an irritant or infectious agent, characterized by swelling of the affected tissue as a result of vascular congestion and exudation of fluid and white blood cells.

inguinal canal (in'gwin-ul) An oblique tunnel in the muscles of the abdominal wall through which the testes and spermatic cords descend into the scrotum.

inner cell mass A group of cells that are derived from the fertilized ovum and are destined to form the embryo.

in situ carcinoma (in-sī'tū kär-sin-ō'muh) A malignant epithelial tumor that is still confined to the surface epithelium and has not yet invaded deeper tissues.

insulin (in'su-lin) A hormone that lowers blood glucose, produced by the beta cells of the pancreas.

interferon (in-tur-fēr'on) A broad-spectrum antiviral agent manufactured by various cells in the body.

interleukin-2 (inter-lōō'kin) A lymphokine that stimulates growth of lymphocytes.

interstitial (in-tur-stish'al) Pertaining to the spaces between the cells.

interver'tebral disk A fibrocartilaginous joint between adjacent vertebral bodies.

intramem'branous bone formation Direct formation of bone by osteoblasts without prior formation of a cartilage model.

intrauterine device (IUD) A small plastic device inserted in the uterus to prevent pregnancy.

intron A noncoding part of a chromosomal DNA chain.

intussusception (in'tus-us-cep'shun) A telescoping of one segment of bowel into an adjacent segment.

ischemia (iss-kē'mē-uh) Reduced blood flow to a tissue or organ.

ischemic heart disease (iss-kē'mik) Used synonymously with coronary heart disease. Designates heart disease as a result of inadequate blood flow through the coronary arteries.

islets of Langerhans (län'ger-hänz) Cluster of endocrine cells in the pancreas.

isoton'ic Having an osmotic pressure (*osmolarity*) equal to that of body fluids.

isotope (ī'sō-tōp) A substance that emits a characteristic radiation, used in medicine to label various substances as a means of determining their uptake and excretion.

J

jaundice (jawn'dis) Yellow color of the skin that results from accumulation of bile pigment within the blood.

juxtaglomerular apparatus (jux'tu-glo-mār'ŭ-lär) A specialized group of cells at the vascular pole of the glomerulus that regulates blood flow through the glomerulus of the kidneys.

K

ker'atin An insoluble sulfur-containing protein that is the principal constituent of the hair and nails.

keratinocyte (ker-u-tin'ō-cyte) A keratin-forming cell in the epidermis.

ke'tone (kē'tone) Any compound having a carbonyl (CO) group.

ketone bodies Various derivatives of acetyl-CoA, resulting from excessive mobilization of fat as an energy source.

ketosis (kē-tō'sis) An excess of ketone bodies (acetoacetic acid, beta-hydroxybutyric acid, and acetone) in the blood resulting from utilization of fat as the primary source of energy.

kinin (kī'nin) A chemical mediator of inflammation formed from components in plasma; same as *bradykinin.*

Klinefelter's syndrome (klīn'felt-er) A congenital syndrome caused by an extra X chromosome in the male. Characterized by testicular atrophy, sterility, feminine body configuration, and subnormal intelligence.

L

latent infection An infection without clinical symptoms.

lecithin (les'ith-in) A phosphorus-containing lipid (*phospholipid*) having detergent properties similar to bile salts.

Legionnaires' disease A type of pneumonia caused by an airborne fastidious bacterium called *Legionella pneumophilia.*

lesion (lē'shun) Any structural abnormality or pathologic change.

leukemia (lōo-kē'mē-yuh) A neoplastic proliferation of leukocytes.

leukocyte (lōo'kō-sīt) A general term for a white blood cell.

leukopenia (lōo-kō-pē'ni-uh) An abnormally small number of leukocytes in the peripheral blood.

leukotriene (lōo-kō-try'-ēn) A prostaglandin-like mediator of inflammation.

LeVeen shunt (le-vēn') A surgical procedure to relieve ascites by shunting the ascitic fluid through a catheter directly into the internal jugular vein.

LH Luteinizing hormone, one of the gonadotrophic hormones.

lipoprotein (li-pō-prō'tēn) A protein that carries cholesterol and other lipids in the blood.

liver lobule A histologic subdivision of the liver in which columns of liver cells converge toward a central vein and portal tracts are located at the periphery.

lithotripsy (lith-o-trip'sē) A method for removing stones from the urinary tract by breaking them into small bits that can be excreted in the urine.

locus The position of a gene on a chromosome. Different forms (*alleles*) of the same gene are always found at the same locus on a chromosome.

low-density lipoprotein (LDL) cholesterol (li-pō-prō'tēn kō-les'ter-all) The fraction of cholesterol carried by low-density lipoproteins, which is correlated with atherosclerosis.

lung acinus (ä-sīn'us) A cluster of respiratory bronchioles and their subdivisions derived from a single terminal bronchiole.

lung lobule A small group of terminal bronchioles and their subdivisions.

lupus erythematosus (lōo'pus er-i-thē-muh-tō'sis) A type\ of autoimmune connective-tissue disease.

luteinizing hormone (LH) One of the gonadotropic hormones secreted by the anterior lobe of the pituitary that regulates growth and function of the gonads (ovary and testis).

Lyme disease (līm) A tick-borne systemic infection caused by a spiral organism, *Borrelia burgdorferi,* characterized by neurologic, joint, and cardiac manifestations.

lymphadenitis (limf-a-den-ī'tis) An inflammation of lymph nodes draining a site of infection.

lymphangitis (limf'an-jī'tis) An inflammation of lymph vessels draining a site of infection.

lymphocyte (limf'ō-sīt) A mononuclear blood cell produced in lymphoid tissue that takes part in cell-mediated and humoral immunity.

lymphokine (limf'ō-kīn) A soluble substance liberated by lymphocytes.

lymphoma (limf-ō'muh) A neoplasm of lymphoid cells.

ly'sosome A small cytoplasmic vacuole containing digestive enzymes.

M

macroglobulin One type of immunoglobulin of high molecular weight.

macrophage (mak'ro-fāj) A wandering phagocytic cell found in the blood tissues.

magnetic resonance imaging (MRI) A diagnostic procedure that yields computer-generated images based on the movement of hydrogen atoms in tissues subjected to a strong magnetic field.

major histocompatibility complex (his-tō'com-pat-i-bil'i-tē) A group of genes on chromosome 6 that determine the antigens on the surface of cells.

Mallory body An irregular red-staining structure in the cytoplasm of injured liver cells, usually resulting from alcohol-induced liver injury.

mammogram (mam'ō-gram) An x-ray of the breast, used to detect tumors and other abnormalities within the breast.

mast cell A specialized connective-tissue cell containing granules filled with histamine and other chemical mediators.

matrix (mā'trix) Material in which connective-tissue cells are embedded.

Meckel's diverticulum (dī-vur-tik'kŭ-lum) A tubular outpouching from the distal ileum; remnant of the vitelline duct.

mediastinum (mē-de-as-tī'num) The central partition that separates the pleural cavities. It contains the heart, major blood vessels, and other midline structures.

mediators of inflammation Chemical agents released from mast cells and certain blood proteins (kinins and complement) in response to tissue injury.

medulla (med-ul'ah) The innermost part of an organ. See also *cortex.*

megaloblast (meg'al-ō-blast) An abnormal red cell precursor resulting from vitamin B_{12} or folic acid deficiency.

meiosis (mī-o'sis) A special type of cell division occurring in *gametes* (ova and sperm), in which the number of chromosomes is reduced by one-half in the ovum and sperm.

mel'anin Dark pigment found in the skin, in the middle coat of the eye, and in some other regions.

melanin-stimulating hormone (MSH) One of the hormones produced by the intermediate lobe of the pituitary. Causes darkening of the skin.

melanocyte (me-lan'o-cyte) Melanin-producing cell in the epidermis.

melanoma (mel-uh-nō'muh) A malignant tumor of pigment-producing cells.

meninges (men-in'jēz) The membranes covering the brain and spinal cord.

meningioma (men-in-jē-ō'muh) A benign tumor arising from the meninges.

meningitis (men-in-jī'tis) Inflammation of the meninges.

meningocele (men-in'go-sēl) A protrusion of meninges through a defect in the spinal vertebral arches.

meningomyelocele (men-ing-gō-mī'el-ō-sēl) A type of spina bifida characterized by protrusion of meninges and cord through the defect in the vertebral arches.

mesangial cell (mes-an'jē-yul) Modified connective-tissue cells at the vascular pole of the glomerulus that hold the capillary tuft together.

mesoderm (me'zō-derm) The middle germ layer of the embryo, which gives rise to specific organs and tissues.

mesothelium (me-sō-thē'li-um) A layer of flat squamous epithelial cells that covers the surfaces of the pleural, pericardial, and peritoneal cavities.

metaplasia (met-uh-plā'sē-yuh) A change from one type of cell to a more resistant cell type.

metas'tasis The spread of cancer cells from the primary site of origin to a distant site within the body.

metastasize (me-tas'tuh-sīz) To spread to distant sites, as applied to the spread of a malignant tumor.

metazoa (me'tuh-zō-uh) Complex multicelled animal parasites, such as worms and flukes.

micelle (mi-sell') An aggregate of bile salt and lecithin molecules by which cholesterol is brought into solution in bile.

microcytic hypochromic anemia (mīkro-sit'ik hī-pō-krō'mik) An anemia characterized by red cells that are smaller than normal and have a reduced concentration of hemoglobin, usually because of chronic iron deficiency.

microglia (mī-kro'glē-yuh) Phagocytic cells of the nervous system comparable to macrophages in other tissues.

miliary tuberculosis (mi'lē-air-ē) Multiple foci of tuberculosis throughout the body as a result of bloodstream dissemination of tubercle bacilli from a primary focus in the lung or peribronchial lymph nodes.

milliosmol (mOsm) (mil ī-oz'mol) A unit of osmotic activity that depends upon the number of dissolved particles in a solution.

mineralocorticoid (min'ril-ō-kor'tik-oid) Adrenal cortical hormone that regulates salt and water metabolism.

mitochondria (mīt-o-kon'drē-uh) Rod-shaped structures in the cell capable of converting foods into energy to power the cell.

mito'sis The type of cell division of most cells in which chromosomes are duplicated in the daughter cells and are identical with those in the parent cell. The characteristic cell division found in all cells in the body except for the gametes.

monocyte (mon'ō-sīt) A leukocyte having a kidney-shaped nucleus and light blue cytoplasm; a phagocytic cell that forms part of the reticuloendothelial system.

monokine A cytokine secreted by monocytes and macrophages.

monoso'my A condition of a cell in which one chromosome of a homologous pair is missing.

monova'lent Having a valence of one.

morphology (mor-fähl'ō-jē) Structure or architecture of a tissue or organ.

mor'ula A mulberry-shaped solid cluster of cells formed by division of the fertilized ovum.

motor neuron A neuron that carries nerve impulses from the brain and spinal cord to muscles and glands.

MRI See *magnetic resonance imaging.*

MSH See *melanin-stimulating hormone.*

multiple myeloma (my-el-ō'muh) A malignant neoplasm of plasma cells.

multiple sclerosis Chronic disease characterized by focal areas of demyelination in the central nervous system, followed by glial scarring.

muscular dystrophy (dis'trō-fē) A hereditary disturbance of a skeletal muscle leading to necrosis and degeneration of muscle.

mutation (mū-tā'shun) An alteration in a base sequence in DNA; may alter cell function. Transmitted from parents to offspring only if mutation is in gametes.

mutator gene A gene that monitors and corrects errors in DNA duplication during cell division.

myasthenia gravis (mī-as-thē'nē-uh grä'vis) An autoimmune disease characterized by abnormal fatigability of muscle and caused by an autoantibody that damages the acetylcholine receptors at the myoneural junction.

mycelium (mī-sē'lē-yum) Matted mass of hyphae forming a fluffy colony characteristic of fungi.

mycoplasma (mī-kō-plas'muh) Small bacteria lacking a cell wall.

myelin (my'e-lin) The fatty insulating material surrounding nerve fibers.

myelitis (mī-el-ī'tis) An inflammation of the spinal cord.

myelodysplastic syndrome (my'elo-displas'tik) A disturbance of bone marrow function that is characterized by anemia, leukopenia, and thrombocytopenia and that may be a precursor to leukemia in some patients.

myelogram (mī'el-'o-gram) A procedure for visualizing the contour of the dural sac surrounding the spinal cord and nerve roots by injection of a radiopaque material into the dural sac.

myocardial infarction (mī-o-kar'dī-ul infärk'shun) Necrosis of heart muscle as a result of interruption of its blood supply. May affect full thickness of muscle wall (*transmural infarct*) or only part of the wall (*subendocardial infarct*).

myoma (mī-ō'muh) A benign smooth-muscle tumor such as commonly develops in the uterus.

myoneural junction (mī-o-nū'ral) The specialized communication between motor nerve endings and muscle cells.

myositis (mī-ō-sī'tis) Inflammation of muscle.

myxedema (mix-uh-de'muh) Mypothyroidism in the adult.

N

necrosis (nek-rō'sis) Structural changes associated with cell death.

Neisseria (nī-sēr′ē-uh) Gram-negative diplococci, some species of which cause meningitis and gonorrhea.

neoplasia (nē-ō-plā′se-yuh) The pathologic process that results in the formation and growth of a tumor.

nephron (nef′rän) The glomerulus and renal tubule.

nephrosclero′sis Thickening and narrowing of the afferent glomerular arterioles as a result of disease.

nephro′sis The renal disease characterized by loss of large amounts of protein in the urine.

nephrotic syndrome (nef-rä′tik sin′drōm) A generalized edema resulting from excessive protein loss in the urine, causd by various types of renal disease.

neural tube The ectodermal tube formed in the embryo that gives rise to the brain and spinal cord.

neurog′lia Supporting cells of tissue of the nervous system.

neuron (nū′ron) A nerve cell, including the nerve cell body and its processes.

neutrophil (nū′trō-fil) A leukocyte having a multilobed nucleus whose cytoplasm is filled with fine granules.

nevus (nē′vus) A benign tumor of pigment-producing cells.

nontoxic goiter Thyroid enlargement not associated with overproduction of thyroid hormone.

noradrenaline (nor-ad-ren′a-lin) Another name for *norepinephrine,* one of the hormones of the adrenal medulla.

norepinephrine (nor′ep-in-ef′rin) One of the compounds (*catecholamines*) secreted by the adrenal medulla.

normocytic anemia (nor-mō-sit′ik) An anemia characterized by red cells having normal size and hemoglobin concentrations.

nucleus polposus (nū′klē-us) The soft elastic center of the intervertebral disk.

O

oligodendroglia (ol′ig-ō-den-drog′li-ah) One type of neuroglia that surrounds nerve fibers within the central nervous system.

oligohydramnios (ol-ig-ō-hī-dram′nē-yus) An insufficient quantity of amnionic fluid.

oncogene (on′-koh-jēn) An abnormally functioning gene that causes unrestrained cell growth leading to formation of a tumor. Results from mutation or translocation of a proto-oncogene.

one-second forced expiratory volume (FEV_1) The maximum volume of air that can be expelled from the lungs in one second.

oocyte (ō-ō-sīt) A developing ovum contained within a follicle in the ovary.

oogenesis (ō-ō-jen′es-is) Formation and development of the mature ovum from the oocyte.

opportunistic infection (op-por-too-nis′tik) An infection in an immunocompromised person caused by an organism that is normally nonpathogenic or of limited pathogenicity.

optic chiasm (kī′asm) The point where the fibers of the optic nerves of each eye cross.

organ A group of different tissues organized to perform a specific function.

organelle A small structure present in the cytoplasm of the cell, such as a mitochondrion.

osmol The standard unit of osmotic pressure. See also *milliosmol.*

osmolar′ity A measure of the osmotic pressure exerted by a solution.

osmo′sis Passage of a solvent, such as water, through a semipermeable membrane from a solution of lesser to one of greater solute concentration.

ossifica′tion The process of forming bone.

osteoarthritis (ä′stē-ō) A "wear and tear" degeneration of the major weight-bearing joints.

osteogen′esis imperfec′ta A congenital disturbance of bone formation characterized by excessively thin and delicate bones that are easily broken.

osteomyelitis (ä′stē-ō-mī-el-ī′tis) An inflammation of bone.

osteoporosis (ä′stē-ō-por-ō′sis) Generalized thinning and demineralization of bone that tends to occur in postmenopausal women.

oxyhemoglobin (ox-ē-hēm′ō-glō-bin) Compound formed by combination of hemoglobin with two atoms of oxygen.

oxytocin (ox-i-to′sin) A hormone that is stored in the posterior lobe of the pituitary gland that causes uterine contractions during labor and ejection of milk from the breast lobules into the larger ducts.

P

panhy′popitu′itarism Failure of secretion of all anterior lobe pituitary hormones.

papilloma (pap-pil-ō′muh) A descriptive term for a benign tumor projecting from an epithelial surface.

Pap smear A study of cells from various sources, commonly used as a screening test for cancer.

parenchyma (par-en′ki-muh) The functional cells of an organ, as contrasted with the connective and supporting tissue that forms its framework.

parenchymal cell (par-en′ki-mul) The functional cell of an organ or tissue.

paresthesia (par-es-thē′ze-ah) An abnormal sensation, such as burning, prickling, or numbness.

Parkinson's disease A chronic disease of the central nervous system characterized by rigidity and tremor, caused by deceased concentration of dopamine in the central nervous system.

partial pressure The pressure exerted by a single gas in a mixture of gases, designated by the letter "P" preceding the chemical symbol for the gas (as in PCO_2).

partial thromboplastin time (PTT) test (throm-bō-plas′tin) A test that measures the overall efficiency of the blood coagulation process.

pathogenesis (path-ō-jen′e-sis) Manner in which a disease develops.

pathogenic (path-ō-jen′ik) Capable of producing disease.

pedicel (ped′i-cel) One of the small terminal processes of the podocytes that cover the glomerular capillaries.

pelvic inflammatory disease (PID) A general term for an infection affecting the fallopian tubes and adjacent pelvic organs.

peptic ulcer A chronic ulcer of the stomach or duodenum related to hypersecretion of gastric juice.

periodontal disease (per-i-ō-don′tal) An inflammation of the gums around the roots of the teeth.

perios′teum The tough, fibrous membrane that covers a bone, except for its articular surfaces.

peristal′sis The wavelike contractions of the wall of the alimentary tract that propel contents through the bowel.

peritoneal dialysis A type of hemodialysis used to treat patients with chronic renal failure, in which dialysate is instilled into the patient's peritoneal cavity and the peritoneum functions as the dialyzing membrane.

peritoneum (per-i-to-nē'um) The membrane that lines the abdominal cavity and also invests the external surfaces of the abdominal organs.

pernicious anemia (per-ni'shus) A macrocytic anemia caused by inability to absorb vitamin B_{12} as a result of inadequate secretion of intrinsic factor by gastric mucosa.

petechia (pe-tē'kēy-uh) A small pinpoint hemorrhage caused by decreased platelets, abnormal platelet function, or capillary defect.

pH Symbol for the negative logarithm of the hydrogen ion concentration—pH 7.0 is neutral; pH less than 7.0 is acid; pH greater than 7.0 is alkaline.

phagocytosis (fag-o-sī-tō'sis) Ingestion of particulate of foreign material by cells.

pheochromocytoma (fē'o-krō'mō-sī-tō'muh) Catecholamine-secreting tumor of the adrenal medulla.

Philadelphia chromosome A chromosomal abnormality found in patients with chronic granulocytic leukemia; abnormality is characterized by a reciprocal translocation of broken end pieces between chromosomes 9 and 22.

phototherapy Fluorescent light treatment of jaundiced babies to reduce the concentration of unconjugated bilirubin in their blood.

pia (pē'yuh) The innermost of the three membranes covering the brain and spinal cord.

pinocytosis (pīn'o-sī-tō'sis) Liquid absorption by cells in which a segment of cell membrane forms small pockets and engulfs the liquid. Similar to *phagocytosis*, except that liquids rather than particulate material are ingested.

pinworm A small parasitic worm infecting humans. Lives in lower bowel and causes perianal pruritus.

placenta Flat disk-shaped structure that maintains the developing organism within the uterus.

placenta previa (prē'vē-yuh) Attachment of the placenta in the uterus such that it partially or completely covers the cervix.

plasma The fluid part of the blood.

plasmid (plas'-mid) A small, circular DNA molecule separate from the main bacterial chromosome.

platelet A component of the blood; a roughly circular or oval disk concerned with blood coagulation.

pleura (plŏōr'äh) The mesothelial covering of the lung (*visceral pleura*) and chest wall (*parietal pleura*).

pneumoconiosis (nōō'mō-kō-nēēiō'sis) An occupational lung disease caused by inhalation of injurious substances such as rock dust.

Pneumocystis carinii (new-mō-cis'tis cär-in'-ē-ī) A protozoan parasite that causes severe pulmonary infections in immuno-compromised persons.

pneumonia (nōō-mōn'yuh) Inflammation of the lung.

pneumothorax (nōō-mō-thor'ax) Accumulation of air in the pleural cavity.

polar body Structure extruded during the meiosis of the oocyte. Contains discarded chromosomes and a small amount of cytoplasm.

poliomyelitis (pō'lē-yo-mī-e-lī'tis) An inflammation of the gray matter of the spinal cord, caused by a virus.

polycythemia (päl-ē-sī-thē'mē-yuh) Increased number of red cells. May be caused by some types of chronic heart or lung disease (*secondary polycythemia*) or to marrow erythroid hyperplasia of unknown causes (*primary polycythemia*).

polyhydramnios (pä-ē-hī-dram'nē-yus) An excess of amnionic fluid.

polyneuritis (päl-ē-nū-rī'tis) An inflammation of multiple nerves.

polyp A descriptive term for a benign tumor projecting from an epithelial surface.

portacaval shunt (por'tuh-kay'vul) Surgically created anastomosis between the portal vein and the vena cava, performed to lower portal pressure in the treatment of esophageal varices.

portal hypertension Elevated pressure in the portal vein and its branches; usually caused by obstruction of blood flow through the liver resulting from cirrhosis.

portal tract Branch of hepatic artery, portal vein, and bile duct located at periphery of liver lobule.

pregnancy test A test performed on blood or urine to detect the presence of human chorionic gonadotropin (HCG) characteristic of pregnancy.

Progestasert (pro-jes'-ta-sert) An intrauterine contraceptive device that liberates progesterone and exerts its effect locally on the endometrium.

proges'terone A steroid hormone that is secreted by the corpus luteum that functions to prepare the endometrium for reception and development of the fertilized ovum.

progno'sis The probable outcome of a disease or a disorder; the outlook for recovery.

prolac'tin Hormone produced by the anterior lobe of the pituitary gland that stimulates milk secretion.

prolactin inhibitory factor (PIF) Hypothalamic hormone that suppresses release of prolactin from the anterior lobe of the pituitary.

prostaglandin (pros-ta-glan'din) A complex derivative of a fatty acid (prostanoic acid) that has widespread physiologic effects.

prostate-specific antigen An antigen produced by prostatic epithelial cells that is often found in higher-than-normal concentrations in the blood of patients with prostatic cancer and other diseases of the prostate.

prothrombin time test A test that measures that phase of the coagulation mechanism after the formation of thromboplastin.

pro'ton A positively charged particle in the nucleus around which electrons rotate.

proto-oncogene (pro-to-on'-koh-jēn) A normal gene that regulates some aspect of cell growth, maturation, or division.

protozoa (prō-t⁻o-zō'uh) Simple one-celled animal parasites, such as the plasmodium causing malaria.

pulp cavity Central cavity in tooth containing nerves, blood vessels, and lymphatics.

purpura (pur'pura) A condition characterized by hemorrhage in the skin and mucous membranes (petechiae and ecchymoses).

pyelogram (pī'el-o-gram) A means for studying the contour of the urinary tract by intravenous injection of radiopaque material or by direct injection of the material into both ureters.

pyelonephritis (pī'el-ō-nef-rī'tis) A bacterial infection of the kidney and renal pelvis.

R

recessive gene A gene that expresses a trait only when present in the homozygous state.

recombinant DNA technology Methods for combining a gene from one organism, such as a gene specifying insulin synthesis, with genes from another organism, such as a bacterium.

Reed-Sternberg cell The characteristic cell of Hodgkin's disease, containing two "mirror image" nuclei with prominent nucleoli.

reflex An automatic action, such as a knee jerk, not under voluntary control.

reflux esophagitis Inflammation of the lining of the esophagus caused by reflux of acidic gastric secretions through an incompetent lower gastroesophageal sphincter.

regional enteritis Chronic inflammation of unknown cause of distal small intestine.

rejection An immunologic process characterized by destruction of a transplanted organ.

releasing hormone Hypothalamic hormone that causes release of hormone from the anterior lobe of pituitary.

renal colic Intense flank pain radiating into the groin, resulting from passage of a renal calculus into the ureter.

renin (ren'in) A humoral substance secreted by the kidneys in response to fall in blood pressure, blood volume, or sodium concentration.

resolution A regression of an inflammatory process without significant tissue destruction and with return of the tissues to normal.

respiratory bronchiole A small bronchiole containing alveoli in its walls.

reticulocyte (rē-tik'ū-lō-sīt) A young red cell that can be identified by special staining procedures.

reticuloendothelial system (rē-tik-ū-lō-en-dō-thē'lē-yul) A system of phagocytic cells distributed throughout the body.

Reye's syndrome (Rīz) A disease characterized by a fatty liver and neurologic disturbances, probably related to aspirin administration in association with a viral infection.

rheumatic fever A disease caused by hypersensitivity to antigens of the beta streptococcus, characterized by fever, joint pains, and inflammation of heart valves and muscle.

rheumatoid arthritis (rōōm'uh-toyd) A systemic disease primarily affecting the synovium with major manifestations in the small joints.

RH immune globulin A gamma globulin containing a high concentration of anti-D (Rh$_o$) antibody; used to prevent Rh sensitization of Rh-negative mothers.

ribosome A small cytoplasmic organelle that serves as the site of protein synthesis.

Ribosomes are usually attached to the endoplasmic reticulum but may be free in the cytoplasm.

Rickettsiae (rik-ket'sē-yuh) Small bacteria-like intracellular parasites that parasitize endothelial cells.

roentgenogram (rent'gen-ō-gram) A photograph taken with x-rays.

rubella (rū-bel'luh) German measles.

S

sarcoma (sar-kō'muh) A malignant tumor arising from connective and supporting tissues.

scabies (skā'bēz) An infestation caused by the small parasite *Sarcoptes scabiei*.

Schwann cell (shwän) An elongated cell that surrounds a peripheral nerve fiber and produces the myelin that insulates the fiber.

sclerotherapy (skler'-o-ther'-a-pē) Treatment of varicose veins in esophagus or elsewhere by injecting them with a solution that scars and obliterates the veins.

sella turcica (sel-la tur'sik-uh) Depression in sphenoid bone at base of skull in which pituitary is located. Also called the *pituitary fossa*.

semilunar valve The cup-shaped valve located between the ventricles and the aorta or pulmonary artery.

seminoma (sem-in-ō'ma) One type of malignant tumor of testis.

sen'sory neuron An afferent neuron that carries impulses into the central nervous system.

septic embolus (sep-tik em'bo-lus) Infected infarct resulting from embolization of blood clot containing pathogenic bacteria.

septicemia (sep-ti-sē'mē-yuh) An infection in which large numbers of pathogenic bacteria are present in the bloodstream.

serotonin (sēr-o-tō'-nin) A vasoconstrictor mediator of inflammation released from platelets.

serum The fluid expressed from clotted blood. It differs from plasma chiefly in the absence of fibrinogen and some other plasma proteins that are consumed in the process of clotting.

sex-linked gene Gene present on the X chromosome.

sickle hemoglobin An abnormal hemoglobin that crystallizes under reduced oxygen tension.

silicosis (sil-ik-ō'sis) A type of occupational lung disease caused by inhalation of rock dust.

sinusoid (sī'nus-oyd) A special type of capillary with a wide lumen of irregular caliber, lined by phagocytic reticuloendothelial cells.

slow viral infection An infection of the nervous system caused by an unusual virus with a very long latent period.

somatotropin (so-ma-to-tro'pin) Another name for growth hormone.

spermatogen'esis Formation of mature sperm from precursor cells.

spina bifida (spī'-nuh bif'fid-duh) Incomplete closure of vertebral arches over the spinal cord, sometimes associated with protrusion of meninges and neural tissue through the defect (*cystic spina bifida*).

splenorenal shunt (splē'no-rē'nul) Surgically created anastomosis between splenic vein and renal vein, performed to lower portal pressure in the treatment of esophageal varices.

spontaneous pneumothorax (nōō-mō-thor'ax) Pneumothorax occurring without apparent cause in healthy young persons.

staghorn calculus (kal'kū-lus) A large renal calculus that has adopted the configuration of the renal pelvis and calyces where it formed.

steroid A complex lipid composed of carbon atoms arranged in a four-ring structure.

stomatitis (stō-mäh-tī'tis) Inflammation of the oral cavity.

stricture (strik'tūre) A narrowing of a tubular channel, usually a result of scarring, such as an esophageal stricture.

stroke Any injury to the brain caused by disturbance of its blood supply.

stroma (strō'muh) The tissue that forms the framework of an organ.

subarachnoid space (sub-är-ak'noyd) The space between the arachnoid and the pia, containing large blood vessels supplying the brain.

subdural space (sub-dōōr'rul) The potential space between the dura and the arachnoid.

surfactant (sur-fak'tant) A lipid material secreted by alveolar lining cells that facilitates respiration by decreasing the surface tension of the fluid lining the pulmonary alveoli.

synapse (sin'aps) Pairing of homologous chromosomes in meiosis.

synovium (si-nō'vē-um) The lining of joint cavities, bursae, and tendon sheaths.

T

tension pneumothorax (nōō-mō-thor'ax) Accumulation of air under pressure in the pleural cavity, with displacement of mediastinum away from the side of the pneumothorax.

teratoma (tār-uh-tō'muh) A tumor of mixed cell components.

tetany (tet'an-ē) Spasm of skeletal muscles caused by subnormal level of ionized calcium in the blood.

thrombin A coagulation factor formed by activation of prothrombin in the process of blood coagulation.

thrombocytopenia (throm'bō-sī-tō-pē'ny-yuh) A deficiency of platelets.

thromboplastin (throm-bō-plas'tin) A component formed during blood coagulation from interaction of platelets and plasma components (*intrinsic system*) or liberated from injured tissues (*extrinsic system*).

thrombosis A blood clot formed within the vascular system.

thyroiditis (thī-roy-dī'tis) Inflammation of the thyroid gland. Term often refers to infiltration of gland by lymphocytes and plasma cells as a manifestation of an autoimmune process.

thyroid-stimulating hormone (TSH) Hormone secreted by the anterior lobe of the pituitary; regulates thyroid function.

thyrotropin (thī-ro-tro'pin) Another name for thyroid-stimulating hormone (TSH).

thyroxine (T₄) (thī-rox'sin) One of the thyroid hormones.

tissue A group of similar cells joined to perform a specific function.

T lymphocyte A type of lymphocyte associated with cell-mediated immunity.

tone The slight continuous contraction of muscles, which aids in the maintenance of posture.

tox'ic goiter (goy'ter) Enlargement of the thyroid gland associated with excessive output of thyroid hormone.

toxic shock syndrome (TSS) A symptom complex in menstruating women who use high-absorbency tampons, caused by a toxin produced by a staphylococcus that grows in the vagina.

Toxoplasma gondii (tähk'sō-plas'muh gän'dē-ī) A small intracellular parasite of birds, animals, and humans. Causes the disease *toxoplasmosis.*

transient ischemic attack (TIA) (iss-kē'mik) Temporary cerebral dysfunction as a result of transient obstruction of a cerebral vessel by a bit of atheromatous debris or blood clot usually embolized from an arteriosclerotic plaque in the carotid artery.

translocation A transfer of a piece of one chromosome to a nonhomologous chromosome.

transurethral resection of prostate (TUR) (trans-yūr-ēth'rul) Removal of prostatic tissue by means of a specially designed instrument inserted into the penis.

Treponema pallidum (trep-pō-nē'muh pal'lid-dum) The spiral organism causing syphilis.

Trichinella spiralis (trik-in-el'luh spī-rä'lis) A parasitic worm that infects humans, causing the disease *trichinosis.*

trichomonad (trik-kō-mō'nad) A small motile parasite of the genus *Trichomonas,* one of which causes vaginitis.

triglyceride (trī-glis'er-īd) A compound composed of three molecules of fatty acid combined with one molecule of glycerol.

triiodothyronine (T₃) (trī'ī-ō-dō-thi'rō-nēn) One of the thyroid hormones.

tri'somy The presence of an extra chromosome within a cell; having three of a given chromosome instead of the usual pair.

tro'phoblast Cell derived from the fertilized ovum that gives rise to the fetal membranes and contributes to the formation of the placenta.

TSH Thyroid-stimulating hormone.

tumor A benign or malignant overgrowth of tissues that serves no normal function.

tumor-associated antigen An antigen associated with growing tumor cells, which serves as an indicator of tumor growth in the body.

tumor necrosis factor A cytokine that can destroy foreign or abnormal cells.

tumor suppressor gene A gene that suppresses cell proliferation.

Turner's syndrome A congenital syndrome usually caused by absence of one X chromosome in the female.

U

ulcer Lesion caused by loss of a portion of a cutaneous or mucous surface, such as a peptic ulcer of the stomach or duodenum.

urea (ū-rē'yuh) The nitrogen waste product derived from protein metabolism and excreted in the urine.

uremia (ur-ē'mi-yuh) An excess of urea and other waste products in the blood, resulting from renal failure.

urinalysis (ur-in-al'i-sis) A commonly performed chemical and microscopic analysis of the urine.

V

va'lence The number of hydrogen atoms with which a single atom of another element can combine.

valve stenosis (sten-ō'sis) Impaired flow of blood through a heart valve that does not open properly.

valvular regurgitation (rē-gurg-i-tā'shun) Reflux flow of blood through a heart valve that does not close properly.

varices (var'i-sēz) Dilated veins (singular term *varix*).

vas def'erens The excretory duct that transports sperm from the testis. Also called *ductus deferens.*

vasoconstric'tion A decrease in the caliber of blood vessels.

vasodilatation Increase in the caliber of a blood vessel.

velamentous insertion of umbilical cord (vel'uh-men-tus) Attachment of the umbilical cord to the fetal membranes rather than to the placenta.

ventricle (ven'tri-kul) A small cavity, especially one in the brain or heart. *Ventricles of brain:* The hollow cavities in the brain. *Ventricles of heart:* The muscular chambers that receive blood from the atria and pump the blood into the aorta (*left ventricle*) or pulmonary artery (*right ventricle*).

ventricular aneurysm (ven-trik'ū-lär an'ur-izm) A localized ballooning out of a scar of the ventricle resulting from a previous myocardial infarction.

ves'icle A small sac filled with fluid or gas.

vesicoureteral reflux (ves'i-kō-ūr-ēt'er-al) Retrograde flow of urine from the bladder into the ureter during voiding.

virulence (vir'u-lenz) The ability of an organism to cause disease.

virus A small infectious particle. An obligate intracellular parasite.

vital capacity The maximum volume of air that can be forcefully expelled after a maximum inspiration.

volvulus (vol'vū-lus) A rotary twisting of the intestine on its mesentery, with obstruction of the blood supply to the twisted segment.

vulvar dystrophy (vul'vär dis'trō-fē) An abnormality of the vulvar epithelium characterized by hyperkeratosis and epithelial maturation disturbances.

W

Wilms's tumor A malignant renal tumor of infants and children.

Y

yolk sac A sac that is formed adjacent to the germ disk and that will form the gastrointestinal tract and other important structures in the embryo.

Z

zona pellu'cida A layer of acellular material surrounding the ovum.

zy'gote (zī'gōt) The fertilized ovum.

Index